Ocular Circulation and Neovascularization

Documenta Ophthalmologica Proceedings Series

Ocular Circulation and Neovascularization

Edited by David BenEzra, Stephen J. Ryan,
Bert M. Glaser and Robert P. Murphy

1987 **MARTINUS NIJHOFF/DR W. JUNK PUBLISHERS**
a member of the KLUWER ACADEMIC PUBLISHERS GROUP
DORDRECHT / BOSTON / LANCASTER

Distributors

for the United States and Canada: Kluwer Academic Publishers, P.O. Box 358, Accord Station, Hingham, MA 02018-0358, USA
for the UK and Ireland: Kluwer Academic Publishers, MTP Press Limited, Falcon House, Queen Square, Lancaster LA1 1RN, UK
for all other countries: Kluwer Academic Publishers Group, Distribution Center, P.O. Box 322, 3300 AH Dordrecht, The Netherlands

Library of Congress Cataloging in Publication Data

```
Ocular circulation and neovascularization.

    (Documenta ophthalmologica.  Proceedings series)
    "International Symposium on Ocular Circulation and
Neovascularization"--Foreword.
    1. Neovascularization--Congresses.  2. Eye--Blood-
vessels--Diseases--Congresses.  3. Diabetic retinopathy--
Congresses.  4. Retrolental fibroplasia--Congresses.
5. Eye--Blood-vessels--Diseases--Animal models--Congresses
I. Benezra, David.  II. International Symposium on Ocular
Circulation and Neovascularization (1st : 1986 :
Jerusalem) III. Series. [DNLM: 1. Eye--blood supply--
congresses.  2. Neovascularization--congresses.
W3 DO637 / WW 103 0213 1986]
RE720.028   1987        617.7            87-11331
```

ISBN 978-94-010-7999-0   ISBN 978-94-009-3337-8 (eBook)
DOI 10.1007/978-94-009-3337-8

Copyright

FOREWORD

Neovascularization is a normal phase of tissue repair mechanism. In the eye, however, sprouting of new vessels within avascular tissues and their greater tendency to bleed have detrimental effects on vision. Diabetic retinopathy, corneal neovascularization, age-related macular degeneration, retinal vein occlusion, and retinopathy of prematurity are major causes of blindness. In all, uncontrolled proliferation of new vessels is the underlying pathological cause leading to the inexorable loss of vision. Development of laser technologies and their wide use in ophthalmology have brought some hope for the treatment of these diseases. However, it became evident that direct closure of the new vessels and/or ablation of large parts of the tissue are not ideal solutions to the problem.

Recent advances in molecular biology and genetic engineering have fostered basic knowledge regarding the growth factors and intercellular messengers and their association with the proliferation of new blood vessels. These latter findings sparked a renewed interest in Michaelson's "X-factor" of ocular neovascularization and opened avenues for possible innovative therapeutic approaches. Therefore, the suggestion to organize an international gathering of clinicians and scientists interested in problems of ocular circulation and neovascularization was received with great enthusiasm. Unanimously, it was decided to dedicate the symposium to Professor I.C. Michaelson, the innovative scientist, the great clinician, the indefatigable teacher, and above all, the wonderful human being.

The meeting was highlighted by the outstanding atmosphere of friendship and scientific exchanges. This book mirrors the information delivered and includes a selection of papers from the scientific program.

The organization of this meeting and the publication of the book would not have been possible without the harmonious team efforts made by the International, Scientific and Local Committees. I am thankful to the chairpersons of the various sessions for their time, keen interest and endeavor for the realization of a high scientific level. I also deeply acknowledge the help and support of Arnall Patz, Bob Murphy, Bert Glaser, Robert Frank, Larry Hjelmeland, Gordon Klintworth, Neville Welsh, Charles Riva, Alec Garner, Desmond Archer, Ephraim Friedman, Myron Yanoff, Moshe Lahav, Willem Manschot, Hans-Walther Larsen and Masanobu Uyama. The powerful stimulus of Hanan Zauberman, Steve Ryan, Gabriel Coscas, Giselle Soubrane, Moshe Ivry, Yuval Yassur and Sue and Peter Ballen was most instrumental in the realization of these "dreams". As always, I was fortunate to have the invaluable collaboration of my loyal assistants:

Evelyne Cohen, Genia Maftzir, Israel Barzel, Arieh Zelikovitch, and Judith BenEzra. The smooth running of the meeting and timely editing of the book could not have been possible without the incalculable help and indefatigable typing and council of Judith Fisher, who seconded me in selecting the papers and editing the book.

I was overwhelmed by the great enthusiasm of all participants and the unanimous decision to perpetuate the International Symposium on Ocular Circulation and Neovascularization. In this first meeting, we have summarized our present knowledge and discussed future trends and concepts. At the second Symposium, which will take place in 1989 in Baltimore, we will hopefully talk about the progress made during the three years between the meetings, and lay the groundwork for the third symposium in 1992 in Paris.

David BenEzra
Jerusalem, 1986

CONTRIBUTORS

S. Abbasi, M.D., Department of Ophthalmology, Scheie Eye Institute, University of Pennsylvania School of Medicine, Philadelphia, PA 19104, USA.

B. Adad-Bensoussan*, M.D., Department of Ophthalmology, Hopital de la Croix-Rousse, 69317 Lyon, France.

R. Adler, M.D., Center for Vitreoretinal Research, Wilmer Ophthalmological Institute, Johns Hopkins University, Baltimore, MD 21205, USA.

G.P. Amato, M.D., Department of Ophthalmology, University of Bologna, Bologna, Italy.

R. Auerbach*, Ph.D., Department of Zoology, University of Wisconsin, Madison, WI 53706, USA.

J.J. Augsburger, M.D., Oncology Service, Wills Eye Hospital, Thomas Jefferson University, Philadelphia, PA 19107, USA.

M. Badarma, M.D., Department of Ophthalmology, Soroka Medical Center, Beersheva, Israel.

G. Baerveldt, M.D., Department of Ophthalmology, USC School of Medicine, Los Angeles, CA 90033, USA.

R. Bellhorn, Ph.D., University of California School of Veterinary Medicine, Davis, CA, USA.

P. Bellio, M.D., Department of Ophthalmology, Groupe Hospitalier Pitie-Salpetriere, 75615 Paris Cedex 13, France.

D. BenEzra*, M.D., Ph.D., Immuno Ophthalmology and Laboratory of Ocular Angiogenesis, Department of Ophthalmology, Hadassah University Hospital, Jerusalem, Israel.

E. Benhamou, M.D., Department of Ophthalmology, Centre Hospitalier Intercommunal, 94010 Creteil, France.

I. BenSira*, M.D., Department of Ophthalmology, Beilinson Hospital, Petach Tikva, Israel.

E. R. Berman*, Ph.D., Department of Ophthalmology, Hadassah University Hospital, Jerusalem, Israel.

D. Berson, M.D., Department of Ophthalmology, Shaare Zedek Hospital, Jerusalem, Israel.

E. Bessler, M.D., Department of Ophthalmology, Soroka Medical Center, Beersheva, Israel.

B.Z. Biedner, M.D., Department of Ophthalmology, Soroka Medical Center, Beersheva, Israel.

J. Bielich, Ph.D., Department of Zoology, University of Wisconsin, Madison, WI 53706, USA.

V. Birkenfeld, Ph.D., Department of Oncology, Hadassah University Hospital, Jerusalem, Israel.

S. Bishara, M.D., Department of Ophthalmology, Hadassah University Hospital - Mt. Scopus, Jerusalem, Israel.

G. E. Blass, M.D., Tennent Institute of Ophthalmology, University of Glasgow, Glasgow, Scotland.

E. Bossi, M.D., Division of Neonatology, Department of Pediatrics, University of Berne, 3010 Berne, Switzerland.

M. Boulton*, Ph.D., Institute of Ophthalmology, London WC1H 9QS, England.

F. Bowen, M.D., Department of Ophthalmology, Scheie Eye Institute, University of Pennsylvania School of Medicine, Philadelphia, PA 19104, USA.

N. M. Bressler*, M.D., Wilmer Ophthalmological Institute, Johns Hopkins University, Baltimore, MD 21205, USA.

S. B. Bressler*, M.D., Wilmer Ophthalmological Institute, Johns Hopkins University, Baltimore, MD 21205, USA.

G.C. Brown, M.D., Retinal Vascular Unit, Wills Eye Hospital, Thomas Jefferson University, Philadelphia, PA 19107, USA.

A.J. Brucker, M.D., Department of Ophthalmology, Scheie Eye Institute, University of Pennsylvania School of Medicine, Philadelphia, PA 19104, USA.

M. Burns, Ph.D., University of California School of Medicine, Sacramento, CA, USA.

P.A. Campochiaro*, M.D., Department of Ophthalmology, University of Virginia School of Medicine, Charlottesville, VA 22908, USA.

B. Cathelineau, M.D., Department of Ophthalmology, Groupe Hospitalier Pitie-Salpetriere, 75615 Paris Cedex 13, France.

B.P. Cats*, M.D., Department of Neonatology, Wilhelmina Children's Hospital, Utrecht, The Netherlands.

G. Chaine, M.D., Department of Ophthalmology, Paris-Val de Marne University Medical School, Paris, France.

T. Chajek, M.D., Department of Internal Medicine B, Hadassah University Hospital, Jerusalem, Israel.

J. Chess*, M.D., Department of Ophthalmology, Albert Einstein College of Medicine, Bronx, NY 10461, USA.

P. Chillemi, M.D., Department of Ophthalmology, University of Bologna, Bologna, Italy.

F.V. Chisari, M.D., Scripps Clinic and Research Foundation, La Jolla, CA 92037, USA.

P. Clark, F.R.C.Path., Institute of Ophthalmology, London WC1H 9QS, England.

E. Cohen, C.O., Department of Ophthalmology, Hadassah University Hospital, Jerusalem, Israel.

S. Cohen, M.D., Department of Ophthalmology, Beilinson Hospital, Petach Tikva, Israel.

G. Coscas*, M.D., Department of Ophthalmology, Centre Hospitalier Intercommunal, 94010 Creteil, France.

G. Costantini, M.D., Department of Ophthalmology, University of Bologna, Bologna, Italy.

R. David*, M.D., Department of Ophthalmology, Soroka Medical Center, Beersheva, Israel.

J.L. Davis, Jr., M.D., Wilmer Ophthalmological Institute, Johns Hopkins University, Baltimore, MD 21205, USA.

E. de Juan, Jr.*, M.D., Duke University Eye Center, Durham, NC 27710, USA.

P. de Souza-Ramalho*, M.D., Ph.D., Department of Ophthalmology, Hospital de Santa Maria, University of Lisbon, 1600 Lisbon, Portugal.

L.A. Donoso, M.D., Ph.D., Research Department, Wills Eye Hospital, Thomas Jefferson University, Philadelphia, PA 19107, USA.

A. Eldor, M.D., Department of Hematology, Hadassah University Hospital, Jerusalem, Israel.

E. El-Hifnawi*, Ph.D., Institute of Anatomy, University of Lubeck, D-2400 Lubeck 1, FR Germany.

J. A. Eliason*, M.D., Department of Ophthalmology, Stanford University School of Medicine, Palo Alto, CA 94305, USA.

R. Epstein*, M.D., Department of Ophthalmology, Rush-Pres.-St. Luke's Medical Center, Chicago, IL 60612, USA.

F. Eyal, M.D., Unit of Neonatology, Hadassah University Hospital - Mt. Scopus, Jerusalem, Israel.

F.L. Ferris III, M.D., National Eye Institute, National Institutes of Health, Bethesda, MD 20205, USA.

A.R. Fielder*, F.R.C.S., Department of Ophthalmology, Leicester Royal Infirmary, Leicester LE2 7LX, England.

S. Fine, M.D., The Retinal Vascular Center, Wilmer Ophthalmological Institute, Johns Hopkins University, Baltimore, MD 21205, USA.

J.L. Fisher, B.S., Department of Ophthalmology, Hadassah University Hospital, Jerusalem, Israel.

H. C. Fledelius*, M.D., Department of Ophthalmology, Central Hospital, DK-3400 Hillerod, Denmark.

J. Folkman, M.D., Departments of Surgery and Anatomy, Harvard Medical School, Boston, MA 02115, USA.

C. Francais, M.D., Department of Ophthalmology, Centre Hospitalier Intercommunal, 94010 Creteil, France.

R. Frank*, M.D., Kresge Eye Institute, Wayne State University School of Medicine, Detroit, MI 48201, USA.

J. Freedman, M.D., Department of Ophthalmology, Kings County Hospital, Brooklyn, NY, USA.

E. Friedman*, M.D., Massachusetts Eye and Ear Infirmary, 243 Charles Street, Boston, MA 02114, USA.

G. Friedman, M.D., Department of Internal Medicine B, Hadassah University Hospital, Jerusalem, Israel.

A. Fuchs, Ph.D., Faculty of Medicine, Israel Institute of Technology, Haifa 31096, Israel.

A. Garner*, M.D., Ph.D., M.R.C.P., F.R.C.Path., Department of Pathology, Institute of Ophthalmology, London EC1V 9AT, England.

N.A. Gilodi, Ph.D., Experimental Ophthalmology Laboratory, University of Geneva, Geneva, Switzerland.

A. Giovannini*, M.D., Department of Ophthalmology, University of Bologna, Bologna, Italy.

B.M. Glaser*, M.D., Center for Vitreoretinal Research, Wilmer Ophthalmological Institute, Johns Hopkins University, Baltimore, MD 21205, USA.

R.E. Goldberg, M.D., Retina Vascular Unit, Wills Eye Hospital, Thomas Jefferson University, Philadelphia, PA 19107, USA.

J.D. Grange, M.D., Department of Ophthalmology, Hopital de la Croix-Rousse, 69317 Lyon, France.

J. E. Grunwald*, M.D., Department of Ophthalmology, Scheie Eye Institute, University of Pennsylvania School of Medicine, Philadelphia, PA 19104, USA.

F. Gumkowski, Ph.D., Department of Zoology, University of Wisconsin, Madison, WI 53706, USA.

D. Guyer*, M.D., Retinal Vascular Center, Wilmer Ophthalmological Institute, Johns Hopkins University, Baltimore, MD 21205, USA.

L.L. Hansen*, M.D., Eye Clinic, Free University, Berlin, West Germany.

S. V. Hansen, M.D., Department of Ophthalmology, Central Hospital, DK-3400 Hillerod, Denmark.

Y. Hayari, Ph.D., Department of Zoology, University of Wisconsin, Madison, WI 53706, USA.

I. Hemo*, M.D., Department of Ophthalmology, Hadassah University Hospital, Jerusalem, Israel.

P. Henkind, M.D., Ph.D., Department of Ophthalmology, Albert Einstein School of Medicine, Bronx, NY 10467, USA.

W. G. Heriot, M.D., Department of Ophthalmology, Albert Einstein School of Medicine, Bronx, NY 10467, USA.

I. Hirsch, M.D., Department of Ophthalmology, Shaare Zedek Hospital, Jerusalem, Israel.

G. Imre*, M.D., D.Sc., Second Department of Ophthalmology, Semmelweis University of Medicine, Budapest, Hungary.

T. Ishibashi*, M.D., Department of Ophthalmology, Faculty of Medicine, Kyushi University 60, Fukuoka, Japan.

T. Itagaki, M.D., Department of Ophthalmology, Kansai Medical University, Moriguchi, Osaka, Japan.

J.A. Jerdan, M.D., Wilmer Ophthalmological Institute, Johns Hopkins University, Baltimore, MD 21205, USA.

L. Johnson, M.D., Departments of Ophthalmology and Pediatrics, University of Pennsylvania, Philadelphia, PA 19104, USA.

P.A. Jorge, M.D., Departments of Ophthalmology and Biochemistry, Hospital de Santa Maria, University of Lisbon, 1600 Lisbon, Portugal.

G. Kaminska, Ph.D., Department of Zoology, University of Wisconsin, Madison, WI 53706, USA.

M. Kaminski, Ph.D., Department of Zoology, University of Wisconsin, Madison, WI 53706, USA.

A.S. Kimmel, M.D., Wills Eye Hospital, Thomas Jefferson University, Philadelphia, PA 19107, USA.

R. Kissun, M.D., Department of Pathology, Institute of Ophthalmology, London EC1V 9AT, England.

M. Klagsburn, Ph.D., Departments of Biological Chemistry and Surgery, Harvard Medical School, Boston, MA 02115, USA.

G. Klintworth*, M.D., Ph.D., Ophthalmology Research, Duke University Medical Center, Box 3802, Durham, NC 27710, USA.

F. Koenig, M.D., Department of Ophthalmology, Centre Hospitalier Intercommunal, 94010 Creteil, France.

F. Koerner, M.D., Eye Clinic, University of Berne, 3010 Berne, Switzerland.

N. Korber, M.D., Department of Ophthalmology, Koln/Merheim, West Germany.

G.E. Korte*, M.D., Department of Ophthalmology, Albert Einstein College of Medicine, Bronx, NY 10467, USA.

I. Kremer*, M.D., Department of Ophthalmology, Beilinson Hospital, Petach Tikva, Israel.

L. Kubai, Ph.D., Department of Zoology, University of Wisconsin, Madison, WI 53706, USA.

L. Kuwashima, M.D., Center for Vitreoretinal Research, Wilmer Ophthalmological Institute, Johns Hopkins University, Baltimore, MD 21205, USA.

M. Lahav*, M.D., Department of Ophthalmology, Veterans Administration Hospital, New England Medical Center, Boston, MA 02111, USA.

W. R. Lee*, M.D., Tennent Institute of Ophthalmology, University of Glasgow, Glasgow, Scotland.

M.I. Levene, M.D., Department of Ophthalmology, Leicester Royal Infirmary, Leicester LE2 7LX, England.

S. Levinger*, M.D., Department of Ophthalmology, Hadassah University Hospital, Jerusalem, Israel.

T. Lifschitz, M.D., Department of Ophthalmology, Soroka Medical Center, Beersheva, Israel.

E.S. Lindenbaum, Ph.D., Faculty of Medicine, Israel Institute of Technology, Haifa, Israel.

W.C. Lu, Ph.D., Department of Zoology, University of Wisconsin, Madison, WI 53706, USA.

G. Maftzir, M.Sc., Immuno Ophthalmology, Department of Ophthalmology, Hadassah University Hospital, Jerusalem, Israel.

L.E. Magargal*, M.D., Retina Vascular Unit, Retina Service, Wills Eye Hospital, Thomas Jefferson University, Philadelphia, PA 19107, USA.

W. A. Manschot*, Ph.D., M.D., Institute of Pathology, Erasmus University, Rotterdam, The Netherlands.

N.G. Maroudas*, Ph.D., Morphological Sciences Research Unit, Faculty of Medicine, Technion, Haifa, Israel.

J. Marshall, M.D., Institute of Ophthalmology, Judd Street, London WC1H 9QS, England.

J. Martins-Silva, M.D., Departments of Ophthalmology and Biochemistry, Hospital de Santa Maria, University of Lisbon, 1600 Lisbon, Portugal.

N. Matamoros, M.D., Department of Ophthalmology, Hadassah University Hospital, Jerusalem, Israel.

E. McLaughlin, Ph.D., Department of Rheumatology, University of Manchester, Oxford Road, Manchester M13 9PT, England.

S. Merin*, M.D., Department of Ophthalmology, Hadassah University Hospital - Mt. Scopus, Jerusalem, Israel.

E. Meyer*, M.D., Department of Ophthalmology, Rambam Medical Center, Haifa, Israel.

J.B. Michelson*, M.D., Scripps Clinic and Research Foundation, La Jolla, CA 92037, USA.

B. Miller, M.D., Department of Ophthalmology, Rambam Medical Center, Haifa, Israel.

H. Miller*, Ph.D., Faculty of Medicine and the Rappaport Family Institute for Research in the Medical Sciences, Technion, Haifa, Israel.

D. Minckler, M.D., Department of Ophthalmology, USC School of Medicine, Los Angeles, CA 90033, USA.

T. Monos*, M.D., Department of Ophthalmology, Soroka Medical Center, Beersheva, Israel.

D. L. Morrison, B.A., Retina Vascular Unit, Wills Eye Hospital, Thomas Jefferson University, Philadelphia, PA 19107, USA.

L.W. Morrissey, Ph.D., Department of Zoology, University of Wisconsin, Madison, WI 53706, USA.

R. P. Murphy*, M.D., Wilmer Ophthalmological Institute, Johns Hopkins University, Baltimore, MD 21205, USA.

Vr. Muthukkaruppan, Ph.D., Department of Immunology, Madurai Kamaraj University, Madurai, India.

M. Nahir, M.D., Department of Rheumatology, Rambam Medical Center, Haifa, Israel.

G.O.H. Naumann, M.D., Department of Ophthalmology, University of Erlangen-Nurnberg, D-8520 Erlangen, Federal Republic of Germany.

Y.K. Ng, M.D., Department of Ophthalmology, Leicester Royal Infirmary, Leicester LE2 7LX, England.

T. Nishimura, M.D., Department of Ophthalmology, Kansai Medical University, Moriguchi, Osaka, Japan.

I. Nissenkorn, M.D., Department of Ophthalmology, Beilinson Hospital, Petach Tikva, Israel.

R. B. Nussenblatt*, M.D., Laboratory of Immunology, National Eye Institute, National Institutes of Health, Bethesda, MD 20205, USA.

H. Ohkuma, M.D., Department of Ophthalmology, Kansai Medical University, Moriguchi, Osaka, Japan.

G. Orr, M.D., Department of Ophthalmology, USC School of Medicine, Los Angeles, CA 90033, USA.

C. Otis, M.D., Department of Ophthalmology, Scheie Eye Institute, University of Pennsylvania School of Medicine, Philadelphia, PA 19104, USA.

A. G. Palestine, M.D., Laboratory of Immunology, National Eye Institute, National Institutes of Health, Bethesda, MD 20205, USA.

A. Patz*, M.D., Wilmer Ophthalmological Institute, Johns Hopkins University, Baltimore, MD 21205, USA.

A. Pazzaglia, M.D., Department of Ophthalmology, University of Bologna, Bologna, Italy.

O. Peleg, M.D., Unit of Neonatology, Hadassah University Hospital - Mt. Scopus, Jerusalem, Israel.

B.L. Petrig, M.D., Department of Ophthalmology, Scheie Eye Institute, University of Pennsylvania School of Medicine, Philadelphia, PA 19104, USA.

S. Pizanti, D.M.D., Department of Oral Medicine, Hadassah University Hospital, Jerusalem, Israel.

A. Pollack*, M.D., Department of Ophthalmology, Kaplan Hospital, Rehovot, Israel.

C.J. Pournaras, M.D., Experimental Ophthalmology Laboratory, University of Geneva, Geneva, Switzerland.

G.E. Quinn*, M.D., Department of Ophthalmology, Scheie Eye Institute, University of Pennsylvania School of Medicine, Philadelphia, PA 19104, USA.

C. Ramahefasolo, M.D., Department of Ophthalmology, Centre Hospitalier Intercommunal, 94010 Creteil, France.

L. Regenbogen, M.D., Department of Ophthalmology, Sheba Medical Center, Tel Hashomer, Israel.

M. Reim, M.D., Department of Ophthalmology, RWTH, D-5100 Aachen, West Germany.

E.B. Ringelstein, M.D., Department of Neurology, RWTH, D-5100 Aachen, West Germany.

C.E. Riva, Ph.D., Department of Ophthalmology, Scheie Eye Institute, University of Pennsylvania School of Medicine, Philadelphia, PA 19104, USA.

I. Rosenblatt*, M.D., Department of Ophthalmology, Soroka Medical Center, Beersheva, Israel.

D. Rosenmann, M.D., Department of Ophthalmology, Shaare Zedek Hospital, Jerusalem, Israel.

E. Rosenmann, M.D., Department of Pathology, Hadassah University Hospital, Jerusalem, Israel.

F. Rousselie, M.D., Department of Ophthalmology, Groupe Hospitalier Pitie-Salpetriere, 75615 Paris Cedex 13, France.

K.W. Ruprecht, M.D., Department of Ophthalmology, University of Erlangen-Nurnberg, D-8520 Erlangen, Federal Republic of Germany.

S.J. Ryan*, M.D., Department of Ophthalmology, USC School of Medicine, Los Angeles, CA 90033, USA.

C. Saldanha, M.D., Departments of Ophthalmology and Biochemistry, Hospital de Santa Maria, University of Lisbon, 1600 Lisbon, Portugal.

M. Sato, M.D., Center for Vitreoretinal Research, Wilmer Ophthalmological Institute, Johns Hopkins University, Baltimore, MD 21205, USA.

J. Scharf, M.D., Department of Ophthalmology, Rambam Medical Center, Haifa, Israel.

Y. Scharf, M.D., Department of Rheumatology, Rambam Medical Center, Haifa, Israel.

R. Schechner, M.D., Department of Ophthalmology, Rambam Medical Center, Haifa, Israel.

A.V.M. Schulte*, M.D., Department of Ophthalmology, Erasmus University, Rotterdam, The Netherlands.

M. Seelenfreund, M.D., Department of Ophthalmology, Shaare Zedek Hospital, Jerusalem, Israel.

L. Shani, M.D., Department of Ophthalmology, Soroka Medical Center, Beersheva, Israel.

A. Shapiro, M.D., Department of Ophthalmology, Hadassah University Hospital - Mt. Scopus, Jerusalem, Israel.

D.E. Shaw, M.D., Department of Ophthalmology, Leicester Royal Infirmary, Leicester LE2 7LX, England.

B.Z. Silverstone*, M.D., Department of Ophthalmology, Shaare Zedek Hospital, Jerusalem, Israel.

S. H. Sinclair, M.D., Department of Ophthalmology, Scheie Eye Institute, University of Pennsylvania School of Medicine, Philadelphia, PA 19104, USA.

N. Sorgente, M.D., Department of Ophthalmology, USC School of Medicine, Los Angeles, CA 90033, USA.

G. Soubrane*, M.D., Centre Hospitalier Intercommunal, 94010 Creteil, France.

K. Strommer, M.D., Experimental Ophthalmology Laboratory, University of Geneva, Geneva, Switzerland.

R.D. Stulting, M.D., Ph.D., Department of Ophthalmology, Emory University, Atlanta, GA 30322, USA.

K. Takahashi, M.D., Department of Ophthalmology, Kansai Medical University, Moriguchi, Osaka, Japan.

K.E.W.P. Tan, M.D., Royal Eye Hospital, Utrecht, The Netherlands.

J. Tauber, M.D., Department of Ophthalmology, New England Medical Center, Boston, MA 02111, USA.

C.M. Taylor, Ph.D., Department of Rheumatology, University of Manchester, Manchester M13 9PT, England.

M. Tsacopoulos, M.D., Experimental Ophthalmology Laboratory, University of Geneva, Geneva, Switzerland.

D. Ucenick, M.D., Department of Ophthalmology, Soroka Medical Center, Beersheva, Israel.

M. Uyama*, M.D., Department of Ophthalmology, Kansai Medical University, Moriguchi, Osaka, Japan.

G.H. van Rens, M.D., Department of Ophthalmology, Erasmus University, Rotterdam, The Netherlands.

I. Vlodavsky*, M.D., Department of Oncology, Hadassah University Hospital, Jerusalem, Israel.

S. Volanti, M.D., Department of Ophthalmology, University of Bologna, Bologna, Italy.

J. Weber, Ph.D., Department of Zoology, University of Wisconsin, Madison, WI 53706, USA.

M. Weiser*, M.D., Department of Ophthalmology, Groupe Hospitalier Pitie-Salpetriere, 75615 Paris Cedex 13, France.

J.B. Weiss*, D.Sc., Department of Rheumatology, University of Manchester, Manchester M13 9PT, England.

M. Wiederholt, Ph.D., Institute of Clinical Physiology, Free University, Berlin, West Germany.

L. Wiek, M.D., Eye Clinic, Free University, Berlin, West Germany.

S. Wolf*, Dipl. Eng., Department of Ophthalmology, RWTH, D-5100 Aachen, West Germany.

H.C. Wong, M.D., Institute of Ophthalmology, London WC1H 9QS, England.

V. Woods, Ph.D., Department of Zoology, University of Wisconsin, Madison, WI 53706, USA.

K. Yamagishi, M.D., Department of Ophthalmology, Kansai Medical University, Moriguchi, Osaka, Japan.

M. Yanoff*, M.D., F.A.C.S., Department of Ophthalmology, Scheie Eye Institute, University of Pennsylvania School of Medicine, Philadelphia, PA 19104, USA.

Y. Yassur*, M.D., Department of Ophthalmology, Soroka Medical Center, Beersheva.

Z. Zagorski*, M.D., Department of Ophthalmology, Medical Academy, 20-079 Lublin, Poland.

H. Zauberman, M.D., Department of Ophthalmology, Hadassah University Hospital, Jerusalem.

A. Zelikovitch, Department of Ophthalmology, Hadassah University Hospital, Jerusalem, Israel.

E. Zmora, M.D., Department of Ophthalmology, Soroka Medical Center, Beersheva, Israel.

S. Zonis, M.D., Department of Ophthalmology, Rambam Medical Center, Haifa, Israel.

* first author

TABLE OF CONTENTS

CHAPTER 9: NEOVASCULARIZATION IV - ANGIOGENESIS MULTIPLE FACTORS

CHAPTER 10:   FUTURE TRENDS AND CONCEPTS

INTRODUCTION OF THE FIRST MICHAELSON MEDAL RECIPIENT

Along with the dedication of the International Symposium on Ocular Circulation and Neovascularization to the memory of Professor I.C. Michaelson, it was decided that the Israel Academy of Sciences and Humanities and the Hebrew University Hadassah Medical School in Jerusalem will award "The Michaelson Medal" once every three years for outstanding contributions to ophthalmology. The task of the nominating committee was to choose the first recipient - an eminent clinician and/or scientist who has contributed most significantly to the field of visual sciences and ophthalmology. Each member was assigned the task of suggesting one name. Although there were six members, only one name was suggested - six times: Arnall Patz. Nonetheless, it was decided to ask a larger International Advisory Board to each suggest three potential candidates with mention of the most worthy among the three. Again, Arnall Patz was on every list. In all, he was the first choice.

Arnall Patz was born in Elberton, Georgia in 1920. He received his M.D. degree in 1945 from the Emory University School of Medicine and served in the U.S. Army Medical Corps. From 1948 to 1950 he did his ophthalmology residency at the General Hospital in Washington, D.C. followed by a fellowship in ophthalmic pathology at the AFIP. Along with his apppointments as senior consultant to the most prestigious medical centers in Maryland and Washington, D.C., he held various academic positions at Johns Hopkins University, where he was appointed Professor of Ophthalmology in 1973. Since 1979 he has been Ophthalmologist-in-Chief to the Johns Hopkins Hospital; Director, Department of Ophthalmology, Wilmer Ophthalmological Institute; William Holland Wilmer Professor of Ophthalmology, Johns Hopkins University and the Seeing Eye Research Professor.

Dr. Patz has authored and contributed to many books and published more than 230 scientific papers. His contributions to modern ophthalmology are innumerable. Outstanding among them are his observations regarding the role of oxygen therapy in the underlying pathology of retrolental fibroplasia (retinopathy of prematurity) and the development of argon laser for ophthalmic use. Both of these contributions propelled clinical ophthalmology and the related visual sciences into the forefront of medicine.

For his unmatched innovative achievements in clinical ophthalmology and the related fields of visual sciences, he has been the recipient of every significant award and/or prize in Ophthalmology, a guest speaker at the most prestigious international meetings and honored by many universities and ophthalmic institutions in the United

2

States and around the world. The University of
Pennsylvania, Emory University and the Thomas Jefferson
University also bestowed upon him an Honorary Doctor of
Sciences. After serving as Vice-President of the American
Academy of Ophthalmology during 1984-86, he was elected its
President in 1986.

In April 1986 I had the privilege of informing
Professor Arnall Patz, M.D., D.Sc. about the unanimous
decision to nominate him as the first recipient of the
Michaelson Medal awarded by the Israel Academy of Sciences
and Humanities and the Hebrew University Hadassah Medical
School in Jerusalem. I am happy that he accepted and agreed
to deliver the Michaelson Lecture.

David BenEzra

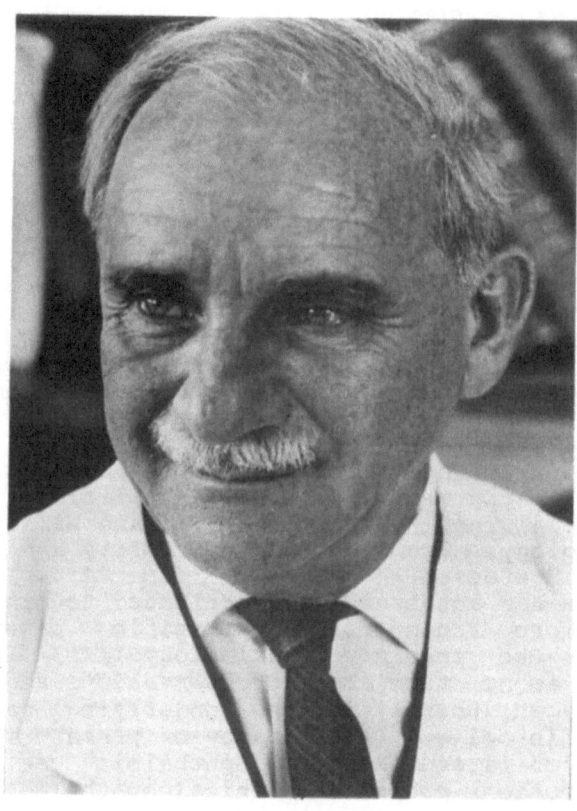

THE ISAAC C. MICHAELSON LECTURE

ARNALL PATZ, MD

Introduction

It is a great privilege to deliver the Isaac Michaelson lecture at this International Symposium on Ocular Circulation and Neovascularization. It is also a very special occasion for me personally because of my long friendship with Professor Michaelson and his family and my great respect for his scientific contributions. As a brilliant clinician and research investigator, he is recognized as one of the leading clinician-scientists of this century. His contributions to basic pathogenetic mechanisms involved in several key retinal vascular disorders provide the ground work and will serve as an inspiration for current and future generations of ophthalmic investigators.

Studies on retinal vascular anatomy

By the late 1930's, Michaelson had already launched a major investigation of the retinal vascular anatomy. In his classic paper with Campbell in 1940, Michaelson reported on the benzidine stain originally developed by Pickworth for the cerebral capillaries. The injection of benzidine was made in the ophthalmic artery post-mortem; after enucleation and fixation flat mounts of the retina were prepared. Michaelson's vivid comparison of benzidine with indian ink injection is noteworthy; with benzidine he noted "the skin of the face around the injected eye appears, of course, considerably congested; but the disfigurement is trivial as compared with the frightening result of injecting such a substance as indian ink." In this study Michaelson demonstrated that both arterial and venous precapillaries run to superficial and deep nets of the retina and there is no arterial or venous predominance in one or the other as had been previously reported. He identified the radially arranged capillaries in the peripapillary area and confirmed the capillary free area in the center of the fovea and around the arterioles.

Michaelson almost invariably examined his experimental findings in the broader perspective of developing concepts of pathogenesis and evolution of disease patterns. For example, in his 1940 paper in the Transaction of the Ophthalmological Society of the United Kingdom when discussing the predilection of the deep (hard) exudates in the outer plexiform layer, he stated "why is the outer capillary network the seat of predilection for the

disfunction? Can anatomical considerations throw any light
on the reason for this localization? In describing the
superficial cotton-wool or soft exudates,
Michaelson stated " white superficial, woolly patches may,
however, be due, not to exudation, but to degeneration of
the fibres in the nerve fibre layer. This degeneration is
found in many conditions - - -. The nerve fibres swell up
and undergo a varicose degeneration."

Michaelson's academic work was interrupted by his
service in the British Army during the second World War.
Continuing these studies on the retinal vascular system, he
culminated his work with the monograph "Retinal
Circulation in Man and Animals" which was published in
1954. In his foreword the late Dr. Jonas S. Friedenwald,
summarizing key points in Michaelson's monograph stated,
"This wide variation in the vascular pattern supplying the
retina is a matter of intrinsic interest from the
morphological and morphogenetic point of view, but has
bearings on many other fields as well. There is hardly a
problem in retinal physiology that cannot be illuminated to
some degree by a consideration of the diffusion gradients
of metabolites in this tissue. The knowledge that these
diffusion gradients are characteristically different in
different species, and even in different portions of the
retina in some animals, can furnish significant clues to
the workers in retinal physiology." Friedenwald continued
by stating, "Dr. Michaelson's thoughtful, scholarly, and
thought-provoking monograph has added much to our knowledge
in these matters and should be useful to the morphologist,
the physiologist and the clinician concerned with retinal
vascular conditions."

Pathogenesis of retinal neovascularization

Michaelson developed a working hypothesis to explain
the normal vascularization of the retina and the
development of pathologic neovascularization. He had
concluded from his studies published in 1948 that in the
developing retinal vasculature a "chemical factor" is
probably responsible for controlling the growth and
development of the retinal vasculature. He further
suggested that this factor had the following properties:(1)
the factor is present in the extra-vascular tissue of the
retina; (2) it is present in the gradient of concentration
such that it differs in arteriolar and venous
neighborhoods; (3) the factor possibly is therefore of a
biochemical nature; (4) its action is on the retinal veins
predominantly; (5) the factor initiating capillary growth
from veins probably determines the distance to which the
capillary growth will extend, the initiation and cessation
of growth depending on variation and concentration of the
factor.

Michaelson further extended his working hypothesis of
a chemical factor being responsible for retinal
neovascularization in human retinal diseases. He pointed

to the frequent formation of neovascularization in the
diabetic retina and also in the vasculitis of young adults
(Eales' disease).

Michaelson suggested that the embryonic capacity for
the development of new vessels from the retinal veins
persisted after the full development of the retinal
vasculature and the pathological formation of new vessels
from the retinal veins resulted from the accumulation of
"an environmental factor in the retina or in the
vitreous." Michaelson logically suggested that the
"environmental factor" that is elaborated by the retina in
chronic retinal diseases, may indeed be the same factor
which he postulated to serve as the stimulus for the
budding from the retinal veins in the normal developing
retina.

There have been extensive studies in recent years
suggesting that a chemical substance is associated with the
development of retinal neovascularization. Furthermore,
the finding of significant retinal vascular closure being
associated with the subsequent development of
neovascularization, has been abundantly documented in
diabetic retinopathy by fluorescein angiography studies.
Relating his embryologic studies to his clinical
observations, Michaelson stated in his 1954 monograph on
the retinal vessels, "With this appreciation of the
epigenesis of new-formed vessels in diabetes and other
conditions comes an understanding of the function which
those vessels are meant to serve. Just as the metabolic
needs of the embryonic retinal tissue demand closer
proximity of capillary vessels, so does the disturbed
metabolism of certain retinal diseases call for the
accession of vessels to insufficiently or non-vascularized
situations, intra-retinal, pre-retinal or vitreous."

Michaelson's comment on the "insufficiently or
non-vascularized situations" is consistent with the well
recognized changes demonstrated by fluorescein angiography
in not only diabetic retinopathy, but branch vein
occlusion, and sickle cell retinopathy. Ashton and
coworkers, whose elegant experimental studies demonstrated
the oxygen induced vascular closure in the young kitten
retina suggested a similar mechanism.

Wise, in 1955 provided a comprehensive review of
retinal neovascularization and designated Michaelson's
chemical factor as factor x". The reader is referred to
Henkind's Krill memorial lecture in 1978 for an excellent
summary of neovascularization. Fundamental to all of these
studies and more recent ones where angiogenic substances
have been identified in retina, Michaelson's original
observations and working hypothesis of a chemical factor
responsible for retinal vascularization and pathologic
neovascularization remain at the core of our understanding
of these disorders.

Bruch's membrane as a barrier

Michaelson's studies for the first time clearly defined the relationship of the choroid in the nutrition of the retina. In a special chapter on the role of the choroid he pointed out in his 1954 monograph that the choroidal vessels supply the nutrition to a part or in some cases all of the retina depending upon the animal species. He considered Bruch's membrane as a semi-permeable membrane, which although permeable to nutrient substances, acted as a physical barrier to capillary growth. In pathological states, Michaelson pointed out that capillaries may pass from the choroidal capillaries into the retina. This barrier effect and break-down of the barrier have been recognized by more recent studies from the eyes of patients with age-related macular degeneration and following laser photocoagulation. Some four decades later, there has been a renewed interest in the role of Bruch's membrane and recent studies have investigated the possibility that endothelial cells may have the ability to degrade Bruch's membrane.

Influence of the choroid on retinal vascularization

Michaelson suggested that the choriocapillaris is apparently capable of supporting nutrition into the outer retina for a distance of approximately 140 microns. In those areas where the retina is not thicker than this amount there appears to be no need for retinal vessels, thus explaining the absence of retinal capillaries in the central foveal area as well as at the periphery in humans. The retinal vessels in the inner retina indeed extend only to the mid-portion of the retina with the outer layers being nourished exclusively by the chorocapillaries.

The relationship of the retinal and choroidal circulations is described in the different vertebrate species examined in Michaelson's 1954 monograph. For example in the eel where there is no choroidal circulation, he noted that the retinal capillaries penetrate through the entire thickness of the retina down to the outer limiting membrane. Michaelson suggests that these vessel patterns are all dependent on the presence of an adequate choroidal circulation to meet the retinal requirements and wherever there is an insufficiency from the choroidal circulation an accumulation of "local intra-retinal factor" is elaborated which stimulates the local development of retinal capillaries.

Textbook of the fundus of the eye

Professor Ballantyne inspired Michaelson's enthusiasm for both the clinical and experimental study of retinal disorders. Their combined efforts culminated in the publication "Textbook of the Fundus of the Eye." This represented a major contribution to the literature and indeed was probably the most authoritative text on retinal diseases at that time. Michaelson's sound background in the pathophysiology of the retinal and choroidal circulations is evident in the lucid discussions of several of the key retinal diseases in this textbook. The text has undergone three revisions, the last appearing under Michaelson's sole authorship, with major collaboration by his son-in-law, Dr. David BenEzra. Each of the three editions have represented significant contributions and are classics in the ophthalmic literature.

The effect of O$_2$ on the immature retina

Shortly after the initial clinical and experimental studies linking oxygen administration to the development of retrolental fibroplasia, Michaelson and coworkers performed a systematic study of the effect of hyperoxia on the developing retinal blood vessels in the mouse eye. This meticulous study extended Michaelson's earlier work on the development of the retinal vasculature and further elucidated the basic pathogenetic changes induced by increased oxygen exposure. The gross decrease in the number of retinal capillaries, particularly in the capillary bed around the disc, was consistent with the vascular closure (vaso-obliteration) first described by Ashton in the experimental kitten model. Michaelson continued his interest in the experimental model of retrolental fibroplasia and he first corresponded with me on this topic in 1955.

Ocular epidemiology

Michaelson was recognized for his leadership in epidemiologic ophthalmology as exemplified by his chairmanship along with Professor Stein of the National Cooperative Study in the prevention of retinal detachment throughout the country of Israel. His epidemiologic interest took on a high priority when he later established the Institute for the Prevention of Blindness in Jerusalem after retiring as chairman of the Department of Ophthalmology at the Hadassah Hospital. Epidemiological contributions are noted throughout Professor Michaelson's career. An excellent example is his Bjerrum Memorial Lecture before the Danish Ophthalmological Society in 1967 where he recieved the distinguished Bjerrum medal. In this lecture he presented a major epidemiological study on systemic hypertension and diabetic retinopathy.

Teaching

Professor Michaelson was not only recognized as an accomplished research scientist and brilliant clinician but a dedicated teacher. His commitment to teaching is evident in the outstanding program he developed at the Hadassah Hospital and the excellence of its graduates, the majority of whom are now senior ophthalmologists throughout Israel. It was a very special opportunity for me to have several of his former residents spend a fellowship in our program on

retinal diseases at the Wilmer Institute.   Professor
Michaelson indicated to me on several occasions his great
pride in the scientific accomplishments of his son-in-law,
David BenEzra who continued his studies after the Hadassah
residency at the National Eye Institute.   Ben Ezra returned
to Israel to take a leadership role on the Hadassah
faculty.   It was gratifying to Michaelson for his former
resident, Hanan Zauberman, to assume the departmental
chairmanship, continuing the tradition of excellence of the
Hadassah program.
     Michaelson's active participation in the development
of ophthalmology in several African countries is most
noteworthy.   He took a key leadership position in providing
training for the physicians and associate staff in these
African units.

The Jerusalem Institute for the Prevention of Blindness
     It is most appropriate that Professor Michaelson
finalized his career by establishing the important
Jerusalem Institute for the Prevention of Blindness in
1973.   Setting the stage for the institute, he organized
the Congress on the Prevention of Blindness in Jerusalem in
1971.   Professor A. Edward Maumenee, who served as honorary
chairman of the congress, praised Michaelson for his
leadership in establishing a dialogue between the
participants from both developing countries and established
programs.
     Professor Michaelson made numerous contributions in
other fields.   His pioneer studies on corneal
neovascularization opened a whole new field of
investigation of this serious disorder.   He reported a pars
plana vitrectomy technique to cut vitreous bands in an
aphakic patient in 19 .   Michaelson, more than any other
scientist, is responsible for the eradication of trachoma
in much of the Middle East and North Africa.
     Professor Michaelson authored over 300 scientific
publications and three major textbooks and monographs.   He
received many distinguished awards.   I have selected
several that give a measure of this 20th Century
physician-scientist, teacher and humanitarian:

Star of Africa
Commander of the Order of St. John of Jerusalem
Grand Commander of the Republic of Liberia
McKenzie Memorial Medal
Israel Prize in Medicine
Mary Hawthorne Prize
Member of the Israel Academy of Sciences and Humanities
Bjerrum Memorial Medal
Charter Member Academia Ophthalmologica Internationalis
Smelser Memorial Medal
Medal of the Academy of Paris

     Professor Michaelson privately published in 1973 a

bound volume of his poems.   These touching verses provide
a picture of his character, giving insight into the breadth
and sensitivity of this individual and of the special
loving relationship he had with his wife, Ora, other loved
ones and close friends.   Ora's great devotion and the
sharing of common goals were a continuing inspiration
thoughout his career. With her permission, I quote two
verses from an unnamed poem written while he was stationed
in Alexandria, March 1944.

> Love is a sea-tide pouring
> And I a waiting shore,
> strange with its long song telling
> and I must listen more.
>
> You are the love presiding
> in sky and air and tide,
> and when by your breast I'm hiding
> they came to us inside.

REFERENCES
1. Michaelson I.C. and Campbell A.C.P.:   The anatomy of the
finer retinal vessels, and some observations on their
significance in certain retinal diseases.   Trans. Ophthal.
Soc. United Kingdom, Vol. LX: 71, 1940.
2. Michaelson I.C.: The mode of development of the vascular
system of the retina, with some observations on its
significance for certain retinal diseases.   Trans. Ophthal.
Soc. United Kingdom, Vol. LXVIII: 137, 1948.
3. Michaelson, I.C.: Retinal Circulation in Man and
Animals, Charles C. Thomas Publishers, Springfield, 1954.
4. Ashton N., Ward B., and Serpell G.: Role of oxygen in
the genesis of retrolental fibroplasia: preliminary report.
Br J Ophthal 37: 513, 1953.
5. Wise, G.N.: Retinal neovascularization.   Trans Am
Ophthalmol Soc 54: 729, 1956.
6. Henkind P.: Ocular neovascularization. The Krill
Memorial Lecture. Am J Ophthal 85: 287, 1978.

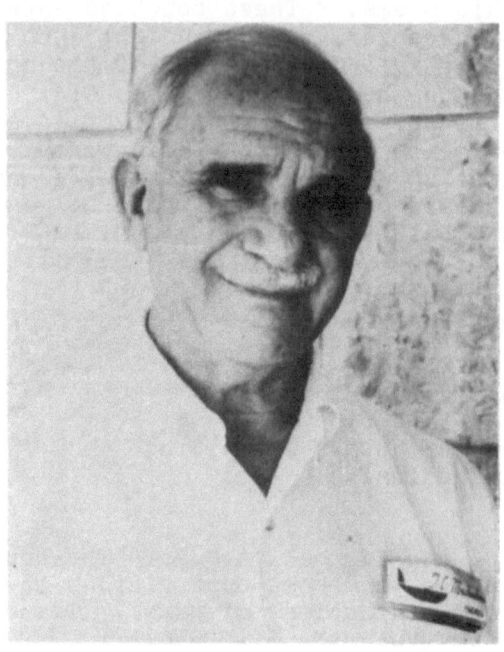

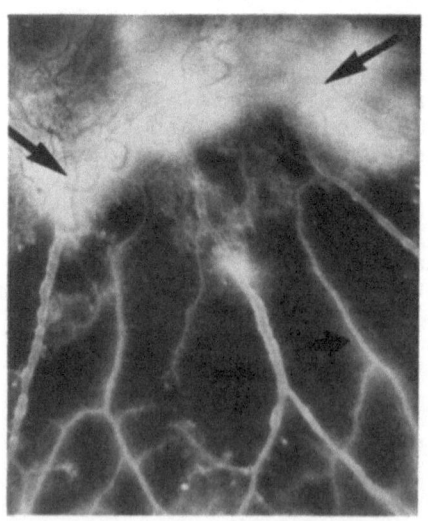
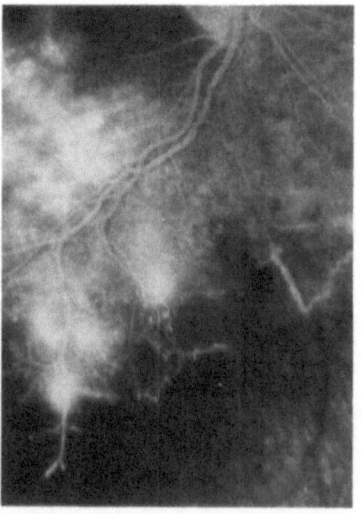

FIGURE 1. Photograph of Isaac C. Michaelson
International Congress on Prevention of Blindness,
Jerusalem 1971.
FIGURE 2. Fluorescein leakage from diabetic disc
neovascularization (long arrows). Extensive capillary
closure and non-perfusion (short arrows).
FIGURE 3. Peripheral capillary closure in occlusive
vasculitis (Eales' disease). Leakage from neovascularization near border of remaining retinal vessels.

RETINAL FLUOROTACHOMETRY (dynamic fluorescein angiography)

A.V.M. SCHULTE M.D. Ph.D., G.H. VAN RENS M.D.
Erasmus University Rotterdam, Department of Ophthalmology, The Netherlands

1. INTRODUCTION

Retinal Fluorotachometry (RFT) is a new clinical method for measurements of retinal blood flow, and in particular retinal capillary perfusion. It visualizes the flow patern in a chosen retinal area and it allows the determination of the velocity of flow in retinal arterioles and capillary beds.

The initial RFT studies were performed on rabbits. Because of the similarity of the monkey retina to the human retina, monkeys (species: macaca fascicularis) were used for further development of RFT techniques. Finally, within the scope of an initial clinical study, a limited number of human recordings was obtained. The purpose of this paper is to describe and discuss the method, and to present some results.

RFT is by this time the only clinically applicable, objective method for measurements on retinal flow at the arteriolar as well as the capillary level.

2. CONCEPT OF RFT

The initial idea was to record the transposition of a well defined front of fluorescein through retinal arterioles and capillaries on cine film, and to quantify retinal blood flow by analysis of these films. For the realisation of this idea, two major problems had to be solved.

The first was the development of a clinically applicable technique to create a high concentration gradient between blood with and without fluorescein (a sharp dye front) in the retinal arterioles and capillaries.

The second was to find a method of high speed cine recording, with high resolution power, of the transposition of this dye front.

3. CREATION OF A SHARP DYE FRONT

3.1. Previous methods

In conventional fluorescein angiography, after intravenous dye injection, the dye front at its entrance in the retinal vessels is poorly defined. By laminar and incidentally turbulent flow during the course from the site of intravenous injection to the retina the dye bolus is stretched out, causing a low gradient of dye concentration at the bolus tip when it reaches the eye. The recording of the transposition of such a vague front is a poor basis for an analysis to quantify flow. For retinal flow measurement a well defined dye front is needed. Previously published techniques for the creation of a sharp dye front in the retina consist of injection of the dye via a catheter into an artery proximal to the central retinal artery (7,12). The closer the tip of the catheter to the central retinal artery, the sharper the dye front at its entrance in the retinal vessels. However, such an intra-arterial injection is less suitable for routine clinical application.

3.2. A new technique

A sharp dye front in the retina after an **intravenous** injection of the dye could be achieved if the entry of the dye into the retinal vessels could be delayed until the concentration of the dye in the ophthalmic artery has reached a level at which maximum fluorescence occurs. The most suitable location to block the entrance of fluorescein into the retinal vessels is in the central retinal artery at its point of entrance in the eye.

A temporary "clamping" of the central retinal artery at this point is achieved by a rapid elevation of the intraocular pressure (IOP) above the systolic pressure in the ophthalmic artery, which causes the central retinal artery (and vein) to collapse at the point of pressure gradient, i.e. at its entrance in the eye. The onset of the IOP elevation is triggered at the time the ultimate tip of the dye bolus enters the choroidal vessels*, which is detected by means of a photomultiplier. The retinal circulation stops abruptly, but the retinal vessels remain filled with blood. Only two small segments at the optic disc, one of the central retinal artery and one of the central retinal vein, collapse.The same is true for the choroidal circulation: it stops after the IOP elevation, but the choroidal vessels remain filled with blood. A few seconds (1.8-2.8 s) after the onset of the IOP elevation the concentration of the dye in the ophthalmic artery has reached a level at which maximum fluorescence occurs. At that time the IOP elevation is released, and the dye enters the retinal vessels with a sharp front. This is the concept of the ocular pressure technique (fig.1).

Understanding this concept requires familiarity with the anatomical site of the central retinal artery, its origin and branches. Both the central retinal artery and the posterior ciliary arteries are relatively long and have few and only smal branches that communicate with the venous system outside the eye (1,2,3,4,5,6). Branches seldom arise from the distal section of the intraneural part of the central retinal artery and never from the part in the lamina cribrosa (5). Consequently, the volume flow into the central retinal artery after "clamping" at the optic disc is quite low, and there is little influx of fluorescein into the central retinal artery. In the case of relatively numerous and/or wide branches the influx of fluorescein will not go beyond the middle section of the intraneural part of the central retinal artery until the IOP elevation is discontinued.

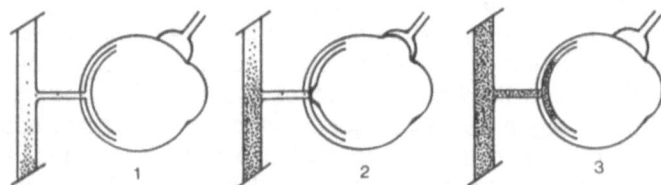

Fig.1
1. The tip of the fluorescein bolus reaches the eye and is detected by the photomultiplier.
2. The signal of the photomultiplier triggers the IOP elevation and the ocular circulation is halted.
3. The IOP elevation is discontinued and the fluorescein enters the retinal vesels with a sharp front.

* More recently, the entrance of dye into the conjunctival and (epi)scleral vessels is used for this triggering procedure.

3.3. Effect of applied IOP elevation on retinal flow

3.3.1. The ocular pressure technique includes an IOP elevation above the systolic pressure in the ophthalmic artery for 1.8-2.8 s. After release of the IOP elevation the transposition of the dye front in the retinal vessels is recorded. The influence of the applied IOP elevation on subsequent retinal flow requires evaluation. Two mechanisms could introduce artefacts.

    a. Reactive hyperaemia, which may be defined as the increase in flow above the control level that occurs if a severe restriction of flow to tissue is suddenly released (14). The applied IOP elevation could cause a restriction of flow, severe enough (in duration) to cause a subsequent reactive hyperaemia.

    b. Acute IOP elevation has been considered to stimulate vagal activity. Vagal stimulation could cause a decrease of heart frequency (and cardiac output) which would affect retinal hemodynamics.

3.3.2. Data from literature on reactive hyperaemia. Riva and Loebl (18) published a study of the relation between IOP elevation and blood flow in the human macular capillaries. The flow of leucocytes was subjectively measured by means of the blue field entoptic phenomenon. It was found that the time lag between the onset of IOP elevation and the beginning of reactive hyperaemia (retinal autoregulatory response) was between 25 s and 67 s. These findings are in concordance with a study by Riehm, Podestà and Bartsch (11). Using the blue field entoptic phenomenon on human subjects they found no autoregulatory response within 30 s following an IOP elevation up to about 40 mm Hg. ffytche, Bulpitt, Kohner, Archer and Dollery (14) measured retinal vessel diameters and fluorescein front velocities at different IOP's in pigs. It was found that reactive dilatation of retinal vessels depended on the duration of the IOP elevation and occurred only if the IOP elevation was maintained for more than 30 s.

3.3.3. Data from literature on vagal stimulation. Ocular pneumo-plethysmography (OPG) is a method for the evaluation of carotid artery obstructive disease in humans, which includes a rapid bilateral IOP elevation until above the pressure in the ophthalmic arteries and subsequent gradual release. Simultaneous recording of OPG curves and pulse frequency revealed no change in pulse frequency induced by the IOP elevation (9,16,17,21).

3.3.4. Data from personal studies on reactive hyperaemia. The blue field entoptic phenomenon has been used to study specifically the effect of the IOP elevation as applied in RFT on the retinal microcirculation in ten healthy humans, in three patients with moderate background diabetic retinopathy, and in three patients with moderate hypertensive retinopathy. These studies were previously described in more detail (28).

During arrest of the intraocular circulation by IOP elevation, normal vision was maintained for at least 3.5 s in all subjects. After 4-6 s visual acuity deteriorated and vision gradually disappeared. The subject was seated in front of a pair of blue field entoptoscopes, which allowed a diffuse illumination of the maculae with blue light (peak: 428 nm, bandwidth: 20 nm). A scleral contact lens with a scleral suction cup attached was placed over the left eye (cf. fig.3). The right eye was used as control. By means of electro-magnetically actuated shutters in both entoptoscopes the fundi could be illuminated alternately, and the subject could compare the speed of the leucocytes in the left macula with the speed of the leucocytes in the right macula. By means of an IOP elevation the intra ocular circulation in the subject's left eye (whiles exposed to the blue light) was halted and the darting spots (leucocytes) were no longer observed. After 3.5 s the IOP elevation was discontinued and immediately the subject again observed the darting spots. An attentive observation was continued for 1 s. Then the right eye was exposed to the blue light. In this manner the speed of the leucocytes in the left eye was compared with the speed of the leucocytes in the right eye. All subjects observed an immediate return to a steady state pulsatile systolic/diastolic speed cycle after release of the IOP elevation, and none of the subjects observed a difference in the speed of the left eye's and right eye's leucocytes.

3.3.5. Data from personal studies on vagal stimulation. The effect of the IOP elevation as applied in RFT on the pulse frequency was measured in ten healthy humans. These experiments were previously described (28). An effect of the IOP elevation on the pulse frequency was not revealed.

3.3.6. These data indicate that the ocular pressure technique as applied in RFT does not introduce an artefact in retinal hemodynamics. Reactive hyperaemia is presumably related to ischaemia giving rise to hypoxia, CO_2 retention, and the accumulation of metabolites. Apparently, the applied IOP elevation is of too short duration to cause such ischaemia.

4.   HIGH-SPEED CINE RECORDING OF THE DYE FRONT TRANSPOSITION
4.1. Excitation of fluorescein with argon laser

Exposures of high quality can be obtained when a 35 mm film with a high resolving power at a frame rate of e.g. 100 frames/s (in our animal experiments up to 150 frames/s) is used. However, a limiting factor for frame size and frame rate is the fluorescence light emitted by the dye in the retinal vessels. Fluorescence light is directly related to excitation light. When using the conventional source of excitation light for fluorescein angiography (the xenon lamp), only a relatively small part of the spectrum of the emitted light consists of efficacious energy for excitation of fluorescein, and only a relatively small portion of that part reaches the retina because of the considerable losses in the fundus camera. Therefore the input of electric energy into the xenon flash lamp in a fundus camera per fluorescein angiographic exposure on 35 mm film is high, and a rate of 100 flashes/s would pose a considerable technical problem.

We expected an argon laser apparatus to be a more effective source of excitation energy because of the following considerations:
- The most effective wavelengths for excitation of fluorescein in blood are in the range of 475-515 nm (8,10,15).
- The argon laser emits monochromatic light mainly of the following wavelengths: 476.5 nm, 488.0 nm, 496.5 nm, 501.7 nm and 514.5 nm; the 488.0 nm and 514.5 nm fractions being the most energetic (about 50% and 35% respectively of total of light energy emitted by the apparatus used in our experiments). These two most powerful emission lines are within the range for

effective excitation of fluorescein in blood.
- The light emitted by a laser is coaxially bundled, which offers the advantage of relatively low losses in its optical pathway to the retina.

The continuous-wave (CW) argon laser was found to be a most suitable source of excitation energy for high-speed fluorescein cinematography in RFT (22,23,25,26,28). We used the Coherent 900, but any other argon laser with equivalent output can be used. A high-speed electronic shutter chopped the CW laser output to cine-camera-synchronized flashes.

4.2. Radiation hazards.

Visible radiation (light) can be damaging to the eye, and the retina is most vulnerable in this respect. Before RFT was considered a safe, clinically applicable method, its potency to cause retinal radiation trauma was evaluated. This evaluation is discussed in detail in a previous publication (28). The retinal radiant exposure in RFT studies on humans was 3 mJ/cm^2 or less per flash; the flash duration was 5 ms; the number of flashes was less than 200; the flash frequency was less than 100 flashes/s; the duration of the flash train was less than 2 s.

Data from other studies and data from personal studies were used for this evaluation. These data indicate that the irradiance and the radiant exposure in RFT are safe for the eye. The level of retinal radiant exposure in relation to maximum permissible exposure is nevertheless high (close to which is employed in standard fluorescein angiography), and patients whose retinas are extremely vulnerable in this respect (e.g. those suffering from retinitis pigmentosa) should not undergo RFT (as they should neither undergo standard fluorescein angiography).

5. INSTRUMENTATION

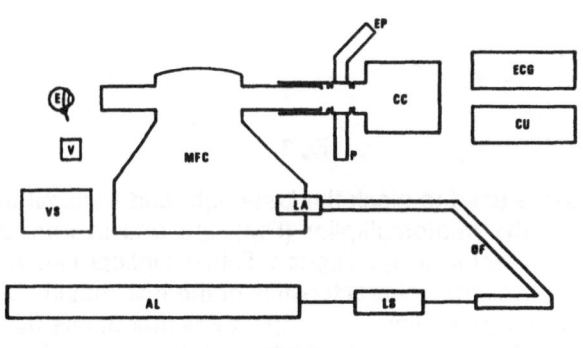

Fig.2

An outline of the RFT set-up is given in fig.2. The Argon laser (AL) offers a light output power of 3 W, consisting for about 50% of 488.0 nm light and about 35% of 514.5 nm light, and for about 95% of light within the 475-515 nm range. An excitation filter is not needed. The high speed laser shutter (SL), with crystal controlled exposure time setting and triggering by a cine camera pulse, chops the laser beam to produce laser flashes. Its operation frequency of up to 100 Hz is adequate for most RFT studies (26L Shutter System manufactured by:

A.W.Vincent Associates Inc., Rochester, NY 14607, USA). An optic fiber (OF) conducts the laser light into the laser adaptor (LA). This adaptor abolishes the coherence of the laser to prevent disturbing interference phenomena, and acts as a diffuser with a small bend angle, which fits the laser into the illumination system of the fundus camera with a minimal loss of light. As a result the ocular fundus is evenly illuminated by the laser light. The retinal field covered by the modified fundus camera (MFC) extends 30°, measured from the nodal point of the eye. The modifications in this camera consist of an improvement of excitation light transmission to the retina and fluorescence light transmission from the retina to the cine film. These improvements allow a decrease in flash duration at the same laser output. The equipment for the IOP elevation should meet the following specific requirements: it should be safe for the eye, have rapid and accurate action, and allow undisturbed optical accessibility of the retina.

In our experiments the most suitable instrument for the human eye (E) was found to be a suction cup at the temporal side of the cornea, mounted in a scleral contact lens (fig. 3), filled with normal saline solution, and coupled via an electromagnetically actuated three-way valve (V) to an accurately adjustable "vacuum" (low pressure) system (VS). [For rabbits we used a cornea covering transparent suction cup, filled with normal saline solution; for monkeys an electromagnetically actuated scleral indentator.]

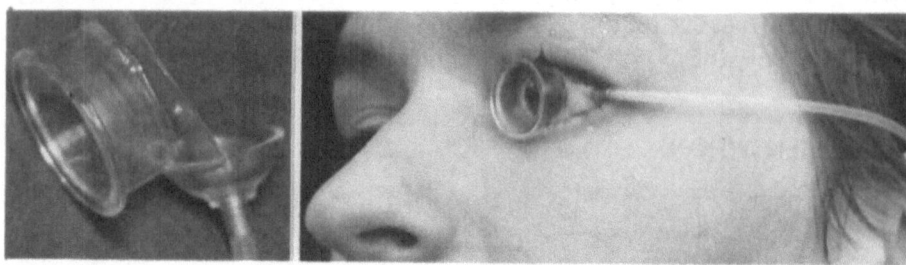

Fig.3

Two barrier filters were used to block the laser light and transmit the fluorescence light: one in front of the photomultiplier (PM) and one in front of the cine film (AMW-FL Filter, manufactured by: Topcon Tokyo Optical Co. Ltd., Tokyo, 174 Japan). The spectral sensitivity characteristics of the PM should cover the 520-620 nm range of the luminescence light. A compact PM that meets this requirement is the XP1911 (Philips, Eindhoven, The Netherlands). The retinal image can be observed via the eye piece (EP), and is focused at the film plane in the cine camera (CC) Arritechno 35 model 150 (Arnold & Richter Cine Technik, München, West Germany), which allows a frame rate up to 150 frames/s. The R-wave of the electrocardiogram triggers the release of the IOP elevation (cf. 6). A standard electrocardiograph (ECG) with an output for triggering a defibrillator was used. Sequence and timing during RFT recordings were programmed with the use of a computer unit (CU). The most appropriate cine film was in our experience the Kodak 35 mm CFE film (= PE 2711). It is an orthochromatic, medium speed,

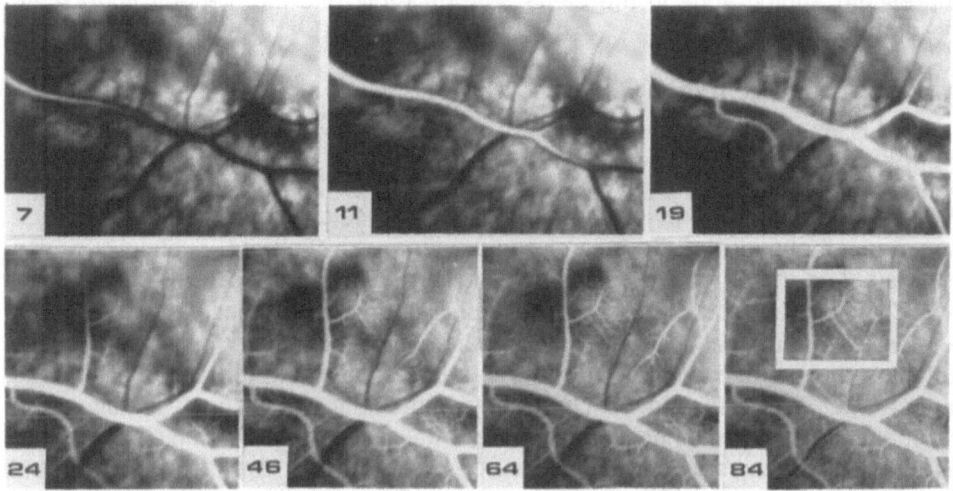

Fig.4

frames/s, which corresponds with a total of 90 frames (1.71 m) to 270 frames (5.13 m) per recording. In humans the frame speed was 50-90 frames/s, which corresponds with a total of 90 frames (1.71 m) to 162 frames (3.08 m) per recording. These lengths do not include the non-exposed beginning (startup) and end (run out) of the film. The recording exhibits subsequent stages of the choroidal filling and of the advancement of the fluorescein front into the retinal vascular bed. A partial reproduction of a monkey RFT recording is given in fig.4 (details of a selection of the frames). Frame 7: a streched, pointed front is seen in the retinal arteriole. Frame 11: the tip of the front advances beyond branches, arising from the arteriole in a perpendicular fashion; the dye does not enter these perpendicular branches yet; at bifurcations the front splits up, and enters both branches simultaneously. Frame 19: fluorescein flows into the perpendicular branches (the fluorescein containing laminae near the wall of the arteriole have reached these branches). Frame 84: a rectangle encloses a retinal capillary bed and its feeding arteriole and draining venules. The frame descriptions hereafter are related to this area, enclosed by the rectangle. Frame 24: fluorescein enters the capillary bed. Frame 46: fluorescein passes the capillary bed. Frame 64: first frame with fluorescein laminae along the walls of the draining venules, i.e. fluorescein enters the post-capillary venules. Frame 84: fluorescein flows into the venules (crescent fluorescent laminae along the walls of the venules). Four succesive frames of a human RFT recording are given in fig.5, showing the inflow of fluorescein in a retinal arteriole.

The time interval between inflow of fluorescein in the choroid and the inflow in the

low-grain, polyester base film, designed to match the P31 green-emitting output phosphor of the caesium-iodide image intensifiers in use in cardiac angiography. The film has adequate sensitivity in the fluorescence range of 520-620 nm, and it offers a relatively high resolving power (100-200 lines/mm). Its thin and strong polyester base has excellent mechanical qualities for high-speed recording.

The set-up allows RFT recording and subsequent conventional (single frame) fluorescein angiography in the same session (only one intravenous fluorescein injection needed).

6. SEQUENCE OF EVENTS AND TIMING

The pupil of the eye to be studied was maximally dilated and the subject was positioned in front of the fundus camera (animal studies were carried out under general anaesthesia). ECG electrodes were connected to the limbs. In monkeys: the scleral indentator was positioned close to the sclera; in humans: the cornea was anaesthetized and the scleral contact lens with temporal suction cup was inserted. The image of the selected retinal area was focused at the film plane. A 10% sodium fluorescein bolus was given by intravenous injection.

After a number of seconds (leg/arm --> choroid circulation time) the photomultiplier detected the entrance of the tip of the dye bolus into the choroidal vessels, and triggered the IOP elevation, which arrested intraocular circulation. The flow in the ophthalmic artery remained unaffected and the fluorescein concentration in that artery gradually increased in the course of about 2 s to a level at which maximal fluorescence occurs. [The action of the IOP elevating device caused a displacement of the eye which brought the retina out of focus.] After a time interval of about 2 s the IOP elevation was released, and the cine camera was started. The fluorescein flowed through the orbital part of the central retinal artery, reached the eye and entered the retinal arterioles (0.6-0.9 ms after IOP release). [By that time the eye movements, caused by this release, were damped, and the retina was back in focus.] Laser flashing and cine recording started 0.5 s after the IOP release and was continued for 1.8 s.

The timing of the IOP release was linked to the cardiac cycle: the IOP elevation was maintained for a set period of 1.8 s; then the next following R-wave of the ECG triggered the release of the IOP elevation. By means of this timing procedure the fluorescein inflow into the retinal arterioles occurred in different recordings in approximately the same phase of the cardiac cycle, which improved the reproducibility, especially with regard to the measurements of flow velocities in the retinal arterioles. The cine camera speed had reached its steady state before the entrance of the fluorescein front into the retinal arterioles. The exposed piece of film was processed in an instant developing machine. Subsequently the quality of the recording was assessed with the use of a 35 mm cine film projecting system. Recordings of sufficient quality were the basis for quantitative flow analysis.

7. RFT RECORDINGS

An RFT recording is an exposed and developed 35 mm cine film, with a length depending on the frame speed (the recording time was a fixed period of 1.8 s, i.e. the time period of laser flashing, cf. 6.). In animals the frame speed was 50-150

retinal arteriole can be accurately measured (in the monkeys: mean 0.43 s, SD 0.03 s; in the humans: mean 0.49 s, SD 0.04 s).

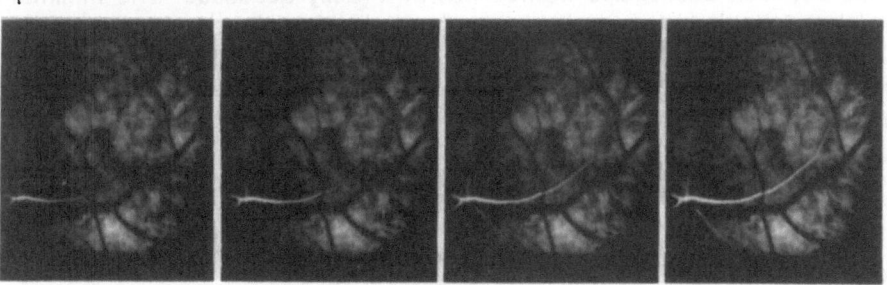

Fig.5

8. MEASUREMENT OF FLOW VELOCITY IN RETINAL ARTERIOLES

A computer assisted analysis of RFT recordings for the measurement of flow velocity in retinal arterioles was previously described (27,28,29). For an objective and reproducible location of the tip of the dye front in the different frames of the RFT cine film, an automated front detecting system has been developed.

According to the nature of the coaxial laminar flow in arterioles, the flow velocity increases from zero at the wall, to a maximum value at the center of the vessel (= V_{max}). The speed of the dye front tip corresponds with V_{max} .

After determination of the cross-sectional area S of the vessel at the measurement site, the volume flow F can be calculated, since $F = 0.63 \, V_{max} \, S$ (13,19,20). [Strictly, this formula should only be used for Poiseuille flow, as occurs in venules. However, in a study by Riva and coworkers this formula provided accurate calculations of pulsatile flow in retinal arterioles as well (24)]. The vessel diameter (D) can be obtained from red-free fundus photographs, and the cross-sectional area can be calculated: $S = 0.25 \, \pi \, D^2$.

To transform the pictorial information from the RFT recording into digital format that can be processed by computer the film was mounted on a specially constructed cine-video converter. The RFT cine frames were projected onto the target of a high-resolution video camera, which was attached to an x-y stage for the selection of the retinal area of interest. The center square of the resulting analog video image was digitized in matrix size of 512 x 512 picture elements (pixels) with eight bits (256 levels) of (photographic) density resolution. This digitized image was displayed on the video monitor. The procedure of dye front location basically consists of the following two steps:

1. detection of centerlines of retinal arterioles and branches by tracing local density maxima (max-tracing); for this purpose a frame is used in which the arteriolar filling is completed;
2. these arteriolar centerlines are used as guidelines for the detection of the dye front position in the frames of the arteriolar filling phase; when tracing in distal direction along these lines, a density drop to zero (relative to the reference density level of non-fluorescent vessels) indicates the position of the tip of the

front.

From these front transpositions the mean flow velocity of the dye front tip in intervals between successive frames can be readily assessed. The minimal (= diastolic) and maximal (= systolic) mean flow velocity of the dye front tip during a cardiac cycle were measured in the inferior temporal retinal arteriole. Nine monkey RFT recordings and three human RFT recordings were used for these measurements. The monkey recordings were carried out on three subjects (three recordings per subject). The frame speed of the monkey recordings was 100 frames/s. The time interval between successive recordings on the same subject was about one week. The human recordings were carried out on three subjects. The frame speed of the human recordings was 60 frames/s. In table 1 the results of these measurements are listed.

Table 1

	diastolic [cm/s]	systolic [cm/s]		diastolic [cm/s]	systolic [cm/s]
Monkey 1					
first recording	1.6	3.6	Human 1	2.2	3.7
second recording	1.5	3.3			
third recording	1.8	3.6			
Monkey 2			Human 2	1.9	3.8
first recording	1.5	3.2			
second recording	1.8	3.4			
third recording	1.7	3.0			
Monkey 3			Human 3	2.4	4.0
first recording	1.5	3.3			
second recording	1.8	3.4			
third recording	1.4	3.1			

9. MEASUREMENT OF RETINAL CAPILLARY TRANSIT TIME

RFT recordings show a dye front which is pointed in the arterioles and in the branches arising from the arterioles. In the precapillaries and capillaries the front is flattened. In the venules the dye flows in laminae near the vessel wall. The pointed shape of the dye front in the arterioles, and the laminar dye stream in the venules are explained by the the nature of the coaxial laminar flow in these vessels. The flattened shape of the dye front in the precapillaries and capillaries is explained by the relation between the sizes of the blood cells and the diameter of the blood column in these small vessels. The flow velocity is in the precapillary vessel relatively high and in the capillaries relatively low, causing the dye front to flow into the different "entrance capillaries" of the capillary bed almost simultaneously. The time interval between entrance into the capillary bed, and entrance into the postcapillary venule is the **capillary transit time**. The quality of the dye front in RFT allows an accurate determination of the capillary transit time. Retinal capillary beds at different locations in the retina are not all the same. For example, there is quite a difference between a peripapillary retinal capillary bed and a peripheral retinal capillary bed. In relation to the capillary transit time, especially the differences of the lengths of the capillary mesh (from the precapillary to the postcapillary vessel) are influential. Therefore, the capillary transit time can be used for flow measurement at the capillary level only if it is linked to equivalent capillary beds (intraindividually and interindividually). In RFT studies on monkeys and on humans it was found that the macular capillary beds in the upper and the lower quadrant, between the superior/inferior temporal artery and the fovea, are the most appropriate for this purpose. In table 2 the measured capillary transit times of a macular capillary bed in the lower quadrant in three monkey and three human RFT recordings are listed.

Table 2

Monkey 1	0.47 s	Human 1	0.52 s
Monkey 2	0.46 s	Human 2	0.54 s
Monkey 3	0.49 s	Human 3	0.48 s

In a first clinical study three young adult patients with diabetes mellitus (young onset type 1 [insulin-dependent]) and with early diabetic retinopathy (vascular changes, including microaneurysms; retinal hemorrhages) were studied. The patients were clearly informed of the procedure and purpose of the study, and gave written consent. The measured capillary transit times were: 0.42 s, 0.43 s and 0.45 s, which is a decrease of approximately16% as compared with the measurements on "normal" young adults.

10. CONCLUSIONS

The RFT recordings demonstrate the efficacy of the ocular pressure technique: a well defined dye front in retinal arterioles and capillaries was obtained after an intravenous injection of fluorescein and a controlled IOP elevation. It is also shown that the use of an argon laser allows high-speed recording on 35 mm cine film of fluorescein inflow in the retina (and choroid). A computer assisted system for the analysis of the arteriolar filling phase of RFT recordings allows automated detection of the position of the dye front tip, and from these data the mean flow velocity of the front tip for each time interval between successive frames can be calculated.

Capillary transit times of macular capillary beds have been measured in monkeys and in humans. In early juvenile diabetic retinopathy a decrease of the capillary transit time of about 16% was found. Further studies are needed to determine the significance of these findings.

References

1. François J. and Neetens A. : Vascularisation of the optic pathway I. Lamina cribrosa and optic nerve. Brit J Ophthalmol 38:472, 1954
2. François J. et al. : Vascular supply of the optic pathway II. Further studies by micro-arteriography of the optic nerve. Brit J Ophthalmol 39:220, 1955
3. François J. and Neetens A. : Vascularisation of the optic pathway III. Study of intra-orbital and intracranial optic nerve by serial sections. Brit J Ophthalmol 40:45, 1956
4. Singh S. and Dass R. : The central artery of the retina I. Origin and course. Brit J Ophthalmol 44:193, 1960

5. Singh S. and Dass R. : The central artery of the retina II. A study of its distribution and anastomoses. Brit J Ophthalmol 44:280, 1960
6. Hayreh S.S. : The ophthalmic artery III. Branches. Brit J Ophthalmol 46:212, 1962
7. Dollery C.T. et al. : Retinal microemboli: cine fluorescence angiography. Trans Ophthalmol Soc UK 85:271, 1965
8. Hodge J.V. and Clement R.S. : Improved method for fluorescence angiography of the retina. Am J Ophthalmol 61:1400, 1966
9. Brockenbrough E.C. et al. : Ocular plethysmography: a new technique for the evaluation of carotid obstructive disease. Review of Surgery 24:299, 1967
10. Baurmann H. : Grundlagen der Fluoreszenzangiographie des Augenhintergrundes. Advances in Ophthalmol 24:204, 1971
11. Riehm E. et al. : Untersuchungen über die Durchblutung in Netzhautkapillaren bei intraokularen Drucksteigerungen. Ophthalmologica 164:249, 1972
12. Hill D.W. et al. : Retinal blood flow measured by fluorescence angiography. Trans Ophthalmol Soc UK 93:325, 1973
13. Baker M. and Wayland H. : On-line volume flow rate and velocity profile measurement for blood in microvessels. Microvasc Res 7:131, 1974
14. ffytche T.J. et al. : Effect of changes in intraocular pressure on the retinal microcirculation. Brit J Ophthalmol 58:514, 1974
15. Delori F.C. and Ben-Sira: Excitation and emission spectra of fluorescein dye in the human ocular fundus. Invest Ophthalmol 14:487, 1975
16. Gee W. et al. : Measurement of collateral cerebral hemispheric blood pressure by ocular pneumoplethysmography. Am J of Surgery 130:121, 1975
17. Gee W. et al. : Noninvasive diagnosis of carotid occlusion by ocular pneumoplethysmography. Stroke 7:18, 1976
18. Riva C.E. and Loebl M. : Autoregulation of blood flow in the capillaries of the human macula. Invest Ophthalmol 16:568, 1977
19. Lipowsky H.H. and Zweifach B.W. : Application of the "two-slit" photometric technique to the measurement of microvascular volumetric flow rates. Microvasc Res 15:93, 1978
20. Damon D.N. and Duling B.R. : A comparison between mean blood velocities and center-line red cell velocities as measured with a mechanical image streaking velocimeter. Microvasc Res 17:330, 1979
21. Eikelboom B.C. : Evaluation of carotid artery disease and potential collateral circulation by ocular pneumoplethysmography. Academic thesis, Leiden, The Netherlands, 1981
22. Schulte A.V.M. : Apparatus for (high-speed) fluorescein angiography. Netherlands Patent Application no 83.01049 , 1983
23. Schulte A.V.M. and De Jong P.T. : Retinal Fluorotachometry. ARVO Abstracts. Invest Ophthalmol Vis Sci 25(Suppl): 7, 1984
24. Riva et al. : Blood velocity and volumetric flow rate in human retinal vessels. Invest Ophthalmol Vis Sci 26:1124, 1985
25. Schulte A.V.M. et al. : Device for retinal or choroidal angiography or hematotachography. European Patent Application no 85200522.2, 1985
27. Schulte A.V.M. et al. : Retinal Fluorotachometry. ARVO Abstracts. Invest Ophthalmol Vis Sci 26(Suppl): 246, 1985
27. Reiber J.H.C. et al. : Quantitative coronary and left ventricular cineangiography: methodology and clinical applications, chapter IX. Martinus Nijhoff Publishers, Dordrecht/Boston/Lancaster, 1986
28. Schulte A.V.M. : Retinal Fluorotachometry. Academic thesis, Rotterdam, The Netherlands, 1986
29. Van Ommeren J. et al. : Artery detection and analysis in cine-angiograms. Pattern Recognition in Practice II, Proceedings of an International Workshop, June 19-21, 1985. Edited by Edzard S.Gelsema, Department of Medical Informatics, Free University, Amsterdam, and Laveen N. Kanal, Department of Computer Science, University of Maryland, College Park, Md,1986

ISOVOLEMIC HEMODILUTION IN ISCHEMIC AND NON-ISCHEMIC RETINAL VEIN OCCLUSION

L.L. HANSEN, I. WIEK, and M. WIEDERHOLT*

Augenklinik und *Institut f. Klinische Physiologie der Freien Universität Berlin im Klinikum Steglitz, Berlin, FRG

Summary. 107 patients with retinal vein occlusion were treated by isovolemic hemodilution (IHD) within the first 8 weeks after appearing of symptoms. Hematocrit was stepwise lowered to 0.3 (to 0.35 in patients older than 75 years) by repeated exchanges of whole blood for plasma and dextran 40. IHD was repeated about 10 times over a period of six weeks. Fluorescein angiograms and rheological measurements (whole blood viscosity, plasma viscosity, red cell aggregability and filtrability) were done before and after IHD. Of 67 patients with central retinal vein occlusion 30 were of the ischemic type ($\geq$ 10 cotton wool spots, arteriovenous passage time $\geq$ 20s). 43 % of this type showed an improvement of visual acuity after IHD, whereas only 17 % of patients with non-ischemic CRVO had a better visual acuity. Of 41 patients with retinal branch vein occlusion (RBVO) 20 were classified as ischemic types ($\geq$ 3 cotton wool spots, defective foveolar arcade). 65 % of these ischemic types of RBVO improved after IHD, however, an increase of visual acuity after 3 months could only be observed in about 15 % of patients with non-ischemic RBVO. Rheological measurements were not different in ischemic and non-ischemic retinal vein occlusion.

1. INTRODUCTION

Central retinal vein occlusion (CRVO) should be divided into two subgroups, an ischemic one with capillary occlusion areas, and a non-ischemic one of a more hyperpermeable character. It is now widely accepted that panretinal photocoagulation reduces neovascular complications of the ischemic type (3,4,5), but it does not improve visual prognosis. Only 10 - 20 % of these patients reach a final visual acuity (VA) of 0.3 or more. The visual outcome of the non-ischemic type of central retinal vein occlusion and of retinal branch vein occlusion (RBVO) with macular involvement is far better. About 50 % of these patients retain a visual acuity of 0.3 and more, however, 20 - 40 % decrease to 0.1 or less. Up to now this visual decay has not been influenced by any treatment if one excludes the prevention of neovascularization and its sequelae by photocoagulation.
For a couple of years we have been applying the new therapeutic concept of isovolemic hemodilution (IHD) in additon to photocoagulation (1,2). This takes into account that, irrespective of the pathogenic process, the outflow obstruc-

tion in retinal vein occlusion (RVO) should result at least in a local disturbance of whole blood viscosity. The reasons for this may be (1) local hemoconcentration by extravasation of plasma constituents, (2) increase of fibrinogen by increased coagulation, (3) enhanced red cell aggregation and (4) reduced flexibility of red cells by local acidification.

In a controlled study it has been shown that IHD improves the visual prognosis in CRVO (1). Furthermore, a pilot study of RBVO disclosed that hemodilution may prevent a serious drop of visual acuity (2). Both studies indicated that there might be differences in the response of ischemic and non-ischemic RVO to isovolemic hemodilution. This preliminary finding was now evaluated in all patients who underwent IHD for RVO in our department during the last 4 years. Furthermore, rheological measurements were done to clarify the role of systemical changes of blood fluidity.

2. PATIENTS and METHODS

107 patients over 50 years with RVO were treated by isovolemic hemodilution within two months after the first symptoms. The patients were divided into groups of 30 patients with ischemic and 37 with non-ischemic CRVO as well as 20 patients with ischemic and 20 patients with non-ischemic RBVO. For ischemic CRVO two of the following conditions had to be fulfilled: (1) the time from the first arterial appearance of the dye to maximal venous filling of the temporal veins in the fluorescein angiogram had to be $\geq$ 20s. (2) Capillary occlusion areas within the posterior pole should comprise at least one PD and/or the fundus show 10 or more cotton wool spots. (3) Corrected visual acuity had to be $\leq$ 0.1. RBVOs were considered to be ischemic with a capillary occlusion area of 1/2 PD and/or 3 or more cotton wool spots. As it is not always possible to assign a patient to the ischemic or non-ischemic group during the first weeks, we completed the allocation after two months.
All eyes were photocoagulated except those with non-ischemic RBVO. The panretinal photocoagulation was done within two days after admission (Xenon-arc or Argon laser), the burns being placed in a scattered manner over the area of occlusion with the exception of the posterior pole. The isovolemic hemodilution was carried out at the same time. The hematocrit was stepwise lowered to 0.3 or 0.35 (in patients older than 75 years) by repeated exchanges of whole blood for plasma and dextran with a molecular weight of 40,000 and held on this low level for about 6 weeks. Our exact protocol as well as the contraindications and the few adverse effects of this therapy have been published elsewhere (1).
Rheological in vitro testing was done for whole blood viscosity (Wells-Brookfield LVT, 230/s-23/s), plasma viscosity (Ubbelohde capillary viscosimeter), red cell filtrability (Myrenne MF4, Nucleopore Filter) and red cell aggregation (photometric, Myrenne).

3. RESULTS and DISCUSSION

In a part of the patients with RVO, we checked the main determinants of blood fluidity and compared them to control
patients of the same age and sex without retinal vascular
diseases (Tab. 1). The plasma viscosity of patients with

| | | Control | Retinal Vein Occlusion | | |
			ischemic	non-isch.	after IHD
Patients	(n)	20	22	19	21
Age	(years)	69.3±1.9	64.5±1.8	68.3±1.6	66.7±1.8
Plasma-viscosity	(cSt)	1.37±0.02	1.34±0.02	1.34±0.02	1.32±0.02
Red cell filtrability	(initial slope)	26.7±1.2	24.7±1.5	22.9±1.1^K	22.2±1.4
Red cell aggregation		22.1±1.3	19.8±1.1	18.8±0.8^K	18.3±0.6
Hematocrit (%)	♀	42.0±0.7	41.2±0.6	43.0±0.9	34.9± .9**
	♂	46.3±1.1*	44.7±1.1*	44.6±1.6	

TABLE 1. Rheological tests in healthy controls and patients
with retinal vein occlusion. Mean ± SE. K: $p < 0.05$ vs control, * $p < 0.05$ vs ♀ ** $p < 0.001$.

RVO was not different from that of control patients and
there were no significant differences between ischemic and
non-ischemic types of RVO. Although there was a slight reduction of red cell filtrability and a decreased tendency
for red cell aggregation in the non-ischemic vein occlusion
compared to controls, these patients did not differ with
respect to their ischemic counterparts. The same applies
for measurements of whole blood viscosity (Fig. 1). The
slight, sometimes significant differences between men and
women are dependent on the higher hematocrit of men. The
formerly demonstrated pathological values of whole blood
viscosity (6,7,9), plasma viscosity (6,7,9) and red cell
filtrability (6) may be dependent on differences in patient
selection, time of testing and in the methodological approach. It certainly requires larger studies to solve these
contradictions. On the other hand, reduction of the hematocrit from values of 43.3 % to 34.9 % by isovolemic hemodilution led to a significant drop of the whole blood viscosity
and hence a higher blood fluidity.

This effect could also be demonstrated in fluorescein angiograms. The time of maximal venous filling is an important
parameter for the severity of CRVO (8) and can be used as an
indicator for blood velocity in retinal veins. It normally
takes 8 - 12 sec from the first arterial appearance of the
fluorescein to complete filling of the veins. This time was
prolonged to 25 sec in ischemic and to 19 sec in non-ische-

26

mic central retinal vein occlusion (Fig. 2). Within two weeks after beginning of hemodilution the passage times could be reduced to 15 and 13 sec respectively. Thus, the significant difference ($p \leq 0.05$) between ischemic and non-ischemic CRVO before IHD was abolished, indicating a somewhat greater effect of IHD in ischemic CRVO.

FIGURE 1: Apparent whole blood viscosity at a shear rate of 23/s of healthy patients (white bars), ischemic and non-ischemic retinal vein occlusion before (dotted bars) and after isovolemic hemodilution (hatched bars) *$p<0.05$ vs ♀.**$p<0.005$.

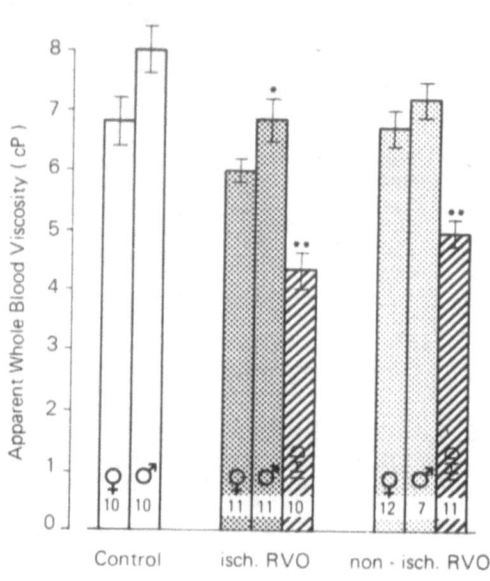

FIGURE 2. Time of maximal venous filling of the temporal veins in patients with CRVO before (white bars) and after hemodilution (hatched bars). Numbers of patiens are given in the bars * $p<0.01$, *** $p<0.001$.

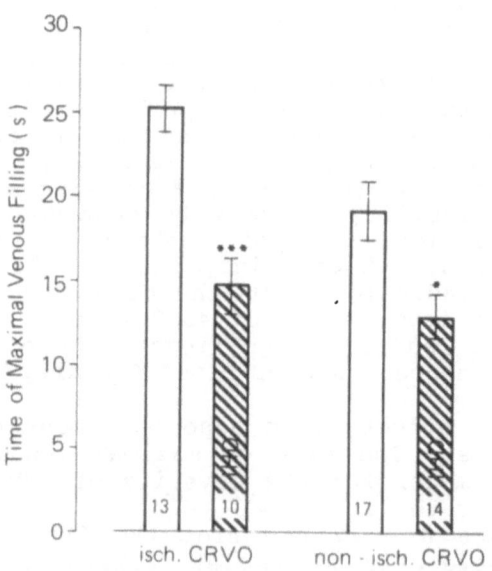

The rates of visual improvement after 3 months attained under different therapies are depicted in Fig. 3. A change in
visual acuity was considered to be present when the patient
could read at least two lines more on the test card. In patients without hemodilution we found no or only few improvements in all forms of RVO (this tells us nothing about final
visual outcome, see Fig. 4). The outcome of hemodiluted non-
ischemic RVO was slightly better; however, the visual improvement of patients with ischemic occlusion was obvious:
43 % of the ischemic CRVO and 65 % of the ischemic branch
vein occlusion had a better visual acuity after hemodilution.

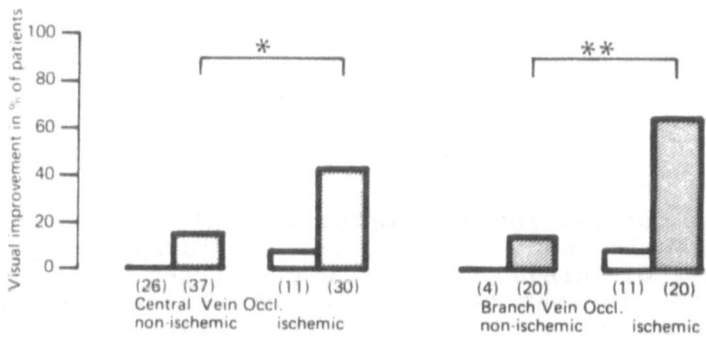

FIGURE 3. Visual improvement of RVO after different therapies. Numbers of patients are given in brackets. White bars:
controls, hatched bars: isovolemic hemodilution. * p<0.05,
** p<0.01.

This significant effect demonstrates that ischemic vein occlusions respond better to isovolemic hemodilution than non-
ischemic types, which may be dependent on the stronger local
disturbances of blood flow found in this type of occlusion.
It has to be mentioned that the visual improvement can be
maintained in nearly all cases even after one year (1).

The final visual acuity may be another indicator for the efficacy of hemodilution. The percentage of patients who are
still able to read with their affected eye is given in Fig.
4. At the first visit only about 15 % of the patients with
ischemic central retinal vein occlusion had a visual acuity
of 0.3 and more compared to about 60 % of the non-ischemic
type. After treatment 43 % of the hemodiluted ischemic patients reached this visual acuity, however, none of the control patients was able to read with the affected eye. In
non-ische-mic central retinal vein occlusions hemodilution
brought about only a small increase, but the decay of the
control group could be prevented.

In conclusion, in our opinion systemic rheological abnormalities do not play an important role in ischemic RVO. Increase of blood fluidity by IHD diminishes local microcirculatory disturbances as indicated by the shortened time of

FIGURE 4: Percentage of patients that are able to read (visual acuity ≥ .3) before (white bars) and 3 months after starting therapy (hatched bars). Numbers of patients are given in brackets. IHD = isovolemic hemodilution.

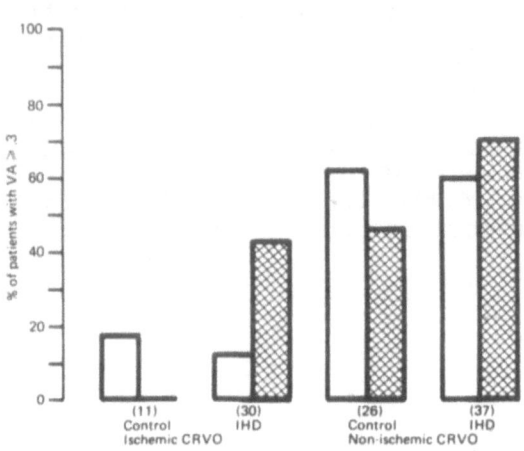

maximal venous filling and improvement of the visual outcome of RVO. In ischemic types of vein occlusion, where microcirculatory disturbances are more pronounced, this effect of hemodilution is even greater. It has to be stressed that the presented data belong to a prospective, non-randomized study. Controlled studies are still under way for patients with non-ischemic CRVO and RBVO with macular involvement.

REFERENCES

1. Hansen, L.L, P. Danisevskis, H.-R. Arntz, G. Hövener, and M. Wiederholt: A randomised prospective study on treatment of central retinal vein occlusion by isovolaemic haemodilution and photocoagulation. Brit. J. Ophthalmol. 69: 108-116 (1985)
2. Hansen, L.L., G. Hövener, C. Mercks, U. Tavakolian, and M. Wiederholt: Isovolämische Hämodilution bei Patienten mit retinalen Venenastverschlüssen. Fortschr. Ophthalmol. 82: 290-292 (1985)
3. Laatikainen, L., E.M. Kohner, D. Khoury, and R.K. Blach: Panretinal photocoagulation in central retinal vein occlusion: a randomised controlled clinical study. Brit. J. Ophthalmol. 61: 741-753 (1977)
4. Margargal, L.E., G.E. Brown, I.I. Augsburger, L.A. Donoso: Efficacy of panretinal photocoagulation in preventing neovascular glaucoma following ischemic central retinal vein occlusion. Ophthalmology 89: 780-784 (1982)
5. May, D.R., M.R. Klein, G.A. Peyman, M. Raichand: Xenon arc panretinal photocoagulation for central retinal vein occlusion: a randomised prospective study. Brit. J. Ophthalmol. 63: 725-734 (1979)
6. Peduzzi, M., A. Debbia, F. Guerrieri, and R. Bolzani: Abnormal blood viscosity and filtrability in retinal vein occlusion. Clin. Hemorheol. 4: 555-561 (1984)

7. Ring, C.P., T.C. Pearson, M.D. Sanders, and G. Wetherley-Mein: Viscosity and retinal vein thrombosis. Brit. J. Ophthalmol. 60: 397-410 (1976)
8. Sinclair, S.H. and E.S. Gragoudas: Prognosis for rubeosis iridis following central retinal vein occlusion. Brit. J. Ophthalmol. 63: 735-743 (1979)
9. Trope, G.E., G.D.O. Lowe, B.M. McArdle et al.: Abnormal blood viscosity and haemostasis in longstanding retinal vein occlusion. Brit. J. Ophthalmol. 67: 137-142 (1983)

O_2 GRADIENTS IN THE MINIATURE PIG RETINA IN NORMOXIA AND HYPEROXIA

C.J. POURNARAS, C.E. RIVA*, K. STROMMER, M. TSACOPOULOS and N.A. GILODI
Experimental Ophthalmology Laboratory and Department of Physiology,
University of Geneva. *On leave from the Department of Ophthalmology,
Scheie Eye Institute, University of Pennsylvania.

1. INTRODUCTION

The inhalation of 100 % oxygen by healthy subjects has been shown to decrease retinal blood flow by approximately 60 % (Riva et al., 1983). Surprisingly, this decrease is accompanied by a 50 % increase in venous oxygen saturation (Hickam et al., 1966), so that the drop in O_2-delivery could be even larger than 60 %.

To explain this apparently exaggerated reactivity, Dollery et al. (1969) have hypothesized on the basis of a simple model of oxygen diffusion that it could be due to a large supply of oxygen from the choroid to the retina.

In recent experimental work on anesthetized miniature pigs using oxygen sensitive microelectrodes, laser Doppler velocimetry and monochromatic 570 nm fundus photography, we found a marked increase in local preretinal periarteriolar PO_2 measured at 50 μm from a retinal arteriole during 100 % oxygen breathing and a 60 % decrease of retinal blood flow. The time course of arterial vasoconstriction and decrease in blood velocity was similar to that of the increase in periarteriolar PO_2. In sharp contrast, the local preretinal PO_2 measured in front of intervascular zones increased very little (Riva et al., 1986).

In this work we further explored the question of what is the source of O_2 which causes vasoconstriction and associated blood flow decrease in the retinal vessels during hyperoxia.

We report here transretinal PO_2 measurements in anesthetized miniature pigs during normoxia and hyperoxia. We show that retinal arteriolar vasoconstriction cannot be due to O_2 diffusing from the choroid, but is probably due to O_2 in the retinal vessels or O_2 which diffuses from the retinal vessels out into the surrounding tissues.

2. MATERIAL AND METHODS

Nine miniature pigs 6-10 kg were prepared according to a procedure described previously (Tsacopoulos, 1975). Systolic and diastolic blood pressure, arterial pH, PCO_2, PO_2, and body temperature were monitored intermittently and kept within physiologcial values.

PO_2 measurements were performed using double-barreled, recess type oxygen sensitive μ-microelectrodes (Tsacopoulos et al., 1977 and 1981) with a tip of 2-4 μm and a recess of 15 to 20 μm. One barrel insured precise localized measurement of the PO_2 with a response time less than 100 msec. The second barrel continuously recorded the extracellular D.C. potential and its modification evoked by light flashes so that the change in shape and amplitude of the local ERG could be recorded. The ERG was used to identify the different retinal layers according to the position of the tip of the μ-electrode (Tsacopoulos et al., 1979).

Transretinal PO_2 measurements were performed starting with the tip of the μ-electrode positioned close to a retinal arteriole (which we will call juxt-arteriolar) and also far away, i.e. at least 5 vessel diameter from an artery.

The Fig. 1 shows a typical transretinal PO_2 recording during 100 % oxygen breathing made close to a retinal arteriole. The microelectrode was moved from the vitreous in steps of 25 μm. We see a progressive increase of the local PO_2 as we approach the arteriole. The PO_2 then decreases as we penetrate into the inner retinal layers. The contact of the μ-electrode tip with the retinal surface is indicated by a negative shift of the D.C. reference signal (arrow R). The arrow (OPL) corresponds to the PO_2 measured in the outer plexiform layer.

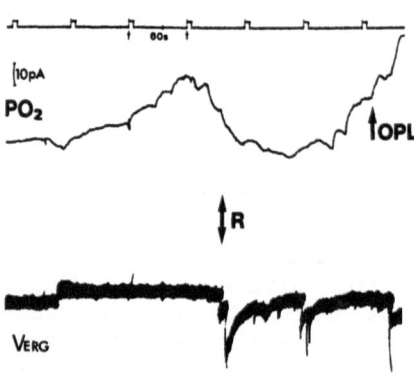

Fig. 1

Simultaneous continuously recorded transretinal juxt-arteriolar PO_2 (middle trace) and D.C. extracellular potential (lower trace).

3. RESULTS

Average values of transretinal PO_2 far from the large retinal vessels (intervascular PO_2).

O_2 gradients in normoxia : In normoxia intervascular PO_2 at 50 μm from the retinal surface was 26 mmHg based on 7 measurements. The local PO_2 progressively decreases when the microelectrode was advanced through the inner retinal layers. The value in the outer plexiform layer (which corresponds to 60 % retinal depth) was 13 mmHg. There was a continuous increase of PO_2 to the outer segment of the photoreceptors, where the local PO_2 was 55 mmHg (Fig. 2).

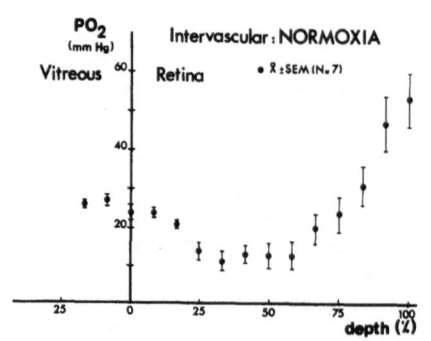

Fig. 2

Intervascular transretinal PO_2 in normoxia.
Average values of 7 measurements ± SE.

Based on 11 measurements, the average periarteriolar PO_2 measured at 50 μm from the retinal surface was 43 mmHg, in contrast to the 26 mmHg measured far from the arteries. The intraretinal PO_2 decrease was steeper in the inner retina in this position. The PO_2 measured in the outer plexiform layer was 24 mmHg while that in the outer segment of the photoreceptors was 47 mmHg (Fig. 3).

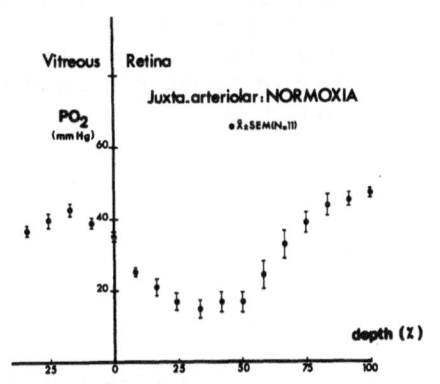

Fig. 3

Juxt-arteriolar transretinal PO_2 measurements in normoxia. Average values of 11 measurements ± SE.

These results indicate that in normoxia, there are O_2 gradients from the retinal surface and the choroid towards the middle of the retina. The PO_2 gradient in the inner retina is steeper when the recording is made close to a retinal arteriole.

O_2 gradient during hyperoxia : The preretinal intervascular PO_2 of 28 mmHg, was not statistically different from that recorded in normoxia, which was in average 26 mmHg.

The PO_2 appeared to decrease slightly from the retinal surface to about 40 % retinal depth and increased markedly from 30 mmHg at 50 % retinal depth to 204 mmHg in the outer segment of the photoreceptors. The gradient of PO_2 in the inner retina was still present but less marked (Fig. 4).

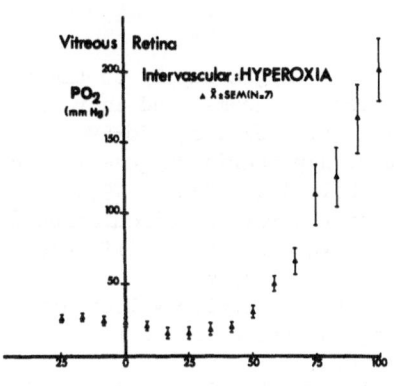

Fig. 4

Intervascular transretinal PO_2 measurements during hyperoxia. Average values of 7 measurements ± SE.

PO$_2$ measurement starting close to the arterioles, during hyperoxia, showed that O$_2$ decreased from 93 mmHg to 35 mmHg at 50 % retinal depth. Then the PO$_2$ increases to 179 mmHg in the outer segment of the photoreceptor layer (Fig. 5).

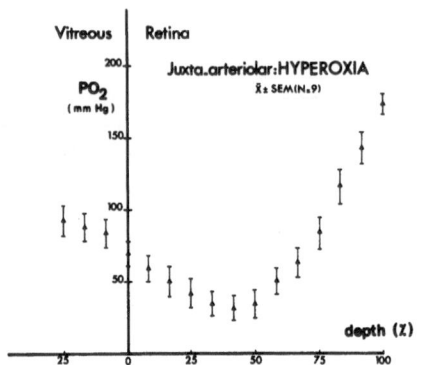

Fig. 5

Juxt-arteriolar transretinal PO$_2$ measurements during hyperoxia.
Average values of 9 measurements $\pm$ SE.

4. CONCLUSION

The transretinal PO$_2$ measurements in intervascular and juxt-arteriolar retinal areas, shows that close to a retinal arteriole, the PO$_2$ gradient towards the inner retina is steeper than that away from the vessel in normoxia as well as in hyperoxia. Since the oxygen flux directly depends on the PO$_2$ gradient, the results presented here demonstrate that the direction of these gradients prevents O$_2$ diffusing from the choroid to reach retinal arterioles.

We conclude that during 100 % oxygen breathing at atmospheric pressure, if O$_2$ is responsible for vasoconstriction of the retinal arterioles, it must be the O$_2$ which is either in the retinal vessels or O$_2$ which diffuses out of the retinal vessels and not O$_2$ which diffuses from the choroid.

Breathing of O$_2$ at hyperbaric pressure might be necessary if one wants to deliver O$_2$ from the choroid to the inner retina as suggested by previous work (Flower and Patz, 1971).

REFERENCES

1. Dollery CT, Bulpitt CT and Kohner EM : Oxygen supply to the retina from the retinal and choroidal circulations at normal and increased arterial oxygen tensions. Invest. Ophthalmol. Vis. Sci. 8, 558-594, 1969.
2. Flower RW and Patz A : The effect of hyperbaric oxygenation on retinal ischemia. Invest. Ophthalmol. Vis. Sci. 10, 605-616, 1971.
3. Hickam JB and Frayser R : Studies of the retinal circulation in man. Observation on vessel diameter, arteriovenous oxygen difference and mean circulation time. Circulation 33, 302-316, 1966.
4. Riva CE, Grunwald JE, Sinclair SH : Laser Doppler velocimetry study of the effect of pure oxygen breathing on retinal blood flow. Invest. Ophthalmol. Vis. Sci. 24, 47-51, 1983.
5. Riva CE, Pournaras CJ and Tsacopoulos M : Regulation of local oxygen tension and blood flow in the inner retina during hyperoxia. J. Appl. Physiol. 61, 592-598, 1986.

6. Tsacopoulos M, Baker R, Levy S and Munoz JL : A versatile system for studying mammalian intraretinal metabolism and function in situ. Exp. Eye Res. $\underline{21}$, 47-57, 1975.
7. Tsacopoulos M and Lehmenkühler A : A double-barreled Pt-microelectrode for simultaneous measurement of PO_2 and bioelectrical activity in excitable tissues. Experientia $\underline{33}$, 1337-1338, 1977.
8. Tsacopoulos M, Poitry S and Borsellino A : Diffusion and consumption of oxygen in the superfused retina of the drone (Apis mellifera) in darkness. J. Gen. Physiol. $\underline{77}$, 601-628, 1981.
9. Tsacopoulos M : Le rôle des facteurs métaboliques dans la régulation du débit sanguin rétinien. Adv. Ophthalmol. $\underline{39}$, 233-273, 1979.

This work was supported by National Eye Institute Grant EY-03242, Swiss National Scientific Foundation Grant 3066-o.84, and the ZYMA Foundation for the Advancement of the Medical and Biological Sciences, Nyon, Switzerland.

Ocular blood supply in internal carotid obstructions

Wolf, S.; Körber, N.[1]; Reim, M.; Ringelstein, E.B.[2]

Dep. of Ophthalmology, RWTH Aachen, F.R.G.
1 Dep. of Ophthalmology, Köln/Merheim, F.R.G.
2 Dep. of Neurology, RWTH Aachen, F.R.G.

1. Introduction

The evaluation of ocular blood flow in patients with internal carotid artery obstructions is of interest for both the ophthalmologists and for neurologists (1,2,7). Deficits in ocular blood flow are supposed to cause neovascularisation, rubeosis iridis and secondary glaucoma.

By means of quantitative video - fluorescenceangiography (3,5,6,9) retinal blood flow parameters were measured in patients with internal carotid artery occlusions. In addition, we quantified the erythrocyte flow velocity by means of video-biomicroscopy in the bulbar conjunctiva (4,10) in patients with hemodynamically significant unilateral internal carotid lesions.

2. Materials and Methods

2.1 Video - biomicroscopy

We used the technique published by Jung et al. (4,10) for the measurement of erythrocyte flow velocity in capillaries of bulbar conjunctiva. The flow velocity was quantified in both eyes under two different perfusion states. After measuring the erythrocyte flow velocity under normal conditions the circulation was measured in a state of reactive hyperaemia. The reactive hyperaemia was provoked by a period of hypoperfusion of 3 minutes. The local hypoperfusion is produced by compression of the eye by means of an occulopressor.

2.2 Video - fluorescence angiography

The complete instrumental set-up is presented in the block diagram in Fig. 1. A Zeiss FK50 funduscamera is linked directly to the low light level TV camera (5). The camera signal is passed through a video time generator and stored on a 3/4" video tape. For the evaluation of the video angiograms a picture analysis system (HP 9826, as control unit for the analyser, Microvideomat 3, C. Zeiss) is used. By means of the picture analysis system dye dilution curves are registered as intensity curves over the time axis from the recordings (3,10).

Areas of measurement (Fig. 2) of any desirable size are positioned on the blood vessels to be investigated. During the registration of the dye dilution curves the measuring areas continuously follow the eye movements of the patient and especially the microsaccades. The grey values of the video points in these areas are summed up and recorded as intensity for each video picture. Thus dilution curves are obtained with a resolution of 1/25 second.

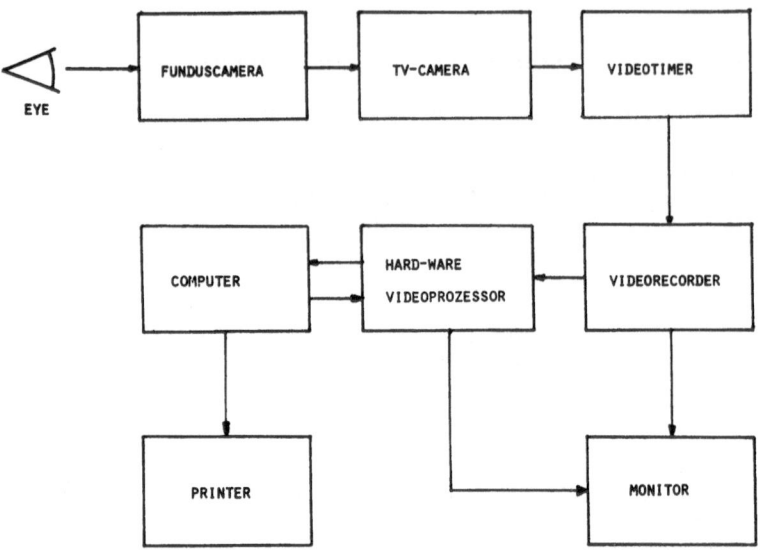

Fig. 1: Block diagram of total instrumental set-up

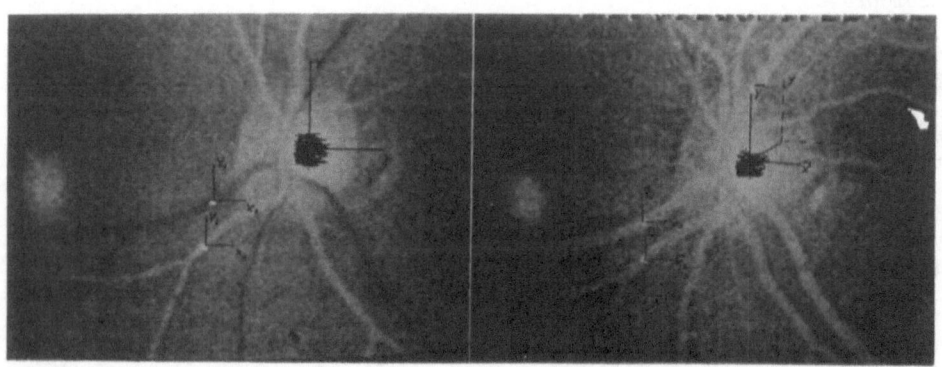

Fig. 2: Picture from the videomonitor with measuring areas

From the dye dilution curves provided by the analyser the following parameters (3,10) are taken:
a) The time required for the dye to appear in the retinal arteriols:
   arm-retina time (ART)
b) The time required for the dye to pass the areas of microcirculation
   between a retinal arteriole and corresponding venule: arterio-venous
   passage time (AVP)
c) The mean dye bolus velocity (MDV) in retinal arteriols. It is
   calculated from the time difference (dt) of the appearance of the dye
   between two areas of measurement on the same arteriole, separated by a
   known distance (s). (MDV = dt/2*s)

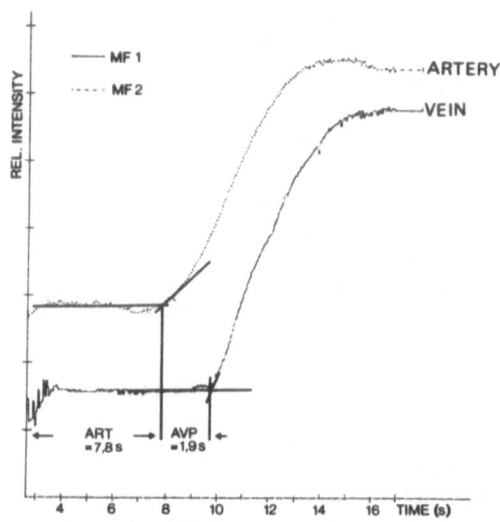

Fig. 3: Dye dilution curve for the evaluation of arterio-venous passage
time (AVP) and arm-retina time (ART)

2.3 Patients
The erythrocyte flow velocity in the conjunctiva was measured in fifteen
healthy volunteers aged 40 to 65 years (mean 57 years) as control group
and in seventeen patients aged 42 to 68 years (mean 56 years) with hemodynamically significant stenosis (more than 90 %) of the internal carotid
artery. All patients were examined in both eyes. The stenoses were
confirmed by Doppler ultrasound examination (1). Video-fluorescenceangiography was not performed in these patients.
In twentythree patients with internal carotid artery occlusion aged 25 to
74 years (mean 59 years) video-fluorescenceangiograms were performed. 14 of
these patients were treated neurologically because of transient ischemic
attacks, amaurosis fugax or lacunar strokes. Ophthalmologically these
patients were normal (normal vision and fundus). In the other 9 patients
an occlusion of the central retinal artery was observed. The occlusion of
the internal carotid artery was confirmed by Doppler ultrasound examination

and by cerebral angiography.

3. Results
3.1 Erythrocyte flow velocity
The results of video-biomicroscopy are shown in Table 1. No differences in erythrocyte flow velocity compared with the control group were found in these patients on the normal side. In both groups the mean velocity was 0.59 mm/s. In the affected side the flow velocity was not significantly reduced under normal conditions. After local hypoxia the erythrocyte flow velocity was significantly reduced compared with the contralateral side (t-test, p 3%). Three minutes after hypoperfusion the velocity in all eyes was similar to the velocity under normal conditions.

Diagnosis	N	Age (years)	v (mm/s) steady state	v (mm/s) reactive hyper	v (mm/s) 3 min. after hypoxia
healthy volunteers	15	57 ± 4	0.59 ± 0.24	0.77 ± 0.24	0.56 ± 0.18
side with a carotis int. obstruction	17	56 ± 8.7	0.53 ± 0.17	0.62 ± 0.15	0.52 ± 0.12
side without obstruction	17	56 ± 8.7	0.59 ± 0.16	0.74 ± 0.15	0.59 ± 0.12

Table 1: Erythrocyte flow velocity in bulbar conjunctiva

3.2 Video - fluorescence angiography
The retinal blood flow parameters in healthy volunteers and in patients with internal carotid artery occlusion are shown in Table 2.

Diagnosis	N	Age (years)	ART (s)	AVP (s)	MDV (mm/s)
healthy voluteers	35	29+/-11	10.5+/-3	1.5+/-6	4,87+/-2.3
internal carotid occlusion	14	60+/-5.7	17.5+/-5	3.3+/-6	1.44+/-3
internal carotid & retinal artery occlusion	9	57+/-6.1	25.7+/-7	very long, not measurable	0.1+/-0.07

Table 2: Retinal blood flow parameters in patients with internal carotid artery occlusion.

In the patients without retinal artery occlusion we found significantly

prolonged retinal blood flow parameters compared to healthy volunteers. In these patients the arm retina time (ART) was 66 %, and the arterio-venous passage time (AVP) 120 % longer compared with healthy volunteers.
Dye velocity was defined as the mean of diastolic and systolic flow velocity. The mean dye bolus velocity was also markedly reduced in these patients. Especially in these patients pulsative changes of dye velocity could be observed.
In the patients with both retinal artery and internal carotid artery occlusion the arm retina time was about 25 seconds. The arterio-venous passage time in these patients was not measured, because of technical problems in measuring longer arterio-venous passage times than 30 seconds. In only two of the nine patients the AVP was shorter than 30 seconds. The mean dye bolus velocity was 0.1 mm/s and about 50 times slower than in healthy volunteers.

4. Discussion
The examination of patients with single sided hemodynamically significant internal carotid artery obstructions clearly demonstrates the feasibility of measuring **erythrocyte** flow velocity in bulbar conjunctiva. We found similar flow velocities on the non-stenosed side as in healthy volunteers. The reduced increase of erythrocyte flow velocity after local hypoxia on the stenosed side demonstrates curtailment of ocular blood supply within the internal carotid artery territory. The erythrocyte flow velocity under normal conditions and the rapid normalisation of erythrocyte flow velocity 3 minutes after hypoxia indicate however that flow changes downstream to the stenosed internal carotid arteries were not critical in these patients.

The prolonged retinal blood flow parameters in patients with occlusion of an internal carotid artery indicate a severely reduced ocular blood flow. The decreased mean dye bolus velocity and the prolonged arterio-venous passage time in these patients presumably are due to a reduced ocular perfusion pressure. These results confirm that changes in ocular circulation can be quantified by means of quantitative video-fluorescenceangiography. We feel that further observations will show a close correlation of ocular blood flow parameters and the genesis of rubeosis iridis or secondary glaucoma in patients with internal carotid artery occlusions. Furthermore, it is hypothezised that video-fluorescenceangiography might provide functional information on collateralisation in cases of internal carotid artery occlusion.

References

1) Bündingen, H.J.; von Reutern, G.M.; Freund, H.J.: Doppler-Sonographie der extrakraniellen Hirnarterien, Grundlagen - Methodik - Fehlermöglichkeiten - Ergebnisse. Thieme, Stuttgart, New York (1982)
2) Deweese, J.A.; May, A.G.; Lipchik, E.O.; Rob, C.G.: Anatomic and haemodynamic correlations in carotid artery stenosis. Stroke (1970) 1: 149 - 157
3) Jung, F.; Kiesewetter, H.; Körber, N.; Wolf, S.; Reim, M.; Müller, G.: Quantification of characteristic blood-flow parameters in the vessels of the retina with a picture analysis system for video-fluorescence angiograms: initial finding. Graefe's Arch Clin Exp Ophthalmol (1983) 211: 133 - 136

42

4) Jung, F.; Körber, N.; Kiesewetter, H.; Prünte, Ch.; Wolf, S.; Reim, M.:
   Measuring the microcirculation in the human conjunctiva bulbi under
   normal and hyperperfusion conditions. Graefe's Arch Clin Exp Ophthalmol
   (1983) 210: 294 - 297

5) Körber, N.; Gesch, M.; Kiesewetter, H.; Reim, M.: Fluoreszenzangiographie der Retina - neue technische Aspekte. Graefe's Arch Clin Exp
   Ophthalmol (1980) 213: 65 - 70

6) Körber, N.; Gesch, M.; Kiesewetter, H.; Reim, M.; Schmid-Schönbein, H.:
   Zur Untersuchung der Retinadurchblutung mittels Fernsehfluoreszenzangio-
   graphie. Ber. Dtsch. Ophthalmol. Ges. 78 (1981)

7) Ringelstein, E.B.; Körber, N.; Zeumer, H.; Hunold, W.:"Die Diagnose der
   Carotisthrombose durch den Augenarzt" (Hager 1962) - Aktualisierung
   dieses Auftrags durch die Doppler-Sonographie. Fortschr Ophthalmol
   (1983) 80: 66 - 69

8) Raitta, Ch.; Eisalo, A.; Folgholm, R.; Takki, K.: The ocular pulse
   wave in health and in occlusive disease of the cervical arteries.
   Graefe's Arch Clin Exp Ophthalmol (1973) 187: 265 - 272

9) Wolf, S.; Jung, F.; Körber, N.; Kiesewetter, H.; Reim, M.: Measurement
   of retinal blood flow parameters by means of image analysis system for
   video-fluorescenceangiography. XXV Acta int. Congress Ophthal. Roma,
   Kugler Publications 1986 in press

10) Wolf, S.; Jung, F.; Körber, N.; Reim, M.: Measurement of erythrocyte
    velocity in the capillaries of human conjunctiva under normal and
    hyperperfusion. Int. J. Microzirculation: Clinical and experimental,
    Vol. 3 NOS 3/4, 1984

RETINAL HEMODYNAMICS IN DIABETES MELLITUS

J.E. GRUNWALD, C.E. RIVA, A.J. BRUCKER, S.H. SINCLAIR, B.L. PETRIG.

1. INTRODUCTION

The retinal circulation and its regulation to 100% oxygen breathing were investigated in patients with diabetes mellitus using bidirectional laser Doppler velocimetry (BLDV) and monochromatic fundus photography.

2. PROCEDURE

Forty three insulin treated diabetics with no diabetic retinopathy (NDR), background diabetic retinopathy (BDR) or proliferative diabetic retinopathy (PDR), and 26 normal subjects with similar ages were included in this study. In addition, in 15 diabetic patients with PDR and high risk characteristics, retinal blood flow and its regulatory response to hyperoxia were investigated just prior to laser panretinal photocoagulation (PRP), and then at about 4 months later. Details of the subjects populations and the techniques used have been described previously[1,2].

V_{max}, the maximum speed of red blood cells, was determined in a major temporal vein in each subject using BLDV. Venous diameter, D, at the site of BLDV measurement was obtained from photographic negatives taken in monochromatic light at 570 nm. Changes in retinal volumetric blood flow rate, Q, were determined from the relationship: $Q = k \cdot D^2 \cdot V_{max}$, where k is a constant of proportionality. The regulatory response to hyperoxia was characterized by the percentage change in blood flow between the baseline value and the value at 5 to 6 minutes of oxygen breathing. All measurements of D were performed by one trained examiner, and all V_{max} determinations were done by another one. Each individual was masked with regard to the results of the other and to the diagnosis of the tested eye. Paired and non-paired t-test were used in the analysis of the data. Results with a probability error smaller than 0.05 were considered as statistically significant.

3. RESULTS

Relative changes in average V_{max}, D and Q from normal, occurring in the different retinopathy groups are shown in Table 1.

Average V_{max} was significantly lower than normal when all diabetic eyes were pooled together. Average V_{max} was also significantly decreased in the BDR and PDR group. D, on the other hand, was significantly increased in the BDR and PDR group. The decrease in V_{max}, which was accompanied by an increase in D resulted in average Q that was not significantly different from normal in any of the diabetic groups.

TABLE 1. Relative changes in V_{max}, D and Q from normal.

	No of Eyes	V_{max}	D	Q
Normal	26	1.00 ± 0.24*	1.00 ± 0.09	1.00 ± 0.30
NDR	12	0.94 ± 0.29	0.99 ± 0.08	0.94 ± 0.28
BDR	20	0.82 ± 0.24	1.10 ± 0.16	1.09 ± 0.49
PDR	11	0.71 ± 0.06	1.12 ± 0.14	0.92 ± 0.27

* Mean ± 1 SD.

In the 15 patients with PDR that were studied before and after PRP, treatment resulted in significant decreases of 7% in average D, 15% in average V_{max} and 17% in average Q (paired t-test). The average regulatory response to hyperoxia which was 20 ± 15% prior to PRP, showed a significant improvement to an average 45 ± 12% following photocoagulation (paired t-test).

4. DISCUSSION

Our results show that V_{max} is decreased in eyes with diabetic retino-pathy. This phenomenon is probably related to the closure of small vessels and to the changes in the rheological properties of blood that are known to occur in diabetes mellitus.

The decrease in average V_{max} is accompanied by an increase in average D, and therefore, average Q is not significantly different from normal in the groups with NDR, BDR or PDR. This does not mean, however, that there are no actual changes in Q in any of these groups. Because of the intersubject variability of Q in each group, the minimum significant change from normal that can be detected is approximately 22% on the average. Therefore, any actual alterations from the normal value smaller than 22% would not be detectable in this study.

PRP treatment, appears to cause a significant decrease in Q. In addition, it improves significantly the retinal blood flow regulatory response to hyperoxia from an average value well below normal to a value that is close to normal[3].

The decreased regulatory response to hyperoxia in eyes with PDR supports the current theory that the retina is hypoxic in these eyes. It is conceivable that the hypoxic retina would react less than a normal retina in response to 100% O_2 breathing, because part of the excess O_2 supplied could be used to satisfy the metabolic demand.

Previous studies in animals have shown that retinal PO_2 increases following PRP[4]. Such an effect could cause the vasoconstriction and decrease in retinal blood flow seen in this study . In addition, the increase in vascular resistance produced by the destruction of small vessels by treatment could also contribute to the decrease in Q. The results showing that the average O_2 regulatory response following PRP is close to normal suggest that PRP may normalize the PO_2 of the remaining retina.

In this paper we have hypothesized that abnormalities in the oxygenation of the retina may cause the changes in retinal blood flow and its regulation. It is possible, however, that abnormal concentrations of other metabolites, which may not be supplied to or removed from the retina at an appropriate rate, may cause the hemodynamic changes detected in this study.

5. REFERENCES

1. Grunwald, J.E., Riva, C.E, Sinclair, S.H., Brucker, A.J. and Petrig, B.L.: Laser Doppler Velocimetry Study of Retinal Circulation in Diabetic Mellitus. Arch Ophthalmol 104: 991, 1986.
2. Grunwald, J.E., Riva, C.E., Brucker, A.J., Sinclair, S.H. and Petrig, B.L.: Effect of Panretinal Photocoagulation on Retinal Blood Flow in Proliferative Diabetic Retinopathy. Ophthalmology 93: 590, 1986.
3. Grunwald, J.E., Riva, C.E., Brucker, A.J., Sinclair, S.H. and Petrig, B.L.: Altered Retinal Vascular Response to 100% Oxygen Breathing in Diabetes Mellitus. Ophthalmology 91: 1447, 1984.
4. Molnar, I., Poitry, S., Tsacopoulos, M., et al. Effect of Laser Photocoagulation on Oxygenation of the Retina in Miniature Pigs. Invest. Ophthalmol. Vis. Sci. 26: 1410, 1985.

Acknowledgment: This work was supported by Grant EY03242 from the National Eye Institute, The Pennsylvania Lions Sight Conservation and by the Vivian Simkins Lasko Retinal Vascular Research Fund.

Retinal Artery Emboli Associated with Mitral Valve Prolapse

Morton H. Seelenfreund, M.D.
Ben Zion Silverstone, M.D.
Israela Hirsch, M.D.
David Rosenmann, M.D.
Shaare Zedek Medical Center, Jerusalem, Israel

Introduction

Mitral valve prolapse (MVP) is the term used to describe an anatomical anomaly of the mitral valve leaflets in which there is a billowing of the mitral leaflets with failure of the leaflet edges to appose normally. Mitral regurgitation occurs, and this is reflected clinically by a mitral systolic murmur and often a mid-late systolic click (1)(2). This entity was first thought to be fairly benign, however, reports of medical complications associated with MVP include sudden death (3), acute myocardial infarction (4), infective endocarditis (5), arrhythmias (6), cerebral ischemic events (7), and agoraphobia (with palpitations) (8).

In 1975 Woldoff described an association between retinal vascular thrombosis and MVP in two patients (9), and other authors have since reported series of cases of retinal emboli in patients with MVP (10)(11). Additional ocular complications associated with MVP are keratoconus (12), progressive external opthalmoplegia (13), and amaurosis fugax (14).

In this report we present a case of papillitis with exudative retinal detachment associated with retinal artery emboli in a young woman with MVP.

Case Report

A 28 year old woman presented with sudden onset of blurred vision of her left eye. She claimed that she had a similar episode several years before and that it had cleared up spontaneously within days. She denied having any significant medical problems and was not taking any medicines including oral contraceptives.

Opthalmologic examination showed a visual acuity of 6/9 in the right eye and 6/24 in the left eye. Intra-ocular tension was right eye 18 mmHg and left eye 16mmHg. Slit lamp exam showed 2+ cells in anterior chamber of the left eye and none in the right eye. The right fundus was normal. The left fundus showed an edematous, slightly pale optic nerve with a markedly blurred nasal border. There was an exudative detachment of the nasal retina adjacent to the disc and extending 2½ disc diameters nasally. There was a whitish choroidal lesion under the area of detachment with sludging of the blood in the nasal arterioles: Fluorescein angiogram showed de - layed filling of the supero-nasal arterioles with diffuse leakage around the optic nerve and nasally.

Visual field showed an enlarged blind spot.

Extensive medical evaluation including complete blood cell count, erythrocyte sedimentation rate, rheumatoid factor, anti-nuclear antibody titer,
VDRL, lupus erythematosis preparation, serum protein electrophoresis,
cryoglobulins and toxoplasmosis titers gave normal findings.

A short trial of 80 mg. of prednison given orally was started and discontinued after a few days when no improvement was seen. Three weeks after
the onset of symptoms, fundus examination showed 2 small yellowish plaques
in the superonasal arteriole. Carotid vessel evaluation by vascular
surgeons showed normal findings (fig. 1).

The cardiologist reported the presence of a loud mid-systolic click and a
late systolic murmur. Echocardiogram showed mitral leaflet displacement
and confirmed the diagnosis of MVP syndrome (fig. 2).

The patient was placed on a regimen of aspirin and dipryidamol. Gradually,
over the next 8 weeks the retinal detachment decreased. The optic nerve
edema subsided. Three months after the initial episode, the patient again
complained of visual changes in her left eye, and a new plaque was found
partially obstructing the inferior branch of the central retinal artery on
the edge of the disc. This Plaque disappeared in 5 weeks. She has been
asymptomatic for the past year.

Discussion

In studying a large series of patients with retinal artery occlusion causing
permanent field defect, Wilson found that young patients with branch retinal artery occlusions were more often found to have underlying carotid
or cardiac disease while patients with central retinal artery occlusion
were more often hypertensive and the occlusion seemed a consequence of
local atheromatous disease (15).

Woldoff first brought attention to the association of MVP with embolic disease to the eye. He suggested that, "...the disturbed laminar blood flow,
a result of mitral valve prolapse, may have resulted in intracardiac
thrombosis and retinal artery embolism " (9).

Wilson (11) described 10 patients with MVP and visual disturbances consistent with embolism in the posterior cerebral ophthalmic circulation.
Although the evidence that MVP caused the embolism was not conclusive,other
sources of the visual disturbances could not be found. Wilson also specu-
lated that small fibrin and platelet thrombi from the mitral leaflets
might have been the source of emboli in those 10 cases.

Caltrider et al described a series of patients with retinal emboli and MVP
in whom there was no evidence of atherosclorotic disease, hypertension,
vasculitis, coagulation defects or ingestion of oral contraceptives. They
also described one patient who developed retinal neovascularization which
was thought to be secondary to recurrent small emboli from prolapsing mitral
valves (10).

The discovery of MVP should not terminate the diagnostic evaluation of
patients with stroke or retinal embolism. Baker has described a patient
with MVP who developed sudden blindness but in whom carotid arteriography
led to the discovery of an ulcerated plaque in the left internal carotid

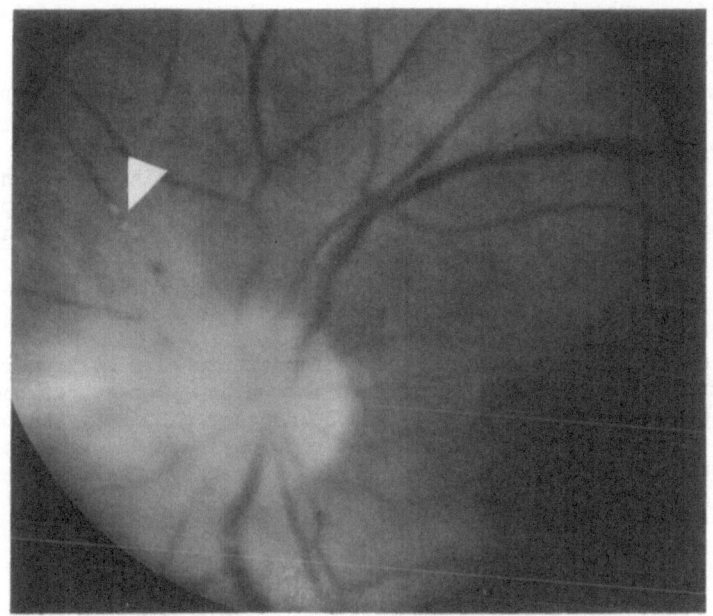

Figure 1. Left fundus 3 weeks after onset of symptoms showing plaques in super-nasal arteriole (arrow).

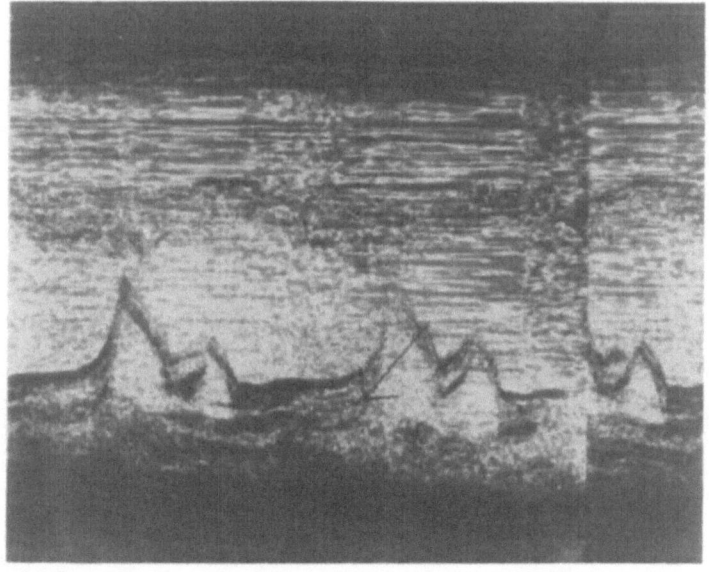

Figure 2. Echocardiogram showing prolapse of mitral valve (arrow).

artery (16), emphasizing that a patient may have more than 1 disease or medical problem.

Several studies have shown a pronounced relationship between MVP and cerebral ischemic events (7)(14). The mechanisms for the cerebral ischemic lesions were thought to be related to either bacterial endocarditis (17), arrhythmias (6), or, most likely, non-infective thromoembolism (7). The focal nature of most clinical presentations plus the angiographic findings of occluded cortical arteries in the absence of other arterial disease are most suggestive of emboli.

Conclusion

In recent years it has become clear that patients with MVP syndrome can present with various severe systemic problems and that ocular complications, especially retinal emboli, can be another manifestation of this syndrome. It is, therefore, important that patients who present with retinal emboli phenomenon be carefully evaluated by a cardiologist for the possibility of MVP syndrome.

References

1. Barlow JB, Pocock WA, Marchand P, and Denny M: The Significance of Late Systolic Murmurs. Am Heart J. 66: 443, 1963.
2. Barlow JB, and Pocock WA: Billowing, Floppy, Prolapsed or Flail Mitral Valves? Am J Cardiol. 55:501, 1985.
3. Pocock WA, Bosman CK, Chesler E, Barlow JB, and Edwards JE: Sudden Death in Primary Mitral Valve Prolapse. Am Heart J. 107:378, 1984.
4. Chesler E. Matisonn RE, Lakier JB, Pocock WA, Obel IW, and Barlow JB: Acute Myocardial Infarction with Normal Coronary Arteries: A Possible Manifestation of the Billowing Mitral Leaflet Syndrome. Circulation. 54:203, 1976.
5. Lachman AS, Bramwell-Jones DM, Lakier JB, Pocock WA, and Barlow JB. Infective Endocarditis in the Billowing Mitral Leaflet Syndrome. Br Heart J. 37:326, 1975.
6. Pocock WA and Barlow JB: Postexercise Arrhythmias in the Billowing Posterior Mitral Leaflet Syndrome. Am Heart J. 80:740, 1970.
7. Barnett HJ, Boughner DR, Tayler W, Cooper PE, Kostuk WJ, and Nichol PM: Further Evidence Relating Mitral-Valve Prolapse to Cerebral Ischemic Events. New Eng J Med. 302:139, 1980.
8. Kantor JS, Zitrin CM, and Zeldis SM. Mitral Valve Prolapse Syndrome in Agoraphobic Patients. Am J Psychiatry. 137:467, 1980.
9. Woldoff HS, Gerber M, Desser K, and Benchimol A: Retinal Vascular Lesions in Two Patients with Prolapsed Mitral Valve Leaflets. Am J Ophthal. 79:382, 1975.
10. Caltrider ND, Irvine AR, Kline HJ, and Rosenblatt A: Retinal Emboli in Patients with Mitral Valve Prolapse. Am J Ophthal. 90534, 1980.
11. Wilson LA, Keeling PWN, Malcolm AD, Ross Russell, RW, and Webb-Peplow MM: Visual Complications of Mitral Leaf Prolapse. Br Med J. 2:86,1977.
12. Beardsley TL and Foulks GN: An Association of Keratoconus and Mitral Valve Prolapse. Ophthalmalogy 89:35, 1982.
13. Darsee JR, Miklozek CL, Heymsfield SB, Hopkins LC and Wenger NK: Mitral Valve Prolapse and Ophthalmoplegia. A Progressive Cardioneuro-logic Syndrome. Am Int Med. 92:735, 1980.
14. Kimball RW and Hedges TR: Amaurosis Fugax Caused by a Prolapsed Mitral Leaflet in the Midsystolic Click, Late Systolic Murmur Syndrome. Am J Ophthalmol. 83: 469, 1977.
15. Wilson LA, Warlow CP, and Ross Russell RW. Cardiovascular Disease in Patients with Retinal Arterial Occlusion. Lancet: 292, 1979.
16. Baker RS, Tibbs PA., and Millett AJ: Carotid-Retinal Embolism with Coexistent Mitral Valve Prolapse. Neurology 31:1192, 1981.

Development of Retinal Neovascularisation in Occlusive Retinal Vascular
Disease in Adults

W.A. Manschot[1], W.R. Lee[2] and G.E. Blass
[1]Institute of Pathology, Eramus University, Rotterdam, The Netherlands
[2]Tennent Institute of Ophthalmology, The University of Glasgow,
Glasgow, Scotland.

Histological studies of the retinal vasculature following central
retinal vein occlusion[1,2,3] have emphasised the close relationship
between central vascular occlusive disease (CRVOD) and 'hyalinisation' of
retinal venules and arterioles. In addition, recent studies[2,3] have
emphasised the frequency of neovascularisation within and around the
walls of hyalinised blood vessels. However the nature of hyalinisation
as part of the primary aging process has not been intensively studied
since the publication of a monograph by Leishman[4]. One electron
microscopic investigation has emphasised atrophy of mural myocytes with
collagenous replacement[5]. Our own recent studies[6], based on material
derived from human eyes (conducted in the same laboratory as those of a
group of distinguished Ophthalmic Pathologists, Michaelson, Loewestein
and Leishman), have shown that simple age related hyalinisation is a
process in which there is gradual 'drop out' of medial myocytes and
thickening of the wall by deposition of layers of basement membrane and
65 nm banded collagen. The endothelium of the retinal vessels retained
intact tight junctions and the subendothelial myocytes showed
morphological evidence of activation: this process has been described
in detail in other sites by Staubesand[7]. When neovascularisation occurs
in CRVO, after the superadded ischaemic insult of central vascular
disease, the process appears to originate in the form of an ingrowth of
endothelial cells and subendothelial myocytes into the acellular vessel
wall (Fig. 1).

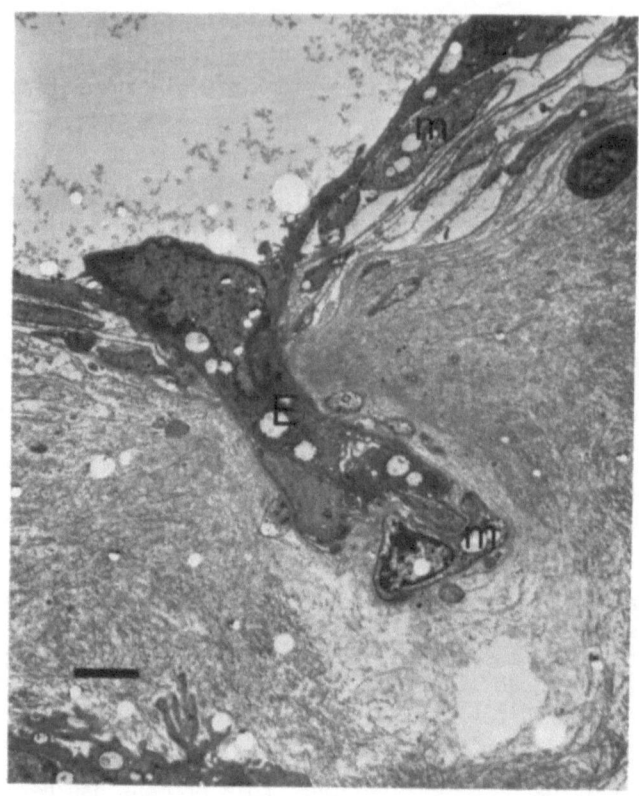

FIGURE 1. Endothelial cell (E) growing into an acellular hyalinised vessel wall with chort myocytes (m)

    Intramural capillaries are always found to consist of endothelial cells surrounded by cohort cells (Fig. 2). In extramural neovascularisation, nodular proliferations of endothelial cells and surrounding cohort cells were a striking feature (Fig. 3).

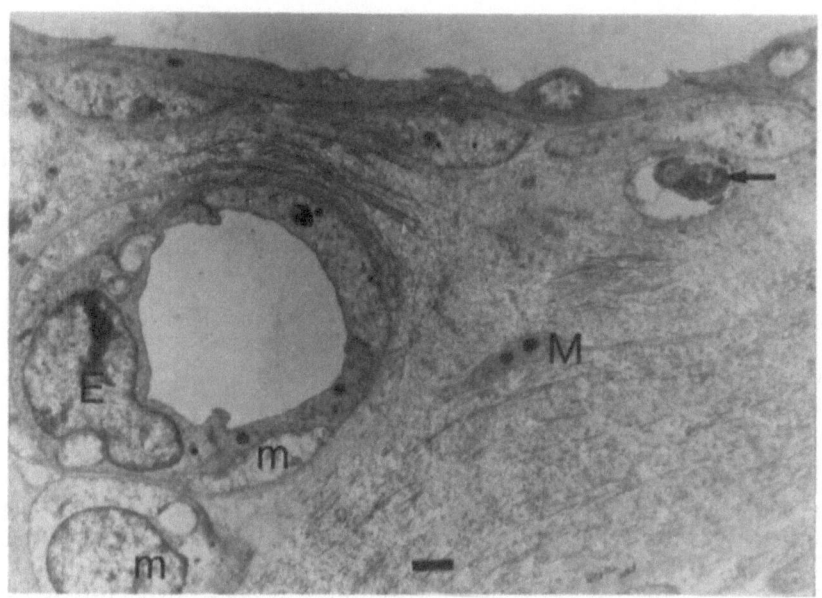

FIGURE 2. Intramural capillary (endothelial cell (E): cohort cell (m))
within hyalinised vessel wall. Note degenerate cell (arrow) and
macrophage (M)

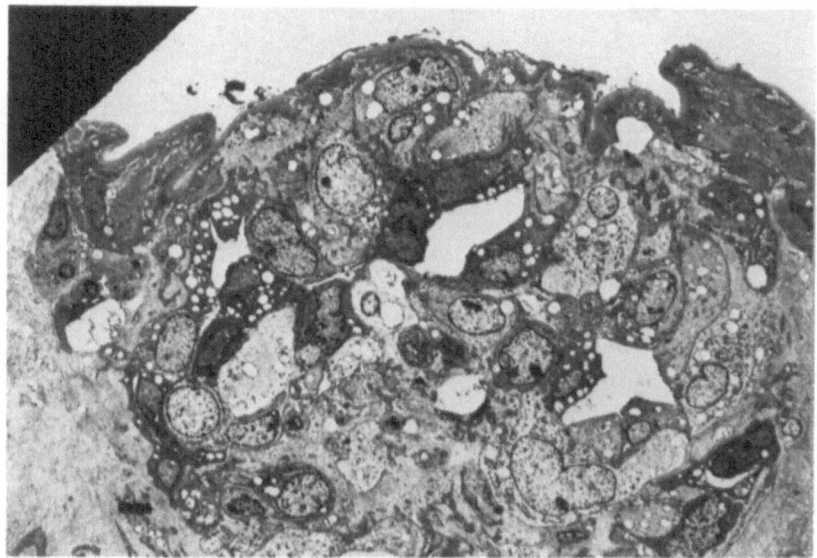

FIGURE 3. A nexus of proliferating endothelial cells and pericytes
located in the inner retina. Note the dimorphic nature of the vascular
cell proliferation.

Future studies should be concentrated on the identification of features within the diseased vessel wall, e.g. fibronectin, or cells, e.g. macrophages, which have the capacity to stimulate endothelial cell proliferation. There is considerable evidence that changes in ground substance in vitro can have profound effects on the behaviour of endothelial cells. What is most striking is the constant relationship in the process of neovascularisation between endothelial cells and cohort cells, probably subendothelial myocytes. This finding is of great relevance to in vitro studies which have concentrated on the behaviour of one cell type in altered environmental situations.

REFERENCES

1. Michaelson IC: Textbook of the Fundus of the Eye. Churchill Livingstone, 3rd Edn. Edinburgh, 1980.
2. Manschot WA, Lee WR: Retinal neovascularisation arising from hyalinised blood vessels. Graefes Arch Clin Exp Ophthal 222: 63-70, 1984.
3. Manschot WA, Lee WR: Development of retinal neovascularisation in vascular occlusive disease. Trans Ophthalmol Soc UK 104: 880-886, 1985.
4. Leishman R: The eye in general vascular disease. Hypertension and arteriosclerosis. Brit J Ophthalmol 41: 641-701, 1957.
5. Kohno T, Ishibashi T, Inomata H. Electron microscopic studies of pipestem sheathed vessels in the human retina. Jap J Ophthalmol 27: 228-235, 1983.
6. Lee WR, Blass GE, Shaw DC: Age related retinal vasculopathy. Eye (previously Trans Ophthalmol Soc UK) 1987 (In press).
7. Staubesand J: Mediadysplasie und Arteriosklerose. Therapie Wache 32: 851-877, 1982

LASER PHOTOCOAGULATION FOR RETINAL VEIN OBSTRUCTION

LARRY E. MAGARGAL, M.D.
DEBRA L. MORRISON, B.A.
ANDREW S. KIMMEL, M.D.
RICHARD E. GOLDBERG, M.D.
LARRY A. DONOSO, M.D., PH.D.

INTRODUCTION

It is well established that the angiographic and pathophysiologic spectrum of retinal ischemia determines the clinical features of retinal vein obstruction.[1-28] It is our purpose to update and review the individual studies we have recently completed,[1-6] and to bring together the information on each type of retinal vein obstruction (RVO) in an effort to enhance understanding of the disease, recognize risk factors, and provide guidelines for management.

Retinal vein obstruction ranges from involvement of the venous drainage of the entire retina when blockage occurs at the level of the lamina cribrosa in central retinal vein obstruction (CRVO), to a small venous tributary either within the major arcades in macular vein obstruction (MVO), or outside the arcades in peripheral vein obstruction (PVO). Intermediate types are the hemispheric or hemi-central retinal vein obstruction (HRVO) which involves the venous return from either the superior or inferior half of the retina, and the branch retinal vein obstruction (BRVO) which involves an entire retinal quadrant, most frequently temporal, and occurs at arterio-venous crossings where a sclerotic artery may compress its companion vein. Visual loss is painless and ranged from minimal to severe reflecting the extent and location of obstruction, typically greatest with CRVO. Funduscopic findings include intraretinal hemorrhage, venous tortuosity and engorgement, retinal edema, and nerve fiber layer infarcts within the distribution of the obstructed vein. These findings vary in occurrence and severity with the type of RVO, the extent of ischemia, and the duration or chronicity of obstruction. Visual impairment may occur due to macular edema and its associated complications, foveal capillary nonperfusion, extensive retinal capillary nonperfusion and its associated neovascular complications, or to a combination of these effects.

Photocoagulation has proven beneficial in the management of both macular edema and neovascularization in selected cases.[1,7,10,11,15,17,20-22] Goals of therapy include the prevention of irreversible structural damage due to persistent macular edema, reduction of vitreous hemorrhage due to neovascularization of the retina and disc, and prevention of neovascular glaucoma due to iris neovascularization. Appropriate classification of RVO according to the severity of retinal capillary damage as demonstrated angiographically is essential for identifying eyes exhibiting favorable characteristics as well as developing a rational therapeutic approach for those eyes progressing in an unfavorable fashion.

THE SPECTRUM OF ISCHEMIA: A BASIS FOR CLASSIFICATION

The ischemic index, as determined by fluorescein angiography, is the degree of capillary nonperfusion calculated as a percentage of the area involved in the venous obstruction.[1,2,3,6] RVO can be classified into three clinically relevant groups based on the ischemic index: hyperpermeable, indeterminate, and ischemic patterns. The hyperpermeable or "edematous group" is characterized by leaking but still perfused capillaries and encompasses the terms venous stasis retinopathy, impending RVO, incomplete RVO, edematous RVO, nonischemic RVO, and papillophlebitis as used by others.[7,9,27] The indeterminate group represents a mixed picture with both intraretinal edema and mild to moderate nonperfusion. The ischemic or preproliferative group exhibits varying amounts of retina edema but is characterized by extensive zones of capillary nonperfusion (an ischemic index of greater than 50%). Ischemic RVO encompasses the terms complete RVO, hemorrhagic RVO and stagnation thrombosis as used by others.[7,9,27] Histopathologic and experimental studies[18,19] have demonstrated that sustained venous obstruction alone is capable of producing progressive capillary nonperfusion and retinal ischemia as observed in clinical studies. It has previously been emphasized that the recognition of these three basic capillary responses – leakage, nonperfusion and neovascularization – is essential in the understanding and management of RVO.[1-7,10,11]

The clinical value of this classification scheme is based on the observation that the degree of retinal ischemia is positively correlated with the risk of developing neovascularization,[1-7,10,11,17,20,21,23,27] therefore correct categorization is essential in the selection of high risk patients for potential treatment. In our Table 1, our natural history studies[1-4] grouped by ischemic pattern for each type of RVO exemplifies the correlation between neovascularization and ischemia. Regardless of type of obstruction, the hyperpermeable and indeterminate groups (less than 50% nonperfusion) represent a low risk of neovascularization, the principle concern being the management of macular edema. In contrast, the ischemic group (greater than 50% nonperfusion) represents a high risk of neovascularization, the principle concern being the prevention of neovascularization (prophylactic approach) or in cases that have already progressed to neovascularization, the prevention of vitreous hemorrhage and/or neovascular glaucoma (therapeutic approach).

Careful analysis of Table 1 reveals other important trends. In the absence of other contributing ischemic factors, eyes with MVO do not develop neovascularization of any kind, presumably on the basis of the small amount of retina involved. Anterior segment neovascularization (NVI/NVG) occurs in only 1-2% of ischemic TBRVO, 14% of ischemic HRVO, and 60% of ischemic CRVO. Since chronic retinal ischemia is a prerequisite for neovascularization,[11,12,23] it is clear that greater areas of retinal ischemia predispose to an increased incidence of developing NVI. It seems that at least one quadrant of retinal capillary nonperfusion or its equivalent is required for NVI to develop following RVO.[10] It has been postulated that when the area and degree of retinal ischemia reaches threshold, angiogenic substances are released which are capable of inducing neovascularization of the iris, disc, and retina.[12,13] There are, however, other variables involved in the neovascular response. Retinal neovascularization occurs in 34% of ischemic TBRVO, 16% of ischemic HBRVO, and only 10% of ischemic CRVO. NVR typically develops at border zones of retinal ischemia where there are intact capillary endothelial cells capable of responding to an angiogenic stimulus. In highly ischemic cases of CRVO there are relatively few viable retinal capillaries remaining that are still capable of proliferation;[14] thus NVR is less frequent than in HRVO and TBRVO. In summary, the progression from branch to hemispheric to central RVO with increasing area of retinal ischemia is characterized by a shift from predominantly posterior segment neovascularization (NVR/NVD) and rare NVI to predominantly

anterior segment neovascularization (NVI/NVG) and relatively less NVR/
NVD. This trend may be explained by the interaction of increasing
amounts of an angiogenic factor sufficient to stimulate neovascularization
and decreasing amounts of retinal vascular substrate capable of responding
to this stimulus. Thus the nature of the neovascular response depends on
both the location and extent of the initial event (nonperfused capillaries)
producing an ischemic condition (retinal hypoxia) and the availability of
receptor tissue to respond to the angiogenic signal (intact capillary endothelial cells).

MANAGEMENT

Treatment of an underlying associated systemic condition is indicated.
Although this is unlikely to reverse the obstruction, it may reduce the risk
of a vein obstruction in the fellow eye or other occlusive vascular
event.[7,27] No medical treatment for RVO has proven beneficial, however,
some advocate the use of platelet inhibitors such as low-dose aspirin (20
mgs daily), Persantine (50 mgs three times daily), or Anturane (200 mgs
four times daily).[7]

Laser photocoagulation has been beneficial in the treatment of macular
edema in BRVO prior to the onset of irreversible degenerative changes.
The Branch Vein Occlusion Study Group showed that photocoagulation significantly improves the visual outcome in eyes with BRVO and macular
edema reducing vision to 20/40 or worse; 60% of treated eyes versus 34% of
untreated eyes were 20/40 or better at 3 year follow up.[15] The treatment
protocol recommended is a light scatter technique (macular debridement or
grid pattern) over the zone of capillary leakage within the vascular arcades
and outside the foveal avascular zone. Our studies also demonstrate a
beneficial effect on visual acuity when treatment was offered at six months
duration but was only of marginal benefit after twelve months in eyes not
pursuing a favorable course.[1,2,7]

Laser photocoagulation has also been advocated for the treatment
(therapeutic approach) and prevention (prophylactic approach) of neovascularization in RVO.[1-8,10,11,17,18] Our protocol utilized a heavy scatter
technique to the zones of capillary non-perfusion (sector treatment for
BRVO and pan retinal photocoagulation for CRVO) and light scatter treatment to areas of leakage within the arcades when concommitant macular
edema was present. The exact mechanism responsible for eliminating the
neovascular drive is not known, however, photocoagulation has been specu-
lated to work by destroying ischemic retina responsible for the angiogenic
substances, facilitating drainage of vasoproliferative factors into the choroidal circulation, and/or enhancing choroidal oxygenation of hypoxic retinal
tissue.[6,7]

Ischemic CRVO carries a high risk (60%) of developing NVI which has
been observed to progress rapidly to intractable NVG. Although most
cases occur within three to five months, it has been reported as early as
two weeks and as late as two years.[3,16,17] In our experience it has
proven difficult to follow these patients clinically and angiographically at
frequent intervals over this time period; untreated patients often return
with severe pain and elevated intraocular pressure when angle closure has
already occurred.[25] Although NVI (early NVG) may regress following pan
retinal photocoagulation (PRP), response to treatment is best prior to extensive angle closure.[3,17,25] Advanced NVG does not respond as well to
any treatment and reasonable goals are usually limited to maintaining comfort and cosmesis in a blind eye. Enucleation for intractable pain is a
last resort, however, as recently as 1978 neovascular glaucoma represented

20% of therapeutic enucleations.[16] With one-third of cases of NVG attributable to ischemic RVO,[23] a potentially preventable cause of NVG terminating in enucleation is evident. In our prospective study of 100 consecutive eyes with ischemic CRVO receiving early argon laser PRP, 3% developed NVI prior to completion of PRP and 2% developed NVG following additional ischemic events.[5] Although laser treatment does not improve visual acuity, utilizing the prophylactic PRP approach is warranted for ischemic CRVO by reducing the risk of neovascular glaucoma from 60% to 2% thereby virtually eliminating the need for therapeutic enucleation in these cases.

Ischemic HRVO eyes carry intermediate risks of both anterior and posterior segment ischemia: 14% NVI, 21% NVD, 16% NVR (Table 1). As part of a retrospective study of 106 eyes with HRVO, 25 eyes were treated prophylactically with sector photocoagulation and demonstrated a significantly reduced risk of neovascularization: 4% NVI, 0% NVD, 4% NVR.[2] It is apparent that prophylaxis is capable of diminishing the risk of both NVG and vitreous hemorrhage, and we felt early treatment should be considered to preserve the maximum visual function, especially for those patients who have a visual impairment in their fellow eyes or are not able to be followed appropriately.

The management of ischemic BRVO is at the center of the controversy over timing of photocoagulation therapy. Since the risk of anterior segment neovascularization and NVG is small, the main concern of management is the problem of chronic macular edema and the danger of posterior segment neovascularization and its complications; principally vitreous hemorrhage and traction retinal detachment. Butner and McPherson found that RVO (mostly BRVO) was the etiology in 13% of cases with spontaneous vitreous hemorrhage, ranking third in their series behind proliferative diabetic retinopathy and retinal tears or retinal detachment.[24] In a recent study[26] of 94 eyes which underwent vitrectomy surgery for non-diabetic vitreous hemorrhage, 38% had an underlying BRVO and 28% had a final visual acuity of less than 20/200.

We found an 89% success rate of preventing vitreous hemorrhage when 75 cases of proliferative TBRVO were treated, although not all cases showed complete regression of neovascular tissue.[1] Thus with treatment there is an 11% incidence of vitreous hemorrhage as compared to a 57% incidence in the natural history of TBRVO.[1] The Branch Vein Occlusion Study has also recently published data in support of photocoagulation for proliferative BRVO.[21]

In determining the merit of early treatment[20,22,27] versus late intervention, several important considerations regarding vitreous hemorrhage must be emphasized. First, although vitreous hemorrhage may clear spontaneously with good final vision, the morbidity of visual impairment during that time period needs to be considered especially in patients with a significant visual impairment in their fellow eye. Second, traction macular detachment represents a severe complication of vitreous hemorrhage requiring prompt vitrectomy which carries additional risks and expense.[1,26] Third, the presence of even small amounts of blood in the vitreous may impede laser treatment of the entire ischemic area for an indefinite time period during which rebleeding may occur thus increasing the prospects of vitrectomy surgery. This is especially true in eyes with involvement of the inferior portion of the retina where vitreous hemorrhage is last to absorb.

Finally, MVO represents no risk of neovascularization and therefore treatment is reserved only for eyes with persistent macular edema as previously described.

Progressive capillary nonperfusion has been observed with serial angiography.[1,2,6,9,27,28] These patients assume the increased risk of neovascular complications as the ischemic index increases and need to be reclassified accordingly. We estimate that at least 10% will convert to an ischemic pattern depending on the type and duration of RVO, the age of the patient and the underlying systemic factors involved.[1,2,6,7,8,23,25,28] Thus an important part of the management of hyperpermeable and indeterminate patterns of RVO includes follow up and appropriate reclassification should an ischemic pattern emerge. In the follow up of the hyperpermeable group, repeat angiography is indicated if vision decreases or ophthalmoscopy shows more prominent hemorrhages and/or the appearance of nerve fiber layer infarcts indicating progression rather than resolution.

SUMMARY

This manuscript represents an update of our experience in the management of over 1500 patients referred with retinal vein obstruction (RVO) to the senior author (LEM) over a ten year period (1976–1986). The site of venous obstruction is always at an arterio-venous crossing where arterial disease impinges on its companion venous wall thus increasing turbulent blood flow culminating in thrombosis. The type of RVO is designated by the area of retina drained into macular (MVO), peripheral (PVO), temporal (TBRVO), hemispheric (HBRVO) and central (CRVO). The degree of retinal capillary damage from increased back up venous pressure as assessed by fluorescein angiography enables classification into three clinically useful groups. Those eyes with leaking but still perfused capillaries represent the hyperpermeable (edematous) group, eyes with extensive capillary nonperfusion are termed ischemic and eyes with mild to moderate capillary nonperfusion are classified as indeterminate (mixed). The main therapeutic concern in "non-ischemic" RVO is management of chronic macular edema to reduce the risk of irreversible macular degenerative changes; whereas, in ischemic RVO a preproliferative stage evolves with the risk of developing neovascular complications the principal threat to vision.

ACKNOWLEDGEMENTS

Supported in part by the Retina Research and Development Foundation of Philadelphia and the Pennsylvania Lions Sight Conservation Corporation.

The authors wish to acknowledge the late Professor I.C. Michaelson and Paul Henkind, M.D., Ph.D. for their pioneering contributions to our current understanding of retina vascular disease and to P. Robb McDonald, M.D., Thomas D. Duane, M.D. and William H. Annesley, Jr., M.D. for their support of the Retina Vascular Unit of the Wills Eye Hospital over the past ten years.

TABLE 1

		Risk of Neovascularization (Percent)		
Study	Pattern	NVI	NVD	NVR
Macular RVO (4)	Overall	0	0	0
Temporal BRVO (1)	Hyper	0	0	2
	Indet	0	0	0
	Ischemic	2.7	17.5	34
Hemispheric BRVO (2)	Hyper	0	0	0
	Indet	3.1	0	3.1
	Ischemic	14.0	21.1	15.8
Central RVO (3)	Hyper	0	0	0
	Indet	3	2	0
	Ischemic	60	24	10

Legend: RVO-Retinal Vein Obstruction, BRVO-Branch Retinal Vein Obstruction, NVI-Neovascularization of the Iris, NVD- Neovascularization of the Disc, NVR-Neovascularization of the Retina, Hyper-Hyperpermeable, Indet-Indeterminate.

REFERENCES

1. Magargal LE, Kimmel AJ, Sanborn GE, Annesley WH, Goldberg RE: Temporal Branch Retinal Vein Obstruction: A Review. Ophthalmology 1986;17:240-246.
2. Sanborn GE, Magargal LE: Characteristics of the Hemispheric Retinal Vein Occlusion. Ophthalmology 1984;91:1616-1626.
3. Magargal LE, Brown GC, Augsburger JJ, Parrish RK: Neovascular Glaucoma Following Central Retinal Vein Obstruction. Ophthalmology 1981;88:1095-1101.
4. Joffe L, Goldberg RE, Magargal LE, Annesley WH: Macular Branch Vein Occlusion. Ophthalmology 1980;87:91-98.
5. Magargal LE, Brown GC, Augsburger JJ, Donoso LA: Efficacy of Panretinal Photocoagulation in Preventing Neovascular Glaucoma Following Ischemic Central Retinal Vein Obstruction. Ophthalmology 1982;89: 780-784.
6. Magargal LE, Donoso LA, Sanborn GE: Retinal Ischemia and Risk of Neovascularization Following Central Retinal Vein Obstruction. Ophthalmology 1982;89:1241-1245.
7. Sanborn GE, Magargal LE, Jaeger EA. Central Retinal Vein Occlusion. In Clinical Ophthalmology, Duane TD (ed) and Jaeger (ed), J.B. Lippincott, Philadelphia, Pennsylvania 1986.
8. Scimeca GH, Magargal LE, Jaeger EA, Robb-Doyle E: Medical Conditions Associated with Retinal Vein Obstruction. Pennsylvania Medicine, November 1985;pp50-52.

9. Hayreh SS, Rojas P, Podhajsky P, Montague P, Woolson RF: Ocular Neovascularization with Retinal Vein Occlusion - III. Ophthalmology 1983;90:488-506.
10. Magargal LE, Brown GC, Augsburger JJ, Parrish RK: Neovascular Glaucoma Following Branch Vein Obstruction. Glaucoma 1981;3:333-335.
11. Brown GC, Magargal LE, Federman JL: Ischaemia and Neovascularization. Trans Ophthalmol Soc U K 1980;100:377-380.
12. Glaser BM, D'Amore PA, Michels RG, Brunson SK, Fensalaw AH, Rice T, Patz A: The Demonstration of Angiogenic Activity from Ocular Tissues. Ophthalmology 1980;87:440-446.
13. Federman JL, Brown GC, Felberg NT, Felton SM. Experimental Ocular Angiogenesis. Am J Ophthalmol 1980;89:231-237.
14. Chan CC, Little HL: Infrequency of Retinal Neovascularization Following Central Retinal Vein Occlusion. Ophthalmology 1979;86:256-262.
15. Branch Vein Occlusion Study Group: Argon Laser Photocoagulation for Macular Edema in Branch Vein Occlusion. Am J Ophthalmol 1984;98: 271-282.
16. Gartner S, Henkind P: Neovascularization of the Iris (Rubeosis Iridis): A Review. Surv Ophthalmol 1978;22:291-312.
17. Tasman W, Magargal LE, Augsburger JJ: Effects of Argon Laser Photocoagulation on Rubeosis Iridis and Angle Neovascularization. Ophthalmology 1980;87:400-402.
18. Green WR, Chan CC, Hutchins GM, Terry JM: Central Retinal Vein Occlusion: A Prospective Histopathologic Study of 29 Eyes in 28 Cases. Retina 1981;1:27-55.
19. Rosen PA, Marshall J, Kohner EA, Hamilton AM, Dollery CT: Experimental Retinal Branch Vein Occlusion in Rhesus Monkeys. II. Retinal Blood Flow Studies. Br J Ophthalmol 1979;63:388-392.
20. Archer DB, Michalopoulos N: Treatment of Neovascularization Secondary to Branch Retinal Vein Obstruction. Int Ophthalmol 1981;3:141-153.
21. Branch Vein Occlusion Study Group: Argon Laser Photocoagulation for Prevention of Neovascularization and Vitreous Hemorrhage in Branch Vein Occlusion: A Randomized Clinical Trial. Arch Ophthalmol 1986; 104:34-41.
22. Morse PH. Prospective Rationale for and Results of Argon Laser Treatment of Patients with Branch Retinal Vein Occlusion. Ann Ophthalmol 1985;17:565-571.
23. Brown GC, Magargal LE, Schachat A, Shah HG: Neovascular Glaucoma: Etiologic Considerations. Ophthalmology 1984;91:315-320.
24. Butner RW, McPherson AR: Spontaneous Vitreous Hemorrhage. Ann Ophthalmol 1982;14:268-270.
25. Magargal LE, Brown GC, Augsburger JJ, Goldberg RE, Donoso LA: Neovascular Glaucoma: Etiologic Factors and Management Considerations. Presented for Publication. The 1986 International Symposium of Ocular Circulation and Neovascularization, 1986.
26. Oyakawa RT, Michels RG, Blase WP: Vitrectomy for Non-Diabetic Vitreous Hemorrhage. Am J Ophthalmol 1983;96:517-525.
27. Sedney SC: Photocoagulation in Retinal Vein Occlusion. Br J Ophthalmol 1976;40:1-241.
28. Kimmel AS, Magargal LE, Morrison DL: Progressive Capillary Nonperfusion in Temporal Branch Retinal Vein Obstruction. Presented at the 1986 American Academy of Ophthalmology Meeting, New Orleans, Louisiana. (Submitted to Ophthalmology, 1986)

PREVENTION OF CLOT FORMATION IN CAT RETINAL VEIN BY SYSTEMIC AND SUBCONJUNCTIVAL UROKINASE

Shmuel Levinger, M.D., Hanan Zauberman, M.D., Amiram Eldor, M.D., Arieh Zelikovitch, and Eliezer Rosenmann, M.D., Departments of Ophthalmology, Hematology, and Pathology, Hadassah University Hospital and Hebrew University Medical School, Jerusalem, Israel

INTRODUCTION

Retinal vein thrombosis is a frequently observed clinical phenomenon often resulting in severe impairment of visual function, and frequently responding poorly to therapy. A rational approach to the treatment of this condition demands the use of the appropriate pharmacological agents, knowledge of the best route of delivery and, perhaps most important, information relating to the maximal time interval after thrombus formation during which the agent can still effectively dissolve the clot.

In order to study these parameters, we have developed a model of laser-induced vein thrombosis in the cat that permits objective evaluation of impaired circulation in the occluded vessel.

Using our model (1), we have investigated the effect of urokinase, a potent plasminogen activator, on the dissolution of the experimentally induced venous thrombus. The drug was administered either intravenously or subconjunctivally in order to determine which was the better route of delivery. The maximal time interval after the onset of vein thrombosis during which the treatment was still effective in preventing permanent occlusion of the vessel was also tested.

MATERIALS AND METHODS

Eighty-nine eyes of 54 adult cats were selected for this study. The animals were anesthesized with ketamine hydrochloride (Ketalar, Parke-Davis, United Kingdom) 30 mg/kg, injected intramuscularly.

In order to occlude a retinal vein, argon laser photocoagulation, using a Lasertek model (Lasertek, USA), was performed (514.5 nm) on the selected vessel with the aid of a fundus contact lens. Twenty-five such spots were delivered to the blood column of the retinal vein, at a distance of one disc diameter from the disc, until the blood flow in the thrombosed vessel was completely arrested.

Fluorescein angiography, performed at the end of each experiment, confirmed total venous obstruction. In order to induce thrombolysis and prevent thrombus organization, cats with occluded retinal veins were treated with urokinase (Ukidan, Serono, Italy) administered either by continuous intravenous infusion or by subconjunctival injection.

Group 1 consisted of 15 cats (28 eyes) which received continuous intravenous infusion of urokinase during a period of five hours. Therapy was initiated at different time intervals after occlusion of the retinal vein, as indicated in Table 1. The therapeutic protocol consisted of a loading dose of 4000 units/kg urokinase, administered intravenously during a period of 10 minutes. This was followed by intravenous administration of 4000 units/kg/hour urokinase during the next four hours and 50 minutes. The control for this group comprised four cats (eight eyes), whose eyes were photocoagulated in the same manner but which received no urokinase.

TABLE 1: Time interval between induction of vein occlusion and intravenous injection of urokinase.

TIME	NUMBER OF EYES	NUMBER OF CATS
5 minutes	4	2
3 hours	2	1
6 hours	2	1
9 hours	2	1
12 hours	2	1
15 hours	4	2
18 hours	3	2
24 hours	7	4
36 hours	2	1
TOTAL	28	15

Group 2 comprised 35 cats (53 eyes); in 35 eyes a total of 50,000 units of urokinase diluted in 2 ml normal saline were injected under the conjunctiva near the fornix, 12,500 units in each quadrant.

In 18 cats the retinal vein was occluded in both eyes: one eye was treated with UK injected subconjunctivally as described above, the fellow eye served as control and was injected subconjunctivally with 2 ml of normal saline, 0.5 ml in each quadrant. The time intervals of urokinase or normal saline administration following venous occlusion are indicated in Table 2.

TABLE 2: Time interval between induction of vein occlusion
and subconjunctival injection of urokinase or normal saline.

TIME	UROKINASE No. of eyes	NORMAL SALINE No. of eyes	TOTAL NO. OF CATS
0 minutes	2	2	2
3 hours	6	2	6
6 hours	2	2	2
9 hours	3	2	3
12 hours	3	1	3
15 hours	1	1	1
18 hours	1	1	1
24 hours	9	2	9
36 hours	6	3	6
48 hours	2	2	2
TOTAL	35	18	35

In selected eyes injected subconjunctivally either with
urokinase or normal saline, the fluorescein angiogram was
repeated seven days after thrombus induction.

Assessment of the effects of thrombolytic therapy:
One week after the induction of retinal vein thrombosis
the animals were anesthesized and indirect ophthalmoscopy
and fluorescein angiography again performed.   Then the eyes
were enucleated leaving an 11 to 13 mm stump of optic nerve
containing the ophthalmociliary artery.   The enucleated eye
was placed on the platform of a special chamber (Fig. 1),
with the corneal surface gently pressing against the concave
surface of a fundus contact lens.

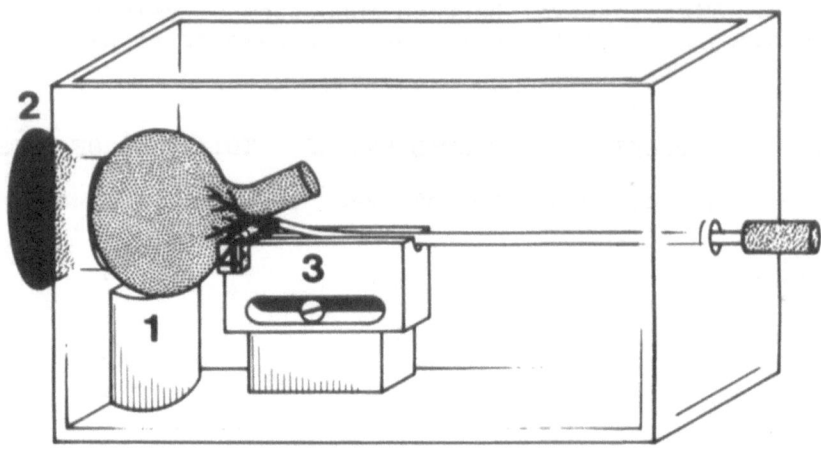

Fig. 1

The ophthalmociliary artery was cannulated according to a technique previously described (1,2). The perfusion chamber was then set up in a vertical position. With the aid of an operating microscope with coaxial illumination, it was possible to observe the fundus of the eye, the focus centered on the area of the occluded retinal vein. The container of perfusate was raised to 5, 15, 40, 50, 100 and 200 cm above the level of the eye.

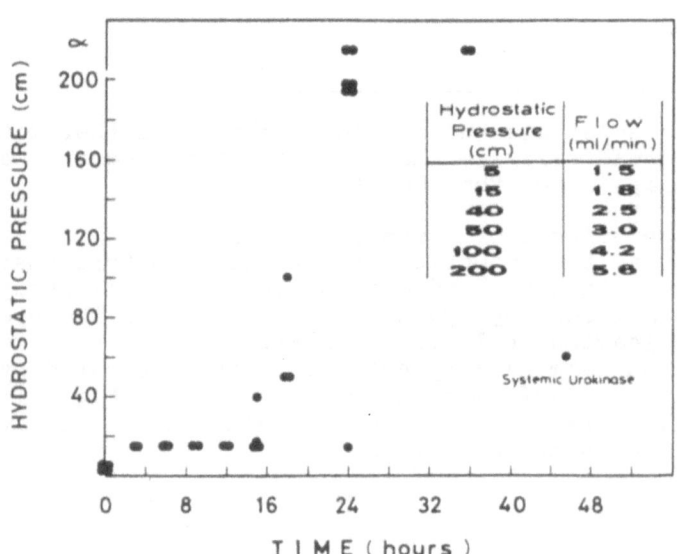

Hydrostatic Pressure (cm)	Flow (ml/min)
5	1.5
15	1.8
40	2.5
50	3.0
100	4.2
200	5.6

Fig. 2

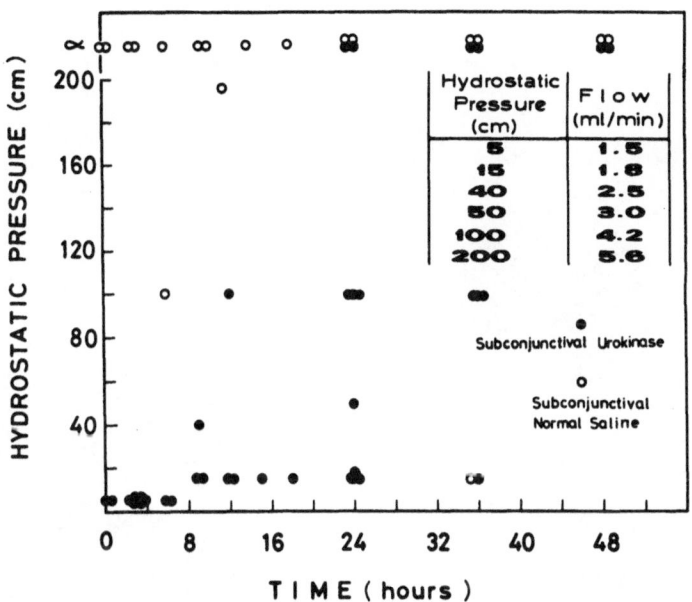

Fig. 3

Measurement of flow rate versus hydrostatic pressure showed that at the lower hydrostatic pressure (5 cm) there was a flow rate of 1.5 ml/min, and at the highest hydrostatic pressure (200 cm) the flow rate was 5.6 ml/min. The correlation between hydrostatic pressure and concomitant flow rate is seen in the insert of Figs. 2 and 3, above.

The minimal hydrostatic pressure and flow rate needed to perfuse the previously thrombosed vessel were monitored visually. The patency of the vessel was confirmed by adding 10% fluorescein to the perfusate and observing its flow through the vessel. Selected eyes were used for histological evaluation of the thrombosed retinal vein. The eyes were fixed in 10% formalin for light microscopy.

RESULTS

Argon laser photocoagulation resulted in the production of a firm thrombus after seven days. Light microscopy of an occluded vessel is shown in Fig. 4. It may be seen that the thrombosed vein and the patent artery are surrounded by glial tissue that replaces the outer and inner nuclear layers.

The presence of an organized clot, seven days after photocoagulation of the vein, which is resistant to the passage of perfusate, made it possible to study the effect of urokinase on the developing thrombus.

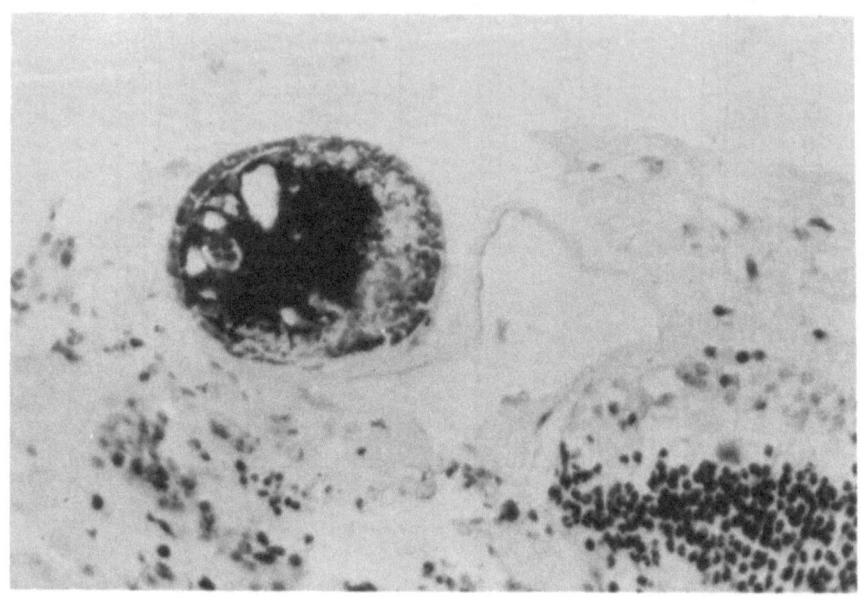

Fig. 4

When urokinase was injected intravenously in the
Group 1 cats within five minutes of induction of the venous
clot, the hydrostatic pressure and flow rate needed to
reestablish the patency of the treated vessel were similar
not only to those necessary to wash out unoccluded retinal
vessels (5 cm, 1.5 ml/min) (1) in the quadrant of the
occluded vessel but also to those in all the other retinal
quadrants. However, when urokinase was injected 3 to 18
hours after vein occlusion, the pressure required was at
least threefold greater than for the unoccluded veins and
the flow rate reached 1.8 ml/min (the upper limit of the
physiological flow rate). When urokinase was administered
24 to 36 hours after occlusion, the pressure needed to
reestablish the patency of the treated vein usually rose to
200 cm and the concomitant flow rate was 5.6 ml/min. In
many instances no flow could be detected through the
occluded retinal vasculature. These results are similar to
those obtained in the control group of eyes with occluded
veins in which no systemic treatment had been given (1).
Fig. 2 shows the hydrostatic pressure and flow rate needed
to reestablish the patency of an occluded cat retinal vein
as a function of time of intravenous UK injection following
onset of thrombosis.

When urokinase was injected subconjunctivally (Group 2)

between five minutes to about six hours after induced
occlusion, the hydrostatic pressure needed to reestablish
vein patency was 5 cm and the concomitant flow rate was 1.5
ml/min. However, when urokinase was injected 3 to 18 hours
following retinal vein thrombosis, the pressure usually had
to be increased to 15 cm with a concomitant flow rate of 1.8
ml/min. In 16 of the 18 eyes injected subconjunctivally
with urokinase 5 minutes to 18 hours after induction of vein
occlusion, the hydrostatic pressure needed in order to
reestablish patency was 15 cm H_2O or less. In the other
two eyes, a hydrostatic pressure of 50 cm was necessary in
one case, and 100 cm in the other. When urokinase was
injected 24 to 48 hours after thrombus induction, in about
50% of this subgroup the perfusion pressure needed to
reestablish patency was 50 to 100 cm and the concomitant
flow rate was 2.5 to 4.2 ml/min. In many instances, the clot
could not be displaced. In the Group 2 control eyes,
injected subconjunctivally with normal saline, patency of
the occluded vein could not be reestablished, even at a
hydrostatic pressure of 200 cm. In only three of the 18
control eyes was patency achieved. One eye required a
hydrostatic pressure of 15 cm, and the other two, 100 and
200 cm, much higher than those needed for the urokinase
treated eyes. Fig. 3 shows the hydrostatic pressure and flow
rates needed to reestablish the patency of an occluded cat
retinal vein as a function of time of subconjunctival UK
injection after the onset of retinal vein thrombosis.

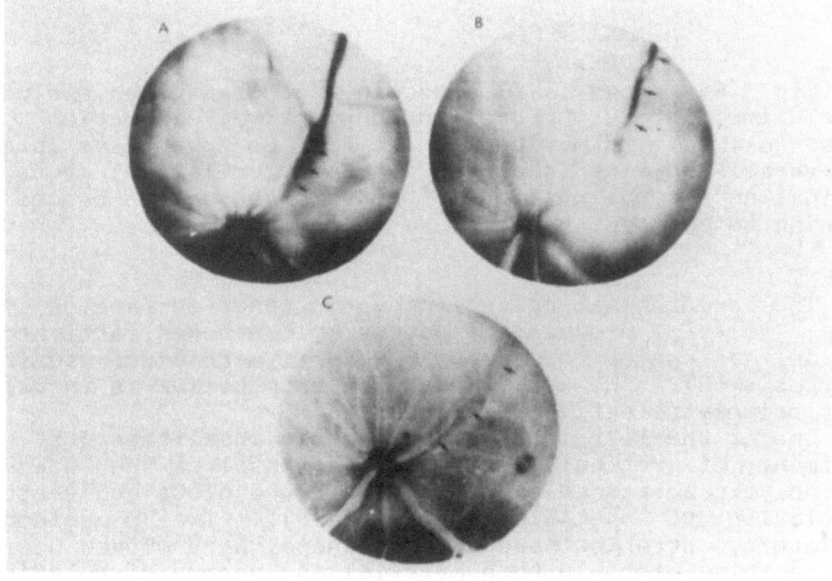

Fig. 5

As may be seen in Figs. 5a and 5b, fluorescein angiograms taken immediately after the induction of retinal vein occlusion reveal that the vessel was impervious to the dye. This eye, belonging to Group 2, was subconjunctivally injected with UK 15 minutes after occlusion. As may be seen in Figure 5c, seven days later the photocoagulated retinal vein showed a delay in fluorescein filling but appeared to be patent, and there were no collateral vessels stemming from the occluded vein.

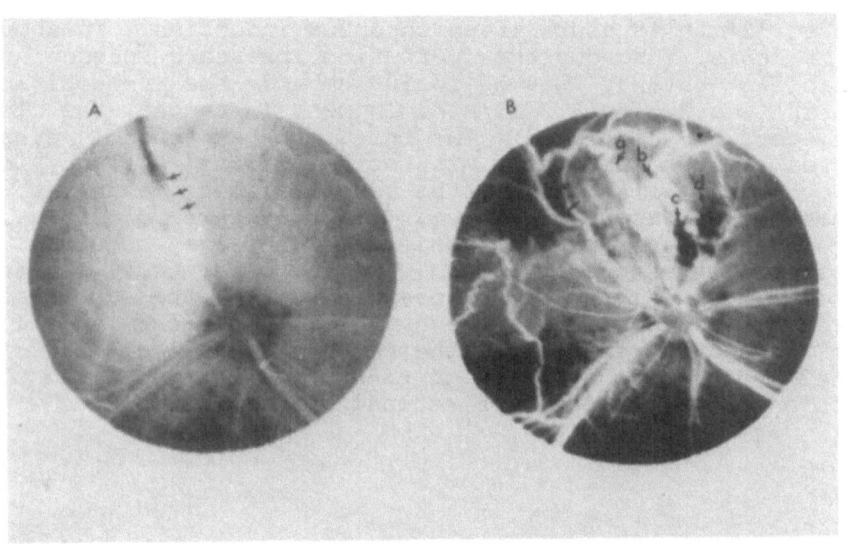

Fig. 6

Fig. 6a shows a fluorescein angiogram of an occluded vessel immediately before subconjunctival injection of normal saline. As may be seen in Fig. 6b seven days later, the vessel remained occluded with many collateral vessels originating in the portion of the vein above the occlusion draining to adjacent vessels.

COMMENT

The endothelial cells lining the inner surface of the blood vessels produce a potent plasminogen activator, regarded as one of the vascular defense mechanisms against thrombosis (3). However, once the endothelium is injured, the fibrinolytic activity is impaired.

One of the most logical therapeutic modalities for the treatment of retinal vein thrombosis involves the use of fibrinolytic agents able to dissolve blood clots and restore circulation to the affected area (4-9). Two plasminogen activators, streptokinase and urokinase, have proved useful in dissolving clots in both arterial and venous circulation. The two agents effect fibrinolysis by activating the body's natural fibrinolytic system. The inactive proenzyme plasminogen is converted to the active enzyme plasmin, fresh fibrin clots are lysed and there is generation of fibrin degradation products. Plasmin, however, exhibits proteolytic activity not only towards fibrin and fibrinogen, but also digests factors V and VIII (10,11). Plasminogen activators have a high affinity for blood clots. Clots, in turn, have a high concentration of plasminogen and a low content of plasmin inhibitors. This means that the plasmin formed within the clot effectively dissolves it.

The efficacy of systemic fibrinolytic therapy has been well documented in clinical practice, although it has been emphasized that aged thrombi are no longer susceptible to lysis (12).

Our study shows that UK is an effective therapeutic agent for experimentally induced retinal vein thrombosis. However, the maximal time interval for the fibrinolytic agent to be optimally effective in restoring the patency of the retinal vein (120 to 150 u diameter) following the thrombotic event is about six hours. When applied after this critical period, the fibrinolytic agent is only partially effective, as evidenced by the progressively increasing hydrostatic pressure and flow rates necessary for perfusion.

Our study also indicates that the subconjunctival route of administration is more efficacious in reestablishing circulation than the intravenous route.

Based on the results of this study which proved the effectiveness of very early administration of a fibrinolytic agent on experimentally induced retinal vein occlusion, we are carrying out a clinical trial.

LEGENDS

Figure 1:

1. Supporting platform
2. Contact lens
3. Movable column
4. Silicone sponge compressing the eye globe against the contact lens

Figure 2: Hydrostatic pressure and flow rate needed to reestablish patency of an occluded cat retinal vein as a function of time of intravenous injection of urokinase following onset of vein thrombosis.

Figure 3: Hydrostatic pressure and flow rate needed to reestablish patency of an occluded cat retinal vein versus subconjunctival urokinase injection following onset of vein thrombosis.

Figure 4: Retinal vein seven days after argon laser photocoagulation. The vein is occluded by an adherent thrombus. The adjacent artery is patent. Phosphotungstic acid hematoxylin stain (x 240).

Figure 5:   Fluorescein angiogram of photocoagulated retinal vein prior to and following subconjunctival treatment of the eye with urokinase.
a.   Eleven seconds after intravenous fluorescein injection. Arrows show occluded vessel.
b.   Seven minutes after intravenous injection of fluorescein.   No dye in occluded area (arrows). Fluorescein is leaking in the photocoagulated portion.
c.   Seven days after subconjunctival injection of urokinase. Dye fills the vein (arrows). No shunt vessels are evident.

Figure 6:
a.   Fluorescein angiogram of photocoagulated retinal vein prior to and following subconjunctival treatment of the eye with normal saline. Arrows show occluded vein.
b.   Retinal vein seven days after subconjunctival injection of normal saline. Vein remains occluded (arrows). Collateral (a and b) connect the vessel with other veins.   Retinal hemorrhages are evident near the optic disc (c and d).

REFERENCES
1.   Zauberman H, Levinger S, Burde RM: Perfusion of occluded retinal vein in the cat's eye.   Br J Ophthalmol 1984; 68:5861.
2.   Gouras P, Hoff M: Retinal function in an isolated, perfused mammalian eye. Invest Ophthalmol 1970; 9:388-399.
3.   Loskutoff DJ, Edgington TE: Synthesis of a fibrinolytic activator and inhibitor by endothelial cells.   Proc Natl Acad Sci USA 1977; 74(9):3903-3907.
4.   Howden GD: The successful treatment of a case of central retinal vein thrombosis with intravenous fibrinolysin. Canad Med Assn J 1959; 81:382 384.
5.   Kwaan HC, Dobbie JG, Fetkenhour CL, et al: Thrombolytic therapy of central retinal vein occlusion, in Martin M, Schoop W, Hirsh, J (eds): New Concepts in Streptokinase Dosimetry.   Bern,   Hans Huber, 1978, pp 221-229.
6.   Kwaan, HC, Dobbie JG, Fetkenhour CL: Thrombolytic therapy of central retinal vein occlusion: an update, in Mannucci PM, D'angelo A (eds):   Urokinase: Basic and Clinical Aspects.   London and New York,   Academic Press, 1982, pp 245-247.
7.   Brancato R, Michelone C. Subconjunctival urokinase for retinal vein occlusion, in Mannucci PM, D'angelo A (eds): Urokinase: Basic and Clinical Aspects. London and New York, Academic Press, 1982, pp 253-258.
8.   Mutlu F: Experimental retinal vein occlusion and treatment with fibrinolysin.   Am J Ophthalmol 1966; 62:282-286.
9.   Kohner EM, Hamilton AM, Bulpitt CJ, et al: Streptokinase in the treatment of central retinal vein occlusion a controlled trial. Trans Ophthalmol Soc UK 1974; 94:599-603.

10. Collen D: On the regulation and control of fibrinolysis. Edward Kowalski Memorial Lecture. Thromb Haemost 1980; 43:77-89.
11. Verstraete M: Biochemical and clinical aspects of thrombolysis. Semin Hematol 1978; 15:35-54.
12. Sasahara AA, Sharma GVRK, Tow DE, et al: Clinical use of thrombolytic agents in venous thromboembolism. Arch Intern Med 1982; 142:684-688.

THE FORMATION AND MAINTENANCE OF NEW BLOOD VESSELS

B.M. Glaser, L. Kuwashima, M. Sato, and R. Adler

INTRODUCTION

Several steps in the formation of new blood vessels
have been elucidated. Among these steps are breakdown of
surrounding extracellular matrix, migration of vascular
endothelial cell to form an advancing new blood vessel
sprout, and endothelial cells proliferation at the base of
the sprout. Two other important events in the process of
new blood vessel formation have yet to receive much
attention. These steps are formation of the new blood
vessel lumen and maintenance of the new blood vessels. The
importance of the maintenance of new blood vessels becomes
apparent when one realizes that new blood vessels regress
rapidly once the stimulating factor or factors are removed.
We will therefore present two sets of studies. The first
set of studies relates to the in vitro formation of
capillary like structures by vascular endothelial cells.
The mechanism of lumen formation in this model is
described. It is not clear whether this mechanism of lumen
formation occurs in vivo. The second set of studies
elucidates some of the factors that may play a role in the
maintenance of new blood vessels and their subsequent
regression upon removal of the angiogenic stimulators.

I. Reaggregated endothelial cells form capillary-like structures in vitro

New blood vessel formation plays an important role in a
variety of phenomena including development, wound healing,
inflammation, recanalization of intravascular clots, tumor
growth, proliferative diabetic retinopathy and the
disciform stage of age-related maculopathies. Endothelial
cells derived from both capillaries and large vessels have
been studied in order to better understand the process of
new blood vessel formation. A new blood vessel begins as a
solid cellular sprout which subsequently becomes hollowed
out to form a tube with a central lumen. However, the way
in which a new vessel forms its lumen is not understood.

We have studied the gyration mediated reaggregation of
fetal bovine aortic endothelial cells and human retinal
capillary endothelial cells grown without tumor conditioned
medium or special substrata. Both types of endothelial
cells (EC) begin to form aggregates within 10 minutes and
were allowed to continue to develop for up to 72 hours. By
light and electron microscopy the EC were found to form
tubular structures closely resembling extracellular

material on the abluminal surface and fenestrae.

Material and methods

Endothelial cells were harvested from fetal bovine aortas and human retinal capillary fragments as previously reported.[1,2] Cells were grown in Eagle's Minimum Essential Medium supplemented with 10% fetal bovine serum (MEM/10) at 37°C in 5% CO_2. These cells formed a characteristic mosaic of nonoverlapping polygonal cells when grown as monolayers. Confluent cells were dissociated with 0.1% trypsin and the trypsin quenched with MEM/10. They were then suspended in MEM/10 containing 20 mM Hepes at a concentration of 8×10^6 cells per ml. Gyration mediated reaggregates were allowed to develop for up to 72 hours at 80 rpm at 37°C. Individual aggregates were examined by light and electron microscopy at various time intervals. As a control, smooth muscle cells were grown from explants of the medial layer of fetal bovine aorta and were treated in the same manner as endothelial cells.

The aggregates were fixed in 1% paraformaldehyde, 1.25% glutaraldehyde, and 0.1 M cacodylate buffer for 2 hours at 4°C, and washed in cacodylate buffer. Aggregates were post-fixed in 1% osmium tetroxide in cacodylate buffer for 2 hours, dehydrated in graded ethanol, stained in block with 1% uranyl acetate in pure ethanol and embedded in Epon. Semithin (1 μm) and thin sections were cut with a Porter-Blum ultra-microtome. Thick sections were stained with 0.1% toluidine blue and studied by light microscopy. Thin sections were stained with uranyl acetate and lead citrate and examined with a JEM 100B electron microscope.

Results

Under these conditions, gyration mediated endothelial cell reaggregates were visible within 10 minutes. Light and electron microscopy of dissociated endothelial cells before reaggregation showed round cells with fine cytoplasmic processes.

After reaggregation for 30 minutes, many vascular endothelial cells developed pseudopod-like cytoplasmic processes and began to surround a neighboring endothelial cell (Fig. 1). Sometimes, a few endothelial cells surrounded only one cell. After 2 hours, some of the central cells began to show signs of degeneration. These central cells did not form junctional complexes with adjacent cells. After 7-12 hours, the central cell had degenerated further and began to separate from the surrounding endothelial cell (Fig. 2). Basement membrane-like extracellular material was found on the abluminal surface of these capillary-like structures. After 24 hours in culture, the central cell died leaving behind a lumen filled with cellular debris . Basement membrane-like extracellular material was found on the abluminal surface between adjacent cells. Electron microscopy of serial thin sections revealed that the structure of most lumina were spherical or ovoid in shape. These lumina interconnect randomly within aggregates to make branching tube-like structures. In contrast, gyration mediated reaggregates of bovine aortic smooth muscle cells failed to show lumen formation.

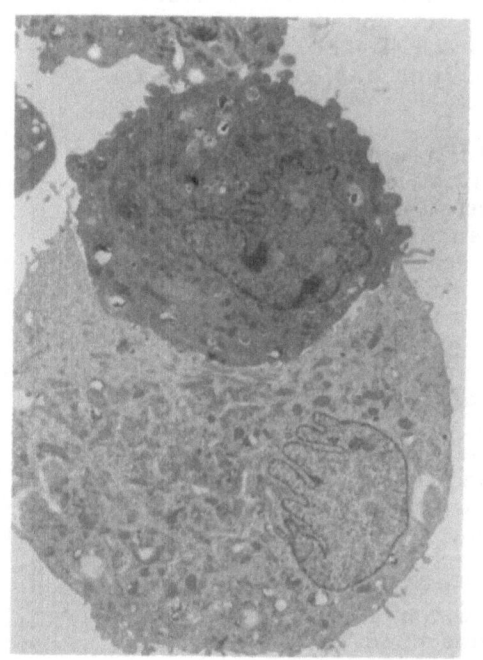 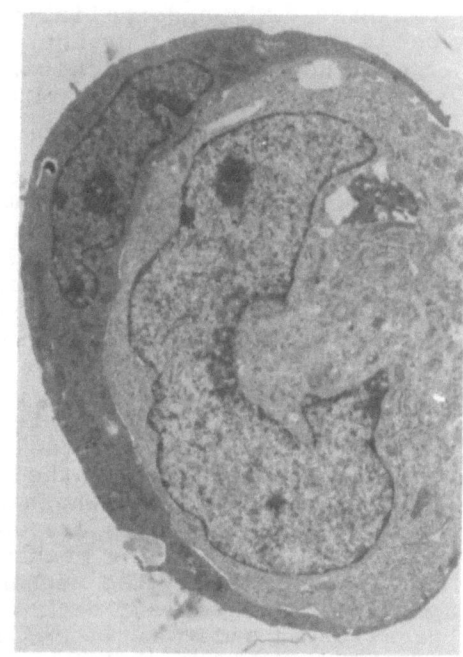

Figure 1. Aortic endothelial cells grown in gyration mediated culture for 30 minutes. Endothelial cells begin to surround a neighboring endothelial cell (a) x3800. (b) X5500.

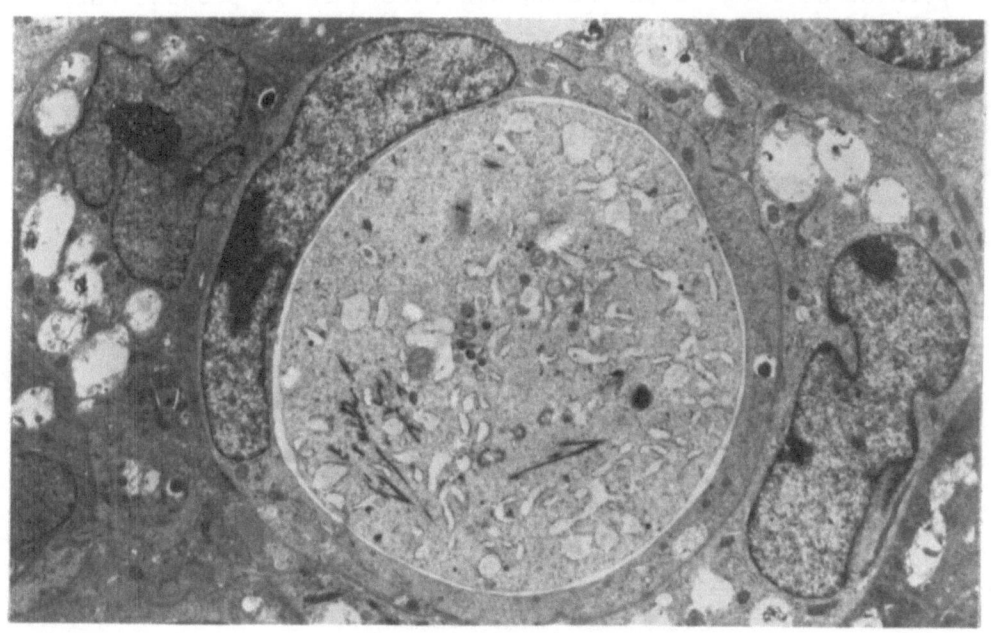

Figure 2. Endothelial cells forming lumen in 7-9 hour
cultures. The endothelial cells surrounded by adjacent
cells show signs of degeneration with markedly swollen
rough endoplasmic reticulum. A slight gap exists between
central and outer cells. X 6500.

Discussion

We have demonstrated that gyration mediated reaggregation
induces endothelial cells to form tubular structures
resembling capillaries. The mechanism of tube formation in
these cultures is as follows: 1) endothelial cells surround
neighboring endothelial cells, 2) the central surrounded
cell degenerates leaving behind a lumen filled with cell
debris, 3) the lumina interconnet to form tubular
structures closely resembling a capillary. These
capillaries-like structures are surrounded by a basement
membrane-like material and occasionally have fenestrated
membranes. These events are seen in experiments using
fetal bovine aortic endothelial cells as well as human
retinal microvessel endothelial cells.

It is still unclear whether a similiar process occurs in
vivo. Further studies are underway to answer this
question. Even if the mechanism of lumen formation does
not follow exactly the mechanism in vivo, the current model
provides a convenient method by which to study the
behavior of endothelial cells under conditions which more
closely resemble conditions within capillaries.

II. Stimulation of vascular endothelial cell prostacyclin release by a retina-derived factor

Maintenance of the newly formed vasculature and
inhibition of vessel regression are vital if new blood
vessels are to persist. New blood vessels typically
persist as long as an angiogenic substance is present but
capillaries regress following removal of that same
angiogenic substance(s). The initial events seen
histologically in regressing vessels are the adhesion of
platelets to the vessel wall accompanied by the formation
of platelet plugs.[3] A significant component of the ability
of an angiogenic substance to stimulate new blood vessel
formation and prevent regression of neovascularization may
therefore depend on its ability to prevent platelet plug
formation and subsequent hemostasis. Prostacyclin (PGI_2),
the predominant prostaglandin produced by endothelial
cells, is a potent inhibitor of platelet aggregation and
also inhibits adhesion of activated platelets to
endothelium.[4] In the present study, the influence of
bovine retinal extract on endothelial cell prostacyclin
production was determined.

Endothelial cells

Fetal bovine aortic endothelial (FBAE) cells were
cultured as previously described.[1] Cells were grown in 75
cm^2 flasks in Eagles minimal essential medium (MEM/0)
supplemented with 10% fetal bovine serum (MEM/10), in 5%
CO_2 at $37^\circ C$. At confluence, the FBAE density was 8.5-9.5 X
10^6 cells per 75 cm^2 flask. Human microvessel endothelial
(HME) cells obtained from retinal capillaries by a

modification of Del Vecchio's method were used at passages 4-8.[5] Bovine retinal extract was prepared as previously reported.[1]

Experimental incubations

FBAE cells were plated in 24-well plates at a density of 4.0×10^4 cells/well and incubated for 24 hours in MEM/10 at 37° C. Following aspiration of MEM/10 and rinsing with MEM/0, test substances were added to a total volume of 1 ml. All dilutions of retinal extract were made in MEM/0. After test substances were added, cells were incubated at 37° C and 5% CO_2 for 24 hours unless otherwise indicated. Media from each well was then removed and centrifuged for 10 minutes to remove cellular debris. Samples were frozen at -20°C until assayed. The number of cells per well was determined in replicate wells using an electronic cell counter.

PGI_2 was quantitated in the endothelial cell conditioned media by radioimmunoassay (RIA) of its stable metabolite 6-keto PGF1alpha as previously described.[6] The level of sensitivity was 5 pg/ml.

Results

With the addition of RE to FBAE, an 8-10 fold increase in PGI_2 occurs at 6 hours which is sustained and augmented through 24 hours of incubation. As previously described, the addition of RE also stimulated FBAE proliferation.[1] Bradykinin's stimulatory effect on FBAE PGI_2 release occurred more rapidly (within 30 minutes) than with RE; however, release of PGI_2 with bradykinin occurred in an initial transient burst which did not continue throughout the incubation period. The stimulatory effect of RE on PGI_2 production is abolished by the cyclooxygenase inhibitor indomethacin. Indomethacin had a similar inhibitory effect on baseline PGI_2 release. Two different FBAE cell lines in addition to human microvessel endothelial (HME) cells responded in a similar fashion to RE, with PGI_2 release routinely stimulated by 6-15 fold over baseline at 24 hours. Stimulation of PGI_2 is dose-dependent with respect to the concentration of RE.

The magnitude of RE stimulation of PGI_2 release was markedly influenced by the cell density of the endothelial monolayer. Sub-confluent cells responded to RE with a 10 to 15-fold increase in PGI_2 release compared to baseline controls. In contrast, confluent endothelial cells increased PGI_2 release by only 2-3 fold in response to RE. As the FBAE monolayer approached confluence there was a concurrent decline in RE-dependent PGI_2 release. Endogenous production of PGI_2 was increased 4-5 fold in sub-confluent cells over their confluent counterparts. The presence of RE is required for the sustained production of PGI_2. Removal of RE from the incubation media results in a rapid decrease in PGI_2 release.

Discussion

A wide range of naturally occurring biological substances are known which stimulate PGI_2 release, among which include mediators of cell damage, bradykinin, arachidonic acid and thrombin. [7-9] This is the first report describing enhancement of PGI_2 release by an extract which also stimulates neovascularization. The time course of retinal extract's effect on endothelial cell PGI_2 release is different in comparison with many of the other substances reported to stimulate PGI_2 production. Whereas maximal PGI_2 release in response to RE requires up to 24 hours, other PGI_2 stimulators such as bradykinin, arachidonic acid, ionophore A23187 and thrombin effect maximal PGI_2 release within minutes. [8,9] Also, release of PGI_2 is a sustained phenomenon in the presence of RE whereas many substances which rapidly stimulate PGI_2 release have a transient, short-acting effect.

Stimulators of vascular endothelial PGI_2 production which also have a time course similar to that of RE include bacterial endotoxin, phorbol acetate, mononuclear cell products (interleukin-1) and platelet-derived growth factor (PDGF). [7,10,11] PDGF is not responsible for the PGI_2 stimulatory ability of RE since PDGF is not inactivated by boiling whereas the PGI_2 stimulatory activity of RE is. It is unlikely that any of the other substances are present in RE at concentrations capable of stimulating PGI_2 synthesis.

PGI_2 is an extremely potent anti-platelet aggregating agent and one of the major prostaglandins produced by endothelial cells. In capillary beds, nonthrombogenicity under normal conditions may be due to a combination of mild platelet inhibition by low levels of PGI_2 along with the innate non-thrombotic property of the endothelial cell membrane. Prostacyclin's role in opposing thrombosis in capillaries may become more important during new blood vessel formation. A histological study by Ausprunk et al[3], the sequence of events in the regression of newly formed blood vessels indicated that the first changes to occur were by the formation of platelet plugs within regressing vessels. The platelet plugs were observed around 24 hours after removal of the angiogenic stimulus from the corneal pockets. It is interesting, in this regard, that removal of RE from culture media also leads to a decline in PGI_2 release within 24 hours. Newly formed blood vessels appear to have intercellular gaps which may expose subendothelial thrombogenic surfaces that act as a nidus for platelet adhesion and aggregation. [12] It is tempting to speculate that the endothelial lining with its many gaps in these immature vessels may have properties similar to that seen in sub-confluent cultures, namely, a greatly increased capacity for PGI_2 release. With time, vessels lose these intercellular gaps and perhaps the need for enhanced PGI_2 production.

References

1. Glaser BM, D'Amore PA, Michels RG, Patz A, Fenselau A: Demonstration of vasoproliferative activity from mammalian retina. J Cell Biology 34:298-304, 1980.
2. Del Vecchio PJ, Sharuk GS, Mac Elroy KF: Isolation and culture of cells from human retinal microvessels. Invest Ophthal. 25:247, 1984.

3. Ausprunk DH, Falterman K, Folkman J: The sequence of events in the regression of corneal capillaries. Lab Invest 28:284-294, 1978.
4. Weiss HJ, Turitto VT: Prostacyclin inhibits platelet adhesion and thrombus formation on subendothelium. Blood 53:244-250, 1979.
5. Del Vecchio PJ, Sharuk GS, MacElroy KS: Isolation and culture of cells from human retinal microvessels. Invest Ophthalmol Vis Sci (suppl.) 25:247, 1984.
6. Branstrom E, Kendahl H: Radioimmunoassay of prostaglandins and thromboxanes. Adv in Prost and Thromb Res 5:119, 1978.
7. Nawroth PP, Stern DM, Kaplan KL, Nossel HL: Prostacyclin production by perturbed bovine aortic endothelial cells in culture. Blood 64: 801-806, 1984.
8. Weksler BB, Ley CW, Jaffe EA: Stimulation of endothelial cell prostacyclin production by thrombin, trypsin and the ionophore A23187. J Clin Invest 62:923-930, 1978.
9. Hong, SL: Effect of bradykinin and thrombin on prostacyclin synthesis in endothelial cells from calf and pig aorta and human umbilical cord vein. Thromb Res 18:787, 1980.
10. Coughlin SR, Moskowitz MA, Zetter BR, Antoniades HS, Levine L: Platelet-dependent stimulation of prostacycline synthesis by platelet-derived growth factor. Nature 288:600-602, 1980.
11. Rossi V, Breviarvo F, Ghezzi P, Dejana E, Mantovani A: Prostacyclin synthesis induced in vascular cells by interleukin. Science 229:174-176, 1985.
12. Schoefl Gl: Studies on inflammation: Growing capillaries. Their structure and permeability. Virchows Arch iv 337:97, 1963.

MECHANISM OF ELEVATED MEMBRANE FORMATION AND
POSTERIOR VITREOUS DETACHMENT IN DIABETES MELLITUS

Eugene de Juan, Jr., M. D.

Duke University Eye Center
Box 3802
Durham, North Carolina   27710

ABSTRACT

Elevated membrane formation in patients with diabetes mellitus can
result in severe visual loss by vitreous hemorrhage and/or traction
retinal detachment. To determine the histologic character of elevated
membranes and propose a mechanism of posterior vitreous detachment we
examined 16 selected autopsy eyes and 34 membranes removed during surgery
for proliferative diabetic retinopathy (PDR). The specimens were studied
by routine histology, immunohistochemistry, and electron microscopy. We
found cells which are positively stained with GFAP and contain large
intracellular filaments present in nearly all types of membranes at the
vitreous surface. We propose that posterior vitreous detachment in PDR is
a cell mediated event.

INTRODUCTION

Diabetic retinopathy is a major cause of visual loss in the United
States.[1]   The most severe visual impairments result from the
proliferative stages of the disease. Clinical observations have
confirmed the role of posterior vitreous detachment in the expression of
the disease.[2-5]   However, most histologic descriptions of proliferative
disease in diabetes have emphasized the vessels and their development
with relatively little description of the formation of elevated
proliferations and posterior vitreous detachment.[6-9]   The purpose of this
communication is to describe the formation of elevated proliferations and
posterior vitreous detachment.

MATERIALS AND METHODS

Postmortem and freshly enucleated eyes from diabetic patients were
obtained from the Duke University Medical Center pathology laboratory
files. Eyes with various stages of development of proliferative membranes
were selected for further studies (16 eyes). The formalin fixed specimens
were prepared for histologic examination after staining with
hematoxylin-eosin and periodic acid-schiff. Phosphotungstic
acid-hematoxylin stain was used to demonstrate the presence of glia.
Immunoperoxidase staining for glial fibrillary acidic protein was
performed on sections from formalin-fixed paraplast-embedded eyes (seven
eyes). Commercially obtained rabbit antibody to human glial fibrillary
acidic protein (Dako) was used with the peroxidase-antiperoxidase (PAP)
technique.[10]   Briefly, 10 μm thick sections mounted on histo-stick coated
slides were deparaffinized in xylene and hydrated in graded alcohol
solutions. The slides were treated with 3% hydrogen peroxide for five

minutes to eliminate endogenous peroxidase activity. The specimens were rinsed in tris buffer and then incubated with rabbit antibody to human glial fibrillary acidic protein for 20 minutes and rinsed in tris buffer for 20 minutes. Swine anti-rabbit IgG antibody was reacted with the specimens for 20 minutes. After rinsing, the specimens were reacted with peroxidase-antiperoxidase immunocomplex for 20 minutes and rinsed. Freshly prepared diaminobenzidine staining solution was reacted with the specimens for five minutes, followed by another rinse in distilled water. The slides were then counterstained with Mayer's hematoxylin. Nonspecific staining was judged by repeating the procedure without the glial fibrillary acidic protein antibody. Positive controls for glial fibrillary acidic protein were taken by using formalin fixed human cerebral tissue.

In addition, 34 epiretinal and preretinal membranes removed during vitreous surgery for proliferative diabetic retinopathy were studied, by light and electron microscopy. The membranes were rinsed in 0.1 M cacodylate buffer with 5% sucrose (pH 7.4) immediately after removal. They were then placed in 2% glutaraldehyde in 0.1 M cacodylate buffer for at least one hour and post-fixed in 2% osmium tetroxide in 0.1 M cacodylate buffer for one hour, rinsed in buffer, and dehydrated in graded ethanol. The membranes were embedded in Spurr low viscosity medium and 1 μm sections stained with toluidine blue and basic fuchsin for light microscopy. Sixty nm sections were cut and stained with uranyl acetate and lead citrate for transmission electron microscopy. When a specimen was large enough, a portion of the specimen was critical-point dried, sputter-coated with gold palladium, and examined with a scanning electron microscope.

RESULTS

In reviewing the available material we identified several types of preretinal membranes. The architecture of the membranes demonstrates specific patterns, but often with several types in a single eye. The emphasis in this study is to categorize these types of membranes in increasing complexity based on light microscopic and immunocytochemical staining appearance.

The simplest proliferative retinal change observed is intraretinal hypercellularity. In these eyes the inner aspects of the nerve fiber and ganglion cell layers appear hypercellular. The cells are spindle shaped and stain positive with antibody directed against human glial fibrillary acidic protein (GFAP). In addition Müller endfeet also stain for GFAP.

The next type of membrane observed is a thin layer (not monolayer) of cells along the retinal surface (Figure 1). These cells stain with antibody to GFAP and have a thin layer of collagen between the cells and the internal limiting lamina. The thin layer of cells is seen in the presence of an attached or detached vitreous. If the vitreous is attached then the epiretinal membrane is thin and the effects on the retinal shape are not dramatic (Figure 1). When the vitreous is detached the epiretinal membrane can cause more prominent surface distortions (Figures 2a and b). The epiretinal membrane may or may not be associated with underlying intraretinal gliosis or Müller endfeet GFAP staining. Vessels are not present in this type of membrane.

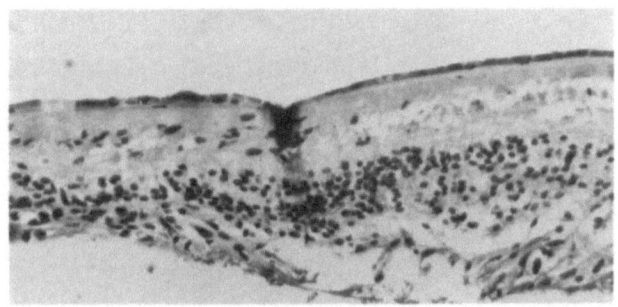

FIGURE 1. Photomicrograph of GFAP positive epiretinal membrane in patient with proliferative diabetic retinopathy.

Figure 2a

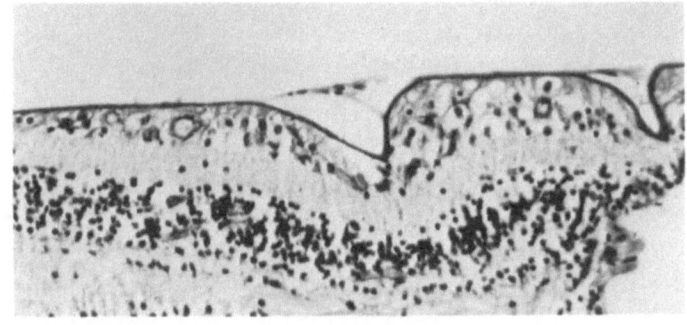

Figure 2b

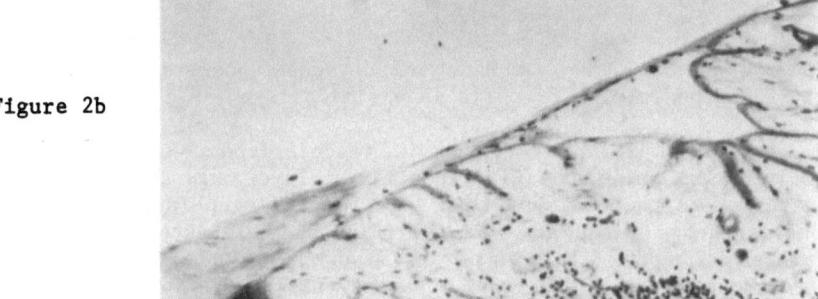

FIGURE 2. a) Photomicrograph of epiretinal glial cells causing folding in internal limiting lamina. Note partial separation of cells from surface of retina. b) Similar appearance in patient with a posteriorly attached vitreous hyloid face.

This thin cellular membrane can separate from the retina but keeps its attachment to the posterior hyaloid face leaving a thin glial membrane on the posterior vitreous surface (Figures 3a and 3b).

Figure 3a

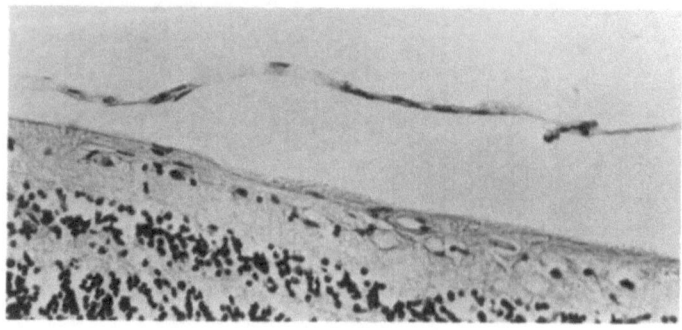

Figure 3b

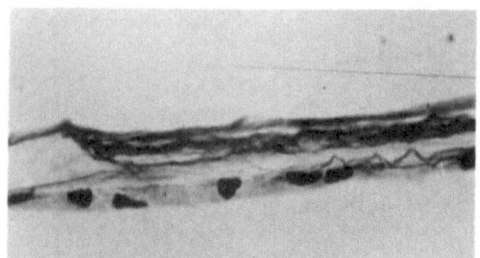

FIGURE 3. a) Fine cellular membrane on detached posterior vitreous surface. b) Higher power view of cells in a similar eye.

A third type of membrane observed is vascularized. This type of membrane has a thin cellular (GFAP positive) layer at the vitreous surface. Posterior to the cells, a thin layer of collagen is present and within the collagenous tissue are vessels (Figure 4). Posterior to the vessels is more collagen. This type of membrane may be attached or separated from the retinal surface. When vessels are present, the preretinal membranes are associated with much greater collagen formation than are the glial avascular membranes. The glial layer at the vitreous border of the membrane remains thin despite increasing vascularity and overall thickness of the membranes (Figure 5).

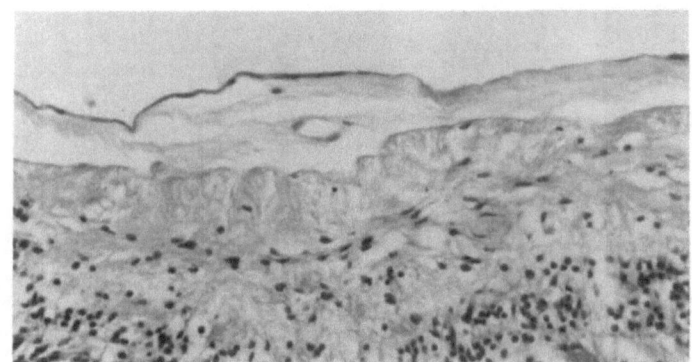

Figure 4

FIGURE 4 Glio-vascular collagenous membrane in patient with proliferative diabetic retinopathy. Vessels are within collagenous matrix. Note thin layer of GFAP positive cells at inner vitreous surface.

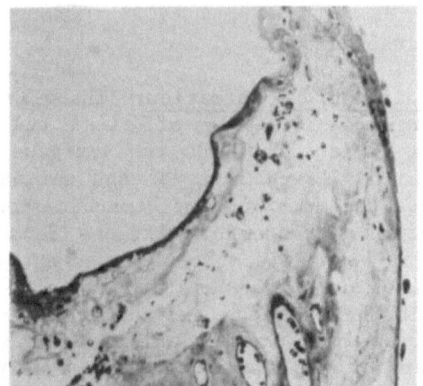

Figure 5

FIGURE 5. Photomicrograph of plastic embedded section demonstrating thickened glio-vascular collagenous membrane and thin layer of glial cells at surface.

This gliovascular-collagenous membrane may be attached or separated from the retinal surface and appears clinically as the typical fibrovascular proliferation along the posterior vitreous surface.

We examined one surgically removed membrane containing only vessels without the glial layer at the surface, however the vitreous surface was not identified.

DISCUSSION

Based on the types of membranes identified in eyes and tissues examined we can propose a mechanism of membrane formation and posterior vitreous separation in proliferative diabetic retinopathy.

Stage I--Intraretinal Gliosis: In this stage glial cells divide and migrate out of the retina onto the retinal surface. The stimulus for this migration may be chronic breakdown of blood retinal barrier and/or growth factors produced from injured retina (Figure 6).

Stage I

**Intraretinal glial
hypercellularity**

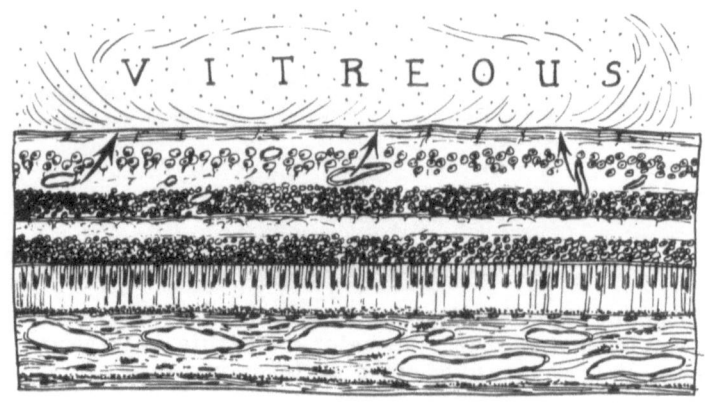

FIGURE 6. Stage I - Intraretinal gliosis.

       Stage II--Epiretinal Glial Membrane Formation: The glia migrate onto the retinal surface and form a thin layer of glial cells which are polarized with the microvilli directed towards the vitreous and basement membrane towards the underlying collagenous layer and retina (Figure 7). At this or any subsequent stage the membrane may separate from the retinal surface giving the appearance of a posterior vitreous detachment (PVD). This could explain why PVD's in young diabetic patients are visible (i.e. because they are avascular-cellular collagenous membranes). We postulate that the glial cells contract the vitreous gel as well as tangentially forcing the membrane to separate from the retinal surface. This process can account for multiple layers of membranes not infrequently seen during vitreous surgery for proliferative diabetic retinopathy. This process is thought to occur in other processes with recurrent membranes.[11]

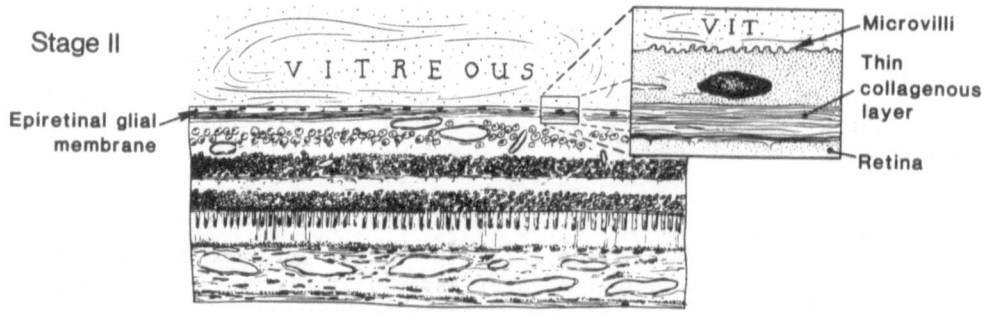

FIGURE 7. Stage II - Thin epiretinal glial membrane.

Stage III: In Stage III (Figure 8) vessels migrate beneath the glial layer and cause a great increase in collagen production. This separates from the retinal surface and produces the typical elevated "fibrovascular" membrane along the posterior hyaloid surface (Stage IV, Figure 9).

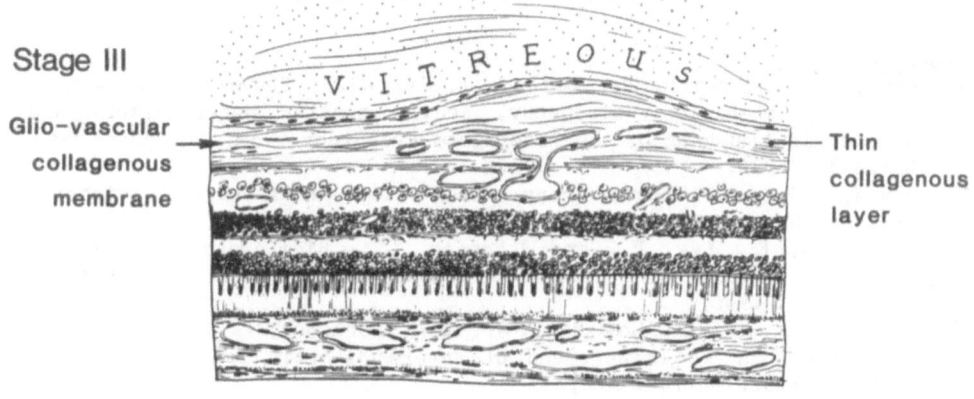

FIGURE 8. Stage III – Attached glio-vascular collagenous membrane.

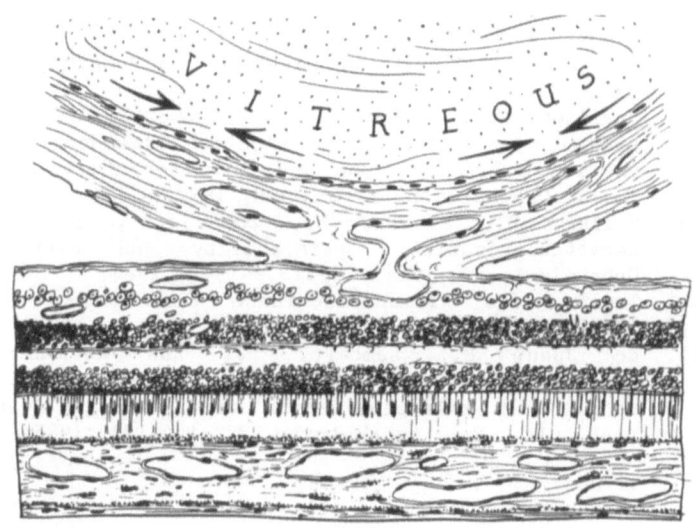

FIGURE 9. Stage IV – Elevated glio-vascular collagenous membrane.

Further cellular proliferation, collagen production and vitreous gel contraction is followed by increased traction on the retina and eventual detachment.

An argument against this hypothesis is in early stages of clinically developing neovascularization in diabetic retinopathy one sees only the vessels. However, it must be realized that the vessels are not seen but simply the blood within the vessel. Vessels do not grow without a surrounding extracellular matrix. The role of the associated tissues in the expression neovascularization should be considered in understanding the process of membrane development in proliferative diabetic retinopathy.

REFERENCES

1. Kini, M., Heibowitz, H., Colton, T., et al.: Prevalence of senile cataract, diabetic retinopathy, senile macular degeneration, and open angle glaucoma in the Framingham Eye Study. Am. J. Ophthalmol. 85:28-34, 1976.
2. Davis, M.: Vitreous contraction in proliferative diabetic retinopathy. Arch. Ophthalmol. 74:741-751, 1965.
3. Tolentino, F., Lee, P., and Schepens, C.: Biomicroscopic study of vitreous cavity in diabetic retinopathy. Arch. Ophthalmol. 75:238-246, 1966.
4. Mandelcorn, M., Blankenship, G., and Machemer, R.: Pars plana vitrectomy for the management of severe diabetic retinopathy. Am. J. Ophthalmol. 81:561-570, 1976.
5. Michels, R.: Vitrectomy for complications of diabetic retinopathy. Arch. Ophthalmol. 96:237-246, 1978.
6. Ashton, W.: Studies of the retinal capillaries in relation to diabetic and other retinopathies. Brit. J. Ophthalmol. 47:521-538, 1963.
7. Kohner, E.M. and Henkind, P.: Correlation of fluorescein angiogram and retinal digest in diabetic retinopathy. Am. J. Ophthalmol. 69:403-411, 1970.
8. Hamilton, C.W., Chandler, D., Klintworth, G.K., and Machemer, R.: A transmission and scanning electron microscopic study of surgically excised preretinal membrane proliferations in diabetes mellitus. Am. J. Ophthalmol. 94:473-488, 1982.
9. Miller, H., Miller, B., Zonis, S., and Nir, I.: Diabetic neovascularization: permeability and ultrastructure. Invest. Ophthalmol. Vis. Sci. 25:1338-1342, 1984.
10. Taylor, C.: Immunoperoxidase techniques. Arch. Pathol. Lab. 102:113-121, 1978.
11. de Juan, E., Lambert, H., and Machemer, R.: Recurrent proliferations in macular pucker, diabetic retinopathy, and retrolental fibroplasia-like disease after vitrectomy. Graefe's Arch. Clin. Exp. Ophthalmol. 223:174-183, 1985.

EARLY PHOTOCOAGULATION OF FOCAL DIABETIC MACULAR EDEMA

M. WEISER M.D., B. CATHELINEAU M.D., P. BELLIO M.D., F. ROUSSELIE M.D.

Department of ophthalmology
Groupe Hospitalier PITIE-SALPETRIERE (Pr.F.ROUSSELIE)
47 - 83, Boulevard de l'Hôpital

75651 PARIS Cédex 13   FRANCE

A - INTRODUCTION

Several studies suggest that argon laser photocoagulation may be helpful in the management of diabetic macular edema, stabilizing visual acuity rather than restoring reduced acuity.

In these studies, treated eyes usually had a low initial visual acuity, and it seemed interesting to try and appreciate photocoagulation's efficiency upon eyes with high initial visual acuity.

Therefore we present a retrospective study of 69 eyes with focal diabetic macular edema, treated by argon laser photocoagulation, whatever the level of initial visual acuity may be.

B - PATIENTS AND METHODS

a) Patients

The study group consisted of 69 eyes in 40 patients ranged in age from 24 to 68 years (mean age = 53 years).
There were 20 women and 20 men.
17 patients had type I diabetes, and 23 patients had type II diabetes.
Mean duration of diabetes was 10 years.

b) Inclusion and exclusion criteria

The only criteria for patient's selection was focal, edematous, diabetic maculopathy defined by presence in the macular area of focal fluorescein leakage from specific capillary lesions such as microaneurysms and dilated capillary segments.

In every eye, ocular media were clear enough to allow photocoagulation and evaluation of its efficiency.

The following data were collected from the clinical records but were not criteria for patient's selection or exclusion :

  . type of diabetes
  . Initial visual acuity
  . Hard exudate rings
  . Cystoid changes.

Were excluded of this study eyes with :

. Macular ischemia
. And with diffuse macular edema, defined by enhanced visibility of the retinal capillary bed and diffuse leakage from extensive areas of the posterior retinal capillary bed.

c) Follow-up

Patients routinely had follow-up visits at one, six months and then every six months.

Fluorescein angiography was repeated at every visit but central visual field documentation could not be available for every eye.

Follow-up always exceeded six months after photocoagulation.

d) Photocoagulation technique

Photocoagulation consisted of focal treatment of the leaky microaneurysms and dilated capillary segments located in the macular area except in the foveal avascular zone.

Photocoagulation was decided after at least six months of follow-up, because of non-regression or aggravation of the pre-defined focal edematous maculopathy, in spite of optimal diabetic control.

Blue-green Argon laser was used. Mild to moderate contiguous burns, spot sizes 100 to 200 microns in diameter, and exposure times 0.05 to 0.10 seconds were placed on the leaky capillary segments.

Treatment of focal macular edema was whenever necessary associated with focal treatment of the leaky capillary segments located in the center of hard exudate rings, and with destruction of peripheral non-perfusion areas in case of ischemic or proliferative retinopathy.

The procedure was performed in one or several sessions, according to the extent of the lesions, and could lead if necessary to foveal avascular zone complete surrounding.

C - RESULTS

a) Presumed duration of maculopathy prior to photocoagulation

The presumed duration of focal macular edema prior to photocoagulation was :

. 6 months to 1 year in 20 patients (50%) ;
. 1 to 2 years in 12 patients (30%) ;
. and more than 2 years in 8 patients (20%).

b) Follow-up

Follow-up ranged from 6 months to 5 years, with a mean of 16 months.

c) Angiographic improvement

Angiographic improvement was defined by resolution of retinal vascular leakage in the macular area.

Resolution of macular edema was achieved in 68 (98.5 %) of the treated eyes :

. totally in 53 eyes (76.8 %)
. partially in 15 eyes (21.7 %)

One eye (1.5 %) did not show any angiographic improvement, but initially had serous retinal detachment in the macular area.

d) Best corrected visual acuity (FIG. 1)

Initial visual acuity was high : 40 eyes (58 %) had 20/30 or better and 52 eyes (75.4 %) had 20/40 or better.

Mean initial visual acuity was close to 20/30.

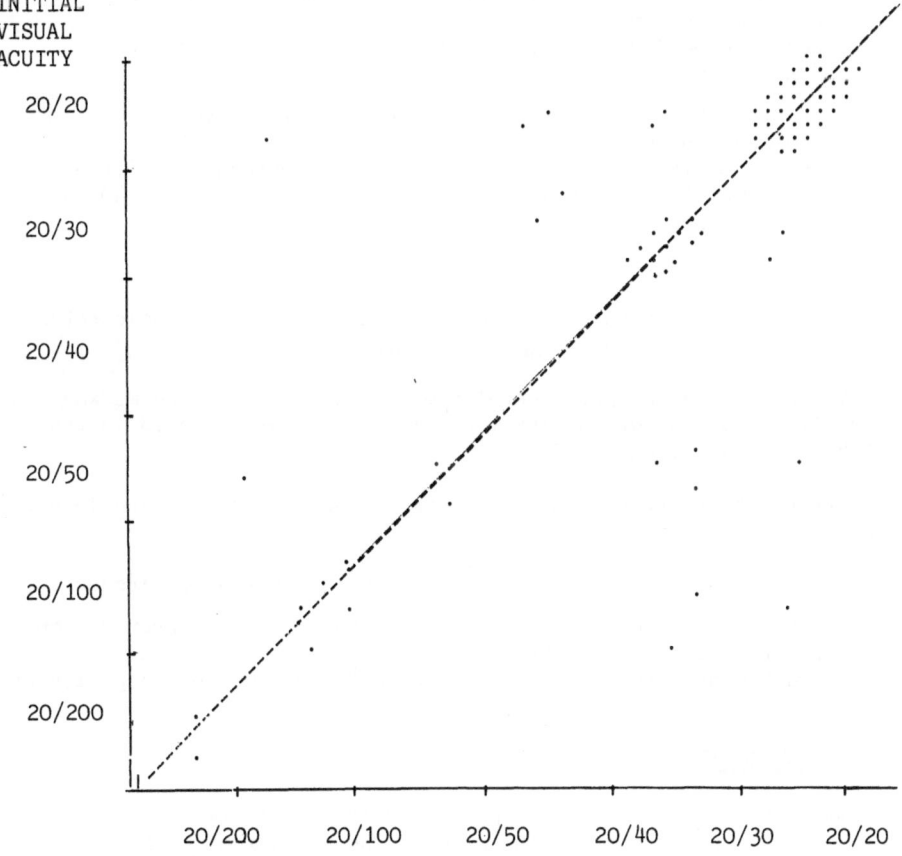

FIG.1 : Best corrected
Visual acuity before and after argon laser photocogulation

After photocoagulation :

. 9 eyes improved (13 %)
. 52 eyes unchanged (75.4 %)
. 8 eyes deteriorated (11.6 %)

Alltogether 88.4 % of the eyes maintained or improved, and mean final visual acuity stayed close to 20/30.

If we consider the 8 eyes that deteriorated, the presumed reason for visual acuity decrease was :

. in 3 eyes : remaining cystoid changes in the center of foveal
                avascular zone
. in 2 eyes : incomplete angiographic resolution
. in 1 eye : misplaced laser burn
. in 2 eyes : unprecised reason

10 eyes had initial visual acuity of 20/100 or lower :

. all 10 eyes had cystoid changes in the macular area and half
  of them had hard exudates
. complete angiographic resolution was achieved in 7 eyes
. visual acuity

  * deteriorated after photocoagulation in 1 eye
  * unchanged in 4 eyes
  * and improved in 5 eyes, sometimes spectacularly (from
    20/150 to 20/30 in one eye and from 20/100 to 20/40 in
    another one).

e) Hard exudates

The 30 eyes with hard exudate rings in the posterior pole before treatment were compared to the remaining 39 eyes.

In these 30 eyes, photocoagulation of focal macular edema was associated with treatment of the leaky capillary segments located in the center of hard exudate rings.

After treatment, resolution of hard exudates was achieved in all eyes.

Visual acuity evolution was not similar in the two groups :

. among the group with hard exudates, only 2 eyes improved compared to 7 eyes in the group without.
. and 6 eyes deteriorated compared to 2 eyes in the group without
  hard exudates.

D - DISCUSSION

Many controlled trials of photocoagulation treatment for macular edema have already been reported. In spite of the variety of pathologic processes that can affect the macula in diabetic maculopathy, the pooled data from these studies, suggest that photocoagulation of macular edema may be a helpful technique.

Our study exclusively concerns focal macular edema. Photocoagulation was performed whatever initial visual acuity might be, because we did not want to let chronic macular edema affect photoreceptors and visual acuity.

This may explain our high initial and final visual acuities compared to other trials, even if photocoagulation rather stabilized than restored visual acuity as previously reported.

Three factors appear to be of major importance upon visual prognosis :

. initial visual acuity
. hard exudates which seems to be a poor prognostic sign
. post-therapeutic angiographic resolution of retinal vascular leakage.

These results lead us to treat such cases of focal diabetic macular edema at an early stage, in order to prevent visual acuity decrease, even if we noticed several spectacular improvements among the ten eyes with a low initial visual acuity.

E - CONCLUSION

Much more needs to be learnt about the physiopathologic mechanisms producing focal macular edema, before therapy can be developed in a rational fashion.

Any-how early treatment of focal retinal vascular leaks combined with optimal diabetic control seems helpful in the management of focal diabetic macular edema, in order to preserve a high level of visual acuity.

Further randomized trials with long follow-up periods will be necessary to demonstrate what only is a clinical impression.

F - REFERENCES

1 - Blankenship GW. Diabetic macular edema and argon laser photocoagulation : a prospective randomized study. Ophthalmology 1979 ; 86 : 69 - 78.

2 - Bresnick GH. Diabetic macular edema. Ophthalmology 1983 ; 93 : 989 - 97

3 - Bresnick GH. Diabetic maculopathy ; a critical review highlighting diffus macular edema. Ophthalmology 1983 ; 90 : 1301 - 17.

4 - Diabetic Retinopathy Study Research Group. Photocoagulation treatment of diabetic retinopathy ; clinical application of diabetic retinopathy study (DRS) findings, DRS report number 8. Ophthalmology 1981 ; 88 : 583 - 600.

5 - Early Treatment Diabetic Retinopathy Study Research Group. Photocoagul. for diabetic macular edema ; Early Treatment Diabetic Retinopathy Study number 1. Arch Ophthalmol. 1985 ; 103 : 1796 - 806.

6 - Ferris FL III, Patz A. Macular edema. A complication of diabetic retinopathy. Surv. Ophthalmol 1984 ; 28 : 452 - 61.

7 - Klein R, Klein BEK, Moss SE, et al. The Wisconsin Epidemiologic Study Of Diabetic Retinopathy. IV. Diabetic macular edema. Ophthalmology 1984 ; 91 : 1464 - 74 .

8 - Klein R, Klein BEK, Moss SE. Visual impairment in diabetes. Ophthalmology 1984 ; 91 : 1 - 8.

9 - Patz A. Schatz H, Berkow JW, et al. Macular edema - an overlooked complication of diabetic retinopathy. Trans Am Acad Ophthalmol Otolaryngol 1973 ; 77 : OP 34 - 42.

10 - Whitelocke RAF, Kearns M, Black RK, Hamilton AM. The diabetic maculopathies. Trans Ophthalmol Soc UK 1979 ; 99 : 314 - 20.

PHOTOCOAGULATION FOR DIABETIC MACULAR EDEMA: RESULTS OF THE EARLY TREATMENT
DIABETIC RETINOPATHY STUDY

R.P. MURPHY, F.L. FERRIS, III, AND THE ETDRS RESEARCH GROUP

From the Wilmer Ophthalmological Institute, The Johns Hopkins Medical
Institutions, Baltimore, Maryland 21205 and The National Eye Institute,
Building 31, Room 6A24, 9000 Rockville Pike, Bethesda, Maryland 20892

Adapted from: Photocoagulation for diabetic macular edema: results of the
Early Treatment Diabetic Retinopathy Study. Contemporary Ophthalmic Forum
4;2:25-31, July-August 1986.

The Early Treatment Diabetic Retinopathy Study (ETDRS) has developed,
tested and proven effective a strategy of photocoagulation that can reduce
the risk of visual loss from diabetic macular edema. The ETDRS is a
randomized clinical trial designed to evaluate photocoagulation and aspirin
treatment in the management of patients with nonproliferative or early
proliferative diabetic retinopathy. A nation-wide, multicentered study
sponsored by the National Eye Institute, the ETDRS continues to follow
patients enrolled in the study to develop information concerning the
following questions about the treatment of diabetic retinopathy:
  1.   When in the course of diabetic retinopathy is it most effective to
initiate photocoagulation therapy?
  2.   Is aspirin treatment effective in altering the course of diabetic
retinopathy?
  3.   Is photocoagulation effective in the treatment of
macular edema?
  To answer these important clinical questions, the twenty-three ETDRS
clinical centers, in collaboration with their administrative and support
facilities (Table 1), recruited and enrolled 3,928 diabetic patients between
1980 and 1985. All patients entering the study had evidence of early
proliferative retinopathy or moderate to severe nonproliferative
retinopathy, and/or diabetic macular edema in each eye. Patients with
"high-risk" proliferative retinopathy (moderate or severe optic nerve
neovascularization or any neovascularization with hemorrhage) were not
entered into the study because immediate photocoagulation has already been
proven beneficial for such patients. (1,2) Patients with visual acuity
worse than 20/200 were also excluded from the study. Written informed
consent was obtained from all patients prior to their entering the study.

STUDY DESIGN
  The complex design and randomization sequence of the ETDRS has been
previously summarized. (3) In December 1985 the ETDRS investigators
published their first report demonstrating that focal photocoagulation for
macular edema was effective.(4) This report was restricted to the subgroup
of eyes which had macular edema and mild to moderate nonproliferative
retinopathy. These eyes initially received either focal photocoagulation
for the macular edema (no panretinal photocoagulation) or no
photocoagulation at all. The published ETDRS results demonstrate that focal
photocoagulation of "clinically significant" diabetic macular edema

substantially reduces the risk of visual loss. Moreover, focal treatment as described by the ETDRS also increases the chance of visual improvement and decreases the frequency of persistent macular edema. During follow-up, the group of eyes assigned to immediate photocoagulation and the group of eyes assigned to deferral of photocoagulation showed some loss of visual field and color vision as measured in the study. However, there were no clinically or statistically significant differences in these parameters of visual function between the two groups.

TABLE 1.   ETDRS Clinical Centers

---

1.   The Johns Hopkins Hospital, Baltimore, MD
2.   Joslin Clinic, Boston, MA
3.   University of Wisconsin, Madison, WI
4.   University of Miami, Miami, FL
5.   University of Minnesota, Minneapolis, MN
6.   University of Southern California, Los Angeles, CA
7.   Good Samaritan Hospital and Medical Center, Portland, OR
8.   University of Illinois at the Medical Center, Chicago, IL
9.   UCLA Center for Health Sciences, Los Angeles, CA
10. Albany Medical College, Albany, NY
11. Zweng Memorial Retinal Research Foundation, Menlo Park, CA
12. Pacific Medical Center, San Francisco, CA
13. Wills Eye Hospital, Philadelphia, PA
14. Holy Cross Hospital, Salt Lake City, UT
15. University of Puerto Rico, Rio Piedras, PR
16. Wayne State University, Detroit, MI
17. Michigan State University, East Lansing, MI
18. University of Washington, Seattle, WA
19. Medical College of Wisconsin, Milwaukee, WI
20. Eye Research Institute of the Retina Foundation/Retina Assoc. Boston, MA
21. Ingalls Memorial Hospital, Harvey, IL
22. Hermann Eye Center, University of Texas, Houston, TX
23. Louisiana State University Eye Center, New Orleans, LA

National Eye Institute, Bethesda, MD

Coordinating Center
     Maryland Medical Research Institute, Baltimore, MD

Fundus Photograph Reading Center
     University of Wisconsin, Madison, WI

Central Laboratory
     Centers for Disease Control, Atlanta, GA

ECG Coding Center
     University of Minnesota, Minneapolis, MN

Drug Distribution Center
     USPHS, Perry Point, MD

ETDRS Report #1 published data on 2244 eyes that had macular edema and mild to moderate diabetic retinopathy. Eyes with "mild" retinopathy had no signs of ischemia (no soft exudates, intraretinal microvascular abnormalities or venous beading) and had no more than moderate intraretinal hemorrhages or microaneurysms. Eyes with "moderate" retinopathy had one or more of the ischemic changes, but not to a severe degree, and were free of neovascularization. At the completion of randomization 754 of these eyes had been assigned to focal argon laser photocoagulation, while 1,490 of these eyes were randomly assigned to deferral of any photocoagulation. Treatment in the former randomization group was limited to direct photocoagulation of macular edema unless severe nonproliferative or proliferative retinopathy developed during follow-up, at which time panretinal photocoagulation was initiated. Photocoagulation in the eyes assigned to deferral of photocoagulation was performed only if "high-risk proliferative retinopathy" developed during follow-up. All comparisons in the first published report were made between these two groups. A more detailed randomization scheme for these eyes is summarized in Figure 1.

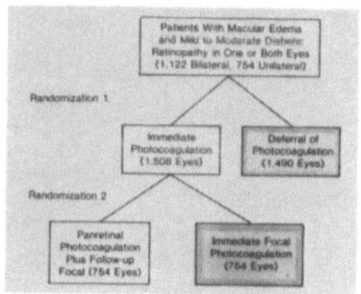

FIGURE 1. ETDRS treatment assignment schedule for patients with macular edema and mild to moderate diabetic retinpathy in one or both eyes.(4)

TREATMENT BENEFIT FOR MACULAR EDEMA

Focal photocoagulation in the study eyes with macular edema and mild to moderate nonproliferative diabetic retinopathy was found to reduce the risk of visual loss (defined as a doubling of the visual angle and equivalent to a loss of 3 lines on the ETDRS visual acuity chart(5) by about 50% (Figure 2). When all eyes with macular edema are considered, 16% of untreated eyes develop this much visual loss in two years, and 24% do so in three years. Visual loss also developed in treated eyes, but in a smaller percentage (7% in two years and 12% in three years). A treatment effect was present regardless of initial visual acuity and regardless of retinopathy severity at entry. The principal benefit of treatment was in reducing the risk of further decrease in visual acuity. Treated eyes were also more likely to have an improvement in visual acuity, but this improvement was rarely more than one or two lines on the visual acuity chart.

The ETDRS also identified a subgroup of eyes with macular edema at higher risk for the development of visual loss - those with "clinically significant" macular edema. The beneficial treatment effect for macular edema is stronger in these eyes. (Fig. 3, top) In untreated eyes with clinically significant macular edema, the risk of a three line loss of acuity was 21% in two years and 30% in three years. The risk of this degree of visual loss was reduced by over 50% with treatment: 8% in two years and 13% in three years.

In contrast, eyes with macular edema which was not "clinically significant" at the time of entry into the study had much lower rates of visual loss, with or without treatment (Fig 3, bottom). After two years of follow-up in these eyes with mild macular edema, there was no clinically or statistically significant difference in the rates of visual loss between the treated and untreated groups. With mild macular edema, eyes randomized to "treatment" received additional photocoagulation if clinically significant macular edema developed; untreated eyes received no treatment, even if macular edema worsened. Clinically significant macular edema did subsequently develop in both "treatment" and "deferred treatment" groups, and appropriate eyes in the "treatment" group did receive focal photocoagulation. The trend for a treatment effect in the latter group of eyes after two years is most likely attributable to the proven beneficial effect of focal photocoagulation for the eyes with clinically significant macular edema.

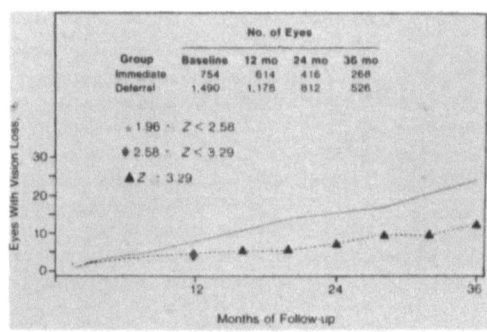

FIGURE 2. Comparison of percentage of treated and untreated eyes with macular edema experiencing visual loss, demonstrating eyes which received immediate focal photocoagulation were half as likely to lose visual acuity as those assigned to deferral of treatment (12% vs 24%). These differences are statistically significant. Broken line indicates treated eyes, solid line indicates untreated eyes. (4) The effects of focal photocoagulation for macular edema were assessed using the 2-sample test of proportions with unequal variances. For monitoring purposes, an observed z value of between +/-1.96 and +/- 2.57 was considered suggestive of a treatment difference, and an observed z value of +/-2.58 or greater (corresponding to a 0.01 level for a single test of significance) was considered a statistically significant difference. Observed z values of +/- 3.29 or greater corresponding to a .001 significance level were also recorded.

Based on these data, the ETDRS investigators recommended that focal photocoagulation be considered (see CLINICAL APPLICATIONS) for all patients with "clinically significant" macular edema. They limited their recommendation to this group because of the clear beneficial treatment effect in this group and a much smaller effect in eyes with macular edema less severe than this.

CLINICALLY SIGNIFICANT MACULAR EDEMA

Because eyes satisfying this definition benefit most from treatment, it is important to know how "clinically significant" macular edema was defined in the ETDRS. The term "clinically significant" macular edema referred

specifically to eyes in which edema was already involving the fovea and
decreasing vision or was threatening vision, even if visual acuity was not
yet reduced. The determination was made by stereo slit lamp examination of
the eye with a contact lens and was confirmed by stereo fundus photographs.
In many of the eyes the diagnosis of retinal thickening could not be made
with non-stereoscopic examinations (as with direct ophthalmoscopy only), and
required stereo slit lamp biomicroscopy. Neither visual acuity nor
fluorescein angiography were used to determine which eyes had "clinically
significant" macular edema although all angiograms were later graded at the
ETDRS Reading Center. Eyes with "clinically significant" macular edema in
the ETDRS had any of the following characteristics:

1. thickening of the retina at or within 500 microns from the center
of the macula,

2. hard exudates at or within 500 microns from the center of the
macula, if associated with thickening of adjacent retina (but not residual
hard exudates remaining after disappearance of retinal thickening),

3. a zone or zones of retinal thickening 1 disc area or larger in
size, any part of which is within 1 disc diameter of the center of the
macula.

For macular edema to be considered as "clinically significant," at
least one of the characteristics listed above had to be present. The
features of clinically significant macular edema are shown in Table 2 and
Figures 4a through 4d.

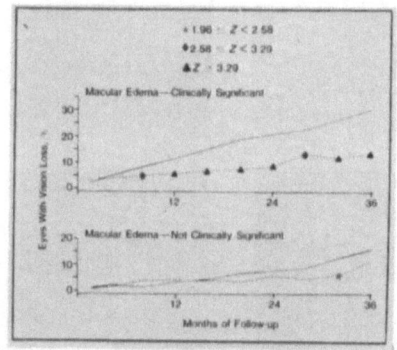

FIGURE 3 TOP. Comparison of percentage of treated and untreated eyes with
"clinically significant" macular edema experiencing visual loss,
demonstrating 13% of treated eyes lost visual acuity while 30% of untreated
eyes lost visual acuity. BOTTOM. Comparison of percentage of treated and
untreated eyes with "non-clinically significant" macular edema experiencing
visual acuity loss, demonstrating a trend toward beneficial treatment
effect. Broken line indicates treated eyes, solid line indicates untreated
eyes. (4)

ETDRS TREATMENT PROTOCOL FOR MACULAR EDEMA

Macular edema in ETDRS patients could be broadly classified into two
common patterns based on the type of leakage found on the fluorescein
angiogram. Localized edema was associated with discrete leakage from
retinal capillaries or microaneurysms with or without the presence of
circinate lipid rings. Localized edema was by far the most common type of
leakage pattern in this group of eyes with mild to moderate nonproliferative
retinopathy. In contrast, diffuse edema was associated with diffuse leakage
from retinal capillaries or diffuse leakage associated with zones of retinal

capillary nonperfusion. Diffuse edema was a less common pattern of leakage in these eyes and was not usually associated with lipid rings.

TABLE 2. Clinically significant macular edema
          (Any of the following characteristics)

Thickening of the retina at or within 500 microns of the center of the macula

Hard exudates at or within 500 microns of the center of the macula, if associated with thickening of adjacent retina (not residual hard exudates remaining after disappearance of retinal thickening)

A zone or zones of retinal thickening 1 disc area or larger, any part of which is within 1 disc diameter of the center of the macula. (4)

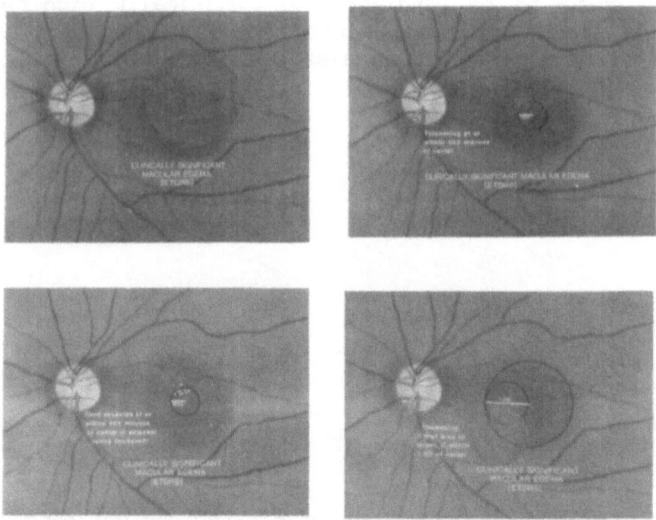

Figure 4. Artist's illustration of "clinically significant" macular edema a) Retinal thickening represented by zone of wavy lines (arrow). The macular edema is "clinically significant" because there is thickening involving the center (small arrow). b) macular edema within 500 microns of center of fovea. c) hard exudates at or within 500 microns of center associated with thickening of adjacent retina. d) zone of retinal thickening 1 DD or larger, any part of which is within 1 DD of center of macula.

There were two types of "treatable lesions" associated with macular edema in the ETDRS. First were focal "leaks" in the retinal vasculature at least 500 microns from the center of the macula which were identified on fluorescein angiography and were thought to be causing retinal thickening. Second were areas of diffuse leakage and avascular zones (with the exception of the normal foveal avascular zone) which were associated with retinal thickening and had not had previous treatment. Additionally, if visual acuity was 20/40 or worse, focal leaks 300 to 500 microns from the center were treated. Lesions this close to the fovea were not treated if the treating ophthalmologist believed that such treatment was likely to destroy the remaining perifoveal capillary network (Table 3).

The treatment strategy for macular edema in the ETDRS consisted of focal (direct) photocoagulation treatment of discrete "treatable lesions" whenever possible. When the leakage was diffuse or associated with avascular zones, a grid treatment was used. Although the ETDRS treatment strategy utilizes a combination of focal and grid regimens, the majority of treatment in the ETDRS was focal, not grid, treatment. A fluorescein angiogram was obtained to identify the lesions to be treated. "Treatable lesions" between 500 microns and two disc diameters (DD) from the center of the macula were considered for treatment. Lesions further than two DD from the center were also considered for treatment if they were thought to be contributing to the macular edema.

TABLE 3. "Treatable lesions" in ETDRS associated with macular edema

---

I.   Focal leaks $\geq$ 500 microns from the center of the macula thought to be causing retinal thickening and/or hard exudates

II. Focal leaks 300 to 500 microns from the center of the macula thought to be causing retinal thickening or hard exudates if visual acuity is 20/40 or less and the treating ophthalmologist believes that such treatment is not likely to destroy the remaining perifoveal capillary network

III. Areas of diffuse leakage not previously treated

IV. Avascular zones (except the normal avascular zone in the fovea) not previously treated

---

In the early part of the study, argon blue-green photocoagulation was used for treatment. However, as argon green photocoagulation became available, it was used by most of the ETDRS ophthalmologists for the treatment of macular edema, because absorption of the blue wavelengths by the xanthophyll in the mid-retina of the central macula made the intensity of the retinal burns difficult to predict.

FOCAL TREATMENT

Discrete lesions between 500 microns and 2DD from the center of the macula were treated with focal treatment as described. Most lesions were treated with 50 micron laser burns, although larger sized burns were allowed. Duration of the applications was 0.1 or 0.05 seconds with sufficient power to coagulate the microaneurysm without excessive "spread" at the level of the retinal pigment epithelium. An attempt was made to coagulate all microaneurysms greater than 40 microns in diameter using 50 micron laser burns (when coagulated the microaneurysm would generally turn either dark or white). Repeated laser burns were usually necessary to change the color of the microaneurysm. Because of the necessity for repeated 50 micron burns, some investigators preferred to use an initial treatment with a mild 100 micron burn to whiten the retinal pigment epithelium under the microaneurysm before switching to the 50 micron spot size and higher power density. Microaneurysm clumps could be treated with multiple 50 micron burns or with 200 to 500 micron applications in an attempt to coagulate the microaneurysms. Confluent treatment was avoided. The strategy for treatment of focal leaks is summarized in Table 4.

GRID TREATMENT

Diffuse leaks and nonperfused capillary zones associated with macular edema were treated with a light scatter pattern of photocoagulation only after focal leaks had been treated as described. Grid treatment for non-focal leaks in the ETDRS consisted of the application of light or mild intensity burns in these areas. The burn size was not to exceed 200 microns. In edematous retina this often required using the 100 or 50 micron spot size. With intense leakage the applications were spaced as closely as one burn width apart. Applications were more widely spaced when leakage was less severe. When indicated, grid treatment was placed as far as two DD from the center of the fovea. When indicated, grid treatment was also placed in the papillo-macular bundle. Grid treatment was never placed closer than 500 microns from the center of the fovea or from the disc margin. ETDRS grid treatment for diffuse leaks and avascular zones is summarized in Table 5.

TABLE 4. ETDRS treatment of focal leaks for macular edema

I.   Laser spot size: 50-micron spot size (protocol allows larger burns but specifies 50-micron spot size within 500 microns of the center)

II. Duration of burn: limit exposure to 0.1 second (within 500 microns of the center, exposure time may be limited to 0.05 second)

III. Power: Vary to obtain an endpoint of whitening around the microaneurysm or leakage site without excessive spreading of the burn

   A.   aneuryms $\geq$ 40 microns: attempt to obtain darkening/whitening of the lesion itself using 50-micron spot size (several applications are usually necessary, sometimes using additional power – survey the macular area at conclusion of the session to make sure this endpoint has been reached and maintained)

   B.   clumps of aneurysms: treat with larger spot sizes (200-500 microns), followed by treatment of the individual microaneurysms with 50-micron spot size to obtain the endpoint

   C.   avoid treatment of nerve fiber layer retinal hemorrhages (although hemorrhages obscuring leaks or aneurysms may be treated)

Patients in the ETDRS were reevaluated every four months. If "clinically significant" macular edema persisted after previous treatment, additional treatment for macular edema was applied according to the same protocol. In more severe cases, two to four additional treatment episodes at intervals of four months were not uncommon. The clinical findings and fluorescein angiogram of an eye with clinically significant macular edema are shown in Figures 5a-5c. The post-treatment appearance of this eye is shown in Figure 5d.

CLINICAL APPLICATIONS

The results of the ETDRS have provided us with the basic information we need to decide whether to treat a patient with diabetic macular edema. We now know that photocoagulation as done in the ETDRS for "clinically significant" macular edema is better than no treatment. We know that nearly one third of eyes with "clinically significant" macular edema and mild to moderate diabetic retinopathy will lose vision equal to or greater than a doubling of their initial visual angle. We know that if treated, we would expect only 13% of these eyes to lose this much vision. Eyes with "clinically significant" macular edema are the most likely to benefit from photocoagulation. To determine whether "clinically significant" macular edema is present it is often necessary to use slit-lamp biomicroscopy with a contact lens.

TABLE 5. ETDRS treatment of diffuse leaks and avascular zones in macular edema

---

I. Laser spot size: use 50-micron spot size (protocol allows 100- or 200-micron spot size, but in no case should spread of burn exceed 200 microns)

II. Power: light to moderate intensity burns

III. Spacing of grid: space burns one burn-width apart, but deviate from even spacing to more completely cover areas of intense leakage or dropout, and to spare as much retina as possible elsewhere

IV. Extent of grid: place grid treatment as far as two DD from the center of the macula

   A. avoid confluent lesions and treatment within 500 microns of the disc margin

   B. do not apply grid treatment within 500 microns of the center of the macula

---

Should all eyes with "clinically significant" macular edema be treated as soon as this edema is noted? Unfortunately, the ETDRS was not designed to determine the best time to apply photocoagulation for diabetic macular edema. There are no study data on a treatment plan which identifies patients with "clinically significant" macular edema, carefully follows them and initiates photocoagulation only if macular edema worsens or vision decreases. The precise timing of initiation of photocoagulation, especially in eyes with better visual acuity, must be made using clinical judgment. Deferral of photocoagulation may be an attractive alternative in eyes with excellent visual acuity because it is reasonable to assume that the short term risks of treatment may be more important for such eyes than for eyes which have already experienced visual loss. However, in the ETDRS, treatment tended to stabilize visual acuity at the pretreatment level, and rarely was there a large improvement in visual acuity after treatment. This suggests that it may be undesirable to wait for visual acuity to decrease very much before initiating treatment.

Two examples help point out the need for clinical judgment in determining when to photocoagulate for macular edema. The potential benefits of immediate treatment probably outweigh the risks for the patient with 20/20 visual acuity, who has lipid encroaching on the fovea and leaking microaneurysms more than 750 microns from the center of the fovea. However, deferral may be the better choice for a patient with excellent visual acuity and leaks only at the edge of the foveal avascular zone. If treatment is deferred in eyes with good vision and clinically significant macular edema, the results of the ETDRS suggest that these patients should have frequent follow-up. If visual acuity decreases, or if macular edema worsens, focal photocoagulation treatment should be initiated.

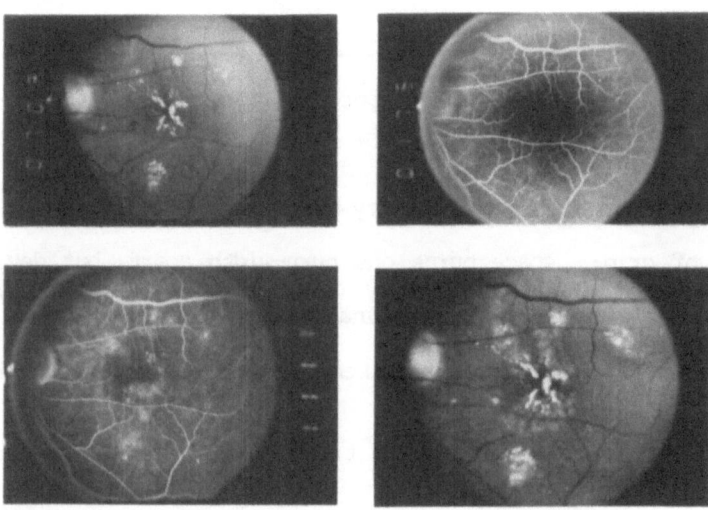

FIGURE 5. a) "Clinically significant" macular edema showing thickening and hard exudates in center of retina. b) Early frame of fluorescein angiogram revealing numerous micro-aneurysms which are contributing to macular edema. c) Late frame of angiogram documenting leakage from micro-aneurysms. d) Immedate post-treatment photograph showing that sites of leakage have been photocoagulated with 50 micron burns.

SUMMARY

The ETDRS has shown that focal photocoagulation can reduce the risk of further visual loss in diabetics with clinically significant macular edema. Diabetic patients should be examined for the presence of this visually disabling complication and treatment should be considered for eyes at risk. Photocoagulation is not the "cure" for diabetes or for diabetic macular edema, but when used judiciously, can further reduce the visual loss caused by this common disease.

REFERENCES

1. Diabetic Retinopathy Study Research Group: Report No. 3: Four risk factors for severe visual loss in diabetic retinopathy. Arch Ophthalmol 97:654-55, 1979.
2. Diabetic Retinopathy Study Research Group: Preliminary report on effects of photocoagulation therapy. Am J Ophthamol 81:383-96, 1976.
3. Murphy RP, Ferris FL: The current status of the Early Treatment Diabetic Retinopathy Study. Ophthalmic Forum 2:149-52, 1984.
4. Early Treatment Diabetic Retinopathy Study Research Group: Early Treatment Diabetic Retinopathy Study: Report No. 1: Photocoagulation for diabetic macular edema. Arch Ophthalmol 103:1796-1806, 1985.
5. Ferris FL, Kassoff A, Bresnick GH, et al: New visual acuity charts for clinical research. Am J Ophthalmol 94:91-6, 1982.

JUXTA-FOVEAL GRID TREATMENT WITH GREEN MONOCHROMATIC ARGON AND WITH RED KRYPTON LASERS FOR DIABETIC MACULAR EDEMA

I. Rosenblatt, MD, Y. Yassur, MD, L. Shani, MD,
T. Lifshchits, MD, D. Uchenic, MD.

Soroka Medical Center and the Faculty of Health Sciences,
Ben-Gurion University of the Negev, Beer-Sheba, and
"Maccabi" Laser Institute, Tel-Aviv, Israel

When diabetic macular edema (DME) affects vision it is due to its being a foveal disease, and any decline of central visual function is a result of the proximity of the edema to the fovea and the duration it is there (1,2). This was the rationale to carry out our present study, because it seemed that it might be reasonable to apply laser treatment as close to the fovea as possible.

Some of the controversy concerning DME laser treatment involves issues such as proximity to the fovea, wavelength and timing of treatment (3-10).

This work included few phases; First, about seven years ago, we limited any treatment with blue-green argon laser to a distance of at least 1 disc diameter from the center of the fovea, due to the absorption characteristics of various tissues and elements of the macula. Within the area of the macula, any treatment, grid or focal, was performed only with mild intensity red krypton laser, because of the special transmission and absorption characteristics of the red light, which is not absorbed by the macular xanthophyl and by hemoglobin and is highly absorbed by the pigment epithel and choroidal melanocytes. A study done by us using that mode of treatment included 112 eyes, which were followed up to 36 months, and compared the results of treatment with blue-green argon alone to the results of treatment with blue-green argon and krypton laser photocoagulation together. (11)

The conclusion of that study was that combined argon and krypton laser treatment was for the long run a little more beneficial for DME than blue-green argon treatment alone.

Being aware of the possible importance of the choroidal blood flow in maintaining good retinal oxygenation, we postulated that monochromatic green argon laser may be theoretically superior to red krypton in treating diabetic foveal edema. We therefore decided to set a study for a DME treatment with that laser.

The idea behind this study was that green argon laser is, like red krypton, not absorbed by the macular xanthophyl, and therefore does not destroy inner retina when mild or moderate intensity applications are used. In addition, as was shown in other studies, the green argon laser has less transmission to the deep layers of the choroid, and therefore it destroys mainly outer retinal layers, RPE and choriocapillaris, and preserves the deeper choriodal vasculature, which later may serve as an oxygen, or other metabolites pool, for the remaining post-photocoagulation thinned retina.

SUBJECTS AND METHODS

In our present study we treated 96 eyes suffering from BDR and macular edema, all of type II diabetics. All patients had a follow up of at least 12 months, and 47 of them had a follow up of 24 months.

The treatment consisted of monochromatic green argon laser photocoagulation, with applications of 100-200μ in a horse-shoe or grid pattern at the posterior pole up to 1 disc diameter from the fovea, and of 50μ spots up to 150μ from the center of the fovea, sparing the fovea itself. The retina over the papilo-macular bundle was spared as well, unless it was severely edematous.

The juxta-foveal applications were of mild to moderate intensity.

R E S U L T S

The visual acuity results after this treatment are shown in graph 1:

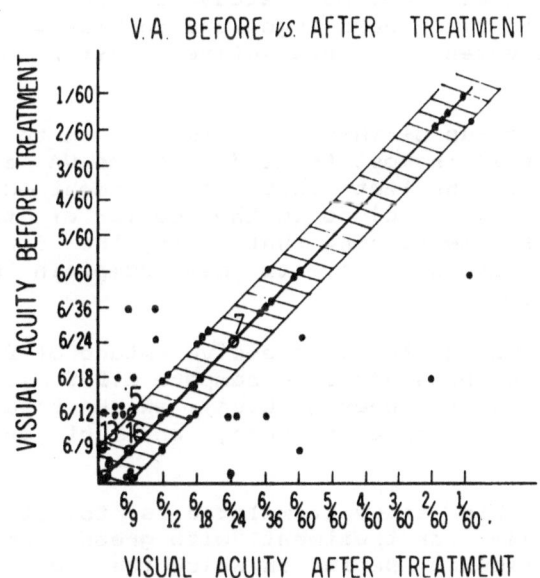

Of the 96 treated eyes, in 10 there was improvement of two lines or more, and in 78 eyes VA remain the same, this included a change of only 1 line. In 8 eyes VA declined 2 lines or more. This means that in 92% of the treated eyes VA remained the same, or improved, and in only 8% of the eyes it declined at the end of the follow-up period. The VA after 18 and 24 months was very similar. Moreover, most of the eyes were treated while they had good vision: Almost half of them (45%) were treated with VA of 6/6-6/9, so that it is difficult to speak about "improvement" in those cases.

In 72 eyes the macular edema decreased or regressed. In 19 it remained about the same and in only 5 eyes the edema increased. In one of these 5 eyes macular SRNV membrane developed in a patient who had drusen; in another eye severe PDR developed, and in another one CME occurred after cataract extraction and posterior lens capsule rupture.

C O M M E N T S

Ferris (13) showed that one year after argon laser treatment in macular edema with central involvement in 33% of the eyes there was a decline of VA of 2 lines or more. Ferenz and Yassur in their previous study (11) showed a 22-34% decline of VA in blue-green argon and in blue-green argon and krypton treated eyes respectively after one year.

Although the follow-up of this study is only up to 2 years, it is obvious that in most treated eyes the VA did not decline in spite of the fact that the treatment was carried in this pattern, so close to the center of the fovea. It is worthwhile mentioning that during the first 2-4 months after treatment patients may complain of temporary blurred vision.

Taking in consideration the progressive nature of DME once it starts it seems reasonable to compare ETDRS (12) protocol to a protocol of the present study, which treats perifoveal elements in a grid pattern, and not only focally.

The results of this study stimulated us to set a randomized control study for treatment with green argon laser for a longer follow-up period in which the control group will be an ETDRS treated modality.

R E F E R E N C E S

1. Patz A, Berbow J.W. Visual and systemic prognosis of patients with Diabetic Retinopathy. Trans. Am. Acad. Ophthal. Otol. 1968, 72:256.
2. Patz A, Schatz H, Gittlesohn A.M. Macular edema, an overlooked complication of Diabetic Retinopathy. Trans. Am. Acad. Ophthal. Otolar. 1973, 77:74.
3. Blankenship G.W. Diabetic macular edema and Argon laser photocoagulation, a prospective randomized study. Tran. Am. Acad. Ophthal. Otolar. 86;69, 1979.

4. Merin S, Yanko L, Ivry M. Treatment of diabetic maculopathy by argon laser. Br.J.Ophthal. 58:85, 1974.
5. Patz A, Fine S. Evaluation and photocoagulation treatment of Diabetic maculopathy. In L'esperance, F.A.fr. editor: Current diagnosis and management of chorioretinal diseases. St. Louis, 1977, The C.V Mosby Co. pp. 256-260.
6. Rubenstein U, Mysku V. Treatment of diabetic maculopathy. Br.J.Ophthal. 56:1, 1972.
7. Marcas D.F., Aberg T.M. Argon laser photocoagulation treatment of diabetic cystoid maculopathy. Ann. Ophthalmology, 1977, 9:365.
8. Wisnia RA. Photocoagulation of nonproliferative exudative diabetic retinopathy. Am.J.Ophthal. 1979, 88:22.
9. Townsend C, Barley J, Kohnek E. Xenon arc photocoagulation for the treatment of diabetic maculopathy. Br.J.Opathal. 1980, 64:385.
10. McDonald H.R., Schatz H. Grid photocoagulation for diffuse macular edema. Retina, 1985, Vol.5, No. 2, p. 65.
11. Ferencz JR, Yassur Y, Veinberer D, Sigal R, Ben-Sira I. The treatment of diabetic macular edema with argon and red krypton laser photocoagulation. Chibret International Journal of Ophthalmology, Vol. 1, No.4, 1984, p. 29.
12. Photocoagulation for diabetic macular edema, early treatment diabetic retinopathy, study report number 1. Arch. Ophthal. Vol.103: Dec. 1985, p. 1796.
13. Personal Communication.

ACUTE DIABETIC RETINOPATHIES

Brigitte ADAD-BENSOUSSAN - Jean-Daniel GRANGE
Hôpital de la Croix-Rousse - Lyon - FRANCE

We want to describe two unusual aspects of the diabetic retinopathy called
Acute diabetic retinopathies.
They are much less known than classic forms (non proliferative and proli-
ferative retinopathies) called chronic retinopathies by contrast.
These acute retinopathies are : -acute oedematous capillaropathies and
acute ischiemic proliferative capillaropathies or florid forms.
They are unusual forms, with an acute start and an acute evolution and
they affect the same category of patients that are :
                 - Young subjects, under 30 years, usually.
                 - Insulin requiring diabetic patients.
                 - With an evolution more than 10 years.
                 - With a poor blood sugar control.
We have to distinguish between them, because therapeutic attitudes will
be different.

1. Acute oedematous capillaropathy.
    Described for the first time by Topilow in 1952, it affects the optic
disc and the macula either separately or simultaneously.
    When only the optic disc is affected we call it diabetic papillar oede-
ma.
    When the macula is affected simultaneously with the papillar we talk
about acute papillo retinopathy.
    When only the macula is affected we call it acute cystoïd maculopathy.

1.1. Clinical signs.
    1.1.1. Diabetic papillar oedema (cf. photos 1 a and 1 b).
    The clinical signs are : - a late fall of visual acuity with sometimes
deterioration of the visual field.
                          - the fundus aspect shows a pinky disc swel-
ling with a dilatation of epi and peripapillar capillaries (network of
Henkind).
                          - On the angiographies,we observe this capil-
lar dilatation with an important leakage of fluorescein out of it, but
there is NO CAPILLAR OCCLUSION on the retina.

    1.1.2. Acute papilloretinopathy.
    Frequently the macula is affected simultaneously with the papilla and,
in these cases clinical signs of macular oedema add themselves to those
of papillar oedema.

    1.1.3. Acute cystoïd maculopathy (cf. photo 2 a)
    The clinical signs are : - an earlier fall of visual acuity.

ACUTE DIABETIC RETINOPATHIES

Photos 1 : <u>Diabetic papillar oedema</u>

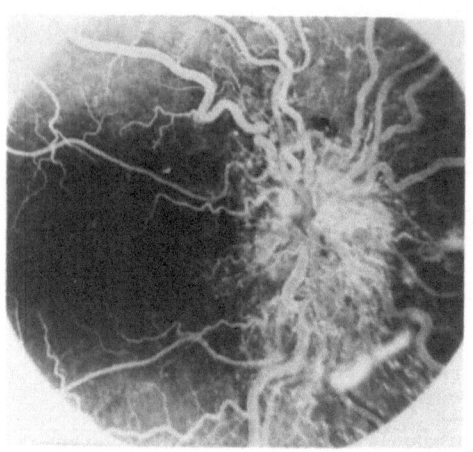 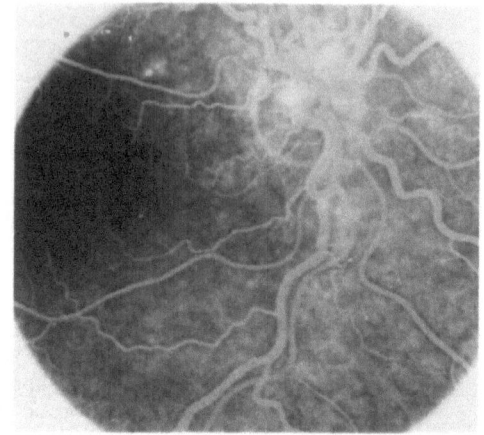

1 a. Acute period   1 b. Six months after : improvement

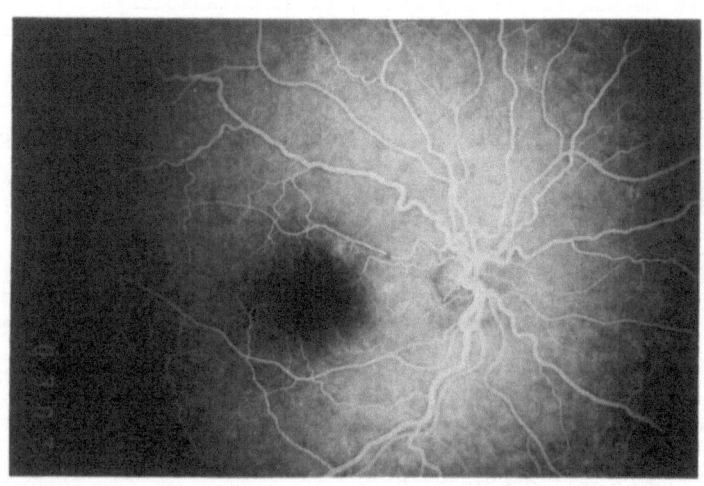

1 c. Two years after : cure

ACUTE DIABETIC RETINOPATHIES

Photos 2 : <u>Acute Cystoïd Maculopathy</u>

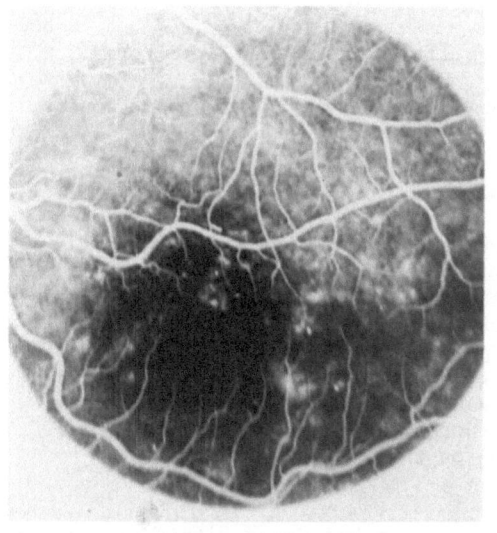 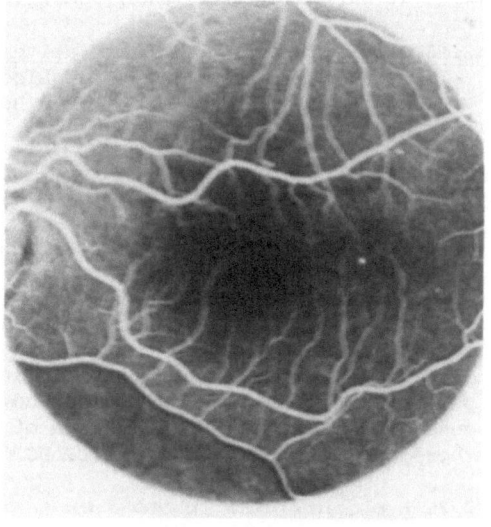

2 a. Acute period   2 b. Six months after : improvement

                      - the fundus aspect is a macular oedema with often associated **exudative** and hemorrhagic macular signs.
                      - on the angiogram we note the dilatation of perimacular capillaries with leakage of fluorescein, but here again there is NO CAPILLAR OCCLUSION on the retina.

1.2. Evolution (cf. photos 1 b, 1 c, 2 b)
    - Usually the cure is observed with solely a good diabetic control within few months, in all those forms of acute oedematous capillaropathies.
    - The second eye is frequently involved, in fifty per cent of cases, within six months, and that, even there is a good diabetic control and an anatomic improvment, in the same time, on the first eye.

1.3. Acute Retinopathies during the pregnancy.
    There is a likeness between those acute oedematous capillaropathies, described before, and a special kind of forms observed during the pregnancy.
    These Acute forms occur during the pregnancy and improve themselves, without any local treatment, after the childbirth.

2. Acute Ischiemic and Proliferative capillaropathies or florid forms.
    They are wellknown as "Rapid, Bloody, Blinding" Forms.
    Described for the first time by BEAUMONT in 1972, they represent one per cent of all the proliferative forms.

2.1. Clinical signs.   (cf. photos 3 a, 3 b)
    The clinical signs are :
    - a late fall of visual acuity but this fall in often sudden by a vitreous hemorrhage.
    - on biomicroscopy, we observe in the first time a dilatation of papillar and macular capillaries but, a short time later, new vessels appear arisen from the optic disc and on the posterior pole principally.
    - on the angiogram, we can note in the first time the dilatation of capillaries on the posterior pole, and, a short time later, numerous new vessels with an important leakage of fluorescein out of them ; but here there are EXTENSIVE CAPILLAR OCCLUSIONS on the retina.

2.2. Evolution   (cf. photo 3 c)
    - Without treatment the evolution results in blindness within six months to two years by repeated vitreous hemorrhages and, secondary, tractus retinal detachment.
    - The treatment consists in Laser Light Coagulation : it will be an early, quick and complete PRP (one session a week, 2500 confluent burns are needed) ; it has to be begun in the same time of the diagnosis and usually the cure is observed with this kind of treatment.

3. Conclusion
    3.1. Acute diabetic retinopathies are unusual forms of the Diabetic Retinopathy, affecting young people and also pregnant women.
    The therapeutic attitudes have to be different :
        - In the first one (Acute Oedematous capillaropathies), there is NO CAPILLAR OCCLUSION and consequently no laser treatment ; only a good diabetic control is needed.
        - In the second (Acute Ischiemic Proliferative Capillaropathies)

ACUTE DIABETIC RETINOPATHIES

Photos 3 : Florid Forms

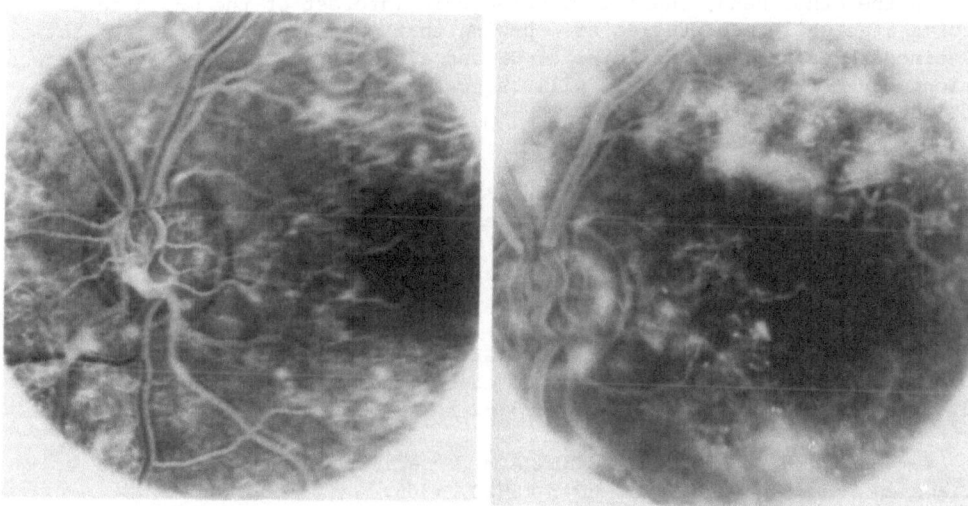

3 a.   3 b.

Acute period

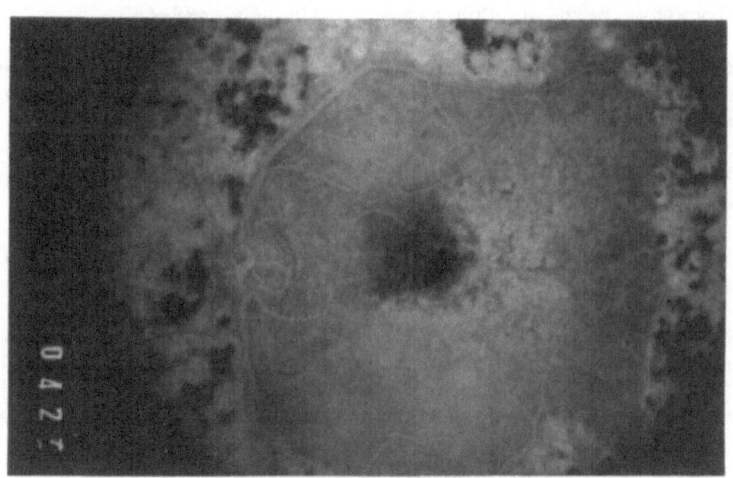

3 c. Two years after : cure after PRP.

there are EXTENSIVE CAPILLAR OCCLUSIONS and, then, Laser Light Coagulation
has to be practiced (In the same time, of course, a good diabetic control
is also needed).

3.2. We would like to recall at last the possible role of the GH.
   The pituitary ablation used few years ago improves the acute forms but
is presently useless.
   On the other hand, there is a pathogenic interest of the GH in these
forms : actually our studies are showing that patients with Acute Diabetic
Retinopathies have a high level of GH and a higher answer to the GRF injection. May be in the future it will be possible to improve these forms by
using somatostatin.

4 . References.

   1 - ADAD-BENSOUSSAN B : place de l'hypophysiolyse dans le traitement
des rétinopathies diabétiques rapidement évolutives - Thesès - LYON 1981.

   2 - BEAUMONT P., HOLLOWS F.C. : classification of diabetic retinopathy
with therapeutic implications - Lancet 1972, February 19, p. 419.

   3 - BONNET M., BENSOUSSAN B., GRANGE J.D., PINGAULT C., FRANCOZ N. ;
capillaropathie oedemateuse aigue du diabetique insulino- dépendant,
J. Fr. Ophtalmol., 1982, 5, 5, 303-316.

   4 - FREUND M., CARMON A., COHEN A.M. : papilledema and papillitis in
diabetes : Am. J. Ophtalmol. 60 : 18-20, 1965.

   5 - GRANGE J.D., BENSOUSSAN B., BONNET M. : Retinopathies diabétiques
rapidement évolutives (approche nosologique et therapeutique). Bull. Soc.
Opht. France, 1983, 11, LXXXIII.

   6 - KEARNS M., HAMILTON A., KOHNER E.H. : excessive permeability in diabetic maculopathy. Brit. J. Ophtalmol., 1979, 63, 489-497.

   7 - KOHNER E., HAMILTON A., JOPLIN, FRASER : florid diabetic retinopathy and its response to treatment by photocoagulation or pituitary ablation. Diabetes 25, 1976, 104.

   8 - LUBOW M., MAKLEY T. : pseudopapilledema of juvenile diabetes mellitus. Arch. OPhtalmol. 1971, 85, 417-422.

   9 - MERIMEE T.J. : A follow study of vascular disease in growth hormone
deficient dwarfs with diabetes. NEJM 298, 1978, 1217-1222.

   10 - PINGAULT C., BONNET M. : Amélioration spontanée d'une rétinopathie
diabétique. Bull. Soc. Ophtalmol. Fr. 1980, 80, 2.

   11 - TOPILOW A., BISLAND T. : Diabetes mellitus as a cause of papillitis.
Amer. J. Ophtalmol. 1952. 35, 855-858.

   12 - YANKO L.,TICHO U., IVRY M. Optic nerve involvement in diabetes.
Acta. Ophtalmol., 1972, 50, 556-569.

ANGIOGENIC FACTORS IN HUMAN VITREOUS

David BenEzra and Itzhak Hemo, Immuno-Ophthalmology and Laboratory of Ocular Angiogenesis, Department of Ophthalmology, Hadassah University Hospital, Jerusalem, Israel

INTRODUCTION

From the study of new blood vessel sprouting within the eye, it became evident that in the retina, hypoxia plays a significant role in this process (1-4). However, the hypoxia theory could not explain all observed phenomena. Michaelson's thorough clinical and experimental observations of ocular neovascularization led him to the assumption that these processes might be regulated via the existence of an "X-Factor" (5,6). Michaelson's outstanding contribution to our present concepts was his early perception of the need for a diffusable chemical factor. In his opinion, this X-factor could be responsible for the sprouting of new vessels during embryogenesis as well as during pathological processes (6). Although innovative and stimulating, Michaelson's ideas, for decades, did not attract the researchers in the field. A renewed interest in "Michaelson X-factor" has been sparked by the discovery of a "Tumor Angiogenic Factor" or "TAF" (7). Following this latter observation, a myriad of neovascular factors have been found (8,9). Although the origins of these factors were different, it was suggested that they may act via a similar final pathway. In this scheme, the pivotal role of the local tissue involved in each instance is emphasized (10,11) (see also chapters on "Angiogenesis - Multiple Factors" and "Future Trends and Concepts" in this book).

In order to evaluate the possible role of the vitreous in ocular neovascularization observed in various clinical conditions, we collected vitrectomy samples and assayed them for their capacity to induce new blood vessel growth.

MATERIALS AND METHODS

Vitrectomy samples: Eighteen random routine vitrectomies performed by various surgeons using the Ocutome system (Storz Instrument Co., U.S.) were included in the study. The first 60 ml of fluid from each vitrectomy were collected, given serial numbers, sent to the laboratory and kept at 4°C.

Processing of the vitreous: All 18 collected samples were processed simultaneously as follows: 1. Centrifugation at 10,000 g in order to remove any gross particles and large collagen fibers. 2. Filtering of the supernatants via 0.45 u pore filters (Nalge). 3. Concentration of the filtered fluid by Amicon UM2 filters (cut-off 1000 molecular weight). 4. Extensive dialysis

against buffered 0.3% NaCl solution pH 7.2. 5. Lyophil-
ization of the dialyzed fluid.
    <u>Preparation</u> <u>of</u> <u>implants</u>:   One mg of each lyophilized
sample was incorporated in Elvax-40 as previously described
(8) (see also chapter on "Corneal Neovascularization" in
this book).   Each implant incorporating 100 to 150 ug of
vitreous lyophilizate was introduced in the mid stroma of a
rabbit cornea and positioned at 2 mm from the limbus.   Six
to seven implants from each vitreous sample were assayed in
a masked manner.   In each experiment "empty" Elvax-40
implants were also included as controls.
    <u>Assessment</u> <u>of</u> <u>neovascular</u> <u>stimulus</u>:   Corneas were
examined daily under the microscope.   The extent   of
neovascularization was recorded on day 6 after implantation.
The length of the leading vessel toward the implant and the
extent of the neovascular bed at the limbus were measured.
From these data, the surface of neovascular budding could be
calculated, taking into consideration that the vascular
tuft forms a triangle with its apex toward the implant (8).
All records were made in a masked manner and uncoded only
upon completion of all experiments.

RESULTS
    Figures 1 - 4 demonstrate some representative samples
of the neovascular stimulus observed on day 6 after the
insertion of implants.

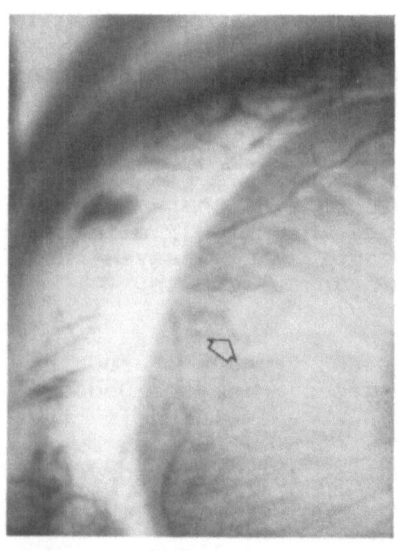 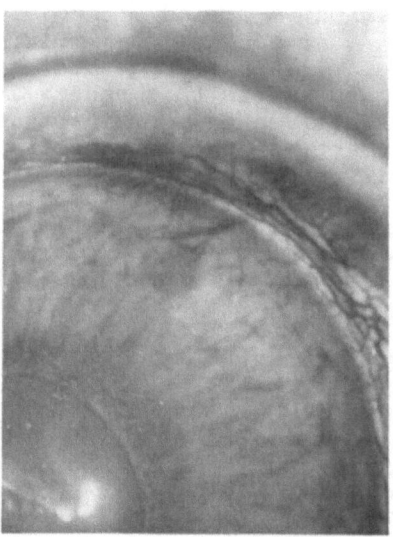

Figure 1 (L).   No neovascularization can be observed.   The
implant (arrow) does not induce any corneal reaction.
Figure 2 (R). Mild angiogenic response. Minimal active base
at the limbus.

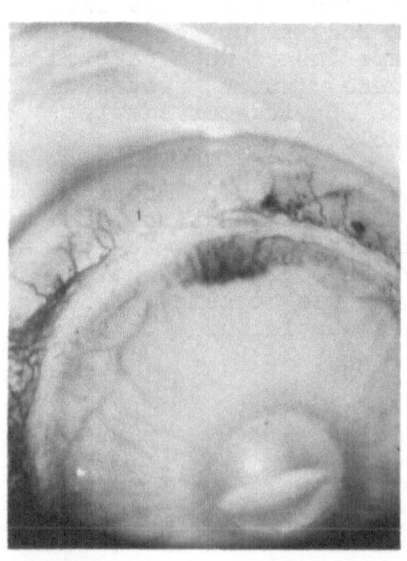 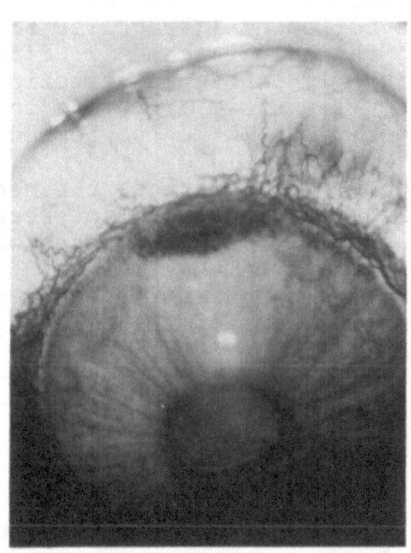

Figure 3 (L).   Moderate angiogenic activity.
Figure 4 (R).   Marked angiogenic activity.   Large active
base with numerous blood vessels directed toward the
implant.

Table 1:   Origin of vitreous samples and number of
experiments carried out.

Diagnosis	No. of samples	No. of experiments
Diabetic Retinopathy	5	31
Trauma (Vitreous Hemorrhage)	5	30
Vitreous organization (non-diabetics)	8	50
Total	18	121

When all data collection was finalized,   the origin of
the   various   vitreous samples was unmasked.   Five   of   the
samples   were   obtained   from   patients   with   severe
proliferative diabetic retinopathy.   From these, 31 corneal
implants were tested.   Five vitreous samples were   obtained
from   non-diabetic   patients   with   vitreous   hemorrhage

following trauma. Thirty corneal implants were assayed from these vitreous samples. Eight additional vitreous samples were obtained from non-diabetic patients with organized vitreous following intraocular foreign body injury or long-standing retinal detachment. Fifty experiments were carried out with implants sequestering these latter vitreous samples. Therefore, from a total of 18 vitreous samples, 121 experiments were performed (Table 1).

Figure 5 illustrates the neovascular stimulus obtained from each individual implant recorded as the length of the leading vessel and the length of the active base at the limbus in front of the implant. From this figure, one can see that some variability of responses was obtained when different implants of the same vitreous sample were tested.

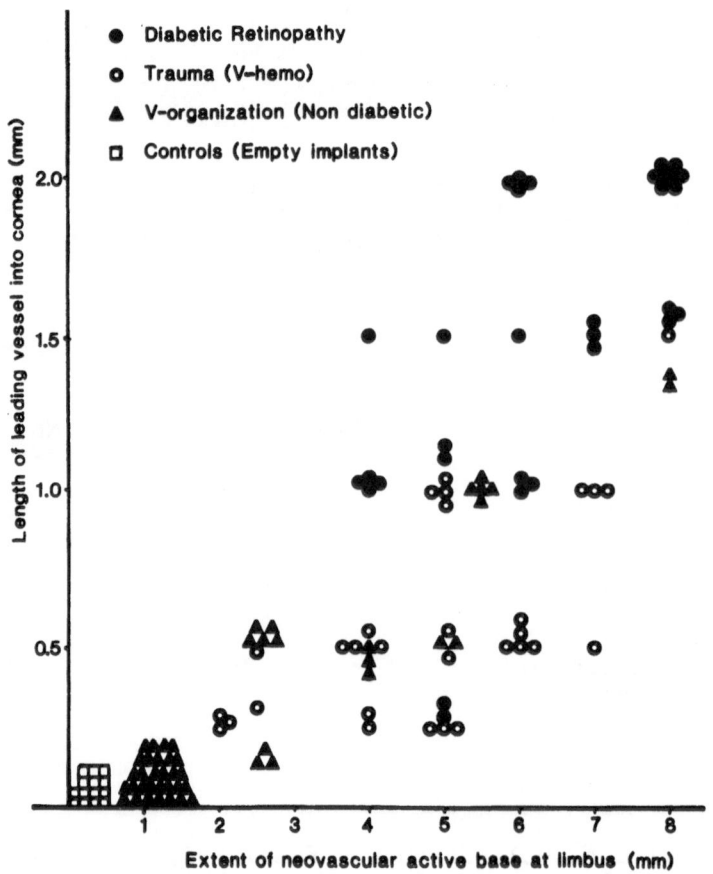

Figure 5. Extent of angiogenic stimulus recorded for each single experiment.

Implants sequestering vitreous obtained from patients with diabetic retinopathy were significantly more angiogenic than vitreous from other origins. The findings that vitreous samples from eyes with diabetic retinopathy induced a stronger neovascular response is reinforced when the data are represented as the recorded mean neovascular surface for each vitreous sample (Figure 6).

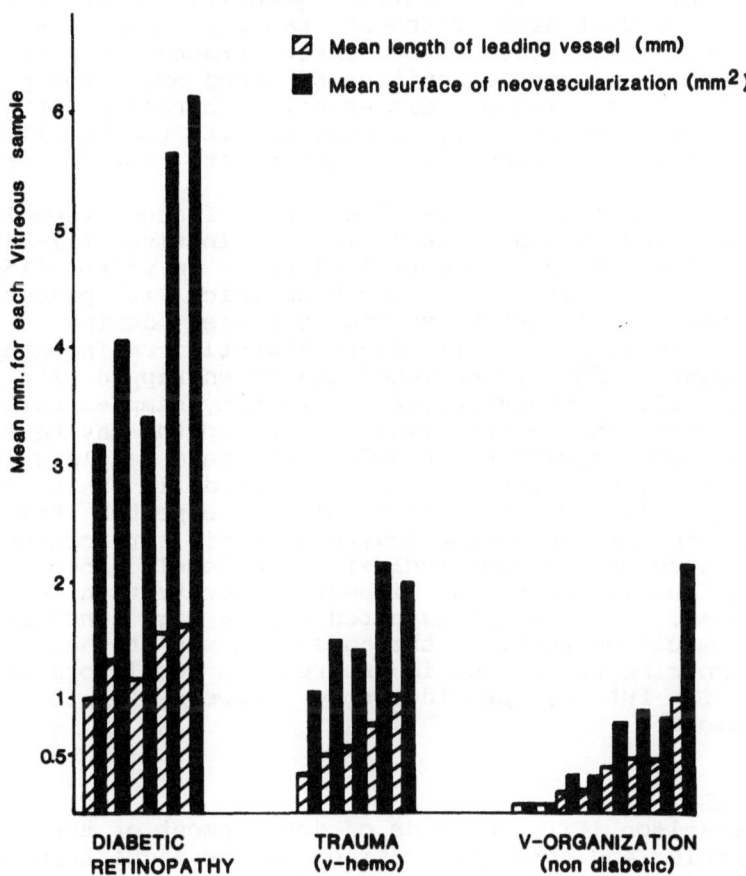

Figure 6. Mean length of leading vessel (mm) and mean neovascular surface (mm²) induced by each vitreous sample.

DISCUSSION

These data clearly demonstrate that angiogenic factors can be sequestered in the vitreous. It is of interest that the five vitreous samples obtained from patients with severe proliferative diabetic retinopathy demonstrated the strongest angiogenic stimulus. On the other hand, little or no attraction of blood vessels was induced when vitreous samples from patients with organized vitreous and longstanding retinal detachment were tested (figures 5 and 6). The nature and origin of the angiogenic factor in the vitreous samples is not clear. It is possible that the level of this vitreous angiogenic factor (VAF) is associated with the blood and/or protein contents of the different vitreous samples, those from the diabetic patients having the highest content of blood and/or other proteins. A thorough investigation to test this assumption was not carried out. However, a similar "quantity" of dry material was used to test each vitreous sample. Also, vitreous samples obtained from cases after trauma and vitreous hemorrhage had larger quantities of blood and serum protein than vitreous samples of diabetics. Therefore, the VAF activity was most probably associated with the "quality" of the vitreous substance rather than its total protein content.

In the retina, a specific growth factor (RDGF) was identified and found to be angiogenic in vivo (12-14) as well as stimulatory to endothelial cells in vitro (15-17). It can be postulated that the RDGF which is present in normal retinas is activated and released during certain metabolic conditions. In severe diabetic retinopathy, a large amount of RDGF is released and is entrapped within the vitreous (15). Therefore,the vitrectomy samples collected from patients with severe diabetic retinopathy may have had a higher concentration of RDGF that could explain their higher angiogenic activity as observed in this study. Following this surmise, it should be expected that the vitreous in patients with severe diabetic retinopathy and those with central venous occlusion who develop neovascular glaucoma should have the highest concentration of VAF. Furthermore, it should be expected that a high concentration of VAF would be found in the aqueous humor of these eyes. These experiments are now in progress in our laboratory and should, in future, provide some answers to the above postulations.

REFERENCES
1. Michaelson IC: The mode of development of the retinal vessels and some observations on its significance for certain retinal diseases. Trans Ophthalmol Soc UK 68:137, 1948.
2. Wise GN: Retinal neovascularization. Trans Am Ophthalmol Soc 54:729, 1956.
3. Ashton N: Oxygen and the growth and development of retinal vessels. In vivo and in vitro studies. Am J Ophthalmol 62:412, 1966.
4. Patz A: The role of oxygen in retrolental fibroplasia. Trans Am Ophthalmol Soc 66:940, 1968.
5. Campbell FW, Michaelson IC: Blood vessel formation in the cornea. Br J Ophthalmol 33:248, 1949.

6.   Michaelson IC: Retinal Circulation in Man and Animals. Charles C. Thomas, Illinois, 1954.
7.   Folkman J, Merler E, Abernathy C, Williams G: Isolation of a tumor factor responsible for angiogenesis. J Exp Med 133:275, 1971.
8.   BenEzra D: Neovasculogenic ability of prostaglandins, growth factors and synthetic chemoattractants.   Am J Ophthalmol 86:455, 1978.
9.   Garner A: Ocular angiogenesis.   Int Rev Exp Pathol 28:249, 1986.
10. BenEzra D: Neovasculogenesis. Triggering factors and possible mechanisms. Surv Ophthalmol 24:167, 1979.
11. Archer D: Retinal neovascularization.   Trans Ophthalmol Soc UK 103:2, 1983.
12. Kissun RD, Garner A: Vasoformative properties of normal and hypoxic retinal tissue. Br J Ophthalmol 61:394, 1977.
13. Federman JL, Brown GC, Felberg NT, Felton SM: Experimental ocular angiogenesis. Am J Ophthalmol 89:231, 1980.
14. Kissun RD, Hill CR, Garner A, Phillips P, Kumar S, Weiss JB: A low molecular weight angiogenic factor in cat retina.   Br J Ophthalmol 66:165, 1982.
15. Glaser BM, D'Amore PA, Seppa H, Seppa S, Schiffman E: Adult tissues contain chemoattractants for vascular endothelial cells.   Nature 288:483, 1980.
16. Glaser BM, D'Amore PA, Michels RG, Brunson SK, Fenselau AH, Rice T, Patz A: The demonstration of angiogenic activity from ocular tissues.   Preliminary report. Ophthalmology 87:440, 1980.
17. Hill CR, Kissun RD, Weiss JB, Garner A: Angiogenic factor in vitreous from diabetic retinopathy. Experimentia 39:583, 1983.

THE ROLE OF ISCHAEMIA IN THE PATHOGENESIS OF RETINAL NEOVASCULARISATION

ALEC GARNER AND RALPH KISSUN
Department of Pathology, Institute of Ophthalmology, University of London,
United Kingdom

Normal retinal vascularisation

The progenitor cells of the retinal vascular system are derived from
the base of the hyaloid artery towards the end of the fourth month of
gestation, fanning out at the level of the optic disc and invading the
inner layers of the developing retina. Progressive differentiation and
organisation of cells in the trailing edge of this vascular primordium
culminates in the formation of endothelium-lined and lumenised capillaries,
whilst subsequent remodelling produces a definitive complex of arterioles,
capillaries and veins. In the human the developing vasculature is preceded
by a vanguard of spindle cells, the nature of which is uncertain: although
commonly assumed to be precursors of the vascular endothelium this is by no
means certain and more recent speculation concerns a putative source of
angiogenic stimulation (Kretzer et al 1986) and an essentially astrocytic
origin serving as an energy source for the emergent vessels (Cogan and
Kuwabara 1986).

One of the determining factors in the vascularising process appears to
be the metabolic needs of the retina. It is claimed, for instance, that the
retina does not start to vascularise until a minimum thickness has been
reached (90-95 μm in the human) (Hittner and Kretzer 1983), lesser thick-
nesses being provided for by diffusion from the underlying choroid. Even
then the retinal circulation is confined to the parts not accessible to the
choroidal source of nutrition. As a corollary, the retina of the guinea-pig
remains thin throughout life and never vascularises.

Further evidence of the intimate relationship between retinal vascularisation and metabolic demand is the capillary-free zone surrounding the
arterioles (Michaelson 1948). Michaelson (1954) suggested that this finding
was a reflection of the relatively high concentration of oxygen in the
tissue adjacent to the arteriole compared with other parts of the circulation and Campbell (1951) showed that the width of the zone could be reduced
by lowering the oxygen concentration in the inspired air. Ashton (1970)
discovered that the paucity of capillaries around arterioles is due to
obliteration of existing vessels, as opposed to a failure to develop, but
only now are some of the intermediate steps relating angiogenesis to metabolic need beginning to be understood. To a considerable degree they
represent a confirmation of a suggestion enunciated by Michaelson (1948)
and fostered by Ashton et al (1954) that the release of a chemical substance with vasoformative properties is involved.

Proliferative retinopathy

Apart from the replacement of effete endothelial cells damaged in
normal wear-and-tear, angiogenesis in the retina in postnatal life is a

pathological process. That which occurs in front of the retina has attracted most attention and, although it can complicate a number of disease entities, the common denominator in most instances is prior reduction in blood flow through the underlying retina (see Garner 1986). For example, diabetic retinopathy is characterised in the early stages by increased retinal blood flow but gradually, as focal areas of capillary closure grow in number and size, the trend is reversed towards an overall reduction and it is at this stage that proliferative activity can be anticipated. Again, central retinal vein thrombosis involving a diminished retinal circulation is commonly followed by a neovascular response. But nowhere is the link between retinal ischaemia and neovascularisation more conspicuous than in the retinopathy of prematurity, wherein damage to recently formed vascular channels and interference with the advance of the still developing retinal vasculature is followed by proliferative activity at the boundary between the intact and avascular regions.

Evidence that the vascularisation in these situations might be mediated by a chemical factor has come from work on retinal and vitreal extracts. On the hypothesis that the factor would diffuse from the ischaemic retina into the vitreous and there, for want of adequate drainage, accumulate until in sufficient concentration to exert a mitotic and chemotactic effect on the underlying retinal vessels (Ashton 1957), vitreal extracts from patients with proliferative diabetic retinopathy were subjected to biochemical analysis. It transpired that the vitreous in this circumstance does indeed contain a moiety with angiogenic properties (Glaser et al 1980, Hill et al 1983). Later studies have shown that this property is not confined to diabetic retinopathy but can occur in a variety of proliferative disorders (Elstow et al, in preparation).

It is presumed that the angiogenic factor reaches the vitreous from the retina and there is evidence from other species that such activity is a function of even the normal retina (Kissun and Garner 1977, Federman et al 1980). This suggests that there is a baseline level of angiogenesis, (concerned, perhaps, with compensating for normal wear-and-tear), which is increased in pathological states to the extent that undue vascular proliferation ensues.

Experimental proliferative retinopathy secondary to ischaemia
       To test the hypothesis that proliferative retinopathy is a response to a quantitative increase in a normal constituent of the retina requires a sufficiently sensitive assay. The commonly employed corneal and chorioallantoic membrane bioassay systems are useful for demonstrating angiogenic activity but do not lend themselves to precise measurement. However, the recognition that tumour angiogenic factor has, in addition to its more obvious properties, a procollagenase-activating capacity (Weiss et al 1983) offered the prospect of a sensitive assay, since it means that angiogenic activity can be measured in terms of the amount of radio-labelled collagen degraded by a given amount of tissue extract. It had already been shown that tumour-derived and retinal angiogenic fractions are closely similar and probably identical (Kissun et al 1982) so that there was good reason to believe that the retinal factor would also have collagenolytic potential.

Newborn kittens were reared in an environment of 80-90% oxygen for 72 hours by which time it was predictable that the entire retinal circulation would have been obliterated (Ashton, et al 1954). Afterwards they returned to normal atmospheric conditions for a further five days before termination of the experiment. Kittens of the same age but reared through-out in normal air were used as controls. The retinas were removed and extracted by a series of purification steps to yield a low molecular size fraction which displayed angiogenic activity when tested on the chick chorioallantoic membrane. Aliquots of the same fraction were then assessed for procollagenase activating capacity and this showed a more than three-fold increase over extracts from the retinas of kittens not subjected to hyperoxia (Taylor et al 1986). It seems, therefore, that there is now direct as well as indirect support for the concept that proliferative retinopathy is a consequence of impaired retinal circulation. The elabor-ation or release of increased amounts of angiogenesis-promoting substances apparently incurs some spillage into the vitreous with a consequent chem-otactic effect on the endothelium of blood vessels lying close to the retinal surface.

What does this tell us about the retinopathy of prematurity? The kitten model has its limitations, as those responsible for its introduction recognised, but it does demonstrate very nicely the link between the damage to the developing retinal circulation and neovascularisation. In the human, although it is the accompanying fibroblastic activity that is responsible for detachment, this never occurs in the absence of vascular proliferation. Consequently, an understanding, leading to control, of the latter process is still central to the problem of the retinopathy of prematurity if de-tachment is to be prevented. One approach to prevention of the vascular activity is to avoid the initial vascular injury but, whether by curtailing the level of oxygen administration, correcting any acidosis or giving vitamin E supplements- this may not always be possible. Another approach is to inhibit the elaboration of angiogenic factor by destroying its putative source through cryopexy or photocoagulation. But to do so presupposes knowledge of its source and, at the present time, this is conjectural. It may derive from the as yet unvascularised retina: an entirely reasonable concept if the stimulus to the normal process of vascularisation is the metabolic need of the retina (Wolbarsht et al 1981). Kretzer et al (1986) suggest that the wall of spindle cells in the vanguard of the developing vasculature is responsible for secreting the angiogenic factor. Alterna-tively, since the factor, in the bovine eye at least, is bound to albumin (Elstow et al 1985) it is possible that the factor is haematogenous and enters the tissues in circumstances which damage the vascular endothelium (Hayreh 1980). Clearly it is important to determine the precise source of the angiogenic stimulus. Other therapeutic prospects based on the angio-genic factor mediation of extraretinal vasoproliferation relate to the development of either pharmacological or naturally occurring inhibitors, and the results of endeavours in this direction are awaited with great interest.

References

1. Ashton N: Retinal vascularization in health and disease. Am J Ophthal-mol 44: 7-17, 1957.
2. Ashton N: Retinal angiogenesis in the human embryo. Br Med Bull 26: 103-106, 1970.
3. Ashton N, Ward B, Serpell G: Effect of oxygen on developing retinal vessels with particular reference to the problem of retrolental fibroplasia. Br J Ophthalmol 38: 397-432, 1954.
4. Campbell FW: The influence of a low atmospheric pressure on the development of the retinal vessels in the rat. Trans Ophthalmol Soc

UK 71: 287-299, 1951.

5. Cogan DG, Kuwabara T: Accessory cells in vessels of the paranatal human retina. Arch Ophthalmol 104: 747-752, 1986.
6. Elstow SF, Schor AM, Weiss JB: Bovine retinal angiogenesis factor in a small molecule. Invest Ophthalmol Vis Sci 26: 74-79, 1985.
7. Federman JL, Brown GC, Felberg NT, Felton SM: Experimental ocular angiogenesis. Am J Ophthalmol 89: 231-237, 1980.
8. Garner A: Ocular Angiogenesis. Int Rev Exp Pathol 28: 249-306, 1986.
9. Glaser BM, D'Amore PA, Michels RG, Brunson SK, Ria T: Demonstration of angiogenic activity from ocular tissues. Ophthalmology 87: 440-446, 1980.
10. Hayreh SS: Ocular neovascularization: an hypothesis. Int Ophthalmol 2: 27-32, 1980.
11. Hill CR, Kissun RD, Weiss JB, Garner A: Angiogenic factor in vitreous from diabetic retinopathy. Experientia 39: 583-585, 1983.
12. Hittner HM, Kretzer FL: Vitamin E and retrolental fibroplasia: ultrastructural mechanism of clinical efficacy. In Porter R, Whelan J, eds. Biology of Vitamin E. London (Ciba Foundation Symposium 101): Pitman Books, pp. 165-185, 1983.
13. Kissun RD, Garner A: Vasoformative properties of normal and hypoxic retinal tissue. Br J Ophthalmol 61: 394-398, 1977.
14. Kissun RD, Hill CR, Garner A, Phillips P, Kumar S, Weiss JB: A low molecular weight angiogenic factor in cat retina. Br J Ophthalmol 66: 165-169, 1982.
15. Kretzer FL, McPherson AR, Hittner HM: An interpretation of retinopathy of prematurity in terms of spindle cells: relationship to vitamin E prophylaxis and cryotherapy. Graefe's Arch Clin Exp Ophthalmol 224: 205-214, 1986.
16. Michaelson IC: The mode of development of the vascular system of the retina, with some observations on its significance for certain retinal diseases. Trans Ophthalmol Soc UK 68: 137-180, 1948.
17. Michaelson IC: "Retinal Circulation in Man and Animals", Thomas, Springfield, Illinois, 1954.
18. Taylor CM, Weiss JB, Kissun RD, Garner A: Effect of oxygen tension on the quantities of procollagenase-activating angiogenic factor in the developing kitten retina. Br J Ophthalmol 70: 162-165, 1986.
19. Wolbarsht ML, Landers MB, Stefansson E: Oxygen and the retinopathy of prematurity: why don't all premature infants develop RLF? Retinopathy of Prematurity Conference, Washington DC, Dec 4-6, 132-148, 1981.

OPTIMAL STRATEGY FOR ROP SCREENING

B.P. Cats and K.E.W.P. Tan, Department of Neonatology, Wilhelmina Children's Hospital, and Royal Eye Hospital, Utrecht, The Netherlands

INTRODUCTION

Nowadays it seems possible that cicatricial ROP will turn out to be a preventable condition; therefore, it is of utmost importance to detect individual cases at a moment when therapy can still be instituted appropriately. To reach this goal, ROP screening has to be carried out in such a way that the chance of detection is maximal. Clinicians should be aware of the incidence and course of ROP in certain patient population. The possible relation with chronological and postconceptual age and with clinical events in the postnatal period which influence the occurrence and extent of ROP should be carefully analyzed.

PATIENTS AND METHODS

Through 1983 we determined the true timely incidence and course of ROP in our population of prematures. All, except four prematures, admitted to the neonatal intensive care unit of our hospital, were subject to a prospective longitudinal weekly ophthalmologic survey. Indirect ophthalmoscopy was performed according to a previously described method (1) in those children surviving beyond two weeks. Four hundred sixty-three fundus examinations were done in 121 children (3.9 $\pm$ examinations per child).

RESULTS

As a result of their longer average hospital stay, younger infants were seen more frequently than older ones (Table 1). ROP was detected in 18 children (of whom one died the week after ROP was found). The incidence of ROP in our premature population therefore can be stated to be 15%. Even in this relatively small sample the increasing risk with decreasing gestational age was apparent (Table 1).

The mean age at which ROP was detected was 35.5 $\pm$ 2.1 weeks postconceptual (p.c.) age and 7.3 $\pm$ 1.6 weeks chronological (chr.) age. Comparing postconceptual and chronological age with regard to all positive ROP findings, there seems to be a larger scatter when using the former (Figures 1a and b).

Table 1.

Gest.age (wks)	(n)	nr. of eye examinations	(mean)	nr. with ROP (%)	
26	7	43	6.1	5 (1†)	50%
27	7	36	5.1	2	
28	14	75	5.4	3	24%
29	15	84	5.6	4	
30	21	78	3.7	1	3%
31	17	45	2.6	-	
32	16	41	2.6	1	12%
33	10	29	2.9	2	
34	9	26	2.9	-	
35	4	13	3.2	-	
36	1	3	3	-	
	121	473	3.9	18	15%

Figure 1a.

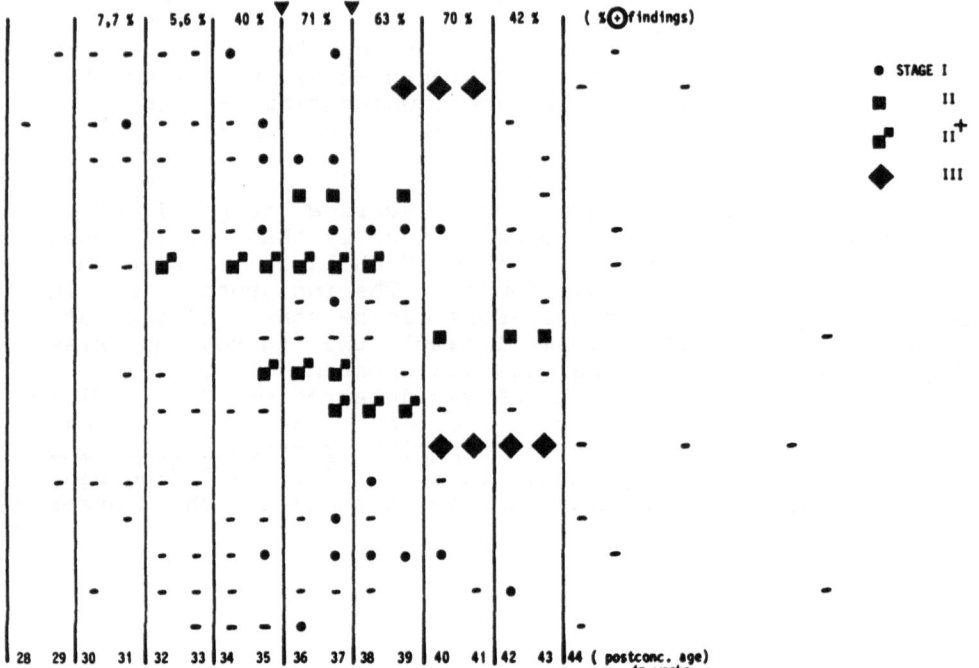

Figure 1b.

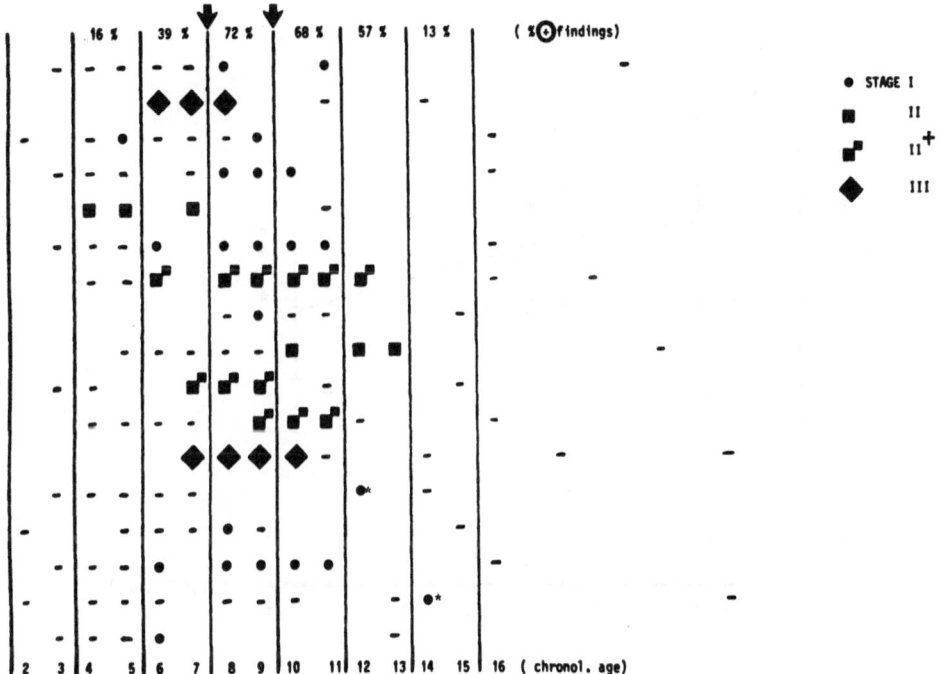

Maximum detection is in the 36 - 37th week of p.c. age (71%) and in the 8 - 9th week of chr. age (72%). Figures 1a and b also show that both stages III and one stage II were present at the first investigation. The mean age at which ROP was seen for the first time is 7.37 ± 1.5 weeks in the children with stage I and 5.75 ± 1.26 weeks in the more advanced stages. The two children with stage I marked with an asterisk (Figure 1b) had first positive ROP findings late. Both had uneventful first weeks; one suffered a sepsis during the eighth week of life and had supplementary O_2 for one week, the other had anesthesia with 100% O_2 and subsequent artificial ventilation for 30 hours (F_iO_2 < 0.35) during the seventh week of life.

Figure 2 shows that with increasing gestational age at birth ROP tends to present earlier. Immatures with a gestational age of 26 - 27 weeks have first positive ROP finding at a mean chronological age of 7.6 weeks, while prematures with a gestational age of 32 - 33 weeks show the first signs at 5.9 weeks.

Figure 2.

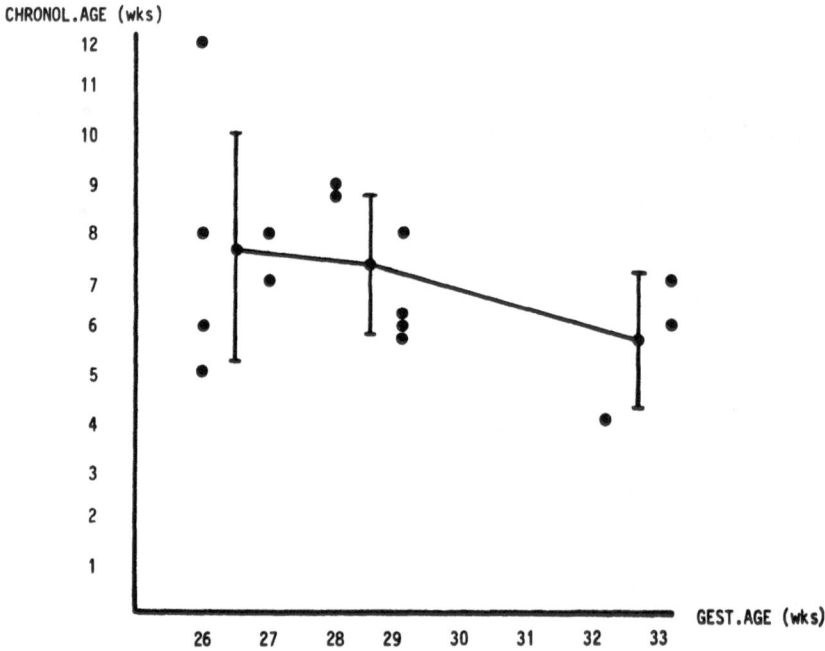

COMMENT
     The exact etiology of ROP remains unknown. Conclusive
data regarding the relative influence of the developmental
stage of the retina at birth, additional exogenous factors
and predisposing ("endogenous") genetic factors on the
extent of ROP are still unclear. Although the natural
course of ROP has been described in detail (2), the data
were collected using widely differing screening procedures.
True incidence studies determining the maximal chance to
detect ROP are scarce. Palmer (3) was the first to
recognize this problem; his recommendations with regard to
an optimal timing to detect active ROP were, however, based
on data collected in retrospect. In 1952 Silverman (4)
noted that ROP seemed to develop later in babies of lower
birth weight and in 1982 Lamberts and colleagues (5) stated
that "the postconceptual age seems to be an important factor
in determining the onset of the retinopathy".
     Recently, Fielder and colleagues (6) have shown that
there seems to be a differential time of onset in children
of differing gestational ages at birth and our data support
their conclusions. However, grouping the positive ROP
findings according to postconceptual and chronological age

shows less scattering when using the latter.

Paradoxically, ROP was detected considerably earlier in those children showing stages II and III as initial finding than in children with stage I. This suggests that early starting cases have more chance to progress beyond stage I. It therefore appears preferable, in our view, not to rely on a single screening moment but to screen at 6/7 weeks and 9/10 weeks of age. However, our data also suggest that a more or less "custom-made" approach has to be adopted in ROP screening. This should take into account chronological as well as postconceptual age. The age at onset of ROP and certain clinical events should subsequently determine the timing of follow-up investigations.

REFERENCES
1. Cats BP, Tan KEWP: Retinopathy of prematurity: review of a four-year period. Br J Ophthalmol 1985; 69 (7):500-503.
2. Flynn JT: Retrolental fibroplasia. In: Wybar K, Taylor D, eds: Pediatric Ophthalmology. New York: Marcel Dekker, 1983.
3. Palmer EA: Optimal timing of examination for acute retrolental fibroplasia. Ophthalmology 1981; 88:662-668.
4. Silverman WA, Blodi FC, Locke JC, Day RL, Reese AB: Incidence of retrolental fibroplasia in a New York nursery. Arch Ophthalmol 1952; 48:698-711.
5. Lamberts, et al: Retinopathy of prematurity: screening of patients at risk. Bull Soc Belge Ophtal 1982; 203:57-70.
6. Fielder AR, Ng YK, Levene MI: Retinopathy of prematurity: age at onset. Arch Dis Child 1986; 61:774-778.

INFLUENCE OF STATISTICAL METHODOLOGY AND CORRELATION OF PATIENT POPULA=
TIONS ON THE CORRELATION OF RISK FACTORS WITH RETINOPATHY OF PREMATURITY

Emilio Bossi, M.D.; Fritz Koerner, M.D.
Division of Neonatology, Dept. of Pediatrics; Eye Clinic, University of
Berne, Switzerland

1. INTRODUCTION

As much as 50 risk factors for the development of ROP have been discussed
since this disease was first observed in 1941 (6). This multitude of factors exemplifies our lack of knowledge of the etiology and of pathogenetic
mechanisms of ROP. The purpose of this study is to show how correlations
between variables considered as risk factors and the development of ROP
may depend on statistical methodology and on the composition of the population chosen for investigation.

2. PROCEDURE

2.1. Patients

Between 1976 and 1981, 639 babies hospitalized in neonatal special and intensive care nurseries were examined by indirect monocular or binocular
ophthalmoscopy. The criteria for selecting infants for routine ophthalmologic examination are listed in table 1.

Birth weight	< 1500 g
Birth weight	$1500-2500$ g $+ FiO_2 \geqslant 0.3$
Birth weight	> 2500 g $+ FiO_2 \geqslant 0.3$ for $\geqslant 48$ hours
At least 1 $paO_2 > 100$ torr	

TABLE 1: Criteria for selection of infants for ophthalmological
examination.

The first examination was done at about 3 weeks of age. The frequency of
follow-up examinations, usually once every 1 to 4 weeks, depended on the
progression rate of fundus abnormalities. A semiquantitative classification of the retinal disease was devised since the new international classification of ROP (ICROP) was not yet available (4). Of these 639 babies,
73 had ROP of all grades (11.4 %). 4 were term newborns, 69 were prematures. 3 of these (0.5 % of all examined babies) were blind. For the statistical investigations presented in this paper, 66 ROP-babies including the
3 blind infants could be matched with 66 controls according to gestational
age, birth weight, birth date and single or multiple birth.

2.2. Variables

The following parameters were chosen as potential risk factors (table 2):

```
No. of paH      < 7.25
No. of paO₂     > 100 torr
Hours FiO₂      > 0.4
No. of paCO₂ - fluctuations¹
No. of paCO₂    < 30 torr
No. of paCO₂    > 50 torr

Days of artificial ventilation
ml of packed red blood cells transfused

Multiple birth
Gestational age²
```

TABLE 2: Parameters investigated. 1) $paCO_2$-fluctuations from va-
         lues ranging between 30 and 55 torr to higher as well
         as lower values or backwards into the original range.
         Magnitude of fluctuations at least $\pm$ 15 torr within
         4 hours.
         2) Used for multivariate analysis only.

2.3. Statistics

An univariate and a multivariate statistical method were applied to the
same data of the same population of infants. The univariate method used
was the Wilcoxon matched pairs signed rank test (2,5). It was used to calculate differences between the frequency of the various variables in the
ROP group versus the control infants. The multivariate method was a multiple linear regression analysis. The severity of ROP served as the dependent variable. The scale of the dependent variable was rather an ordi-
nal one. Linearity of the dependency of ROP from various risk factors is
unlikely. Therefore, any regression functions calculated can only be crude
approximations. The backward elimination procedure was utilized: it eliminates non-significant variables in a stepwise manner. In contrast to univariate analysis, which considers each variable individually, multivariate
analysis considers interrelationships between variables (3).

3. RESULTS

The correlations between risk factors and ROP, as determined by univariate
analysis, are shown in table 3.

"Risk factor"	ROP-group (mean)	Control-group (mean)	P
No. of paH < 7.25	5.5	1.4	< 0.002
No. of paO$_2$ > 100 torr	7.7	4.0	< 0.02
Hours FiO$_2$ > 0.4	25.3	18.7	< 0.02
No. of paCO$_2$ - fluctuations	2.2	0.8	< 0.02
No. of paCO$_2$ < 30 torr	3.4	2.5	NS
No. of paCO$_2$ > 50 torr	6.8	1.9	< 0.001
Days of artificial ventilation	6.7	2.8	< 0.01
ml of packed rbc transfused	82	45.2	< 0.001

TABLE 3: Correlations as calculated by univariate analysis (Wilcoxon matched pairs signed rank test). NS=non significant

The group of babies who had ROP had experienced a mean of 5.5 episodes of pH values below 7.25, as compared to a mean of 1.4 such episodes in the group of control. The difference is statistically significant. The following parameters also correlated at statistical significance with ROP when univariate statistics were used: hyperoxemia, oxygen treatment with more than 40 % concentrations, paCO$_2$-fluctuations as defined, hypercarbia, artificial ventilation and blood transfusions.

Table 4 shows which parameters maintained their significant correlation with ROP when a multivariate statistical method was used on the whole population of ROP-babies and controls.

"Risk factor"	Univariate analysis. Whole population.	Multivariate analysis. Whole population. (Partial regression)
No. paH < 7.25	+	+
No. paO$_2$ > 100 torr	+	
Hrs. FiO$_2$ > 0.4	+	+
No. paCO$_2$ - fluctuations	+	
No. paCO$_2$ < 30 torr		+ (neg.)
No. paCO$_2$ > 50 torr	+	
Days of artificial ventilation	+	+
ml packed rbc transfused	+	
Multiple birth	+	+
Gestational age	(matched)	

TABLE 4: Parameters correlating with ROP when calculated by multivariate analysis as compared to univariate analysis. +: correlation statistically significant. (neg.): negative partial correlation (see text).

Only acidosis, treatment with $O_2 > 40$ %, artificial ventilation and
multiple birth   remained significant predictors. High $paCO_2$-values
were not significant but the number of episodes of $paCO_2$-values below 30
torr gained a negative partial correlation.

The different results of univariate and multivariate testings show that
statistical correlations between so-called risk factors and ROP are influenced by the statistical method used.

Table 5 demonstrates the importance of the composition of the population
chosen for investigation. For this purpose, the total population of patients was broken down into two groups with a gestational age below 32
weeks, and 32 weeks and more respectively. Data were analyzed with multiple linear regression and the correlations were compared with those of
multiple regression analysis of the whole population. The results of univariate analysis of the whole population are included for comparison (table 5).

"Risk factor"	Univariate analysis. Whole population	Multivariate analysis (Partial regression)		
		Whole population	25-31 w. gest.age	32-40 w. gest.age
No. paH < 7.25	+	+++	+	+
No. paO_2 >100 torr	+		+++	
Hrs. FiO_2 >0.4	+	+		
No. $paCO_2$ - fluctuations	+		+	
No. $paCO_2$ <30 torr		+ (neg.)	+ (neg.)	
No. $paCO_2$ >50 torr	+			
Days artificial ventilation	+	+		
ml packed rbc transfused	+			
Multiple birth	+	+		+++
Gestational age	(matched)		++	
Multicorrelation coefficient R^2		0.43	0.62	0.61

TABLE 5: Comparison of correlations between "risk factors" and ROP in the
whole patient population and in subdivisions of this population
as calculated by MLR. The correlations obtained by univariate
analysis of the whole population are included for comparison.
+: correlation statistically significant. ++,+++: magnitude of
partial F values (reflects the strength of each single variable
within the context of all variables in multivariate analysis).
(neg.): negative partial correlation.

Acidosis was the only variable found to correlate with ROP in all three
groups. High paO_2, $paCO_2$-fluctuations, rare occurrence of low $paCO_2$ values
and gestational age correlated only in the very immature group. Multiple

birth was a strong predictor in the more mature babies, but did not correlate in the most immature ones.

4. DISCUSSION

The clinical parameters investigated in this study were chosen for pathophysiologic considerations. Tissue hyperoxia will inhibit a normal development of retinal vessels. Hyperoxia can be potentiated by an acute displacement of the HbO_2-dissociation curve to the right, e.g. by elevated
DPG-concentrations in transfused adult erythrocytes, by elevated pCO_2,
and by acidosis. In this context, we have demonstrated that a simultaneous
combination of elevated paO_2 and $paCO_2$ in the first seven days of life is
more frequent in babies developing ROP than in controls, being most marked
in those babies who later became blind (1). In a later phase, when the
energy demand of the developing retina increases, a local oxygen or energy deficiency builds up at the zone of maturation, leading to vasoproliferation (7). At this stage, hypercapnia could promote vasoproliferation
by provoking vasodilatation, thus inducing an increased transmural pressure leading to a flattening of epithelial cells which is followed by an
increased mitotic rate.

Furthermore, the results of this investigation indicate that the weight
of certain predictors in multiple regressions with ROP highly depends on
the developmental state of the retinal vasculature: most variables correlate significantly only in infants with gestational ages below 32 weeks
of birth (4).

The results presented in this study clearly imply that statistical methodology and the composition of the population investigated, as far as gestational age is concerned, exert an important influence on correlations
between so-called risk factors and ROP. These facts could explain in part
the conflicting results of studies on risk factors.

5. CONCLUSIONS

The results of clinical investigation aimed at defining risk factors for
the development of ROP must be interpreted with caution. Direct conclusions for deriving pathogenetic models or for instituting specific prophylactic measures have to be carefully balanced. Bearing this in mind,
the data of the literature and of this study still give an overwhelming
evidence for the assumption that retinal immaturity and oxygen are determinant for the development of ROP. Other factors like acidosis, pCO_2
and multiple birth deserve further attention.

6. REFERENCES

1. Bossi, E.; Koerner, F.: Patterns of simultaneously measured paO_2- and
   $paCO_2$-levels in newborns developing retinopathy of prematurity. Pediatr. Res. 19: 1128, A (1985)

2. Conover, W.J.: Practical nonparametric statistics. John Wiley and Sons,
   New York (1971).

3. Flury, B.: Frühgeborenen-Retinopathie: Gedanken zur Anwendung statis-
   tischer Methoden. In: F. Körner, E. Bossi (eds): Die Retinopathie des
   Frühgeborenen. Fischer, Stuttgart, New York, p. 201 (1984)

4. Koerner, F.; Bossi, E.; Wetzel, C.; Flury, B.: Retinopathy of prematurity: the influence of gestational age and retinal maturity on the

statistical behaviour of risk factors. Graefe's Arch.Clin.Exp.Ophthal-
mol. 224: 40 (1986)

5. Siegel, S.: Nonparametric statistics. McGraw-Hill, New York (1956)

6. Silverman, W.A.: Retrolental fibroplasia. A modern parable. Monographs
in neonatology, T.K. Oliver (ed) Grune and Stratton, New York (1980)

7. Wolbarsht, M.L.; Landers, M.B.III: The rationale of photocoagulation
therapy for proliferative diabetic retinopathy: a review and a model.
Ophthalmic Surg.11: 235 (1980)

RETINOPATHY OF PREMATURITY: AGE AT ONSET AND THE INITIAL SITE
OF RETINAL INVOLVEMENT.   A PRELIMINARY REPORT.

A. R. Fielder, Y. K. Ng, M. I. Levene and D. E. Shaw

INTRODUCTION
The postnatal age at which acute retinopathy of
prematurity (ROP) develops appears to be negatively related to
the gestational age of the infant (1).   Thus, the very small
premature infant develops ROP later postnatally than his
larger, more mature counterpart.   But, when the degree of
prematurity is corrected for, the first ophthalmoscopically
visible signs of acute ROP are seen over a relatively narrow
postmenstrual age range.   These findings suggest that the
onset of acute ROP is governed predominantly by the
postmenstrual age of the infant, rather than by events in the
neonatal period.   In other words, a certain stage of
development, probably at a retinal level, has to be reached
before ROP can develop.
In this article we present our preliminary findings of an
ongoing prospective study of ROP in the East Midlands of
England.   We will concentrate on two aspects: the age at which
acute ROP becomes ophthalmoscopically visible and the initial
site of retinal involvement.

PATIENTS AND METHODS
An ongoing prospective study into ROP in an area of the
East Midlands of England was started at the beginning of July
1985.   This area is served by five neonatal intensive care
units in the cities of Derby, Nottingham and Leicester.
All babies with birth weight ≼1700 gm irrespective of
oxygen treatment have been included.   Also included were twin
siblings of study babies.   Ophthalmological examinations
commenced in the third postnatal week and were performed
weekly, clinical condition permitting, until twelve weeks of
age.   Those infants discharged from hospital before this age
were seen as outpatients at two weekly intervals .   After this
age, follow-up was as clinically indicated, with a final
examination at the corrected age of six months.   All
ophthalmic examinations have been performed by ARF.   Pupils
were dilated with 0.5% cyclopentolate eye drops instilled 60
and 30 minutes before examination.   Topical anaesthetic
(oxybuprocaine 0.4%) was instilled immediately prior to the
examination by indirect ophthalmoscopy, using a 28 dioptre
lens, an eyelid speculum and scleral indentation.   Retinal
findings were recorded according to the International
Classification of Retinopathy of Prematurity (2), but in this

analysis neither the initial nor the peak stage of acute ROP has been reported.

For the purpose of this preliminary report, the criteria for inclusion were: ophthalmic examinations completed up to the age of eight weeks. However, babies who developed ROP before this time but with shorter periods of follow-up have also been included.

RESULTS

227 infants satisfied the selection criteria. Gestational ages ranged from 25.0 to 40.0 weeks (median 31.0 weeks). Seven infants with birth weights ⩾1700 gm were included as they were twins of study babies. Two of these developed ROP. No infant received vitamin E supplementation.

139 of 227 infants developed ROP, i.e. 61.2%. The median gestational ages of infants with ROP (139 infants) and without ROP (88 infants) were 30.0 and 32.0 weeks respectively (Mann-Whitney U test P <0.0001). Infants were divided into two groups according to their gestational age; <28 weeks (34 infants) and ⩾28 weeks (193 infants). Retinopathy developed in 32 of 34 <28 and 107 of 193 ⩾28 weeks. Broken down, according to gestational age, ROP was seen in: 32 of 34 infants <28 weeks; 53 of 70, 28-30 weeks; 38 of 77, 31-33 weeks, and 16 of 46, 34+ weeks gestational age.

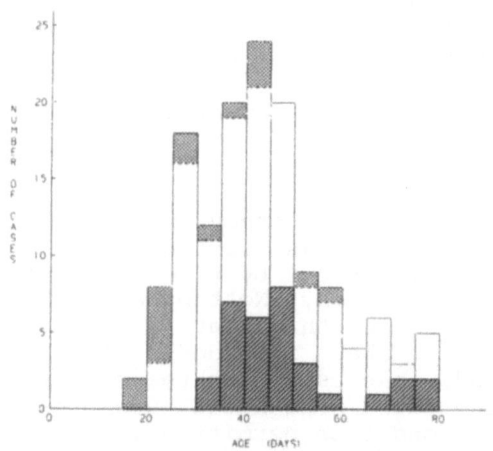

Figure 1. Postnatal age (in days) at the onset of ROP. Except for 15 babies, stippled areas (all ⩾28 weeks gestation), all had at least one normal eye examination prior to the onset of ROP. Hatched area denotes infants <28 weeks. *, one infant who did not develop ROP until 102 days of life.

The postnatal age at which ROP was first noted is shown in the frequency histogram (Fig. 1) and ranged from 18 to 102 days, median 42 days. 124 of the 139 affected infants had at least one normal ophthalmic examination prior to the development of

ROP, but in 15 (all with gestational ages >28 weeks) retinal changes were noted on the first examination (stippled areas at the top of the histograms in Fig.1). Infants with gestational ages <28 weeks developed ROP later than those ≥28 weeks (hatched areas at bottom of histograms in Fig. 1). The median postnatal age at onset for infants <28 weeks was 45 days and for those ≥28 weeks was 40 days, this difference being significant (Mann-Whitney U test P=0.013). The median postnatal age at onset of ROP in the temporal region of the retina for <28 and ≥28 weeks was 48 and 40 days respectively, this difference being significant (Mann-Whitney U test P=0.004).

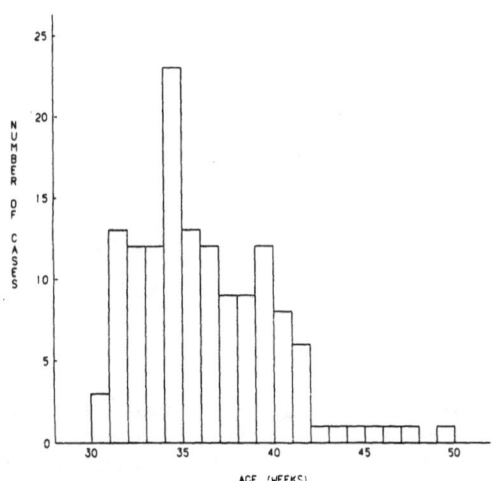

ACE (WEEKS)

Figure 2. Postmenstrual age (in weeks) at the onset of ROP. 75.5% ROP was first seen between 31.0 and 39.0 weeks and 83.4% between 31.0 and 40.0 weeks postmenstrual age. 19 of 20 infants with onset after 40.0 weeks had gestational ages ≥28 weeks.

The postmenstrual age at which ROP developed was calculated by adding the postnatal age at onset to the gestational age at birth and the results plotted as a histogram (Fig. 2). The postmenstrual age at onset ranged from 30.5 to 49.5 weeks, and in 20 infants this was after term. Of these 20, 19 had gestational ages ≥28 weeks, the one exception was an infant with a gestational age of 27 weeks who developed ROP at 41.5 weeks. 75.5% of all ROP was first observed between 31.0 and 39.0 weeks, and 83.4% between 31.0 and 40.0 weeks postmenstrual age.

The retinal region in which ophthalmoscopic signs were first observed in the 139 affected infants has been determined. This was nasal in 19, temporal in 80 and simultaneously in both nasal and temporal regions in 40 infants. These results have been further broken down according to gestational age (Fig. 3). The proportion of infants who developed ROP first

in either the nasal or simultaneously nasal and temporal
retinal regions, within each gestational grouping, was as
follows:- 25-27 weeks, 68.8%; 28-30 weeks, 41.5%; 31-33 weeks,
29.0%; 34 weeks and over, 25.0%. Infants with changes first
in the temporal region were, for the same groupings: 31.2%,
58.5%, 71.0% and 75.0%. Thus with increasing gestational age
there was an increasing tendency for the first signs of acute
ROP to involve the temporal retina.

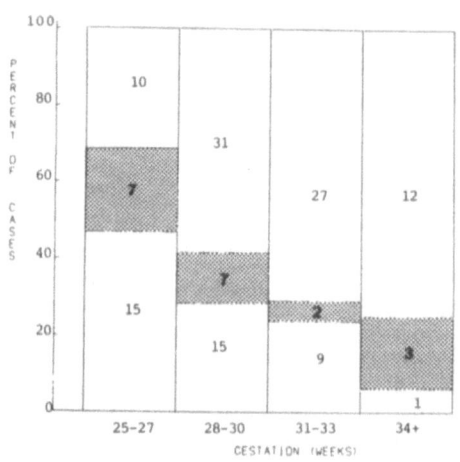

Figure 3. Gestational age and the initial retinal site
at the onset of ROP. Areas within each column denote the
retinal region first involved by acute ROP: top area =
temporal retina, stippled = nasal, bottom = nasal and temporal
regions involved simultaneously. Numbers in each section
indicate the number of cases and the y axis, the percentage.
Thus of 32 infants <28 weeks gestational age, the initial
retinal site was: temporal 10 infants (31.2%), nasal 7
(21.9%), nasal and temporal 15 (46.9%). For the other
gestational age groupings the corresponding figures were: 28-
30 weeks, 31 (58.5%), 7 (13.2%), 15 (28.3%); 31-33 weeks, 27
(71.0%), 2 (5.3%), 9 (23.7%); 34+ weeks, 12 (75.0%), 3(18.7%),
1 (6.2%).

DISCUSSION
    In this prospective study we have analysed both the age
at onset of acute ROP and the initial site of retinal
involvement. These results broadly confirm our previous
findings, obtained retrospectively, that the onset of acute
ROP is significantly later in infants born at <28 weeks
gestational age compared to those born at ≥28 weeks. In all
but 15 of 139 affected infants, eye examination had been
normal at least once before the onset of ROP. These 15
infants could have been omitted from analysis as the precise
time of onset is unknown. However, all 15 came from the ≥28
week group and for 9 of these the onset could be stated to be
25 days or less. As discussed previously (1) several studies

in the 1950's (3,4,5) reported later onset in smaller babies, but only Silverman and co-workers noted a negative correlation between the onset of retrolental fibroplasia and birth weight (3). As the premature population, methods of neonatal management and ophthalmological diagnostic criteria have all changed over the past 25 years, the results of early studies are not directly comparable to more recent reports.

Also as mentioned previously (1) there are inevitable inaccuracies in these data, both in the assessment of gestational age at birth and the identification of ocular signs. Ophthalmological examination in the very small preterm infant is potentially hazardous, the media are hazy and examinations are performed, in this study at least, only on a weekly basis on babies whilst on the neonatal unit and every fortnight after discharge from hospital. Despite these inaccuracies we consider that these results do indicate the time of onset of acute ROP as closely as is clinically possible. Another possible inaccuracy of our retrospective study (1) could have been failure to appreciate that ROP may first involve the nasal retina. Unfortunately it cannot be categorically stated that, in that study, the nasal retina was never identified as the initial site of ROP, but on the general assumption that this was the case, we have compared the age at onset for ROP in the temporal retina, in the present study, in infants <28 weeks and ⟩28 weeks gestational age. This difference was significant (P=0.004) and for the reasons stated may correlate more closely with our previous results (1). This particular aspect cannot be unravelled further but does indicate the need to carefully examine the entire retinal circumference, and the inadequacy of some previous classification schemes which stressed that the first signs of acute ROP were confined to the temporal retina (6,7).

The results of this study also confirm our previous retrospective observation (1) that acute ROP develops over a relatively narrow postmenstrual age range and although in the present prospective study, the data scatter is greater, this spread is at the upper end. This may be due to two factors; first and probably the most important, this scatter came from larger babies who were discharged to home very early on and would not have been identified in our previous study, which concentrated predominantly on infants whilst they were on the neonatal unit. Second, due to the two week delay in seeing these larger babies as outpatients, the time of diagnosis may be less precise.

Perhaps the most intriguing result of this survey is the finding that the first visible changes of acute ROP are not always in the temporal retina. For those infants with gestational ages of 25-27 or 28-30 weeks the likelihood of retinopathy developing first in the nasal retina, or simultaneously in both nasal and temporal regions is 68.8% and 41.5% respectively, whereas for those over 31 weeks this is approximately 28%. From another viewpoint, the likelihood of ROP being seen first in the temporal retina ranges from 31.2% at 25-27 weeks to 71.1%-75.0% after 31 weeks gestation. This aspect of ROP has received little attention apart from a number of anecdotal comments such as "can be present temporally, ---if not present temporally, it is usually not seen elsewhere" (8), or "the earliest signs of RLF are seen in the temporal periphery" (7). Patz in a review of retrolental fibroplasia (9) stated that "there is a predilection for RLF in the temporal periphery ---but with current paediatric practices, the changes are primarily confined but not always, to the temporal periphery". Similar comments were made by Biglan (10) and Kingham (6) who both noted that acute changes were usually in the temporal retina but could also sometimes be seen nasally. To the best of our knowledge this present investigation is the first in which the retinal region first involved by acute ROP has been systematically studied.

What are the implications of our findings? First; they indicate that nasal changes in acute ROP are common, particularly in the very small preterm infant and consequently during examination the entire retina should be examined. Secondly, whilst the pathogenesis of ROP remains a mystery and it is beyond the scope of this preliminary report to consider this subject in detail, a few points can be made. ROP is a condition of developing retinal vessels: the more premature the infant the less well developed will this vascular system be and the more posterior the signs of acute ROP (11). The incidence of ROP rises with decreasing gestational age; in this study retinopathy was seen in 94% of infants with gestational ages 25-27 weeks, 76% of infants in the 28-30 gestational age group and 35% in those born at 34 weeks and over. But there is a significant negative relationship between the onset of ROP and gestational age and this condition develops over a relatively narrow postmenstrual age range. This suggests that a certain stage of development has to be reached, probably at a retinal level, before the response can develop and this stage is achieved earlier by the nasal than the temporal regions of the retina. The upper postmenstrual age limit beyond which ROP cannot develop is not known precisely, and cannot be answered by this present study, but as the incidence of nasal changes falls with increasing gestational age, it is likely to be lower for the nasal than the temporal retina.

Acknowledgements

We are pleased to acknowledge the help and encouragement of paediatrician and nursing colleagues of the neonatal units of Leicester, Derby and Nottingham. Our thanks to Mrs. Marjorie Hopson who typed the manuscript. Dr. Y. K. Ng is supported by the Medical Research Council.

References
1 Fielder AR, Ng YK, Levene MI. Retinopathy of prematurity: age at onset. Arch Dis Child 1986: 61: 774-8
2 An international classification of retinopathy of prematurity. Br J Ophthalmol 1984: 68: 690-7
3 Silverman WA, Blodi FC, Locke JC, Day RL, Reese AB. Incidence of retrolental fibroplasia in a New York nursery. Arch Ophthalmol 1952: 48: 698-71

4   Report to the Medical Research Council by their council on
    retrolental fibroplasia. Retrolental fibroplasia in the
    United Kingdom. Br Med J 1955: ii: 78-82
5   Kinsey VE, Retrolental fibroplasia: cooperative study of
    retrolental fibroplasia and the use of oxygen.   Arch
    Ophthalmol 1956: 56: 481-529
6   Kingham   JD.   Acute   retrolental fibroplasia.   Arch
    Ophthalmol 1977: 95: 39-47
7   Keith CG. Retrolental fibroplasia, a new classification of
    the developing and cicatricial changes. Aust J Ophthalmol
    1979: 189-94
8   Flynn JT, O'Grady GE, Herrera J, Kushner BJ, Cantolino S,
    Milam   W.   Retrolental   fibroplasia.   1.   Clinical
    observations. Arch Ophthalmol 1977: 95: 217-223
9   Patz   A.   Retrolental fibroplasia (retinopathy of
    prematurity). Trans Ophthalmol Soc N.Z. 1980: 32: 49-54
10 Biglan AW.   Update on retrolental fibroplasia.   Trans PA
    Acad Ophthalmol Otolaryngol 1984: 37: 39-43
11 Flynn JT.   An international classification of retinopathy
    of prematurity: clinical experience.   Ophthalmology 1985:
    92: 987-994

RETINOPATHY OF PREMATURITY: TREATMENT APPROACHES

ARNALL PATZ, MD

Introduction

There has been a significant increase in the survival
of infants with birthweights up to 1500g since the original
epidemic of the Retinopathy of Prematurity (ROP) in the
early 1950's with a 4-5 fold increase in survival of
infants with birthweights less than 1000g, those with the
highest risk of developing ROP. The increased survival of
these high risk infants is probably responsible for the
significant increase in cases of ROP in recent years.

The new international classification of the acute
stages of ROP provides photographic standards and permits a
localization of the zone of the retina involved and the
extent of the changes in the fundus by the meridians
involved. The abnormal vascular changes in the new
international classification are divided into four stages
starting with the demarcation line in Stage I to retinal
detachment, stage 4. "Plus" disease represents a more
florid retinopathy. The photographic standards used in the
classification will foster the development of natural
history and collaboratiive therapeutic trials.

Current therapy and prophylaxis of acute ROP

Cryotheraphy and vitamin E prophylactic therapy have
been extensively investigated in recent years, but still
remain controversial at this time. Before discussing
cryotherapy, it is appropriate to mention briefly the use
of photocoagulation for ROP. Several investigators in
Japan and other countries noted that photocoagulation
appeared beneficial in treatment of the acute proliferative
stage of ROP, but treatment proved difficult in many cases
because of inadequate pupillary dilatation and vitreous
haze. Cryotherapy has gradually replaced photocoagulation.
Cryotherapy has frequently been used to treat the
neovascular ridge and the adjacent area anteriorly in an
ablative pattern. Several reports in this symposium have
provided additional information on the advantages and
limitations of this procedure.

As in most conditions where there is significant
spontaneous regression inherent in the natural history, a
large sample size and a randomized controlled treatment
protocol appear needed to document conclusively the role
of the therapy being employed. Because of the variation in
treatment methods and the lack of a standardized

classification it is impractical to combine the
cryotherapyresults from published reports and the careful
studies reported in this meeting.

A collaborative clinical trial testing cryotherapy has
been recently instituted in twenty-four centers in the
United States. Hopefully, by utilizing a standardized
protocol and the new international classification, this
prospective randomized and controlled study with the
inherent large sample size available can further define the
risks and benefits of cryotherapy.

Vitamin E and retinopathy of prematurity

There have been several controlled clinical trials
reported on the role of Vitamin E in the prevention of
ROP. An update on the Philadelphia study, the largest of
these trials, was presented in this symposium. The reader
is referred to the June 1986 publication of the Institute
of Medicine which provides an excellent summary of these
published studies. The Institute of Medicine's current
report provides the following conclusion and recommendation: "Vitamin E as prophylaxis for retinopathy of
prematurity was subject to a detailed analysis. This
committee found no conclusive evidence either of benefit or
harm from vitamin E administration. Risks from vitamin E
appear to be minimal for premature infants provided that
doses are kept moderate to achieve a blood level no higher
than 3 mg/dl."

Summary

Cryotherapy for acute proliferative ROP has been
evaluated by several investigators. Additional very useful
information was presented in this symposium. These pioneer
studies require further documentaton. A major
collaborative study now underway in the U.S. should provide
an adequate sample size in a randomized controlled study.
A recent review of Vitamin E studies for the prevention of
ROP indicates that its role is still controversial.

REFERENCES

1. Vitamin E and Retinopathy of Prematurity, Institute of
Medicine, Nat. Acad. Press: Washington, D.C., June 1986.

VITAMIN E AT PHARMACOLOGIC SERUM LEVELS AND INCIDENCE,
PROGRESSION AND CICATRICIAL RESIDUA OF RETINOPATHY OF
PREMATURITY

G. QUINN, L. JOHNSON, S. ABBASI, C. OTIS AND F. BOWEN

The purpose of this chapter is to present an overview of
our recent experience with vitamin E and ROP at University of
Pennsylvania. Our interest in the vitamin for the prevention
and treatment of retinopathy of prematurity (ROP) at
Pennsylvania Hospital goes back to the early 1970's when one of
us (LJ) began a randomized trial in premature infants with
birthweight (BW) $\leq$2000g of supplemental E to raise serum
levels to the physiologic range (target serum level 1.5mg/dl).
David Schaffer M.D. who had been doing ROP screening
examinations in the nursery at Pennsylvania Hospital since 1968
was masked from treatment group assignment as were the parents
and medical staff. The hypothesis which the protocol was
designed to test was based on the presence of E deficiency at
birth in premature infants and the fact that E is a potent
antioxidant which theoretically should act to decrease damage
from oxygen free radicals at several points on the pathway to
cicatricial disease (1).

After promising preliminary studies suggested a benefit on
incidence, severity and visual outcome from using the vitamin
at physiologic serum levels (1,2), a randomized, double blind
clinical trial was designed to look at several endpoints:
initiation of disease, progression of disease, and visual
outcome (both cicatricial disease at a one year examination and
visual acuity at 3 years). The goal of the study medication
(vitamin E free alcohol, Hoffman LaRoche) was to achieve and
maintain, by oral, intramuscular, and/or intravenous routes, a
serum level of 5mg/dl during the period of retinal vascular
immaturity or until the acute phase disease had regressed.
This target level was chosen because of encouraging results (2)
obtained with treatment at the diagnosis of severe ROP with
serum levels in this range (14 C, 10 E, p<0.02).

An ROP classification had been developed to include far
peripheral disease (3). After clarification of the contribution
of plus disease (4), this schema closely corresponded to the
International Classification of ROP published in 1984 (5). It
takes into account degree, extent and location of retinopathy
and the presence or absence of plus disease. For the purposes
of this presentation, ROP has been divided into categories of
increasing severity of ROP: mild (up to ridge without plus
disease), moderate (up to 2 quadrant extraretinal
neovascularization and/or plus disease in the presence of a

ridge) and severe (four quadrant extraretinal neovascularization and plus disease, grade 3+ ROP). This categorization
has been adopted by the Cryotherapy/ROP study group to record
incidence of ROP and to define prethreshold (moderate) and
threshold (5 or more clock hours of Grade 3+ROP) disease for
randomization to treatment (6,7).

914 premature infants were admitted and randomized within
4 BW groups of whom 545 were in the ≤1500g BW group. As
randomized to placebo (P) or vitamin E (E) treatment group, the
755 infants with complete acute phase data were closely matched
for demographic variables such as sex and race and for known
risk factors for ROP except as noted below. With ROP
categorized as none, mild, moderate and severe, a significant
difference between treatment groups was seen for the total
population. There was no difference for ROP as a yes/no
variable.

Fifty babies developed moderate to severe disease of whom
9 P and 3 E had severe ROP. More P than E infants had mild and
severe ROP but more E than P had no or moderate ROP (see Table
1). Significantly more placebo progressed from moderate to
severe disease then E treated infants.

TABLE 1. RETINOPATHY OF PREMATURITY INCIDENCE AND SEVERITY IN
INFANTS LESS THAN 1500G AT BIRTH WITH COMPLETE ACUTE PHASE DATA

	NO ROP	MILD ROP	MOD ROP*	SEV ROP*
PLACEBO (n)	107	84	16	9
VIT E (n)	113	70	22	3

MOD = MODERATE, SEV = SEVERE

Since, in our early work (1), almost all infants were
enrolled by 24 hours of age (mean age at entry 11.3 ± 10.4
hours), we looked at the prospectively recorded date of entry
to the study as a determinant of treatment effect. Other
investigators, notably Finer (8) and Hittner (9,10), have
emphasized that early administration of the vitamin might be
crucial in decreasing the overall incidence of disease.

Admission up to age 5 days was allowed in our clinical
trial so that most of the population at risk for ROP at the
three participating hospitals of the University of Pennsylvania
Neonatal Complex would be included. One of the hospitals
serves an entirely outborn population which is often
transported without family. If signed consent by age one day
had been required, important information on many infants would
have been lost. Overall 67.6% of infants were enrolled by age
1 day. For that hospital, only 47% were enrolled by age one
day. Early and late enrolled infants were not different with
regard to ROP risk factors at any of the hospitals.

Considering only infants enrolled by age one day, a beneficial effect of Vitamin E was seen on incidence of ROP as a yes/no variable in the clinically important ≤1500g BW group (p<0.05). Benefit was also seen in this BW group when ROP was categorized as none, mild, moderate, and severe (p<0.05).

Interpretation of an effect of vitamin E on cicatricial disease is complicated by a protocol which required discontinuation of study medication and treatment using E at pharmacologic serum levels at the diagnosis of severe disease. Therefore, to the extent that this treatment was effective, differences between treatment groups would be minimized. One P infant with severe disease treated in this manner with vitamin E had no visible residua at the one year follow-up examination; 2 had only peripheral scarring (grade 1 cic).

Cicatricial disease as seen at follow-up at age one year has been previously reported (11). Cicatricial sequelae were confined to infants with BW ≤1500g and were rare after mild disease. A total of 23 infants (11 P and 12 E) showed some degree of retinal residua at the one year examination. Among these, cicatricial disease, categorized as the presence or absence of macular heterotopia (grade 1 cic vs ≥ grade 2 cic in the worse eye), was more severe in placebo infants (p<0.02). 5 P vs 1 E had grade 3 cic or worse. Considering the population as a whole, which is essential when making recommendations for a prophylactic therapy, only a trend toward benefit is seen (11)

TABLE 2. GRADE OF CICATRICIAL DISEASE FOR EACH EYE OF THE PLACEBO (P) AND VITAMIN E (E) TREATED INFANTS

	A	B	C	D	E	F	G	H	I	J	K	L
						SUBJECT						
P-Rx												
OD	0	1	1	1	2	2	3	2	1	5	5	–
OS	1	1	1	2	1	2	1	3	5	1	5	–
E-Rx												
OD	1	1	1	1	1	1	1	1	1	1	2	3
OS	0	1	1	1	1	1	1	1	1	2	2	5

Three infants with severe ROP (2 P, 1 E) who died before age one year (ages 5,6, and 9 months) had clear cicatricial disease at an examination near the time of their death. Grade 1 cic was observed in two and grade 2 in the other. Cicatricial outcome was clear even though these infants did not survive to complete the one year study endpoint. They will, therefore, be included in the cicatricial disease data base for subsequent reports.

Since GQ joined this study group in 1978 , LJ and GQ have been particularly interested in plus disease as defined by rapid progression of retinopathy and dilation and tortuosity of posterior pole vasculature. In this study, which enrolled infants from 1979-1981 and followed them through a three year examination, there were 47 infants with plus disease. This accounted for almost all disease in the moderate ROP category and all in the severe. Progression to severe disease was more frequent in placebo treated infants (9 P, 3 E, $p<0.05$). Of infants with plus disease, 85% survived long enough for a cicatricial grading.

Three infants with mild ROP developed grade 1 cic at the one year examination. Otherwise, cicatricial residua were confined to infants with plus disease ($p<0.0001$), regardless of treatment group. There appears to have been an important decrease in severity of cicatricial disease in association with E treatment (see Table 2). Macular heterotopia or worse seemed to be more common in the placebo treatment group, while scarring confined to the periphery seemed to be more common in the E treatment group. However the number of infants with plus disease was small, even though 914 infants were enrolled. As mentioned above, treatment group differences were probably minimized because the protocol required intervention at the stage of severe ROP.

Regardless of the above, prophylactic vitamin E at pharmacologic serum levels cannot be recommended because a serious side effect was found to be associated with pharmacologic serum levels used from birth on. Among E treated infants there was an increased incidence of sepsis and late onset necrotizing enterocolitis (NEC) which is primarily of infectious etiology at this age. We believe this relates to decreased intraphagocytic killing of bacteria because of excessive free radical scavenging by vitamin E (12). The increased incidence of sepsis and NEC was seen only in infants $\leq1500g$ BW and was not associated with an increase in mortality.

TABLE 3. CASES OF CULTURE PROVEN NEONATAL SEPSIS AND NECROTIZING ENTEROCOLITIS IN INFANTS ON STUDY MEDICATION EIGHT DAYS OR MORE

	SEPSIS AND NEC*	SEPSIS	NEC	NEITHER
PLACEBO	4	18	18	192
VITAMIN E	4	40	32	155

$P<0.01$, * NEC and sepsis episodes are widely separated in time.

The E effect on progression of disease which was demonstrated in this study has considerable theoretical importance. It may also have clinical significance since the risk benefit ratio for treatment with pharmacologic serum levels once clinically significant disease has occurred is different from that for prophylaxis.

Risk factor analysis showed progression of disease to be highly correlated with degree of illness as reflected in the number of ventilator days, days of oxygen therapy, days in the hospital, and measured exposure to hypoxia, hypercarbia and

hyperoxia during the period of indwelling arterial lines.
Since significant hypoxia and hyperoxia both result in
increased production of oxidant radicals and ROP appears to
reflect neonatal as well as perinatal events, then the free
radical quenching ability of vitamin E may offer an important
additional treatment option, especially in the case of Zone I
disease ("rush" type) (13). In any event, an E related
decrease in progression of plus disease and its residua
supports the concept that oxidant damage is involved in the
initiation, progression and scarring phases of ROP.

ACKNOWLEDGEMENTS: The authors would like to thank
David Schaffer M.D. for reviewing the manuscript and making
helpful suggestions.

REFERENCES

1. Johnson L, Shaffer DB, Boggs TR. Vitamin E deficiency and
    retrolental fibroplasia. Am J Clin Nutr. 1974;27:1158-73.
2. Johnson L, Schaffer D, Quinn G, et al. Vitamin E
    Supplementation and the retinopathy of prematurity. Ann NY
    Acad Sci. 1982;393:473-95.
3. Schaffer DB, Johnson L, Quinn G, Boggs TR. A classification
    of retrolental fibroplasia to evaluate vitamin E therapy.
    Ophthalmol.1979;86:1749-60.
4. Quinn GE, Schaffer DB, Johnson L. A revised classification
    of retinopathy of prematurity. Am J Ophthalmol. 1982;94:
    744-49.
5. The Committee for the Classification of Retinopathy of
    Prematurity. An international classification of retinopathy
    of prematurity. Arch Ophthalmol.1984;102:1130-1135.
6. Manual of procedure: Muliticenter cryotherapy for
    retinopathy of prematurity, funded by National Institute of
    Health grant EY 06315-02.
7. Palmer EA, Biglan AW, Hardy RJ. Retinal ablative therapy
    for active retinopathy of prematurity: History, current
    status and prospects. In: Retinopathy of Prematurity,
    Silverman WA and Flynn JT, eds. Blackwell Scientific
    Publications, Inc. Boston, Mass.
8. Finer NN, Schindler RF, Grant G, et al. Effect of intra-
    muscular vitamin E on frequency and severity of retrolental
    fibroplasia; a controlled trial. Lancet. 1982;1:1087-91.
9. Hittner HM, Godio LB, Rudolph AJ, et al. Retrolental fibro-
    plasia: efficacy of vitamin E in a double-blind clinical
    study of preterm infants. N Engl J Med. 1981;305:1365-71.
10. Hittner HM, Speer ME, Rudolph AJ, et al. Retrolental
    fibroplasia and vitamin E in the preterm infant-Comparison
    of oral versus intramuscular:Oral administration.
    Pediatrics. 1984;73:238-49.
11. Schaffer DB, Johnson L, Quinn GE, Weston M, Bowen FW.
    Vitamin E and retinopathy of prematurity. Follow-up at one
    year. Ophthalmol. 1985;92:1005-11.

12. Johnson L, Bowen FW, Abbasi A, et al:Relationship of
    prolonged pharmacologic serum levels of vitamin E to
    incidence of sepsis and necrotizing enterocolitis in
    infants with birth weight 1,500 grams or less. Pediatrics
    1985;75:619-38.
13. Uemura Y. Current status of retrolental fibroplasia.
    Japanese J Ophthalmol. 1977;21:366-378.

DOES VITAMIN E HAVE A PROTECTIVE ROLE IN THE RETINA AS AN ANTI-OXIDANT AND
FREE RADICAL SCAVENGER?

E.R. BERMAN

Vitamin E (α-tocopherol) and/or lipid peroxidation have long been implicated in the pathogenesis of a broad range of human diseases, some of
which are listed in Table 1. The relatively large number and variety of
ocular disorders included in this listing may not be entirely fortuitous
since most ocular tissues are either highly oxygenated and/or exposed to
varying intensities of light. Both of these factors are the principal
known predisposing conditions in the initiation of free radical-induced
lipid peroxidation. The common denominator in this wide variety of disorders may be related to the principal known biological function of vitamin E, namely a free radical scavenger that protects cell membranes from
damage caused by lipid peroxidation. The clinical expression of oxidative
damage is highly variable since these disorders bear little similarity to
one another.

TABLE 1. Human disorders in which vitamin E and/or lipid
peroxidation may be involved

Generalized neuromuscular disorders
    Abetalipoproteinemia
    Cystic fibrosis

Ocular disorders
    Cataract
    Ocular inflammation
    Photic retinopathy
    Retinopathy of prematurity (ROP)
    Ocular siderosis
    Senile macular degeneration (SMD)

Lipid peroxidation is not spontaneous; it is initiated by free radicals
that are present at low concentration in virtually all oxygenated cells.
A brief review will be given of current thinking on how these free radicals
are produced under normal physiological conditions, and how vitamin E is
believed to modulate lipid peroxidation in biological membranes (the so-
called antioxidant effect of vitamin E).

Endogenous generation of free radicals

As shown in Fig. 1, the key "substrates" for free radical production are
polyunsaturated fatty acids (PUFA) which are the principal (if not only)
molecules susceptible to peroxidation. These fatty acids are not in the
free state in biological membranes, rather they are for the most part in

a bound (esterified) form, as components of complex lipids such as phospholipids and neutral lipids. Peroxidation of the polyunsaturated fatty acids is initiated when a free radical (e.g., superoxide anion $[O_2^-]$) attacks a lipid PUFA and abstracts the allylic hydrogen atom (Fig. 1). This causes a rearrangement of the unsaturated double bonds to a form called a conjugated diene, which itself is a free radical ($[L\cdot]$ in Step 1 of Fig. 1).

At this point, the important question arises: where do the free radicals (superoxide anions) come from in the first place? A complete explanation is beyond the scope of the present discussion, but the principal sources of free radicals may be summarized as follows: (a) xenobiotics, i.e. toxins such as tar, singlet oxygen, benzo $[\alpha]$ pyrene, etc., and (b) intracellular enzymatic one-electron reduction of oxygen, a process which occurs normally in almost all aerobic cells. Considering the one-electron reduction of oxygen (which is probably the main source of free radicals), one of the products known to be produced is superoxide anion $[O_2^-]$. This highly reactive species is partially destroyed, i.e. converted to H_2O_2, by a very well known enzyme, superoxide dismutase (SOD). This reaction was first described by Fridovich and coworkers more than a decade ago (1,2), and has since been confirmed in many other laboratories. However, SOD in many cases does not destroy all of the $[O_2^-]$ produced in the cell; some of this free radical, albeit in very low concentrations, remains unchanged and in this highly reactive form is able to attack directly the PUFA molecules in the cell membranes. The retinal photoreceptors are especially vulnerable to attack by free radicals because of their high content (40-50%) of a highly unsaturated fatty acid, docosahexaenoate (22:6).

Once the free radical attack on a PUFA occurs and another free radical $[L\cdot]$ is formed, the next step, in the presence of oxygen at concentrations as low as 10^{-4} M, is rapid. It should be noted that this is the concentration of dissolved O_2 in aqueous media under normal atmospheric pressure. As shown in Fig. 1, the free radical formed in the presence of O_2 is a lipid peroxide ($[LOO\cdot]$), which then interacts with another molecule of PUFA (LH). This is the chain-propagating step, the sine qua non of lipid peroxidation; if there were no autooxidative chain reaction, lipid peroxidation would stop after only one hypothetical molecule of PUFA (LH) had been oxidized, a condition which could never cause measurable membrane damage. Lipid hydroperoxides, as shown in Fig. 1, can either be converted to harmless hydroxy fatty acids by the Se-containing enzyme, glutathione peroxidase, or can interact with free radicals in the biological membrane ($[L\cdot]$ or $[LOO\cdot]$), ensuring a continued chain reaction, especially if metal cations such as Fe^{2+} are present. It is in this part of the autooxidative chain reaction that Vitamin E is thought to act, by scavenging free radicals, and thus interrupting the continued production of the radicals from PUFA molecules.

There is extensive experimental evidence, both in vivo and in vitro, supporting the above concept. Photoreceptor damage and ERG disturbances can be demonstrated as a consequence of lipid peroxidation induced either by oxygen (3), light (4,5) or vitamin E deficiency (6). The latter manifests itself as a dramatic accumulation of lipofuscin in the pigment epithelium of experimental animals (7,8). These and other aspects of oxygen toxicity have been previously discussed by Feeney-Burns and Berman (9,10).

Retinopathy of prematurity

Turning to retinopathy of prematurity (ROP), the deleterious effects of oxygen (11,12) have been known for more than a quarter of a century; how unfortunate that the observations of Owens and Owens (13) many years ago,

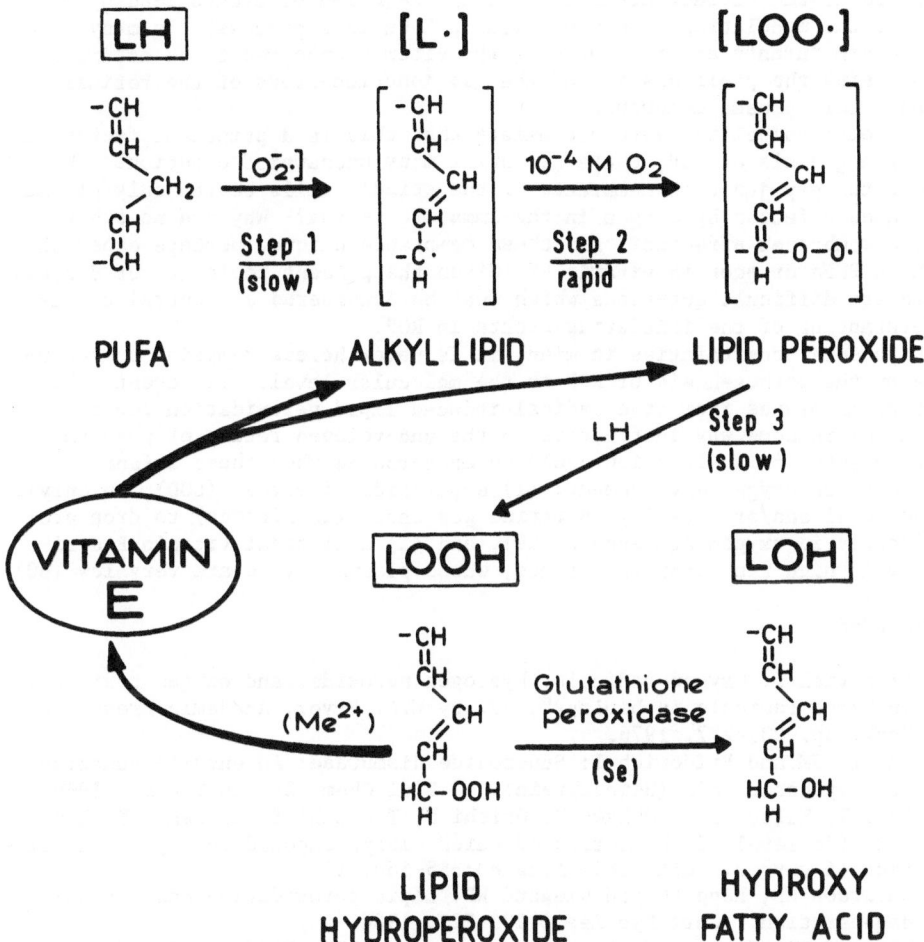

FIGURE 1. Abbreviated scheme of autooxidative chain reaction for lipids, showing initiation by superoxide anion (step 1), propagation (steps 2 and 3) and termination either by the action of Se-glutathione peroxidase or by the intervention of vitamin E.

on the decreased severity of ROP in preterm infants receiving vitamin E supplementation, went largely unnoticed! It was not until the 1970s that two unrelated events occurred: (a) there was a renewed interest in the role of vitamin E as a free radical scavenger in biological systems in general and (b) there was a striking resurgence of ROP owing to the increased number of very-low-birth-weight (VLBW) infants born and surviving. These events led to a reexamination of the possible therapeutic benefits of vitamin E with, for the most part, encouraging results from Johnson and coworkers (14-18) and other investigators (19-22), although less positive results have recently been reported by Bremer et al (23). Hittner, Kretzer and their coworkers (24-28) have confirmed the beneficial effects of vitamin E therapy in minimizing the severity of ROP and, most importantly, observed at the ultrastructural level the sequelae of events leading to ROP and the modulating effect of vitamin E on this process. In many cases of preterm infants at risk for ROP, the vitamin appeared to be acting by suppressing the proliferation of the gap junction areas of the retinal spindle cell plasma membranes.

Although compelling evidence exists that this is a principal factor in the pathogenesis of ROP, there are still many unanswered questions. Why should the gap junction membranes of the spindle cells be the only plasma membranes affected by oxygen in the immature retina? Why are no other plasma membranes affected? Are these membranes unique, perhaps especially rich in PUFA or poor in vitamin E? Given the present tools at our disposal, these are difficult questions which must be considered as central to our understanding of the initiating events in ROP.

With some uncertainties in mind, it is nevertheless tempting to specu-late on the pathogenesis of ROP at the molecular level. Two agents that protect membranes from free radical-induced lipid peroxidation could be absent or in some way ineffective in the undeveloped retina of preterm VLBW infants; this situation could be exacerbated when these infants are placed in an oxygen environment: (1) superoxide dismutase (SOD), an enzyme whose level and/or activity in retina was shown (in kittens) to drop pre-cipitously in oxygen atmosphere (29), and (2) a clinical vitamin E defi-ciency in high risk preterm infants, whose plasma levels are very low (30).

REFERENCES

1. Fridovich I: Oxygen radicals, hydrogen peroxide, and oxygen toxicity. In "Free radicals in biology", ed. by W.A. Pryor, Academic Press, New York, pp. 239-277, 1976.
2. McCord JM and Fridovich I: Superoxide dismutase: An enzymic function for erythrocuprein (Hemocuprein). J Biol Chem, 244:6049-6055, 1969.
3. Yagi K, Matsuoka S, Ohkawa H, Ohishi N, Takeuchi Y and Sakai H: Lipo-peroxide level of the retina of chick embryo exposed to high concentra-tion of oxygen. Clin Chim Acta 80:355-360, 1977.
4. Anderson RE, Rapp LM and Wiegand RD: Lipid peroxidation and retinal degeneration. Curr Eye Res 3:223-227, 1984.
5. Wiegand RD, Giusto NM, Rapp LM and Anderson RE: Evidence for rod outer segment lipid peroxidation following constant illumination of the rat retina. Invest Ophthalm Vis Sci 24:1433-1435, 1983.
6. Amemiya T: Effect of vitamin E administration on photoreceptor outer segment and retinal pigment epithelium of vitamin E deficient rats. Int J Vit Nutr Res 51:114-118, 1981.
7. Katz ML, Stone WL and Dratz EA: Fluorescent pigment accumulation in retinal pigment epithelium of antioxidant deficient rats. Invest Ophthalm Vis Sci 17:1049-1058, 1978.
8. Robison WG Jr, Kuwabara T and Bieri JG: Deficiencies of vitamin E and A in the rat. Retinal damage and lipofuscin accumulation. Invest Ophthalm Vis Sci 19:1030-1037, 1980.
9. Feeney L and Berman ER: Oxygen toxicity: Membrane damage by free ra-dicals. (Editorial on Recent Advances). Invest Ophthal 15:789-792 1976.
10. Feeney-Burns L, Berman ER and Rothman H: Lipofuscin of human retinal pigment epithelium. Amer J Ophthal 90:783-791, 1980.
11. Ashton N, Ward B and Serpell G: Role of oxygen in the genesis of retro-lental fibroplasia. Br J Ophthalmol 37:513, 1953.

167

12. Patz A, Eastham A, Higgenbotham MS and Kleh T: Oxygen studies in retrolental fibroplasia. II. The production of the microscopic changes of retrolental fibroplasia in experimental animals. Am J Ophthalmol 36:1511, 1953.
13. Owens WC and Owens EU: Retrolental fibroplasia in premature infants. II. Studies on the prophylaxis of the disease: The use of alpha tocopheryl acetate. Amer J Ophthalmol 32:1631, 1949.
14. Johnson L, Schaffer D and Boggs TR: The premature infant, vitamin E deficiency and retrolental fibroplasia. Am J Clin Nutr 27:1158-1173, 1974.
15. Johnson LH, Schaffer DB, Rubinstein D,et al: The role of vitamin E in retrolental fibroplasia. I. Pediatr Res 10:425, 1976.
16. Johnson LH, Shaffer DB, Goldstein DE,et al: Influence of vitamin E treatment and adult blood transfusions on mean severity of retrolental fibroplasia in premature infants. Pediatr Res 11:535, 1977.
17. Johnson L, Schaffer D, Boggs T,et al: Vitamin E treatment of retrolental fibroplasia (RLF) grade III or worse. Pediatr Res 14:601, 1980.
18. Johnson L, Schaffer D, Quinn G, et al: Vitamin E supplementation and the retinopathy of prematurity. Annals New York Acad Sci 393:473-495, 1982.
19. Finer NN, Grant G, Schindler RF, et al: Effect of intramuscular vitamin E on frequency and severity of retrolental fibroplasia: A controlled trial. Lancet 1:1087-1091, 1982.
20. Puklin JE, Simon RM and Ehrenkranz RA: Influence on retrolental fibroplasia of intramuscular vitamin E administration during respiratory distress syndrome. Ophthalmology 89:96-102, 1982.
21. Phelps DL and Rosenbaum AL: Vitamin E in kitten oxygen-induced retinopathy: II. Blockage of vitreal neovascularization. Arch Ophthalmol 97:1522-1526, 1979.
22. Phelps DL: Vitamin E and retrolental fibroplasia in 1982. Pediatrics 70:420-425, 1982.
23. Bremer DL, Rogers GL, Bell H and Lytle R: The efficacy of vitamin E in retinopathy of prematurity. J Pediat Ophthal & Strab 23:132-136, 1986
24. Hittner HM, Godio LB, Rudolph AJ, et al: Retrolental fibroplasia: efficacy of vitamin E in a double-blind clinical study of preterm infants. N Engl J Med 305:1365-1371, 1981.
25. Hittner HM, Godio LB, Speer ME, et al: Retrolental fibroplasia: Further clinical evidence and ultrastructural support for efficacy of vitamin E in the preterm infant. Pediatrics 71:423-432, 1983.
26. Kretzer FL, Mehta RS, Johnson AT, et al: Vitamin E protects against retinopathy of prematurity through action on spindle cells. Nature 309:793-795, 1984.
27. Kretzer FL, Hittner HM, Johnson AT, et al: Vitamin E and retrolental fibroplasia: Ultrastructural support of clinical efficacy. Annals New York Acad Sci 393:145-166, 1982.
28. Hittner HM and Kretzer FL: Vitamin E and retrolental fibroplasia: Ultrastructural mechanism of clinical efficacy. Biology of Vitamin E, Pitman, London, pp. 165-185, 1983.
29. Bougle D, Vert P, Reichart E, et al: Retinal superoxide dismutase activity in newborn kittens exposed to normobaric hyperoxia: Effect of vitamin E. Pediatr Res 16:400-402, 1982.
30. Farell PM: Vitamin E deficiency in premature infants. J Pediatr 95:869-872, 1979.

RETINOPATHY OF PREMATURITY, PAST AND RECENT EXPERIENCE IN DENMARK

HANS C. FLEDELIUS AND SVEND ERIK HANSEN

The presentation deals with two aspects of retinopathy of prematurity (ROP) pertaining to quite different parts of the disease spectrum.

First a survey is given of severe visual handicap due to retrolental fibroplasia (RLF), the cicatricial sequel to progressive ROP. Apparently, Denmark is one of the very few countries with a valid compulsory nationwide registration of visual handicap in children. Further, diagnostic dropouts are unlikely, due to the organization of the Danish Health system. Therefore, solid epidemiological facts can be presented, and not merely deductions from neonatal center reports (cf. Phelps 1979), implying selected or sporadic material.

Next, experience with the new international ROP classification is reported, analysing all low birth weight children seen by the paediatric ophthalmologist serving the neonatal department of a Danish county hospital. This way an epidemiological small-scale survey - considered complete, however - is obtained regarding early retinal changes in prematures at risk, born 1982-84.

Visual handicap due to RLF in Denmark 1948-85

Fig. 1 shows the annual number of Danish children registered as having significant visual handicap due to RLF, from the first known case with birthyear 1948 till now. The graph comprises children with a corrected visual acuity of 6/18 (0.3) or less at their disposal. - Obviously, we are dealing with minimum figures for the last two years, since there is no guarantee of all recent cases having been recorded yet.

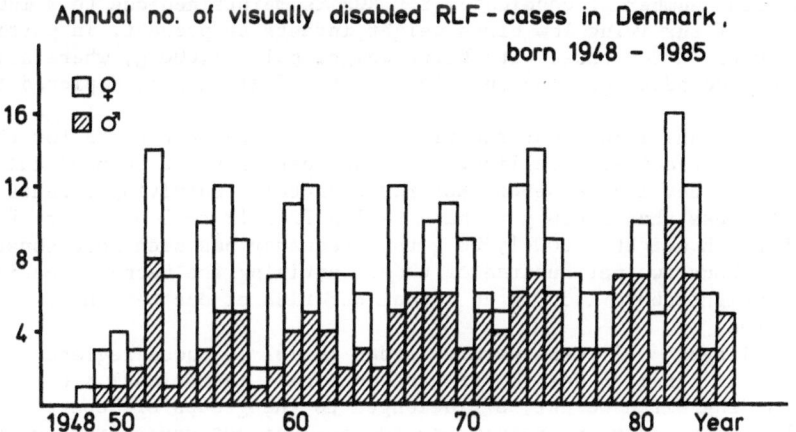

Fig. 1. Danish RLF statistics 1948-85, comprising all cases registered due to significant visual handicap.

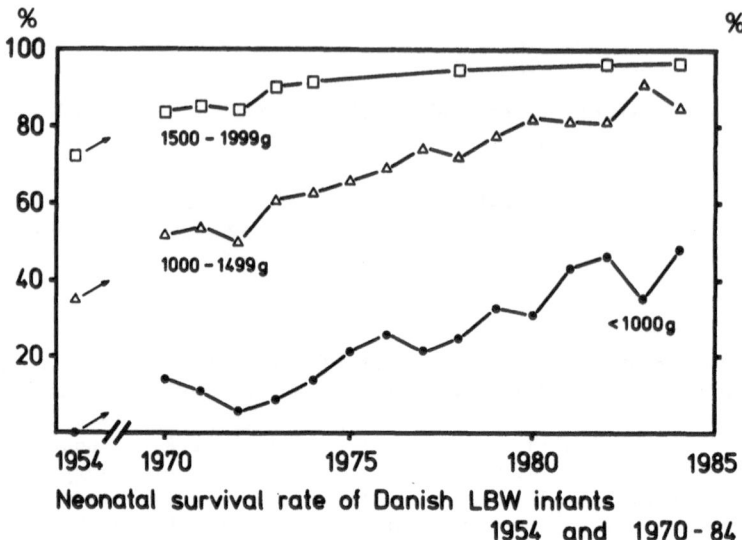

Fig. 2. Diagram illustrating the improvement in neonatal survival rate
(in %) for various birth weight groups in Denmark 1970–84, with the
year of 1954 serving as reference.

The profile of the graph suggests a slight increase in annual number of
visually disabling RLF. In a five million population we are now expecting
8–10 cases a year. Over the same period we have faced a significant decline in birth rate, from about 80,000 to 52,000 liveborn a year. A direct
comparison of these figures indicates an alarming increase in the frequency of RLF with visual handicap, from about 9 per 100,000 liveborn to about
the double value.

This may seem paradoxical, because all other parameters of perinatal
health care have indicated increasing efficiency. At the same time, however,
this is the key to the paradox. Stillbirth rate and neonatal mortality rate
have been reduced so markedly that, in spite of the falling birth rate, a
rather constant number of candidates for ROP is maintained due to a much
higher share of surviving low birth weight infants at present. In particular, this is valid for those with birth weight below 1,000 g, where almost
all died some decades ago. The numerical state of affairs is depicted in
Fig. 2 and 3.

It is worth emphasizing that the risk of developing severe RLF for those
mostly at risk is actually falling. Over the last 15 years we have calculated the risk of developing severe RLF for neonatally surviving infants with
birth weight less than 1,000 g to have fallen from 13 to 3 per cent. For
those with birth weight 1,000–1,500 g the frequency has been more constant,
fluctuating about two per hundred of those surviving the neonatal period.
With birth weight above 1,500 g an actual RLF risk of one per thousand has
been estimated.

Gestational ages < 31 weeks were recorded in 73% of those registered because of visual handicap due to RLF, and none had gestational age above 36
weeks. Regarding birth weight, 87% belonged to the groups of less than
1,500 g, both data sets pertaining to the analysis of cases from the recent 15 years. Going longer back in time, gestational age estimates were

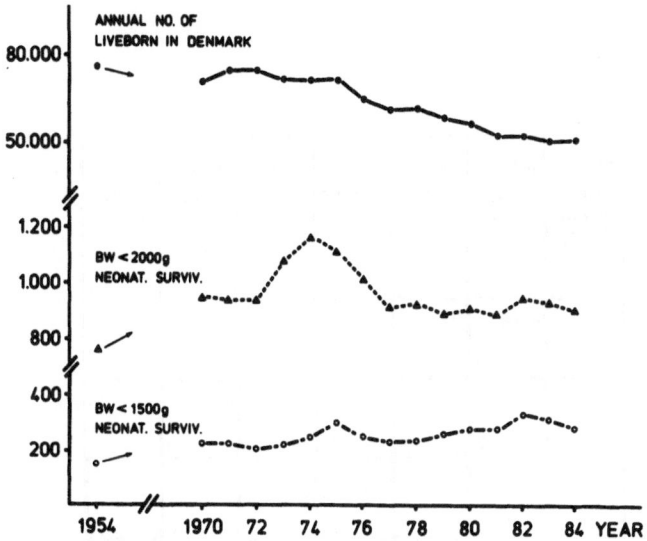

Fig. 3. Annual number of liveborn in Denmark (for the same years as in Fig.
2, at top) and actual number of low birth weight infants surviving
the neonatal period, with 2,000 g as upper limit (in the middle)
and with 1,500 g as upper limit (at bottom).

available only occasionally. Birth weight data from earlier RLF victims,
however, showed distributions almost as now, except that fewer with extremely low birth weight survived at that time.

Survival statistics may also have relevance for the changes in sex ratio
apparent from the Danish RLF sample. From the first part of the period, only 40% of those registered were boys, possibly to be explained by the higher mortality of the male sex, leaving relatively fewer boys as candidates
for developing RLF. At present, boys make up 60% of the registered RLF-ca-
ses, a shift that is statistically significant. Probably this is due to increased survival rate of fragile boys. A parallel indicator is provided by
the birth weight distribution of RLF children according to sex. Considering
birth weight groups above 1,250 g a significant predominance of the male
sex indicates survival of boys that had probably died in an earlier era.
Below the birth weight limit of 1,250 g the two sexes appeared equally frequent.

Finally a remark about degree of visual handicap in the registered RLF
group. Two thirds had no or doubtful light sense, and only 27% belonged to
the best group, i.e. those registered as weaksighted (corrected visual acuity between 0.1 and 0.3). Indeed those visually impaired by RLF constitute a heavy group. Otherwise childhood visual handicap in Denmark is characterized by 2/3 belonging to the weaksighted subgroup.

Retinopathy of prematurity in a Danish County Hospital 1982-84

From the discussions held in the international ROP classification workshop I adjusted my examining routines as paediatric ophthalmologist in an
800-bed regional hospital serving a population of 350,000. The neonatal
unit of the paediatric department takes care of those prematurely born, but
very frail and ill neonates are transferred to the University Center of
nearby Copenhagen. When the need of specialized treatment is over, the in-

	BW ≤1000g	1001– 1250	1251– 1500	1501– 1750	1751– 2000	2001– 2500	2501– 3000
GA ≤28 W	♂♂♂♀ 5	■♂■♂ 7	♀ 1				
29 – 30		■♂♂♀ 9	♂♀ 5	■♂♀ 4	1		
31 – 32		♀♀ 2	■♀ 8	♂ 11	15	♂ 3	
33 – 34		4	5	♀♀ 15	♂♀ 22	16	1
35 – 36		1	4	♂ 7	●♂ 7	18	5
37 – 38				1	4		

Fig. 4. The 1982–84 sample of premature infants of Frederiksborg County, examined at Hillerød Central Hospital for ROP. Open circles = ROP with regression. Filled circles = ROP leaving myopia of prematurity. Filled squares = ROP having progressed to RLF.

fants are returned to the county department. This implies that eventually I examine all neonates at risk of developing ROP. All infants with birth weight < 2,000 g and/or gestational age < 36 weeks are eye-examined from the age of one month, plus bigger infants who had oxygen treatment for respiratory trouble. All cases have been followed till the age of 4-6 months.

The results are condensed in Fig. 4, a diagram showing 185 infants born 1982-84, subdivided by birth weight and gestational age. The number of infants belonging to each subgroup is shown in the lower right corner. 28 (15%) showed ROP changes, however with regression in 24; five of these had developed myopia of prematurity, a state compatible with normal visual acuity later on. In four the ROP progressed to severe RLF, with blindness of both eyes. Three of the 4 were boys; birth weights ranged from 1,100 to 1,520 g, gestational ages from 29 to 31 weeks.

The diagram allows calculation of retinal morbidity risk in various subgroups. For gestational age ≤ 30 weeks ROP thus appeared in 44%. For birth weights ≤ 1,250 g the corresponding figure was 38%. By increasing gestational age and birth weight the ROP incidence was falling throughout.

As for sex, 17 out of the 28 with ROP were boys. Clinically, the ROP-group was loaded according to several parameters, e.g. prolonged oxygen treatment, severe anaemia/blood transfusions, and convulsions in the first weeks of life.

Comments

Regarding the ROP analysis 1982-84, four cases of blindness due to RLF appears a high number for one county, but so far they have not been followed by new cases in 1985-86.

Regarding treatment our attitude has been conservative. Two of the blind children had been treated with cryotherapy and cerclage operation, without improvement, however. We are still waiting for large controlled treatment series with significant documentation of therapeutic efficiency.

The above figures illustrate that it is difficult for a small nation to provide sufficient material for evaluating treatment modalities in an eye disease with a marked tendency of spontaneous regression, unless the efforts are concentrated in a few neonatal units with a high number of infants. And even then, a 5 million population with a low birth rate may prove too small. - This is also the reason for the focussing on the nationwide RLF-statistics in the first part of the above presentation. Obviously, epidemiological research of this kind is best performed in a small country with a stable population, an effective registration of all citizens, and free access to hospital facilities.

REFERENCES

1. Fledelius H (1976): Prematurity and the eye. Acta Ophthalmol (Copenh) Suppl 128
2. Holm E (1949): Retinopathia praematurorum. Acta Ophthalmol (Copenh) 27, 623-31
3. International classification of retinopathy of prematurity, prepared by an international committee (1984) Brit J Ophthalmol 68, 690-697
4. Phelps DL (1979)Retinopathy of prematurity. An estimate of vision loss in the United States. Pediatrics 67, 924-25
5. Seedorff T (1968): Retrolental fibroplasia. Acta Ophthalmol (Copenh) 46, 500-506

"RUSH TYPE" RETINOPATHY OF PREMATURITY (ROP) - A REPORT OF
THREE CASES

I. BEN-SIRA, I. NISSENKORN, I. KREMER, S. COHEN

"Rush type" ROP is characterized by markedly dilated and
tortuous vessels in the posterior pole and limited vascularization of the retina in an area corresponding to Zone I-II
according to the International Classification of Retinopathy
of Prematurity (1). It takes a rapid course within the first
month of life and appears only in infants of extremely low
birth weight (2-5).

The fibrovascular proliferation (FVP) involves the entire
circumference of the posterior retina and in most cases
retinal detachment develops within a short period from the
onset of retinopathic changes, without progressing through
sequential stages of ROP (2-5).

We present three infants with "Rush type" ROP in whom
treatment by cryoablation and photocoagulation yielded good
results.

CASE REPORTS

Case 1 - a female infant born in the 26th week of gestation
with a birth weight of 950 gr. Assisted ventilation was
started with 100% oxygen and continued for 3 weeks. PO_2
was maintained between 50-70 mm Hg.
Eye examination at four weeks revealed congestion of iris
vessels and rigidity of pupils. Fundus examination showed
360° of severe ROP, Stage III, in Zone I in both eyes.
Under general anesthesia a conjunctival incision of 3-4 mm
was made in each quadrant and a cataract cryoprobe was
inserted into each incision well behind the equator. Cryoablation of the avascular retina was performed through 360°.
The avascular retina close to the macula was photocoagulated
with xenon light photocoagulation because the inferior
oblique muscle interfered with the cryoprobe.
Twenty four hours after the procedure the iris vessels were
less engorged, the pupils were less rigid and the FVP had
begun to disappear. Three weeks later a progression of the
retinal vessels between the cryoablation scars was observed.

Case 2 - a male born in the 26th week of gestation with a birth weight of 800 gr. Assisted ventilation was started because of respiratory distress syndrome. PO2 ranged between 50-70 mm Hg. Oxygen was given for ten days.

Eye examination at four weeks showed pupillary rigidity and engorgement of iris vessels. Fundus examination showed severe active ROP, Stage III, in Zone I-II, 360°, similar in both eyes.

Under local anesthesia with oxybuprocaine 0.4% and four injections of lignocaine 2% into the subtenon space, cryoablation was performed on the avascular retina anterior to the FVP. The technique of treatment was similar to that used in Case No. 1.

Two weeks after cryoablation there was a disappearance of all signs of "plus" disease. Two weeks later there was a resolution of all the FVP.

Case 3 - a female infant born in the 26th week of gestation with a birth weight of 870 gr. Assisted ventilation was given for 12 days. PO2 was in the range of 70 mm Hg.

Fundus examination at the age of five weeks showed severe active ROP, Stage III, 360°, with signs of "plus" disease in the anterior segment and fundus in both eyes.

Following local anesthesia as in Case 2, cryoablation was performed on the avascular retina, 360°. One week later there was a disappearance of all signs of "plus" disease. Two to three weeks later there was a regression of FVP.

COMMENT

Treatment of such small babies weighing less than 1000 gr who require oxygen and whose general condition is unstable is particularly difficult and a neonatologist should be in attendance throughout the procedure (6,7).
Particular care should be taken not to press too vigorously on the eye during cryoablation and to keep the central retinal artery under continuous observation (5).

In conclusion we should like to stress the importance of ophthalmological examination in premature infants from the age of three weeks and prompt initiation of treatment when Stage III ROP is diagnosed (2,3,5,8-11).

REFERENCES

1. Committee for the classification of retinopathy of prematurity. An International Classification of Retinopathy of Prematurity. Arch Ophthalmol 102:1130-35, 1984.
2. Yamashita Y: Studies on retinopathy of prematurity. III. Cryocautery for retinopathy of prematurity. Jpn J Clin Ophthalmology 26:385-93, 1972.
3. Nissenkorn I, Kremer I, Gilad E, et al: "Rush type" retinopathy of prematurity, a report of three cases. Brit J Ophthalmology (in press)
4. Majima A: Studies on retinopathy of prematurity. I. Statistical analysis of factors related to occurrence and progression in active phase. Jpn J Ophthalmol 21:404-20, 1977.
5. Tasman W: Zone I retinopathy of prematurity. Arch Ophthalmol 103:1693-4, 1985.
6. Clark WN, Hodges E, Noel LP, et al: The oculocardiac reflex during ophthalmoscopy in premature infants. Am J Ophthalmol 99:649-51, 1985.
7. Frishberg Y, Amir J, Nissenkorn I, Ben-Sira I, et al: Severe bradycardia and nodal rhythm complicating cryopexy for ROP. Pediatrics & Strabismus J Ophthalmol 23:5:258-260, 1986.
8. Sasaki K, Yamashita Y, Mackawa T, Adachi T: Treatment of retinopathy of prematurity in active stage by cryotherapy. Jpn J Ophthalmol 20:384-395, 1976.
9. Hindle NW: Cryotherapy for retinopathy of prematurity timing of intervention. Br J Ophthalmology 70:269-276, 1986.
10. Mousel DK: Cryotherapy for retinopathy of prematurity. Ophthalmol 92:375-378, 1985.
11. Tasman W, Brown GC, Schaffer DB, et al: Cryotherapy for active retinopathy of prematurity. Ophthalmology 93:580-585, 1986.

A CONTROLLED STUDY ON THE USE OF CRYOTHERAPY IN PREVENTION OF RETROLENTAL FIBROPLASIA (RETINOPATHY OF PREMATURITY)

S. Merin, S. Bishara, M. Ilsar, A. Shapiro, F. Eyal and O. Peleg, Units of Ophthalmology and Neonatology, Hadassah Mt. Scopus Hospital, Jerusalem, Israel

INTRODUCTION

Cicatricial retrolental fibroplasia resulting in blindness or severe decrease in vision continues to be a serious threat to premature infants undergoing intensive care in order to save their lives. In fact, the number of affected infants may be on the increase due to improved methods of neonatal care and greater survival rates of smaller infants.

The efficacy of preventive treatment by cryotherapy is still a controversial subject. BenSira and co-workers (1) claimed that no child became bilaterally blind since they started with routine preventive cryotherapy. Less spectacular but still beneficial results were claimed by others, such as Hindle and Leyton (2), Mousel and Hoyt (3), Stark and co-workers (4), and Hindle (5). No beneficial effects were reported by Harris and McCormick (6), Keith (7), and Kingham (8).

Most studies claiming beneficial results were uncontrolled. We started therefore a controlled and prospective study at the Hadassah Mt. Scopus Neonatal Intensive Care Unit (NICU), in 1980. The study was triggered by an outbreak of an "epidemic" of five infants severely affected by cicatricial RLF, in the course of the six months preceding the study.

MATERIALS AND METHODS

The NICU of Hadassah Mt. Scopus is a large unit for care of premature infants. In the five years of the study about 500 admissions were recorded with a tendence to increase from year to year. Table I indicates the number of admissions in each birth weight group and the survival rates.

Table I: Admissions of low birth weight premature infants during six years (1980 - 1985) and their survival rates.

Birth weight (grams)	<750	750-999	1000-1499
Total admissions	47	147	296
Survivors	5	51	233
% survivors	11	37	79

The eye examination was performed routinely in all babies starting at the age of one month. It was done weekly except in cases of: (1) rapid changes, when the examination was done every day or every second or third day; (2) stable condition, when we examined once in two weeks; (3) regression, when we examined once a month until total vascularization of the retina.

The pupils were dilated by Mydriacil 1% and Phenylephrine 2.5% applied twice. A nurse was always present and the examination was performed using an Alfonso speculum, indirect ophthalmoscopy and indentation.

Patients were considered for preventive treatment if they reached stage III of our former classification, in which stage III A had also localized retinal hemorrhages and stage III B had some localized vitreous hemorrhages'. This stage is closest to stage 3 of the 1984 International Classification, but does not take into account the location and extent in hours of peripheral neovascularization. The majority, however, had an extent of about 5 - 6 hours affected, continuous or cumulative. Once the infant reached the stage of possible surgical intervention, the findings and the available knowledge on the subject were explained to the parents and their consent achieved. The actual treatment was performed if during the next day, or days, progression in the form of increasing neovascularization was noted.

For the preventive treatment, we used general anesthesia, the cataract cryopencil and indirect ophthalmoscopy. Cryo was applied from neovascular ridge to ora on the ischemic area in affected zones or 360^{0} if more than half of the circumference was affected. The right eye was treated and the left eye remained as a control.

RESULTS

During the six years of the study, 18 infants were found eligible for preventive treatment. Table II lists the results in these 18 infants.

Table II: Comparison of results in the two eyes of 18 infants included in the study in the course of six years.

No. of infants	Results
13	same in both eyes
3	better in treated eye
1	better in untreated eye
1	treated in both eyes

Of the 13 patients who were the same in both eyes, two were blind and 11 recovered. Of the three who were better in the treated eye, two had a retinal detachment in the untreated eye and a cicatricial RLF in the treated eye. One had cicatricial RLF stage I in the untreated eye and recovered in the treated eye. One patient had cicatricial RLF in the treated eye and recovered in the untreated eye. In one case both eyes were treated at the insistence of the parents.

DISCUSSION

During the study period, fewer cases of cicatricial RLF or blindness from RLF were encountered when compared to the pre-study period. This could result from a variety of causes, such as improved neonatal care or the routine administration of supplemental vitamin E to all low-weight premature infants.

Comparing the treated eye with the natural history of the disease in the control eye, this study could not confirm or refute the effectiveness of preventive cryotherapy. In more cases the treated eye was better but in the vast majority both eyes were finally similar. Our conclusion from this study is, therefore, that one of several possibilities exists: First, that cryotherapy is not effective. Second, that cryotherapy is effective if used earlier than we did, which means to treat many cases unnecessarily. To obtain three eyes better in treated eyes, we had to treat 18. To treat earlier means that 90% or even more will be treated unnecessarily. Third, that cryotherapy has limited value in prevention of RLF, and that it is effective in a small percentage of patients for reasons unknown. In this case, we have to compare such statistical value with the possible statistical risks of the treatment. Fourth, that cryotherapy is effective in a proportion of patients, who may have certain predisposing conditions. These could presumably be a "plus disease", some other danger signs such as dense neovascular nodes, a very large ischemic area up to the posterior pole or rapid progression of signs.

Comparison of our criteria for eligibility for treatment with the threshold stage used by the Multicenter Trial of Cryotherapy for Prevention of ROP now conducted in the United States, shows clear similarities. We must wait for the results of this large scale, well-controlled, clinical study, to resolve the continuing controversy on the subject of the effectiveness of cryotherapy in prevention of ROP.

REFERENCES
1. BenSira I, Nissenkorn I, Grunwald E, Yassur Y: Treatment of acute retrolental fibroplasia by cryopexy. Br J Ophthalmol 64:758-762, 1980.
2. Hindle, NW, Leyton J: Prevention of cicatricial retrolental fibroplasia by cryotherapy. Can J Ophthalmol 13:277-282, 1978.
3. Mousel DK, Hoyt CS: Cryotherapy for retinopathy of prematurity. Ophthalmology (Rochester) 87:1121-1127, 1980.
4. Stark DJ, Manning LM, Lenton J: The incidence and results of active treatment of acute retrolental fibroplasia. Aust J Ophthalmol 10:1935, 1982.
5. Hindle NW: Cryotherapy for retinopathy of prematurity: timing of intervention. Br J Ophthalmol 70:269-276, 1986.

6. Harris, GS, McCormick AQ: The prophylactic treatment of retrolental fibroplasia. Mod Probl Ophthalmol 18:364-367, 1977.
7. Keith CG: Visual outcome and effect of treatment in stage III developing retrolental fibroplasia. Br J Ophthalmol 66:446-449, 1982.
8. Kingham JD: Acute retrolental fibroplasia. II. Treatment by cryosurgery. Arch Ophthalmol 96:2049-2053, 1978.

THE EFFECT OF CRYOTHERAPY ON OXYGEN-INDUCED RETINOPATHY IN THE NEWBORN
KITTEN

I. Kremer[1], R. Kissun[2], I. Nissenkorn[1], I. Ben-Sira[1], A. Garner[2], Department of Ophthalmology, Beilinson Medical Center, Petach Tikva, Israel[1] and
Department of Pathology, Institute of Ophthalmology, London, England[2].

ABSTRACT
      In fourteen kittens with experimental oxygen-induced retinopathy,
partial cryotherapy was performed in the right eye of each kitten, while
the left one was left untreated as a control. Subsequent fundoscopic
examination and histopathological studies showed no significant difference
between the treated and untreated eyes.
      We attribute these unsatisfactory results mainly to the fact that
the cryoablation of the kittens' retina was incomplete and additionally
to the fact that oxygen-induced retinopathy of the kitten and human
retinopathy of prematurity (ROP) are two different entities and therefore
cryotherapy may yield positive results only in the latter.

INTRODUCTION
      The first reports (1-3) of the use of cryotherapy in the control of
the proliferative phases of retinopathy of prematurity (ROP) varied in
their conclusions regarding the advantages and limitations of this form
of treatment. In 1979, Kingham published (4) his disappointing clinical
results obtained in 14 cryotreated eyes; in only two of those eyes was
the treatment considered to be of positive value.
      In the same year, Hindle and colleagues reported their successful
clinicopathological results in the treatment of active ROP by cryotherapy
(5). Their method of treatment was similar to that used in the previously
mentioned reports (1-4), and consisted of direct freezing of the developing fibrovascular ridge and the adjacent areas anterior and posterior
to it, by one to two circular rows of cryoapplications (5). Hindle showed
that in most of the treated eyes the mesencymal ridge disappeared and
no cicatrization developed. Keith, using the same direct method of cryoablation of the arteriovenous shunt but not the avascular retina anterior
to it, found no beneficial effect in nine infants with active ROP (6).
      In contrast to the above-mentioned method of treatment (1-6), Ben-Sira
and colleagues described an indirect treatment scheme involving cryoablation of the avascular retina just anterior to the ridge, while avoiding
direct treatment of the ridge and the neovascular growths posterior to it
(7). Nissenkorn and co-workers later reported a clinicopathological case
which showed almost complete regression of the disease in the areas
posterior to the cryo scars and low-grade active disease between the
scars (8).
      Nagata (9) and Majima and colleagues (10), in addition to other
Japanese investigators, have employed a similar indirect method for the
treatment of ROP, involving xenon light photocoagulation of the anterior
aspect of the ridge and of the avascular retina just contiguous with it,
while avoiding any damage to the extraretinal fibrovascular proliferations

which they reckoned would induce vitreous hemorrhage. Most of the above mentioned authors (5-10) recommend that treatment should be withheld until Stage III of ROP (according to the international classification) (11). Recently, additional reports (12-14) have been published presenting the results of the two different patterns of cryotherapy.

Because of the diversity of opinion about long term results of cryotherapy, the different modes of cryo treatment (direct versus indirect), and the lack of adequately controlled studies, we decided to study the effect of this treatment on oxygen-induced retinopathy in the newborn kitten model. As vaso-obliteration with subsequent peripheral retinal ischemia have already been suggested to be the inducing factor of preretinal vasoproliferation in the oxygen-treated kitten (15-17), we had to apply the indirect method of cryotherapy, and therefore we planned to ablate as much ischemic retina as possible.

MATERIAL AND METHODS

Nineteen kittens aged between 3 and 10 days were reared with their mothers in 80% oxygen, within a large incubator especially designed for this experiment, in which CO_2 concentration, humidity and temperature were fully controlled. The kittens were kept in these conditions for a period of 65-72 hours, after which they were removed from the incubator and returned with their mothers to normal oxygen concentration in air. Between several hours and four days after being returned to air, the kittens were anaesthetized with intraperitoneally administered pento-barbitone sodium (6 mg per 200 gr body weight) and mydriasis was obtained with cyclopentolate hydrochloride 1.0% and phenylephrine hydrochloride 5% drops. Fundus examination of both eyes was done with an indirect ophthalmoscope, in order to confirm the constrictive effect of the oxygen therapy on the retinal vasculature. After the fundus examination, each kitten's right eye was treated by cryotherapy following instillation of several drops of a local anaesthetic (Ametho-cain-1%), while the left eye remained untreated as a control. The cryotreatment was performed by approximately 360^0 transconjunctival applications of 1 mm cataract probe connected to an ACU-22 cryounit (Keeler-Amoils), delivering nitrous oxide to the probe. The cryoprobe was applied to the sclera radially and circumferentially as far posteriorly as possible, each application lasting 6 seconds. The cryoablation was performed without directly visualizing the treated area of the retina because it was impossible to see the fundus anterior to the equator through the dense tunica vasculosa lentis, even with an indirect ophthalmoscope equipped with a Helium light bulb. Since the scleral thickness of the Guinea pig's eye is quite similar to that of the kitten, the exact time needed for freezing the kitten's retina was studied histopathologically in a preliminary experiment on Guinea pigs. As this experiment was done without directly visualizing the retina while performing the cryotreatment, the procedure was subsequently repeated in two 30 day-old kittens in which direct visualization of the cryotreated areas using the indirect ophthalmoscope was possible. It was found that the time taken by the latter kittens' retina to whiten (freeze) was six seconds, while using the same cryoprobe as was employed in the subsequent kitten experiments. It was possible to apply the above mentioned cryoprobe as far posteriorly as the equator only, because of the small orbits and short fornices. We avoided surgical opening of the conjunctival sac, which could have caused bleeding and endangered the kittens' life, should the mother cat see or smell it. Therefore, the cryopexy was confined to the retina anterior to the equator, except for the medial aspect of the eye, where the nictitating membrane interfered with the treatment. The distance between each cryo application was between 1.5-2.0 mm. The kittens subsequently underwent funduscopic examination of both eyes one, four, seven and eight days after the treatment, and fundus photography was done in three animals. After a final funduscopic examination they were killed between 14 and 19 days following the cryotreatment. India ink injection was performed in one of the kittens. The eyes were enucleated, fixed in buffered formaldehyde and processed in the conventional way for hematoxylin-eosin (H.E.) and periodic-acid-Schiff (P.A.S.) staining, except for the two eyes pretreated with India ink, which were fixed in buffered formaldehyde only.

RESULTS

All 19 kittens showed complete obliteration of the retinal vasculature and even optic disc vessels after 3 days of oxygen therapy. This finding was identical in both eyes of each kitten. Five kittens died within the first 24 hours after the cryotherapy and so were excluded from the experiment. The remaining 14 kittens developed retinal new vessels in both the treated and untreated eyes as early as 8 days after being returned from oxygen to air breathing. The new vessel formation started by budding from the optic disc vasculature and subsequently spread circumferentially as small tufts growing into the vitreous from the retina. In the same period, although starting a few days earlier, apparently normal intraretinal vessels were seen growing from the optic nerve head centrifugally. Two weeks after oxygen therapy the posterior poles of both eyes were completely vascularised with slightly dilated and engorged intraretinal vessels. At that time, the border between the avascular and vascular retina in all cases was located quite posteriorly, within a radius of about 5 disc diameters (D.D.) away from the optic disc in both eyes, and was characterized by dilated brush-like vascular endings (Fig. 1). The arborizing glomerular tufts of new vessels were actually seen growing forwards at random in both eyes from the whole area of the vascularized retina but were clinically most conspicuous in the posterior region (Fig. 2). Additionally, small to medium vitreous haemorrhages were found at the posterior poles of both eyes in all the kittens. We could not find any clinically significant difference between the two eyes of each kitten, although atrophic chorioretinal cryoscars were clearly seen in the retinal periphery and equatorial areas 8 days post treatment. Only a few of these scars were found to be close to the border between the vascular and avascular zones 14 days after oxygen therapy (Fig. 3).
The histological sections stained with H.E. and P.A.S. confirmed the above clinical findings and showed well developed preretinal new vessels (Fig. 4), growing in diffuse pattern into the vitreous from the retina of the posterior pole and from the optic disc (Fig. 5-6). It is important to note that no spindle cells were seen near the anterior border of the growing vessels. The new vessels were seen in both the treated and untreated eyes, without any significant difference between the two. Atrophic chorioretinal scars were seen in the equatorial and peripheral areas, where most of the retinal nuclear layers had been destroyed and replaced by fibrous tissue infiltrated by pigment-laden macrophages (Fig. 7). The sclera overlying these chorioretinal scars

was found to be very thin. The posterior edges of the majority of cryoscars and anterior border of the proliferating preretinal new vessels were separated by a zone of intact avascular retina, between 1-2 D.D. wide.   The eyes pretreated with India ink injection also showed the same extent of neovascular growths in the treated and untreated eyes (Fig. 8-9).

Figure 1

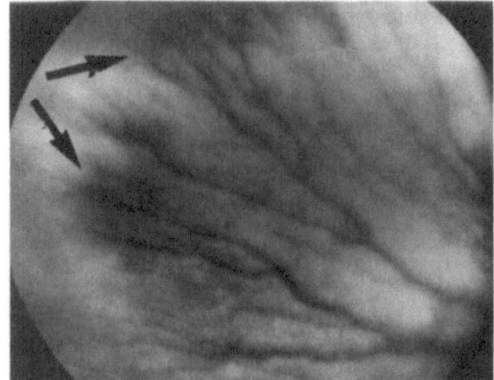

Figure 2

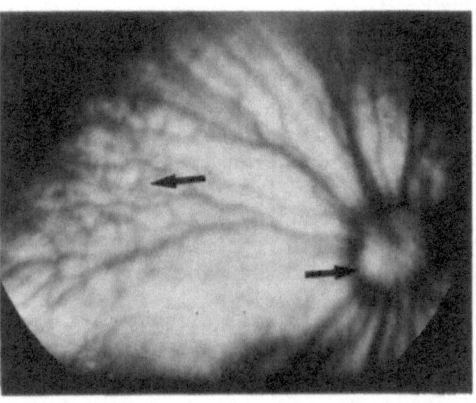

Figure 3

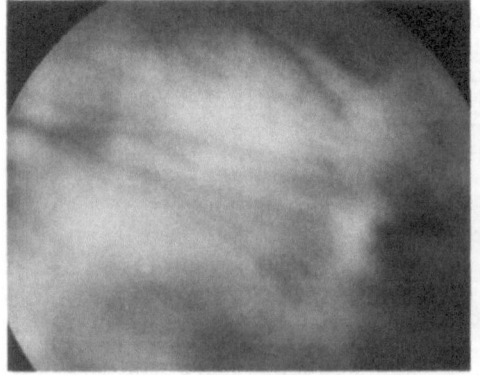

Figure 4

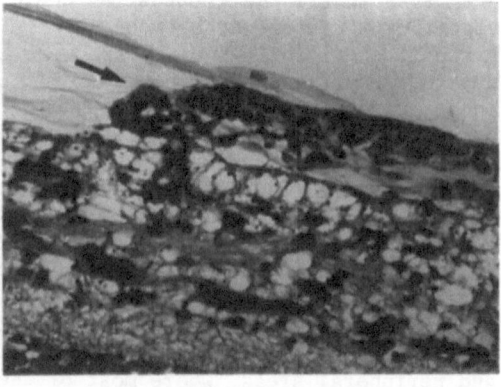

Figure 5

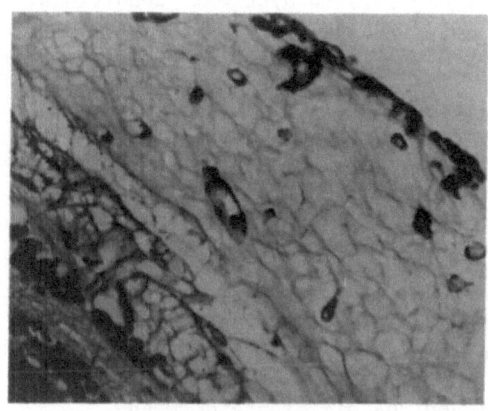

Figure 6

Figure 7

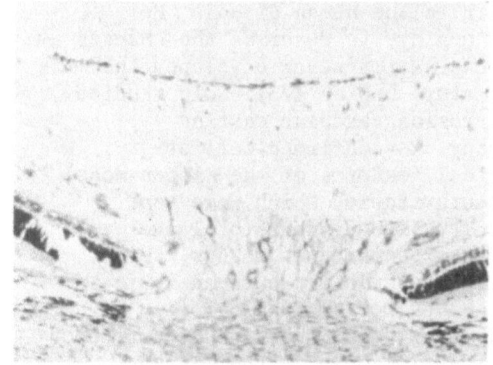
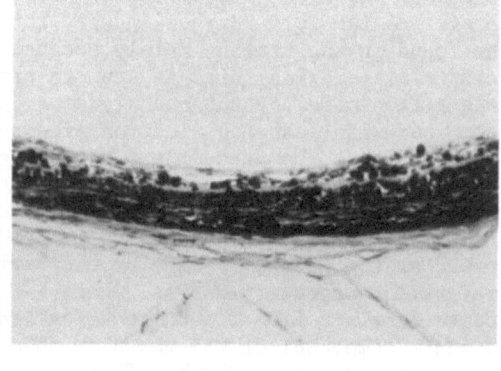

Figure 8

Figure 9

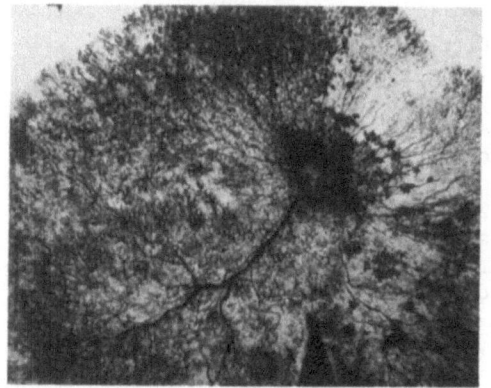
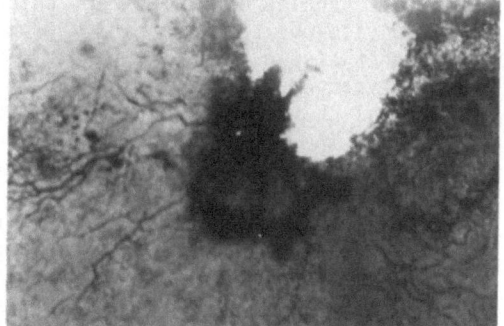

DISCUSSION

Ashton and co-workers (15) and Patz et al (16), working independently, produced vasoproliferative changes in the retinas of newborn animals of several species, including kittens, by exposure to hyperoxic conditions. The events observed in the kitten model were considered to reflect the early stages of ROP. They proved that the developing retinal vasculature of the kitten responds in a biphasic way: (a) initial vasoconstriction of major vessels and subsequent vaso-obliteration of the capillary bed and rest of the vascular tree in the presence of raised arterial oxygen levels and (b) on return to room air, by peripheral retinal ischemia with consequent neovascular proliferation, possibly due to secretion of a vasoproliferative substance by the ischemic retina (15-17). Evidence that a vasoproliferative factor is released under these conditions has recently been demonstrated (18). As regards to histologic changes seen in the immature retina after oxygen exposure and transfer to air, Ashton et al (17) showed, in kittens, that an intense angioblastic activity developed in the inner layers of the retina with extension of delicate new vessels into the vitreous (17-22).

Ashton himself, in 1954 (20), mentioned the difference between the experimental and human disease and stated that, while the vasoproliferations in premature infants may progress to cicatrization and traction retinal detachment, in the animal eye they regress and traction retinal detachment never occurs in the kitten. Gole et al (23) re-examined the kitten model and compared it to the human disease. He preferred the term "oxygen-induced retinopathy" to describe the changes he found in the kitten, mainly because the kitten never developed the cicatricial retinal disease seen in premature babies (23). Gole studied the kitten model by the technique of corrosion vascular casting combined with scanning electron microscopy. He confirmed earlier findings that the predominant morphological features of the kitten model were preretinal and intraretinal neovascularization which were more numerous posteriorly than anteriorly. Only a few networks of large calibre vessels, which appeared to act as arteriovenous shunts, were noted at the advancing edge of the retinal vasculature between intra-retinal neovascular lobules. These A-V shunts were morphologically quite distinct from the human so-called mesenchymal shunt and constituted a minor component of the vascular abnormalities seen in the kitten. Flynn in 1979 published his fluorescein angiographic findings (24) in premature babies with ROP, demonstrating that the extent of the vaso-obliteration occurring in the presence of raised arterial oxygen levels is quite small and confined to the retina immediately behind its advancing vascular border, a fact which is in sharp contrast to the complete vaso-obliteration seen in the kitten (17). Flynn et al (25) concluded that the advancing vasoformative mesenchymal tissue survives during oxygen breathing and subsequently changes into a so-called mesenchymal shunt, which acts as a focus for scarring and traction retinal detachment. The other factor which is contributing to the scarring process is the neovascular fronds developing posterior to the mesenchymal shunt (24-25). A study by Foos (26-27) of autopsy eyes with ROP, showed that the "shunt" consists of a vanguard area composed of spindle-shaped cells and a separate rearguard zone in which vascular endothelium and definitive capillaries can be identified. The rearguard endothelial proliferation gives rise to the subsequent extraretinal fibrovascular activity. In 1983, Kretzer et al (28) described a theory for the induction of ROP according to which nascent retinal blood vessels are formed, in normal conditions, by canalization of spindle cells behind the migrating mesenchymal apron of the immature retina. They suggested that elevated oxygen tension may trigger extensive gap junction formation between the spindle cells and so interfere with their subsequent migration and canalization (28-29). Kretzer's group also confirmed Ashton's observation that the embryonic kitten's retinal vasculature, lacks| mesencymal spindle cells and develops through a process of vascular budding, and therefore is not comparable to the human system (29).

If we postulate that Ashton's biphasic theory (17-19) according to which oxygen-induced retinal ischemia triggers neovascularization in active ROP, is correct, we should aim the cryoablation to those ischemic retinal areas, which probably secrete the vasoproliferative factor (18). But if on the other hand it is assumed that the Kretzer-Hittner spindle cell theory (28-30) is correct, one should then treat the disease by cryoablation of the total spindle cell apron. Therefore, by choosing the kitten, we had necessarily to apply the indirect method of treatment, i.e. to destroy the majority of the ischemic retina of the kitten by cryotherapy, shortly after it had returned from oxygen to air breathing, in order to decrease the relative amount of vasoproliferative factor-producing tissue. This treatment was ineffective in the above kitten experiments, as no difference has been detected either clinically or histologically between the treated and untreated eyes from the point of view of retinal neovascularization. We consider that the principal reason for this finding may have been the difficulty encountered in ablating sufficient ischemic retina, especially as the degree of vaso-obliteration induced by hyperoxia in the kitten extends all the way back to the optic disc and is not limited to the immediate vascular frond as in the human ROP. The additional reason is that oxygen-induced retinopathy of the kitten and the human ROP are most probably two different diseases. Therefore it is not possible to draw any conclusions from our experiments carried out on the kittens with regard to the effect of cryotherapy on the human disease, in which this treatment seems to yield positive results (12,14).

LEGENDS TO FIGURES

Figure 1 - a fundus photograph showing the dilated brush-like vascular endings of the developing intraretinal vessels, 12 days post oxygen therapy. At the bottom, two pigmented cryoscars are seen.
Figure 2 - a fundus photograph showing new vessels on the disc and surrounding it.
Figure 3 - pigmented cryoscars seen near the border between vascular and avascular retina.
Figure 4 - the advancing edge of the dense network of preretinal new vessels growing in the vitreous. No spindle cells are seen in the retina anterior to it.
Figure 5 - delicate preretinal new vessels coming out through the internal limiting membrane of the posterior pole retina, growing into the vitreous, and forming a confluent preretinal neovascular membrane.

Figure 6 - a dense network of preretinal new vessels is seen covering the disc and the retina of the posterior pole.

Figure 7 - an area of a cryoscar, where the retina and choroid have been replaced by a fibrous scar invaded by pigment-laden macrophages and most probably also by pigment-epithelial cells.

Figure 8 - a photograph of formalin fixed retina after premortem India Ink injection, showing the intra and extraretinal new vessels of an untreated eye.

Figure 9 - an area of peripheral retina, showing persistence of neovascular growth near the cryoscars.

REFERENCES

1. Payne J, Patz A : Treatment of acute retrolental fibroplasia. Trans Am Acad Ophthalmol 1972; 76:1234-1246.
2. McCormick AQ : Retinopathy of prematurity; Current Problems in Pediatrics 1977; 7:11.
3. Harris GS : Retinopathy of prematurity and retinal detachment. Canad J Ophthalmol 1976; 11:21-95.
4. Kingham JO : Acute retrolental fibroplasia II. Treatment by cryo-surgery. Arch Ophthalmol 1978; 96:2049-2053.
5. Hindle NW, Leyton J : Prevention of cicatricial retrolental fibroplasia by cryotherapy. Canad J Ophthalmol 1978; 13:277-282.
6. Keith CG : Visual outcome and effect of treatment in stage III developing retrolental fibroplasia. Br J Ophthalmol 1982;66:446-449.
7. Ben-Sira I, Nissenkorn I, Grunwald E, Yassur Y : Treatment of acute retrolental fibroplasia by cryopexy. Br J Ophthalmol 1980;64:758-62.
8. Nissenkorn I, Kremer I, Ben-Sira I, Cohen S, Garner A : A clinico-pathological case of retinopahy of prematurity (ROP) treated by peripheral cryopexy. Br J Ophthalmol 1984; 68:36-41.
9. Nagata M : Treatment of acute proliferative retrolental fibroplasia with xenon-arc photocoagulation; its indications and limitations. Jpn J Ophthalmol 1977; 21:436-459.
10. Majima A, Takahashi M, Hibino Y, Karnao N, Takai M : Clinical obser-vation of photocoagulation on retinopathy of prematurity. Jpn J Clin Ophthalmol 1976; 30:93-97.
11. An international classification of retinopathy of prematurity. Br J Ophthalmol 1984; 68:690-697.
12. Topilow HW, Ackerman AL, Wang FM : The treatment of advanced retinopathy of prematurity by cryotherapy and scleral buckling surgery. Ophthalmol 1985; 92:379-387.
13. Mousel DK : Cryotherapy for retinopathy of prematurity. Ophthalmol 1985; 92:375-378.
14. Tasman W : Management of prematurity. Ophthalmol 1985; 92:995-999.
15. Ashton N, Ward B, Serpell G : Role of oxygen in the genesis of retrolental fibroplasia; a preliminary report. Br J Ophthalmol 1953; 37:513-520.
16. Patz A, Eastham A, Higginbotham DH, Kleh T : Oxygen studies in retro-lental fibroplasia II. The production of the microscopic changes of retrolental fibroplasia in experimental animals. Am J Ophthalmol 1953; 36:1511-1522.
17. Ashton N, Ward B, Serpell G : Effect of oxygen on developing retinal vessels with particular reference to the problem of retrolental fibroplasia. Br J Ophthalmol 1954: 38:397-432.

18. Taylor CM, Weiss JB, Kissun RD, Garner A : Effect of O$_2$ tension on the quantities of procollagenase activating angiogenic factor present in the developing kitten retina. Br J Ophthalmol(in press).
19. Ashton N: Donders lecture - some aspects of the comparative pathology of oxygen toxicity in the retina. Br J Ophthalmol 1968; 52:505-531.
20. Ashton N : Animal experiments in retrolental fibroplasia. Trans Am Acad Ophthalmol Otolaryngol 1954; 58:51-53.
21. Ashton N : Experimental retrolental fibroplasia. Annual Review of Medicine 1957; 8:441-454.
22. Ashton N : Oxygen and the growth and development of retinal vessels. Am J Ophthalmol 1966; 62:412-435.
23. Gole GA, Gannon BJ, Goodyer AM : Oxygen induced retinopathy; the kitten model re-examined. Austr J Ophthalmol 1982; 10:223-232.
24. Flynn JT et al : Fluorescein angiography in retrolental fibroplasia; Experience from 1969-1977. Ophthalmol 1974; 86:1700-1823.
25. Flynn JT, O'Grady GE, Herrera J, Kushner BJ, Cantolino S, Milam W : retrolental fibroplasia I. Clinical observations. Arch Ophthalmol 1977; 95: 217-223.
26. Foos RY : Acute retrolental fibroplasia. Albrecht von Graefes Arch Klin Exp Ophthalmol 1975; 195: 87-100.
27. Foos RY : Chronic retinopathy of prematurity. Ophthalmol 1985; 92:563-574.
28. Kretzer FL, Hittner HM, Johnson AT, Metha RS, Godio LB : Vitamin E and retrolental fibroplasia; ultrastructural support of clinical efficacy. Ann New York Acad Sci 1982; 393: 145-166.
29. Kretzer FL, Metha RS, Johnson AT, Hunter DG, Brown ES, Hittner HM : Vitamin E protects against retinopathy of prematurity through action on spindle cells. Nature 1984; 309:793-795.
30. Kretzer FL, McPherson AR, Rudolph AJ, Hittner HM : Pathogenic mechanism of retinopathy of prematurity; a controversial explanation for the efficacy of oral and intramuscular vitamin E supplementation and cryotherapy. Bull New York Acad 1985; 61:883-900.

ROP IN SOROKA MEDICAL CENTER NEONATAL I.C.U.

T. Monos, M.D., Y. Yassur, M.D., T. Lifshitz, M.D., L. Shani, M.D.,
E. Zmora, M.D., M. Karplus, M.D.

Soroka University Hospital, Ben Gurion University, Beer-Sheva, Israel.

According to data from all around the world we are now facing a new
ROP epidemic. This might very well be due to the significant rise of the
survival rate of low birth weight premature babies. ROP is a multi-
factorial disease, in which one of the most important risk factors is the
newborn's prematurity level. Certainly increased awareness of the
disease, more sophisticated diagnostic tools, more intensive follow-up of
early signs - all contributed to the rising number of diagnosed cases of
the different stages of this disease.

The rising interest in this subject urged many authors to look into
the relative contribution of the various factors in the pathogenesis and
severity of the disease.

Follow-up of prematures at the Soroka Medical Center of the Ben-
Gurion University during the last three years urged us to consider a few
risk factors which seemed particular to this specific nursery, this being
according to changing concepts now-a-days.

There are two prominent populations in our premature nursery: two-
thirds are Jews and one-third are Beduins. The Beduin population has a
much darker skin, hair and fundus pigmentation than the Jewish population.

It is also worthwhile noting that all the prematures routinely receive
for pediatric reasons Vit. E according to the following protocol: Starting
on the first day of life 5 mg/kg/d IV until oral supplementation can be
tolerated; then 15 mg/kg/d per os until the age of three months. The
monitoring of the various accepted risk factors for ROP in the nursery is
sophisticated and tight.

The prematures of birth weight of 1750 gr and less go through their
first ophthalmic examination at the age of four weeks. Those in which no
ROP is found are being examined thereafter in two to four week intervals
until the retinal vascularization up to the ora serrata is completed.
Those in which ROP is diagnosed are being seen once a week, or more
frequently as indicated by the severity of the disease. Our findings are
now graded according to the international classification recommended in
1984 (1).

PATIENTS, METHODS AND RESULTS

Our present series includes 271 prematures who were born between the
years 1983-1985 and who survived for at least 6 months. Table 1
demonstrates that 169 prematures were Jews and 102 were Beduins.

TABLE 1. Survivors in 1983 - 1985 (Related to birth weight)

Birth weight (grams)	Jews n	Beduins n	
750 - 1000	8	5	13
1001 - 1250	40	16	56
750 - 1250	48	21	69
1251 - 1500	57	26	83
1501 - 1750	64	55	119
Total	169	102	271

Table 2 presents the prevalence of acute ROP in the various weight groups:

TABLE 2. Prevalence of ROP in survivors (related to birth weight)

Birth weight (Grams)	Stage 1 %	n	Stage 2 %	n	Stage 3 %	n	Total %	
750 - 1000	38	5	46	6	15	2	100	13/13
1001 - 1250	27	15	9	5	4	2	39	22/56
750 - 1250	29	20	16	11	6	4	51	35/69
1251 - 1500	17	14	2	2	0		19	16/83
1501 - 1750	4	5	0		0		4	5/119

It is evident that all babies less than 1000 gr had some degree of ROP and half of all babies less than 1250 gr had it. In bigger prematures it was to a great extent less. This percentage is in accordance with that from most other centers in the world (2). However the percentage of severe ROP (more than Stage 2) is low in our series.

Table 3 presents the prevalence of acute ROP in Jewish and Beduin babies.

TABLE 3. Prevalence of ROP in Jews and Beduins.

	Jews n	%	Beduins n	%	
ROP	40	24	16	16	$X^2 = 2.47$
No ROP	129	76	86	84	$P > 0.1$
Total	169		102		

It is clear that the prevalence of ROP among the Jews is higher - 24%, in comparison to 16% in the Beduins.

Table 4 demonstrates that there are twice as many Stage 1 ROP in Jewish babies than in Beduin (19% versus 9.5%).

TABLE 4. Prevalence of ROP stage 1 among Jews and Beduins

	Jews		Beduins			
	n	%	n	%		
ROP Stage 1	30	19	9	9.5	$x^2 = 4.038$	
No ROP	129	81	86	90.5	$P < 0.05$	
Total	159		95			

It is important to notice that this difference is statistically significant. Such a difference between the two groups was not demonstrated in Stages 2 and 3.

COMMENTS
The main points to be emphasised in our study population are as follows:
First, ROP is more prevalent in lower birth weight groups, a well known observation elsewhere, this being true for Jewish and Beduin babies.
Secondly, the absolute number of severe cases of ROP Stage 3 is very small, this being true even for the low birth weight babies. This cannot be explained only by the survival rate if compared to statistics from other nurseries. We raise the question as to whether this could not be influenced by the routine admission of Vit. E from the first day of life, even if the dosage is below what is reported in most of the Vit. E studies to be a therapeutic dosage (3,4). It was already claimed by Finer et al. (5) that even half of the reported necessary dosage of Vit. E is also effective. Recently, Shaeffer et al. (6) reported, in a controlled study, of the beneficial effect of Vit. E which was administered in the same dosage and route that we administered. May be that even a lower dosage has some protective effect if given from the first day of life.
Thirdly, it is obvious that the prevalence of ROP is higher in Jews than in Beduins when Stage 1 is considered. It is worthwhile here to mention Dr. Glaser's and others' concept (7) that RPE cells serve as an inhibitor to retinal neovascularization and an attractor to astroglia. The role of RPE cells in causing gliosis and fibrosis in retinal diseases is well appreciated now-a-days. The lower prevalence of disciform SMD lesions in more pigmented eyes than in less pigmented is already reported (8,9). It may be that the darker pigmentation of the Beduins, as compared to Jews, plays a protective role in the development of ROP, perhaps by attraction of astroglia at the very early stage of the retinal ischemia in the irritated undeveloped retina of the premature. The fact that in stages 2 and 3 there was no difference in the percentage of ROP between Jews and Beduins may be explained by counteraction of other risk factors in those babies, postulating that if ROP has already started, the

protective effect of pigmentation cannot anymore overcome the other potent
risk factors.

Therefore, this observation requires more attention, and we do
recommend to investigate it in other white and black populations, and to
assess the relative importance of this factor to other risk factors. Also
laboratory studies on dark-and light-pigmented eyes are necessary.

REFERENCES
1. International classification of ROP. Arch. Ophthalmol. 1984; 102:1130.
2. Campbell PB et al: Incidence of retinopathy of prematurity in a
   tertiary Newborn Intensive Care Unit. Arch. Ophthalmol. 1983; 101:1686
3. Hittner MM, Godio LB, Rudolph AJ, et al: Retrolental fibroplasia:
   Efficacy of Vitamin E in a double-blind clinical study of preterm
   infants. N. Engl. J. Med. 1981; 305, 1365.
4. Hittner MM, Speer ME, Rudolph AJ, et al: Retrolental fibroplasia and
   vitamin E in the preterm infant: a comparison of oral versus intramuscular: Oral administration. Pediatrics 1984; 73: 238.
5. Finer NN, Grant G, Schindler RF, et al: Effect of intramuscular
   Vitamin E on frequency and severity of retrolental fibroplasia. A
   controlled trial. Lancet 1982; 1: 1087.
6. Shafer DL, Johnson L, Quinn GE, et al: Vitamin E and retinopathy of
   prematurity: The Ophthalmologist's perspective. In: Flynn JT, Phelps
   DI, Eds. Birth defects original article series: Retinopathy of
   prematurity: Update 1985. New York: Alan R. Liss, 1986. In press.
7. Rowen SL, Glaser BM: Retinal RPE cells release a chemoattractant for
   astrocytes. Arch. Ophthalmol. 1985; 103, 704-707.
8. Hyman LA, Lilienfeld AM, Ferris FL, III and Fine SL: Senile macular
   degeneration: A case control study. Am. J. Epidemiol. 1983; 118: 213.
9. Weiter JJ, Delori FC, Wing GL, Fitch KA: Relationship of senile
   macular degeneration to ocular pigmentation. Am. J. Ophthalmol. 1985;
   99: 185.

SCLERAL RIGIDITY, VENOUS OBSTRUCTION, AND AGE-RELATED MACULAR DEGENERATION:
A Working Hypothesis

Ephraim Friedman, M.D.
MASSACHUSETTS EYE & EAR INFIRMARY - BOSTON, MASSACHUSETTS

ABSTRACT:

It is proposed, as a working hypothesis, that age-related macular degeneration is caused by a progressive increase in the rigidity of the sclera, gradual obstruction the vortex veins, and decompensation of the choroidal venous system of the posterior pole. The hypothesis accounts for all of the clinical signs characteristic of the disorder and defines its relationship to senescence. The biophysical, epidemiologic and therapeutic implications are assessed.

Figure 1

Diagrammtic representation of the sequence of pathologic events beginning with a progressive increase in scleral rigidity and culminating in the characteristic signs of age-related macular degeneration.

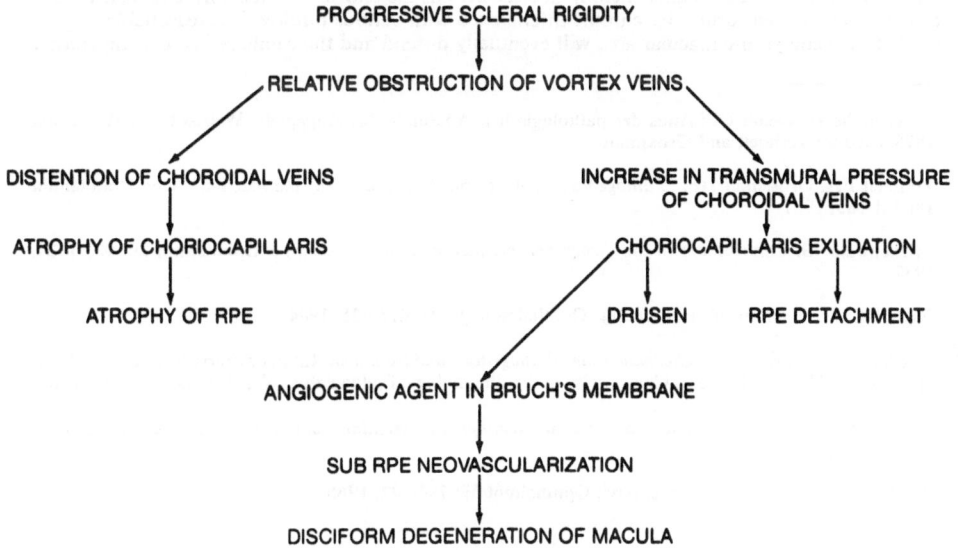

PATHOGENESIS OF AGE RELATED MACULAR DEGENERATION: A WORKING HYPOTHESIS

More than a century has passed since the entity called senile or age-related macular degeneration (AMD) was first described.[1] We have, in the interim, learned much about its natural history but identification of its cause has eluded us. It is the thesis of this paper that a plausible cause can be synthesized by linking together two well established but heretofore unconnected ideas. Half a century ago two giants of American ophthalmology, Frederick H. Verhoeff and Jonas Friedenwald, each published a classic monograph, ostensibly on different subjects, which, when cojoined, provides a framework for understanding the pathogenesis of AMD.

Verhoeff and Grossman,[2] reported in 1937 that " ... *disciform degeneration of the macula is due to some disturbance in the choriocapillaris. Since the disorder is most commonly a senile disease, localized angiosclerosis is probably the usual cause of this vascular disturbance."* Friedenwald[3] in the same year noted that *"in the aged and in extreme myopia the rigidity of the eye is increased".* What has since been missing is the connection between a *"rigid eye"* and a *"disturbance in the choriocapillaris."*

The purpose of this paper is the advancement of the concept that the rigid sclera causes obstruction of the vortex veins, decompensation of the choroidal venous system at the posterior pole, and a *"disturbance in the choriocapillaris"* of the macular area. The *"localized angiosclerosis"* is phlebosclerosis of the vortex veins.

This proposal is made with the knowledge that it runs counter to the currently fashionable theories. For example, an otherwise excellent recent review[4] of pathogenetic mechanisms of maculopathy includes the following assertions: *"the sclera probably is of little importance in the pathogenesis of macular disease"* and *"The choroidal vasculature once was thought to play a major role in the pathogenesis of macular disease, particularly senile macular degeneration."*

I. THE VULNERABILITY OF THE MACULA

It is proposed that the pathologic process causing AMD tends to affect the macula preferentially because the venous pressure is higher there than elsewhere in the choroid. This is the inevitable concomitant of the evolution of the concurrent vascular system, a unique adaptation of the terrestrial vertebrate eye to enhance its thermo-regulatory capacity.[5] [6] The pressure in the vortex vein has been found to be close to intraocular pressure.[7] Direct measurement of venous pressure in the posterior pole has not been reported, but as the choroidal veins in the macular area are the most distal the pressure must be higher there than elsewhere in the choroid. If this normally high venous pressure is raised even further by chronic interference with venous outflow it is reasonable to propose that the veins of the macular area will eventually distend and the capillary bed decompensate.

[1] PagenstecherH, Genth CP: Atlas der pathologischen Anatomie des Augapfels, Weisbaden, CW Kteidal 1875; cited by Verhoeff and Grossman

[2] Verhoeff FH, Grossman HP: *Pathogenesis of disciform degeneration of the macula.* Arch Ophthalmol 18: 561-585, 1937

[3] Friedenwald JS: *Contribution to the theory and practice of tonometry.* Am J Ophthalmol 20: 985-1024, 1937

[4] Eagle RC: *Mechanisms of maculopathy.* Ophthalmology 91: 613-625, 1984

[5] Friedman E: *Central serous choroidopathy: Pathogenesis and treatment.* In: Brockhurst RJ, Boruchoff SA, Hutchinson BT, Lessell S, eds. Controversy in Ophthalmology, Philadelphia: WB Saunders 1977; 706-709

[6] Schollander PF, Krog J: *Countercurrent heat exchange and vascular bundles in sloths.* J Applied Physics 10: 405-411, 1957

[7] Bill A: *The uveal venous pressure.* Arch Ophthalmol 69: 780-782, 1965

The probable effects of this elevated pressure on the vortex veins have been learned by studying the vortex veins of senile eyes, the eyes of patients with AMD and other choroidopathies.[5] While the extrascleral portion of the vortex vein was invariably found to be normal, nonspecific intimal thickening, similar to early atherosclerosis, was observed in the intrascleral portion of the veins. A review of the pertinent literature[8] reveals that phlebosclerosis, largely restricted to the splenic, portal, and pulmonary veins, typically follows the prolonged venous hypertension of congestive failure.

A phenomenon which appears inconsistent with this hypothesis is the failure of surgical or experimental[9] [10] occlusion of vortex veins to cause anything resembling AMD. Closure of one or two veins causes acute congestion, with flow returning to normal in one to two weeks. Occlusion of three or four veins typically causes choroidal detachment or other severe ocular injury. Apparently transient closure of the vortex system over a period of weeks should not be expected to mimic chronic obstruction over a period of decades.

II. RELATIONSHIP OF AMD TO SENESCENCE

AMD is, by definition, a disorder associated with age. In the Framingham Eye Study[11] 28% of those between 75-85 years of age were found to be affected. Yet the elderly of some populations have a remarkably low prevalence rate and AMD does not appear to be the inevitable consequence of senescence of any of the tissues directly involved in the disorder. The RPE Bruch's membrane and choriocapillaris have been shown[12] [13] to be only minimally affected by age alone. AMD is related to senescence to the degree that something happens to the sclera of the eyes of some elderly which causes it to become rigid and interfere with the flow of blood through the vortex vein.

The concept of ocular or scleral rigidity is at least as old as "sclera" (from the Greek skleros for hard), but it was Friedenwald who first devised a clinically practical way of measuring it and

8   Moschcowitz E: *Studies in phlebosclerosis VI The immunity from phlebosclerosis in the coronary vein.* Am J Cardiol 13: 495-497, 1964

9   Zauberman H, Livini N: *Experimental vascular occlusion in hypercholesterolemic rabbits.* Invest Ophthalmol Vis Sci 21: 284-255, 1981

10 Hayreh SS, Baines JAB: *Occlusion of the vortex veins.* Br J Ophthalmol 57: 217-238, 1973.

11 Kahn HA, Leibowitz HM, Ganley JP, et al: *The Framingham eye study II. Association of ophthalmic pathology with single variables previously measured in the Framingham heart study.* Am J Epidemiol 106: 33-41, 1977

12 Friedman E, Tso MON: *The retinal pigment epithelium II. Histologic changes with age.* Arch Ophthalmol 79: 315-320, 1968

13 Friedman E, Smith TR, Kuwabara T. *Senile choroidal vascular patterns and drusen.* Arch Ophthalmol 69: 220-230, 1963

demonstrated its increase with age, hyperopia and high myopia. Subsequent studies[14] [15] [16] have validated the method and, with two exceptions,[17] [18] confirmed his findings.

The precise reason for the increase in rigidity is not known, but among the histopathologic changes observed in the aging human sclera are a decrease in cellularity, accumulation of cholesterol esters and sphingomyelins, and degenerative changes involving collagen[19] and elastic fibers.[20] The pattern of age related change in the lipids of the human sclera is strikingly similar to that found in other connective tissues such as the cornea and aorta, and to atherosclerosis.[21] Friedenwald has suggested that the measurement of ocular rigidity might provide an index of the degree of senescence of the connective tissues of the body as a whole. Whether the scleral lipid accumulates because of a specific disease process such as atherosclerosis or as a result of "normal" senescence is unknown at this time.

III. CLINICAL & MICROSCOPIC CHARACTERISTICS OF AMD

RPE atrophy, drusen, RPE detachment, and choroidal neovascularization, are the clinical hallmarks of the disorder which is frequently divided into "dry", predisciform or "wet", exudative, disciform stages. While there is general agreement that the disciform stage is dominated by exudation from the choriocapillaris and new vessels, opinions differ widely as to the primary cause of the RPE atrophy and drusen.[22] [23] [24]

A. RPE ATROPHY

Disease or aging of the RPE, ischemia, heredity and thickening of Bruch's membrane have

---

[14] Becker B, Gay AJ: *Applanation tonometry in the diagnosis and treatment of glaucoma. An evaluation of decreased scleral rigidity.* Arch Ophthalmol 62: 211-215, 1959

[15] Singh YP, Goel SK, Misra RN: *Scleral rigidity in emmetropes.* J All India Ophthalmol Soc 18: 167-169, 1970

[16] Kornzweig AL, Feldstein M, Schneider J: *The eye in old age IV. Ocular survey of over one thousand aged persons with special reference to normal and disturbed visual function.* Am J Ophthalmol 44: 29-37, 1957

[17] Schneider J, Feldstein M, Kornzweig AL: *Scleral rigidity and tonometry in the aged.* Am J Ophthalmol 48: 643-647, 1959

[18] Perkins, ES. *Ocular volume and ocular rigidity.* Exp. Eye Res 33: 268-279, 1981

[19] Vanna S, Teir H: *Observations on structures and age changes in the human sclera.* Acta Ophthalmol 38: 268-279, 1960

[20] Kanai A, Kaufman HE: *Electron microscopic studies of the elastic fiber in human sclera.* Invest Ophthalmol Vis Sci 11: 816-821, 1972

[21] Broekhuyse RM; *The Lipid composition of aging sclera and cornea.* Ophthalmologica 171: 82-85, 1975

[22] Gass JDM: *Pathogenesis of disciform detachment of the neuroepithelium I. General concepts and classification.* Am J Ophthalmol 63: 573-585, 1967

[23] Tso MOM: *Pathogenetic factors of aging macular degeneration.* Ophthalmolgy 92: 628-635, 1985

[24] Garner A: *Pathology of macular degeneration in the elderly.* Trans Ophthalmol Soc UK 95: 54-61, 1975

all been incriminated as causes of drusen and atrophy of the RPE. Noell's[25] surprising demonstration that the rodent retina was exquisitely sensitive to the damaging effects of low levels of illumination has stimulated strenuous efforts to ascertain whether light might cause AMD.[23][26] Though intriguing, neither the epidemiologic nor experimental evidence is compelling thus far as an explanation for AMD.

A simpler explanation, and one which is consistent with the idea of venous obstruction, is that RPE atrophy is a consequence of compression of the choriocapillaris by large distended vessels.[27][28] The posterior pole of the aging eye was found to be characterized by isolated, randomly distributed, clinically insignificant bands of atrophic choriocapillaris corresponding to the imprint of large choroidal vessels. The adjacent non-compressed choriocapillaris was relatively intact. It is proposed that this process is exaggerated in AMD and the atrophic zones involving the choriocapillaris and RPE become confluent and clinically significant.

B. DRUSEN

The literature contains many detailed descriptions of the morphology of drusen[29][30] but no consensus as to their origin. Of the many mechanisms proposed as the cause of drusen, the one most consistent with this hypothesis is that drusen are manifestations of an imbalance between the rate of secretion by the RPE on the one hand and the rate of removal of these metabolic products by the venous system on the other.[13] The rationale for emphasizing the role of the choroidal venous system in the pathogenesis of AMD is based on the observation made on flat preparations of the aging choroid that drusen tend to form in relation to the capillaries of the collecting venules.

C. RPE DETACHMENT

If it is acknowledged that some drusen are the result of exudation of the choriocapillaris, it is reasonable to conclude that RPE detachments, large or small, early or late, are but extreme manifestations of the exudative process.[31] The uveal effusion seen in nanophthalmos has been postulated to be the result of impaired venous drainage through the thick sclera characteristic of the nanophthalmic eye[32]; this view is compatible with the thesis of this paper.

[25] Noell WK, Walker VS, Kang BS, et al: *Retinal damage by light in rats.* Invest Ophthalmol Vis Sci 5: 450-473, 1966

[26] Weiter JJ, Delori FC, Wing GL, et al: *Relationship of senile macular degeneration to ocular pigmentation.* Am J Ophthalmol 99: 185-187, 1985

[27] Friedman E, Smith TR: *Senile changes of the choriocapillaris of the posterior pole.* Trans Am Acad Ophthalmol Otolaryngol 69: 652-661, 1965

[28] Bischoff PM, Flower RW: *High blood pressure in choroidal arteries as a possible pathogenetic mechanism in senile macular degeneration.* Am J Ophthalmol 96: 398-399, 1983

[29] Green WR, Key III SN: *Senile macular degeneration: a histopathologic study.* Trans Am Ophthalmol Soc LXXV: 180-254, 1977

[30] Sarks SH: *Drusen and their relationship to senile macular degeneration.* Aust J Ophthalmol 8: 117-130, 1980

[31] Friedman E, Van Buskirk EM, Fineberg E, et al: *Pathogenesis of senile disciform degeneration of the macula.* Proceedings of the XXI International Congress, Mexico, D.I. 8-14 March 1: 454-458, 1970

[32] Brockhurst RJ: *Vortex vein decompression for nanophthalmic uveal effusion.* Ophthalmology 98: 1987-1990, 1980

D. CHOROIDAL NEOVASCULARIZATION

New vessels between Bruch's Membrane and the RPE in the region of the ora serrata and the optic nerve are ubiquitous in the aging eye and relatively benign.[13] Essentially identical vessels develop under the RPE of the macular area in the later stages of AMD but their presence is ominous. It is the appearance of these vessels in the posterior pole and the subsequent leakage and bleeding which signals the impending disciform stage of AMD. Much is known of the microscopic and flourescein angiographic appearance of these new vessels, but their pathogenesis remains obscure.[33] [34]

The idea advanced here is that chronic exudation from the choriocapillaris associated with these three most distal portions of the choroidal venous system results in the deposition of an angiogenic substance in Bruch's membrane.

IV. EPIDEMIOLOGY OF AMD

Over the past 50 years our understanding of the pathogenesis of AMD has remained relatively unchanged in its essentials. We have, however, learned much about the natural history of the disorder, particularly its epidemiology.

A. THE ASSOCIATION WITH REFRACTIVE ERROR

Other than age the characteristic most consistently associated with AMD in case-controlled epidemiologic studies is hyperopia.[35] [36] [37] [38] Hyperopes are more likely to develope AMD and myopia appears to afford protection. No explanation for this association has surfaced thus far.

Friedenwald found that *"the coefficient of rigidity in normal eyes is inversely proportional to the volume of the eyeball,"*[3] and I propose that it is the high scleral rigidity in hyperopia that is responsible for its association with AMD, and the low scleral rigidity of myopia that is protective. The physical basis for the difference in rigidity between hyperopia and myopia is not known but is likely to be related to the difference in the thickness and elasticity of the sclera.

Friedenwald found a marked and significant depression of the coefficient of scleral rigidity in moderate myopia, but in extreme myopia it was increased. He attributed this to stretching of the sclera beyond its elastic limit. While there is a negative association between AMD and moderate myopia due, presumably, to the low scleral rigidity, highly myopic eyes, spared typical AMD, have been found to be associated with a high incidence of choroidal neovascularization.[39] This

[33] Gass JDM: *Pathogenesis of disciform detachment of the neuroepithelium IV.Flourescein angiographic study of senile disciform macular degeneration.* Am J Ophthalmol 63: 645-659, 1967

[34] Lewis H, Straatsma BR, Foos RY, et al: *Reticular degeneration of the pigment epithelium.* Ophthalmology 92: 1485-1495, 1985

[35] Ferris FL: *Senile macular degeneration: review of epidemiologic features.* Am J Epidemiol 118: 132-151, 1983

[36] Maltzman BA, Mulvihill MN, Greenbaum A. *Senile macular degeneration and risk factors: A case-control study.* Ann Ophthalmol 11: 1197-1201, 1979

[37] Delaney WV, Oates RP: *Senile macular degeneration: a preliminary study.* Ann Ophthalmol 14: 21-24, 1982

[38] Hyman LG, Lilienfeld AM, Ferris FL, et al: *Senile macular degeneration: a case-control study.* Am J Epidemiol 118: 213-227, 1983

[39] Hotchkiss ML, Fine SL: *Pathologic myopia and choroidal neovascularization.* Am J Ophthalmol 91: 177-183, 1981

predisposition may be more a function of the high venous pressure associated with the large axial length than the rigid sclera. At the other refractive extreme, the uveal effusion characteristic of the extremely hyperopic eye in nanophthalmos is attributable to the venous obstruction caused by the thick, and presumably rigid, sclera.[32]

B. THE ASSOCIATION WITH RACE

South African[40] and Rhodesian[41] blacks have a remarkably low prevalence rate of AMD in comparison to that of whites in North America, England, and Wales.[35] Reports from China[40] and Japan[42] indicate that AMD is also rare in those countries. While this distribution is consistent with either an environmental or genetic cause, the equal prevalence of AMD among blacks and whites in the United States[43] suggests that the environment of western societies should be examined for risk factors. Indeed, there appears to be a correlation between the prevalence of AMD and atherosclerosis in the racial groups studied to date. In this is confirmed, more extensive investigation of possible relationships among diet, lipid metabolism, and AMD would be justified.[44] [45] [46] [47]

C. THE ASSOCIATION WITH SYSTEMIC DISORDERS

Prominent among the associations with AMD identified by recent epidemiologic studies are systemic hypertension, and other cardio-vascular and pulmonary diseases.[50] In the case of systemic hypertension such an association might be explained by the hydrostatic effect of an elevated arterial blood pressure on the macular choriocapillaris.[28] It is noteworthy that the strongest association between AMD and systemic hypertension is between AMD and elevated blood pressure measured years earlier,[48] suggesting that both share a common etiology rather than a direct causal relationship.

Elevated serum cholesterol has recently been found to be significantly associated with the presence of drusen in eyes of participants in the Framingham Eye Study.[44] The same study also yielded an association of drusen with glucose intolerance which, interesting enough, decreased in significance with time. An explanation for this phenomenon may reside in the report that the scleral

[40] Gregor Z, Joffe L: *Senile macular changes in the black African.* Br J Ophthalmol 62: 542-550, 1978

[41] Chumbley LC: *Impressions of eye disorders among Rhodesian blacks in Mashonaland.* S Afr Med J 52: 316-318, 1977

[42] Hoshino M, Mizuno K, Ichikawa H: *Aging alterations of retina and choroid of Japanese: light microscopic study of macular region of 176 eyes.* Jpn J Ophthalmol 28: 89-103, 1984

[43] Ganley J, Roberts J: *Eye conditions and related need for medical care among persons 1-74 years of age. United States, 1971-72.* Vital and Health Statistics, Series 11, no. 228, DHHS Publication no. (PHS) 83-1678. Washington DC: GPO, March 1983

[44] Hirsch RP, Seddon JM, Milton RC: *Risk factors for drusen in the Framingham Eye Study.* Abstract, Supplement to Invest Ophthalmol Vis Sci 27: 120, 1986

[45] Vidaurri JS, Peer J, Halfon ST, et al: *Association between drusen and some risk factors for coronary artery disease.* Ophthalmologica 188: 243-247, 1984

[46] Landolfo V, Albini L, DeSimone S: *Senile macular degeneration and alteration of the metabolism of the lipids.* Ophthalmologica 177: 248-253, 1978

[47] Kini MM, Leibowitz M, Colton T, et al: *Prevalence of senile cataract, diabetic retinopathy, senile macular degeneration, and open angle glaucoma in the Framingham Eye Study.* Am J Ophthalmol 85: 28-34, 1978

[48] Sperduto RD, Hiller R: *Systemic hypertension and age-related maculopathy in the Framingham study.* Arch Ophthalmol 104: 216-219, 1986

rigidity in diabetes mellitus is decreased.[49] At an earlier age drusen and diabetes are independently associated with an abnormal lipid metabolism but the decrease in scleral rigidity attributable to the diabetes mellitus could decrease the tendency for drusen to form.

According to Verhoeff and Grossman[2] :"*the fact that the disorder most commonly occurs in patients of advanced age suggests that general angiosclerosis is a predisposing factor or that some condition associated with angiosclerosis is often an important factor in producing changes in the choriocapillaris."* But they were also quick to point out that there was "*no support for the view that general angiosclerosis is always the cause of the disorder*", and that still remains the case. There is no evidence that either atheromatosis or arteriosclerosis of the retinal or choroidal vasculature is the cause of AMD, but there is a deposition of lipid in the sclera[19] and other ocular tissues.[50] [51] The subsequent increases in the rigidity of the sclera produces "*changes in the choriocapillaris"*[2] by obstructing venous outflow.

VALIDATION OF THE HYPOTHESIS:

The optimal epidemiologic approach to validation of this working hypothesis is a prospective natural history study of patients with elevated scleral rigidity. The most accurate method of measuring it is probably that described by Anderson and Grant.[52] They recommended comparing a recumbent applanation pressure with a Schiotz reading plotted graphically on the Friedenwald 1955 nomogram.[53]

It has not escaped my notice that if this hypothesis is validated, AMD could be expected to respond favorably to decompression of the vortex veins.[32] Pending such validation, however, any such surgery would have to be considered premature.

In the interim, non surgical methods of decreasing the choroidal venous pressure should be evaluated, such as sleeping in the sitting position, and also increasing the tissue pressure, i.e. the intraocular pressure, pharmacologically. More important, in the long run, is the possibility that AMD may well be a largely preventable condition.

* * * *

Acknowledgement: This manuscript was typed by Marcia Shapiro and technical assistance was given by Susan M. Oak. I acknowledge both gratefully. This work was supported by gifts from the Silverman and Friedman family.

---

[49] Czechowicz-Janicka K, Janik J, Kjos, et al: *Scleral rigidity in certain endocrinological diseases: I.E Index in healthy subjects and diabetics.* Klinika Oczna 82: 307-309, 1980

[50] Friedman E, Smith TR: *Clinical and pathological study of choroidal lipid globules.* Arch Ophthalmol 75: 334-336, 1966

[51] Fraunfelder FT, Hanna C: *Subconjunctival and episcleral lipid globules.* Am J Ophthalmol 79: 262-270, 1975

[52] Anderson DR, Grant WM: *The influence of position on intraocular pressure.* Invest Ophthalmol Vis Sci 12: 204-212, 1973

[53] Friedenwald JS: *Tonometer calibration an attempt to remove discrepancies found in the 1954 calibration scale for schiotz tonometers.* Trans Am Acad Ophthalmol Otolaryngol 61: 108-123, 1957

SUBFOVEAL CHOROIDAL NEOVASCULAR MEMBRANES SECONDARY TO AGE-RELATED MACULAR DEGENERATION: A REVIEW

D. GUYER, R.P. MURPHY, S.L. FINE

From the Wilmer Ophthalmological Institute, The Johns Hopkins Medical Institutions, Baltimore, Maryland 21205

INTRODUCTION

Age-related macular degeneration is a major cause of blindness in the Western world. The two forms of this condition are an atrophic type and an exudative or neovascular type. While only 10% of AMD patients have the exudative form, 88% of the severe vision loss (legal blindness or worse) attributable to this disease is due to this type.[1] This neovascular maculopathy is characterized by the presence of choroidal neovascular membranes (CNVM) which are proliferations of the choriocapillaris through a defect in Bruch's membrane. These CNVM leak blood and lipid, which leads to the development of disciform scars. CNVM can be subdivided according to location. Extrafoveal CNVM are located 200-2500 microns from the center of the foveal avascular zone (FAZ) (Figure 1). The efficacy of laser photocoagulation for extrafoveal CNVM has been demonstrated by the Macular Photocoagulation Study Group (MPS).[2] Juxtafoveal CNVM are found 1-200 microns from the FAZ (Figure 1). The possible beneficial role of laser photocoagulation for juxtafoveal membranes is presently being evaluated by the Krypton Photocoagulation Study (KPS), a multi-center prospective randomized controlled clinical trial supported by the National Eye Institute. Finally, CNVM directly under the center of the FAZ are termed subfoveal (Figure 1). The purpose of this article is to review the natural history, treatment, and pathology of subfoveal CNVM secondary to AMD.

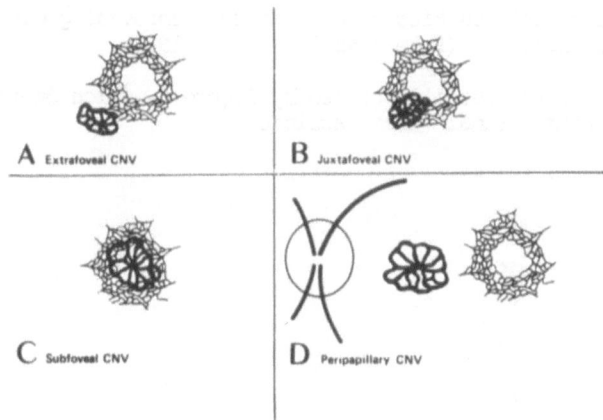

FIGURE 1 A-D. Diagram of foveal avascular zone. A represents an extrafoveal membrane, where the new vessel lies completely outside the zone. B represents a juxtafoveal membrane where the new vessel is within, but not under, the geometric center of the zone. C represents a subfoveal membrane where the new vessel lies under the geometric center of the zone. D represents a peripapillary membrane where the new vessel lies in the papillomacular bundle. (From Bressler et al, 1983)

206

NATURAL HISTORY

The first study designed to determine the visual prognosis of patients with subfoveal CNVM secondary to AMD was performed in 1982 by Bressler et al:[3],[4] After an average follow-up interval of 21 months, 18 (31%) out of 58 eyes with subfoveal CNVM had improved or the same visual acuity, while 40 (69%) had lost two or more lines of vision. Legal blindness, 20/200 or worse, was present in 41 (70%) of the patients at final follow-up.

Figure 2 subdivides this group of 58 eyes on the basis of initial visual acuity. Of the 19 eyes with initial visual acuities of 20/200 to 20/400, only one eye (5%) improved, while eighteen eyes (95%) remained legally blind. Thirteen eyes had initial visual acuities between 20/125 and 20/160. None of these eyes improved, four (31%) had unchanged visual acuities, and nine (69%) deteriorated to legal blindness. Therefore, of the subgroup of 32 eyes with initial visual acuities of 20/125 or worse, 27 (84%) were legally blind at follow-up.

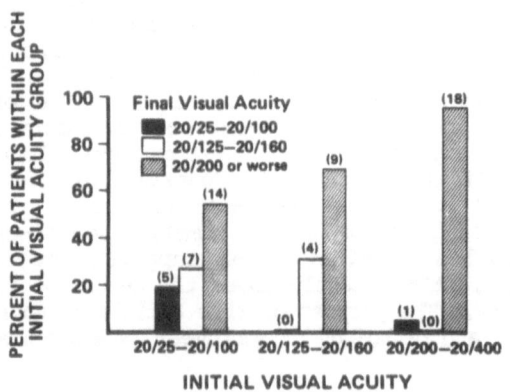

FIGURE 2. Final visual acuities of eyes in the subfoveal group with respect to initial visual acuities (from Bressler et al, 1982).

This poor prognosis is also illustrated by Figure 3, which depicts a scatter plot of initial versus final visual acuities.

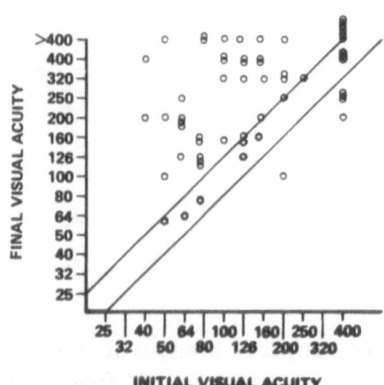

FIGURE 3. Change in visual acuities for the 58 eyes in the subfoveal group that had new vessels directly under the center of the foveal avascular zone. (From Bressler et al, 1982).

Furthermore, for the patients in the Bressler series with initial visual acuities of 20/125 or worse the visual prognosis was not statistically significantly influenced by initial CNVM size.

The visual prognosis of the subgroup of patients with subfoveal CNVM and relatively good initial visual acuity (20/100 or better) is similarly poor. In the Bressler series, only five (19%) out of 26 such eyes had the same or better vision at follow-up, while 21 (81%) lost two or more lines of vision (Figures 2 and 3). Fourteen (54%) of the eyes progressed to legal blindness. In this subgroup initial CNVM size did have an influence upon visual prognosis. The visual acuity was the same or improved in five (38%) out of thirteen eyes with small CNVM (<1500 microns in diameter), but in none (0%) with large CNVM (>1500 microns in diameter) (P< 0.02) (Figure 4).

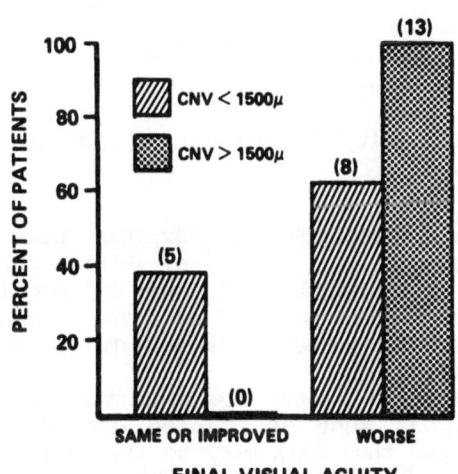

FIGURE 4. Percentages of eyes with subfoveal membranes with an initial visual acuity of 20/100 or better whose visual acuity at follow-up remained the same or improved, or whose visual acuity at follow-up deteriorated two or more lines on the Snellen chart. The hatched columns represent eyes with membranes less than 1500 microns. The stippled columns represent eyes with membranes greater than 1500 microns. (From Bressler et al, 1983)

In conclusion, these patients have a poor visual prognosis, and as expected, those patients with large CNVM at initial examination have an especially unfavorable natural history.

This finding of poor visual prognosis for patients with subfoveal CNVM and relatively good initial visual acuities was recently confirmed by Guyer et al.[5], using a larger study group (N=92). Of the patients who were reexamined 24 months following their initial presentation, 77% had lost at least four lines of vision and 64% had lost at least six lines. Even estimation of the visual loss using a conservative assessment procedure showed a four-line loss in 65% of the patients and a six-line loss in 50%. At 24 months, twelve (55%) had two-year visual acuities of 20/400 or worse, and eighteen (82%) had two-year visual acuities of 20/200 or worse. A scatterplot of the data emphasizes this unfavorable natural history (Figure 5).

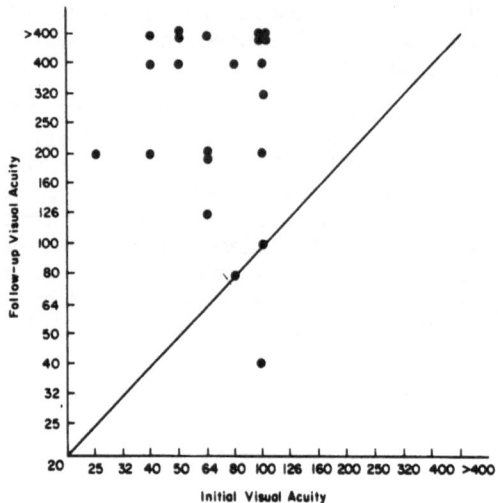

FIGURE 5. Initial visual acuity vs follow-up visual acuity at 24 months. (From Guyer et al, 1986).

The change in visual acuity over time for subgroups based upon age, sex, initial findings in the fellow eye, CNVM size, initial visual acuity, and the presence of blood at the initial examination did not differ among the subgroup categories in the series reported by Guyer et al. However, the small sample sizes of these subgroups may have permitted modest effects of these factors to escape detection.

While the studies discussed above are consistent in demonstrating a poor visual prognosis, it must be pointed out that they are all retrospective in nature, and thus fall prey to the weaknesses inherent in retrospective evaluations. Hopefully a prospective study, such as the one described below, will soon confirm or refute the retrospective findings.

As to the possible location of origin of subfoveal CNVM within the retina, several findings suggest that at least some such CNVM may originate in an extra-foveal location and progress toward the center of the FAZ over time. It has been shown, for instance, that subfoveal CNVM are in general larger than extra-foveal CNVM.[3] In the series by Bressler et al.[3], 66% of the subfoveal CNVM were greater than 1500 microns in diameter, while only 12% of the extrafoveal CNVM were of this diameter (p<0.000001). In addition, MPS data show that 36 (73%) of 49 untreated extrafoveal CNVM involved the FAZ at one-year follow-up.[2] Finally, the average age of patients in the subfoveal CNVM series by Guyer et al was 74 years[5], while in the MPS untreated extrafoveal CNVM group the average age was considerably younger.[2]

TREATMENT

At first glance, it may seem daring to photocoagulate at or near the center of the FAZ. However, the dismal visual prognosis for untreated patients with subfoveal CNVM may justify more radical treatment. If a subfoveal CNVM can be photocoagulated and destroyed early, a smaller final scotoma size may result. Thus photocoagulation, in tandem with the use of low vision aids, could theoretically improve the visual prognosis for these patients.

Several studies involving small groups of patients have reported attempts at the treatment outlined above. Yassur et al.[6] performed a randomized prospective trial of eyes with CNVM located inside the FAZ. They found that visual acuity deterioration was worse for untreated eyes. However, this study is not useful in evaluating possible therapies for truly subfoveal CNVM, since many of the CNVM were poorly defined. No distinction was drawn between CNVM extending into the FAZ but not directly under the center of the FAZ (most of their cases) and CNVM present directly under the FAZ; by MPS standards the latter are subfoveal but the former are juxtafoveal.

Similarly, the series reported by Jalkh et al.[7] suffers from the same CNVM classification problem. Those authors classified "foveal CNVM" as being less than 200 microns from the FAZ center, while the MPS would classify some of those CNVM as juxtafoveal and some as subfoveal. Consequently, these treatment data are not truly comparable to the retrospective natural history data for subfoveal CNVM which was discussed above.

A somewhat more useful study was performed by Decker et al.[8], who treated 25 truly subfoveal CNVM patients with krypton red laser photocoagulation. Post-operatively only seven (28%) out of 25 eyes had the same (six eyes) or improved (one eye) vision (Figure 6).

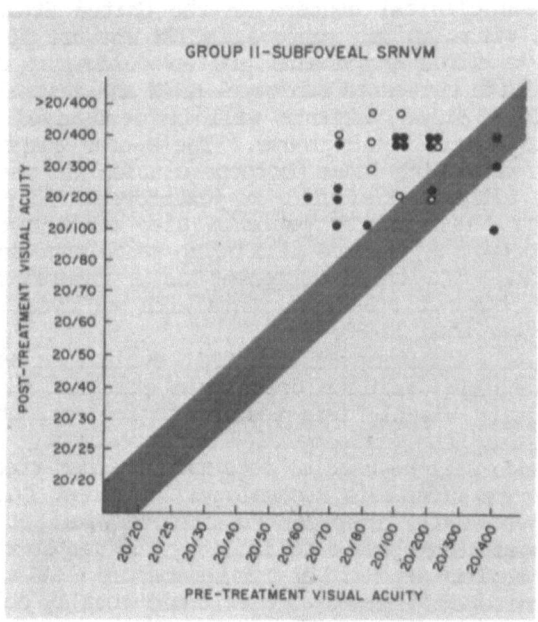

FIGURE 6. Visual acuity pre- and post-photocoagulation of 25 eyes with subfoveal neovascular membranes. Successful closure of neovascular membrane (solid circle). Nonclosure of neovascular membrane (open circle). (From Decker et al, 1984).

Sixteen of their patients had subfoveal CNVM and relatively good initial visual acuities of 20/100 or better. Of these, only two (12%) retained this level of vision or improved at a mean follow-up of ten months (range eight to 18 months). The CNVM were totally obliterated in 17 (68%) of 25 eyes. Of these 17 eyes, two improved, four stayed the same, and twelve decreased in visual acuity by two or more lines of vision. Three eyes had final visual acuities of 20/100, but no eye had a better than 20/100 final outcome. Since these authors had no concurrent control group they compared their findings with the natural history study findings of Bressler et al.[3,4] The authors concluded that laser photocoagulation for subfoveal CNVM is not indicated unless the initial visual acuity is 20/100 or worse. Unfortunately, as Decker et al themselves suggested, this comparison of entirely different patient groups at different institutions can only yield conclusions of limited value, especially given the extremely small size and limited follow-up of both study groups.

Since the poor natural history for patients with subfoveal CNVM is now apparent, a controlled clinical trial of laser photocoagulation is indicated. The few reported series of laser photocoagulation for subfoveal CNVM are flawed, however, as discussed above. Clearly, a multi-center prospective randomized controlled clinical trial is needed to determine the possible impact of laser photocoagulation upon subfoveal CNVM. Fortunately, such a study, the Foveal Photocoagulation Study (FPS), was begun in February of 1986.

The FPS is being organized by the MPS and funded by the National Eye Institute. Thirteen clinical centers in the United States are currently enrolling patients with AMD and subfoveal CNVM who are 50 years of age or older. The study's three components are as follows. One component is enrolling patients with untreated subfoveal CNVM and initial visual acuities of 20/80 to 20/400. These patients will be randomized to either laser photocoagulation or nontreatment groups. The second component is studying patients already treated with laser photocoagulation who have recurrent CNVM that originated as either extrafoveal or juxtafoveal and now progressed to the center of the FAZ. These patients also must have initial visual acuities of 20/80 or worse, and are also being randomized into treatment and nontreatment groups. The third component is a natural history registry which will observe, but not treat, patients with subfoveal CNVM and initial visual acuities better than 20/80.

For all three components of the FPS, evaluation will include best corrected visual acuity, complete ophthalmic examination, and fluorescein angiograms as needed. Visual field testing to follow scotoma size will be crucial in determining the efficacy of laser treatment. In addition, low vision aid assistance will be used to determine whether treated or untreated patients benefit more from this technology. Contrast sensitivity testing will be performed as well, in order to discover earlier and less severe visual acuity changes than those obtainable by the use of the Snellen chart. Finally, both the ability to totally obliterate the CNVM and the recurrence of CNVM will be monitored. Decker et al.[8] could totally obliterate only 68% of the subfoveal CNVM in their series. The CNVM recurrence rate data will be important in evaluating the benefits of laser therapy as well. As an example, the efficacy of laser treatment for extrafoveal CNVM was somewhat moderated by the recent MPS report that 70 (59%) of treated eyes later had a recurrence of their CNVM.[9] If the patient recruitment goals for the FPS are met, the ophthalmic community could anticipate an answer to this important therapeutic dilemma within the next several years.

We are reminded by the CNVM recurrence problem discussed above, as well as the pre-operative visual morbidity caused by the CNVM, that laser photocoagulation can only mitigate AMD, but not arrest or prevent it. Future research must focus upon the prevention of this disease. Recent work by several authors suggests the possible role of chronic light exposure[10,11], vitamin levels[12-14], cigarette smoking[9,15-17], and vascular disease[15,16,18-20], among other factors, in the pathogenesis of AMD. While these findings are presently preliminary, hopefully further work will conclusively determine the actual pathogenesis of AMD, and thus assist in its prevention.

PATHOLOGY

The pathology of AMD and CNVM has already been extensively reviewed by other authors.[22-25] In addition, a clinicopathologic correlation was recently described which sheds more light upon our subject.[26] The case involved a patient with a subfoveal CNVM secondary to AMD that was treated two times each with both argon green and krypton red laser photocoagulation. The patient was first treated when his visual acuity was 20/100. Immediately following the first laser photocoagulation his vision decreased to 8/200; he never attained better than 20/160 vision and eventually deteriorated to 20/400 vision within one year post-operatively. Subsequent pathologic examination revealed an extensive macular scar of a maximum length of 4 mm. This scar consisted of two components: an intra-Bruch's membrane fibrovascular section, and a section from Bruch's membrane through the neurosensory retina. Areas treated with the krypton red laser showed inner retinal sparing, while those regions treated with the argon green laser showed transretinal effects. In addition, neovascularization extended under the retinal pigment epithelium in the nasal aspect of the lesion. Thus it is apparent in this case that CNVM recurrences were a major problem. The CNVM recurred three times clinically, requiring three more laser treatments, and neovascularization was still present on pathologic examination. The visual loss from 20/100 to 20/400 in only one year was similarly disappointing. It is possible, however, that the multiple treatments required for this patient were a reflection of the fact that this patient was one of the first to be treated for a subfoveal CNVM. There was understandable reluctance because of the subfoveal position to employ the power settings which eventually proved necessary in order to clinically obliterate the CNVM.

Only further study by the FPS will determine if the visual outcome and CNVM recurrence rates will be such that laser photocoagulation becomes the recommended treatment for these patients.

CONCLUSION

The visual prognosis of patients with subfoveal CNVM secondary to AMD is dismal, according to retrospective studies. Therefore, a multi-center prospective randomized controlled clinical trial will be important in determining the possible role of laser photocoagulation for these patients. Such a trial, the Foveal Photocoagulation Study, is currently underway and will hopefully soon provide an answer to this important therapeutic dilemma.

REFERENCES

1. Hyman LG. Senile macular degeneration: an epidemiologic case control study, thesis. The Johns Hopkins University, Baltimore, 1981.
2. Macular Photocoagulation Study Group. Argon laser photocoagulation for senile macular degeneration: results of a randomized clinical trial. Arch Ophthalmol 1982; 100:912-918.

3. Bressler SB, Bressler NM, Fine SL, et al. Subfoveal neovascular membranes in senile macular degeneration: relationship between membrane size and visual prognosis. Retina 1983; 3:7-11.
4. Bressler SB, Bressler NM, Fine SL et al. Natural course of choroidal neovascular membranes within the foveal avascular zone in senile macular degeneration. Am J Ophthalmol 1982; 93:157-163.
5. Guyer DR, Fine SL, Maguire MG, et al. Subfoveal choroidal neovascular membranes in age-related macular degeneration: visual prognosis in eyes with relatively good initial visual acuity. Arch Ophthalmol 1986; 104:702-705.
6. Yassur Y, Axer-Siegel R, Cohen S, et al. Treatment of neovascular senile maculopathy at the foveal capillary free zone with red krypton laser. Retina 1982; 2:127-133.
7. Jalkh AE, Avila MP, Trempe CL, et al. Choroidal neovascularization in fellow eyes of patients with advanced senile macular degeneration: role of laser photocoagulation. Arch Ophthalmol 1983; 101:1194-1197.
8. Decker WL, Grabowski WM, Annesley WH. Krypton red laser photocoagulation of subretinal neovascular membranes located within the foveal avascular zone. Ophthalmol 1984; 91:1582-1586.
9. Macular Photocoagulation Study Gruop. Recurrent choroidal neovascularization after argon laser photocoagulation for neovascular maculopathy. Arch Ophthalmol 1986; 104:503-512.
10. Guyer DR, Alexander MF, Auer CL, et al. A comparison of the frequency and severity of macular drusen in phakic and non-phakic eyes. ARVO Abstracts. Invest Ophthalmol Vis Sci 1986; 27(Suppl):20.
11. Blumenkranz MS, Russell SR, Robey MG, et al. Risk factors in age-related maculopathy complicated by choroidal neovascularization Ophthalmol 1986; 93:552-557.
12. Noel WK, Albrecht R. Irreversible effects of visible light on the retina: role of vitamin A. Science 1971; 172:76-80.
13. Tso MO. Pathogenetic factors of aging macular degeneration. Ophthalmol 1985; 93:628-635.
14. Robison WG, Kuwabara T, Bieri JG. The role of vitamin E and unsaturated fatty acids in the visual processes. Retina 1982; 2:263-281.
15. Hyman LG, Lilienfield AM, Ferris FL, et al. Senile macular degeneration: a case control study. Am J Epidemiol 1983; 118:213-227.
16. Delany WV, Oates RP. Senile macular degeneration: a preliminary study. Ann Ophthalmol 1982; 14:21-24.
17. Paetkau ME, Boyd TAS, Grace M, et al. Senile disciform macular degeneration and smoking. Can J Ophthalmol 1978;13:67-71.
18. Kahn HA, Leibowitz HM, Ganley JP, et al. The Framingham eye study II: association of ophthalmic pathology with single variables previously mentioned in the Framingham heart study. Am J Epidemiol 1977; 106:33-41.
19. Vidaurri J, Pe'er J, Halfon S, et al. Association between drusen and some of the risk factors for coronary artery disease. Ophthalmologica 1984; 188:243-247.
20. Kornzweig AL. Changes in the choriocapillaris associated with senile macular degeneration. Ann Ophthalmol 1977; 9:753-764.
21. Sperduto RD, Hiller R. Systemic hypertension and age-related maculopathy in the Framingham Study. Arch Ophthalmol 1986; 104:216-219.
22. Green WR. Clinicopathologic studies of senile macular degeneration. In: Nicholson DH, ed. Ocular Patholgoy Update. New York: Masson, 1980; 115-144.

23. Green WR. Senile macular degeneration: a histopathologic study. Tr Am Ophthalmol Soc 1977; 75:180–254.
24. Green WR, McDonnell PJ, Yeo JH. Pathologic features of senile macular degeneration. Ophthalmol 1985; 92:615–627.
25. Sarks SH. Aging and degeneration in the macular region: a clinicopathological study. Br J Ophthalmol 1976; 60:324–341.
26. Guyer DR, Fine SL, Murphy RP, et al. Clinicopathologic correlation of krypton and argon laser photocoagulation in a patient with a choroidal neovascular membrane. 1986 (submitted for publication).

ZINC AND COPPER METABOLISM STUDY IN PATIENTS WITH HIGH MYOPIA
AND SENILE MACULAR DEGENERATION

Ben-Zion Silverstone, M.D., Morton H. Seelenfreund, M.D. & David BersonMD.
Department of Ophthalmology, Shaare Zedek Medical Center,
Jerusalem.

Introduction:

It is well accepted that some retinal disorders affecting the Retinal
Pigment Epithelium (RPE), are related to changes in the zinc and cooper
metabolism (1,2,3).

In previous studies carried out in different groups of patients with high
myopia, and in a group of patients with senile macular degeneration (SMD),
these changes in the metabolism of these metals were found (4,5).

The association between high myopia and SMD is infrequent (5), and we,
therefore, found of interest to compare the metabolism of these metals
in these two groups.

Material and Methods:

Two groups of patients were included in the present study. Each group was
previously compared to a control group (4,5).

1.- A high myopic group that includes 25 patients. Age range was from
    20 to 70 years. All patients had myopia higher than -6.00, with
    typical myopic changes in the fundi.

2.- A Senile macular degeneration group of 16 patients. Age range was
    between 50 to 84 years. The degree of the macular abnormality was
    classified according to Zweng Classification (6).

Results:

The results of serum zinc in copper in both the high myopic group and
senile macular degeneration group, are summarized in Tables I and II.
In Table II a further subclassification in Myopes and Hyperopes with
senile macular degeneration is included as well.

On the basis of the results, when the senile macular degeneration group
was compared to the high myopic group, high values of statistical significance of serum zinc and copper were found in the former group.
(zinc, $p < .005$., copper, $p < 0.25$).

Discussion:

There are many investigations that support the concept of significant
interaction between zinc and copper alterations and structural changes

in the RPE (1,2,4,5,6). It is not clear whether these changes are secondary
to a basic inherited metabolic disorder or connected to a progressive disease that affects the RPE and choroid. This last possibility might be
supported by our recent findings of changes in the metabolism of these
metals, after a mechanical damage to the RPE - Choroid complex by argon
laser photocoagulation (7).

Our preliminary observations in different groups of high myopic patients
showed alterations in the serum zinc and copper, among many of them
(3,4,5). Since an infrequent association between SMD and high myopia is
well known, we compared our results in these two groups of patients.

In both disorders changes in the RPE are present. However, their pathogenesis seems to be different. Bass and Chandra and associates (7,8)
have described in patients with SMD degenerative or aging changes in the
choriocapillaries bed, and thickening of the Bruch's membrane. On the
other hand, in high myopia the degenerative changes are present mainly in
the RPE and outer retinal layers (9). In the present study when the group
of patients with SMD was compared to the high myopic group, both serum
zinc and copper were found elevated, and of statistical significance
(zinc., $p < .005.$, copper $p < 0.25$). (Table I). The SMD hyperopic
group clearly showed statistical significant elevated values of the serum
zinc and copper (zinc, p. $< .0005.$, copper p $< .005$, Table II).
The SMD myopic group showed elevated serum zinc of low significance
(zinc, $p < .025$ Table II).

In a previous work carried out among high myopic patients, high serum
zinc and low serum copper were found (4). In the present work, hyperopic
patients with SMD showed elevated serum zinc and copper levels, which is
intertesting, and suggest a possible difference in the pathogenesis or
both disorders, as previously mentioned.

Whether the difference in the results obtained in both groups is attributable to a genetic difference, or to an abnormality in the RPE - Choroid
complex of different amount, or possibly to both, must be clarified in
future studies.

TABLE I

The results are in μ mol/L.

	HIGH MYOPIA	SENILE MACULAR DEGEN.
SERUM ZINC	20.26 ± 5.87	28.48 ± 9.54
SERUM COPPER	17.05 ± 5.15	21.17 ± 7.49

ZINC   p   < .005

COPPER p   < .25

TABLE II

The results are in μ mol/L.

	HIGH MYOPIA	SMD MYOPIA	SMD HYPEROPIA
SERUM ZINC	20.26 ± 5.87	26.0 ± 10.27	31.67 ± 8.11
SERUM COPPER	17.05 ± 5.15	19.0 ± 9.19	23.96 ± 3.43

HIGH MYOPIA / SMD (MYOPIA)

SERUM ZINC : p   <   0.25

SERUM COPPER: No significance.

HIGH MYOPIA / SMD   HYPEROPIA)

SERUM ZINC: p   <   .0005

SERUM COPPER: p   <   .005

REFERENCES

1. Ghalot DK, Khosla PK: Copper metabolism in retinitis pigmentosa. Br J Ophthalmol 1976; 60:770.

2. Silverstone BZ, et al: Plasma zinc levels in high myopia and retinitis pigmentosa. Metab Pediatr Ophthalmol 1981; 5:187.

3. Silverstone BZ et al: Copper metabolism changes in pigmentary retinopathies and high myopia. Metab Peditr Ophthalmol. 1981; 5:11.

4. Silverstone BZ et al: A metabolic aspect of high myopia. Ann Ophthalmol 1985; 17:546.

5. Silverstone BZ et al: Zinc and copper metabolism in patients with senile macular degeneration. Ann Ophthalmol. 1985; 17, 419.

6. Chandra, SR et al: Natural history of disciform degeneration of the macula. Am J Ophthalmol. 1974; 78:579.

7. Silverstone BZ et al: Copper and zinc levels after external damage by laser photocoagulation to the retinal pigment epithelium. Preliminary reports. Metab Pediatr Ophthalmol. 1985; 8:61.

8. Gass JDM: Stereoscopic Atlas of Macular Diseases. Diagnosis and Treatment. 2nd ed. St. Louis, CV Mosby, 1977; 19-21.

9. Schie HG, Albert DM: Textbook of Ophthalmology. Chapter 12. London, WB Saunders, 1977: 271.

NATURAL HISTORY OF OCCULT SUBRETINAL NEW-VESSELS IN AGE-RELATED MACULAR
DEGENERATION

G. SOUBRANE, G. COSCAS, F. KOENIG, C. FRANCAIS - CRETEIL (France)

The neovascular or "wet" form, of age related macular degeneration
encompasses a wide spectrum of clinical features. Subretinal new
vessels that appear well defined on fluorescein angiography portend a
poor visual prognosis without treatment, but the results of three
randomized controlled trials have demonstrated the therapeutic value of
argon blue-green photocoagulation on visual outcome (1-3). However, in
many cases, subretinal neovascularization may not be clearly visible on
fluorescein angiography, although it is suspected clinically. Little
information is available (4,5) on the natural history of subretinal new
vessels not clearly outlined on fluorescein angiography, so-called
"occult" subretinal neovascularization.
      Therefore, we designed this study to define the clinical features
and to assess the visual prognosis of patients with occult subretinal
neovascularization in an attempt to determine the possible
effectiveness of treatment methods.

PATIENTS AND METHODS

      Patients selected for this retrospective study were 55 years or
older, had evidence of age-related macular degeneration, and had been
followed for more than one year. In addition, the eyes being evaluated
satisfied the following criteria : (1) visual symptoms considered due
to biomicroscopically identified neovascular macular degeneration and
not to any other ophthalmic disease ; (2) initial visual acuity of 6/60
or better; and (3) a serous detachment of the retina associated with
hemorrhages and/or lipid deposits at time of presentation. Eyes with
detachment of the retinal pigment epithelium were excluded from the
study.
      Of 302 eyes examined at the University Eye Clinic of Creteil and
diagnosed as having occult subretinal neovascularization in age-related
macular degeneration, 50 eyes (47 patients) met the inclusion criteria
of this study. All eyes underwent a complete ocular examination,
stereoscopic fundus photography, and fluorescein angiography initially
and at each follow-up examination thereafter.

RESULTS

      The 47 patients in our study had an average age of 72 years
(range, 56 to 85 years) ; 80% were between 65 and 80 years. Age-related
macular degeneration was bilateral in 38 patients, three of whom had
both eyes evaluated in the study. The visual symptoms were long-term
(mean time, 35 weeks) and 16 patients complained of metamorphopsia.

220

Follow-up varied from one to eight years (mean follow-up period, 27 months) (Table I).

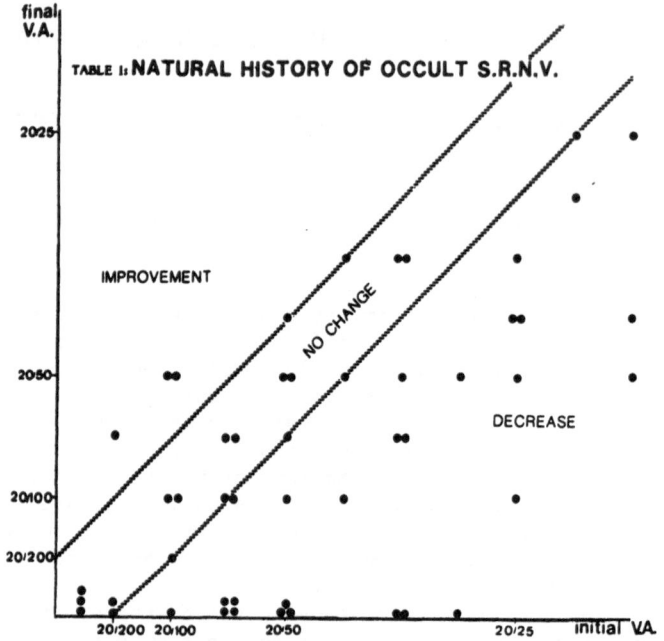

Visual acuity, (6/60 or better), was initially quite fair : 31 eyes (62%) had 20/50 or better, and 42 (84%) had normal near vision. At the end of the follow-up period, 17 eyes (38%) had retained a good distance visual acuity (20/50 or better) and 26 (52%) maintained normal near visual acuity (Table 1). In general, visual acuity progressively decreased throughout the follow-up period. After 3 years, 45% of the patients had a visual acuity better than 20/50. After 5 years, this percentage had dropped to 20%. Thus, the long-term trend was for gradual, progressive deterioration of visual acuity.

At presentation, biomicroscopic examination showed retinal serous detachment in all 50 eyes, associated with retinal or subretinal blood in 21, and with hard exudates in 16 ; 38 eyes of 50 had drusen ; and 28 showed pigment epithelial mottling. During follow-up all eyes demonstrated some degree of bleeding, usually mild. In most of the cases, the exudative lesion remained the same, although some progressed to fibrosis or atrophy.

Even on good quality angiograms, the features of occult subretinal new vessels were very subtle and often difficult to analyze, although their presence was clinically obvious. Leakage of fluorescein, considered a constant and diagnostic feature of subretinal new vessels growth, was sometimes the only angiographic sign of occult neovascularization. Usually, a zone of irregular hyperfluorescence showed late leakage. A peripheral uneven zone was suspected of containing some developing subretinal neovascularization. The hyperfluorescence was occasionally delayed, but the late leakage of dye was helpful for the diagnosis.

In some cases (six eyes), an early sea fan-like hyperfluorescence was observed, which faded on the late venous phase of the angiogram.

In the area of a suspected neovascular membrane many hyperfluorescent dots appeared and showed late staining in 32 eyes. This angiographic feature appeared a good sign associated with occult subretinal neovascularization.

During the follow-up period, the angiographic pattern of the macular lesion remained approximately the same in 28 eyes, without visible and definite subretinal vessel growth, although there was some extension of the lesion. In 22 eyes, the angiographic appearance changed : in seven eyes, one or usually more buds of new vessels became visible, and in 15 eyes the classical sea fan pattern developed.

DISCUSSION

We presumed that neovascular tissue was present in the macular disciform lesions when blood existed beneath the retina, when exudative deposits occurred on the limits of the serous retinal detachment, and when an irregular pattern of hyperfluorescence developed in the subretinal and subpigment epithelial spaces. However, good quality fluorescein angiography failed to show the typical neovascular pattern. Moreover, fluorescein angiography and fundus photography were clearly inaccurate tools to predict the location and the extension of occult subretinal neovascularization in our patients.

Goss (4) and Sarks (6) suggested that hemorrhage and exudate may arise from vessels already established on the inner surface of Bruch's membrane. Futhermore, Green and associates (7) showed that the neovascularization can be located beneath the retinal pigment epithelium without subsequent disciform degeneration.

Numerous factors may be responsible for the lack of visibility of the neovascular network. The pigment epithelial cells may not be completely atrophic and actually may be hypertrophic, allowing the pigment to hide the subpigment epithelial changes. As Miller and co-workers (8) showed in an experimental model, the retinal pigment epithelium proliferates around neovascular tufts. A gradual degeneration in the metabolism of the retinal pigment epithelium leading to the accumulation of metabolic waste products in Bruch's membrane would decrease its permeability, as Hogan (9) suggested.

The variation of leakage from the capillaries could reflect a different exudative nature in the neovascular tissue according to ensuing stages of evolution. The experimental model of Ryan (10) supports this hypothesis. The small size of these vessels and subsequently the reduced blood flow could also be responsible for the failure of fluorescein angiography to demonstrate their presence.

Although our knowledge of the morphologic changes of age-related macular degeneration is incomplete, the data accumulated during our study to document the natural history in this disease of occult subretinal new vessel growth may provide a baseline for prognosis and for the evaluation of an effective time of therapy. Although severe visual loss occurs during follow-up, the rate at which visual acuity decreases appears slower than in the typical neovascular form. In our series, half of the eyes retained useful and reasonably fair central vision during the first three symptomatic years.

REFERENCES

1.Coscas, G., and Soubrane, G. : photocoagulation des néo-vaisseaux sous rétiniens dans la dégénérescence maculaire sénile par le laser à argon. Résultats de l'étude randomisée de 60 cas. Bull. Soc. Ophthalmol. Fr. 88 : 102-106, 1982.
2.Macula Photocoagulation Study Group : Argon laser photocoagulation for senile macular degeneration. Résults of randomized clinical trial. Arch. Ophthalmol. 100 : 912-918, 1982.
3.Moorfields Macular Study Group : Treatment of senile disciform macular degeneration. A single blind randomized trial by argon laser photocoagulation. Br. J. Ophthalmol. 60 : 745-753, 1982.
4.Gass, J.D.M. : Pathogenesis of disciform detachment of the neuro-epithelium. Am. J. Ophthalmol. 63 : 573-660, 1967.
5.Gass, J.D.M. : Serous retinal pigment epithelial detachment with a notch. A sign of occult choroïdal neovascularization. Retina 4 : 205-220, 1984.
6.Sarks, S.H. : New vessel formation beneath the retinal pigment epithelium in senile eyes. Br. J. Ophthalmol. 57 : 951-965, 1973.
7.Green, R., Mc Donnell, P., and Yeo, J.H. : Pathologic features of senile macular degeneration. Ophthalmology 92 : 615-627, 1985.
8.Miller, H., Miller, B., and Ryan, S.J. : Newly-formed subretinal vessels : Fine structure and fluorescein leakage. Invest. Ophthalmol. Vis. Sci., in press.
9.Hogan, M.J. : Role of the pigment epithelium in macular diseases. Trans. Am. Acad. Ophthalmol. Otolaryngol. 76 : 64-80, 1972.
10.Ryan, S.J. : Subretinal neovascularization. Natural history of an experimental model. Arch. Ophthalmol. 11 : 1804-1809, 1982.

ABSTRACT
    Natural history of occult subretinal neovascularization has not yet been assessed although subretinal new vessels clearly defined on the angiogram were shown to carry a poor visual prognosis in age-related macular degeneration.
    To precise the clinical features and the visual prognosis of occult S.R.N.V., we studied 50 affected eyes, in 47 patients of 55 years of age or more, with a clinical and although, decrease of visual acuity was relatively slow.
    Biomicroscopic clues of occult SNRV were a serous retinal detachment, hemorrhages, hard exudates and pigment epithelial mottling. The angiogram showed either a delayed hyeprfluorescent area, progressively enlarging during the examination with late leakage, either a sea fan-like pattern which faded thereafter or hyperfluorescent dots on the border of a suspected zone.
    During follow-up, 22 eyes showed a bud or a typical S.R.N.V. that revealed itself outwardly, in the previous area. In the remaining 28 eyes, there were no visible S.R.N.V. and the angiographic pattern remained the same but with extension of the oozing lesion. 62% had an initial V.A. of 20/50 or better. At the end of the follow up period 38% had retained this level of acuity.

MONOCHROMATIC ARGON GREEN LASER IN THE TREATMENT OF JUXTAFOVEAL SUBRETINAL NEOVASCULARIZATION (SRNV) IN AGE RELATED MACULAR DEGENERATION (ARMD).

Y. Yassur, MD, I. Rosenblatt, MD, D. Ucenick, MD.

Soroka Medical Center and The Faculty of Health Sciences, Ben-Gurion University of the Negev, Beer-Sheva and "Maccabi" Laser Institute, Tel-Aviv, Israel.

The data concerning the incidence, prevalence, and natural history of legal blindness due to SRNV in ARMD in the first and in the fellow eye are not completely solid until today. However, there is no doubt anymore concerning few facts: first that the visual prognosis of eyes with SRNV is poor (1,2). Secondly, that most of the fellow eyes are affected within five years. Thirdly, that visual prognosis of the fellow eye, if it has SRNV, is very poor, and that if the SRNV is juxta-foveal or sub-foveal, the prognosis is even worse.

Various fundamental questions have not yet been answered by proper controlled studies: Is treatment better than natural history? When is the best time to treat - early or late? Should treatment be applied when visual acuity is still good or only when it declines? How intense and where to treat? The answers to each of these questions is controvertial and some of the answers are eventually conected to the issue of the wavelength (3,4,5,6).

The tendency to use pure wavelength laser is based on the fact that the different layers of the fundus absorb, transmit, and reflect differently various wavelengths (6,7,8), and that in order to achieve destruction of a lesion at any layer of the fundus we should aim that the neighboring layers should be damaged as less as possible. Also when using monochromatic laser, less total energy and lower power density are required for the same therapeutic effect.

In the late seventies, before monochromatic green laser was commercialy available, our group was among those who recomended treatment with red krypton laser, which seemed to be a better solution for ARMD (4,9). However, it was clear that even that laser was not the ultimate answer to ARMD lesions although superior to blue-green laser.

In recent years monochromatic green argon laser (540nm) has become commercialy available. This pure green argon laser seemed theoretically to have advantages for treatment of SRNV: it is highly absorbed by blood, and therfore by SRNV membrane, with minimal absorbtion by the inner retina, a fact that enabls us to treat very close to the fovea. In addition it is also highly transmited to the sub retinal space, where most of the pathology in SRNV exists. This laser has one main limiting factor which is the difficulty in treatment when there is blood in the retina itself.

MATERIAL AND METHODS

We treated 23 eyes of 23 patients suffering from ARMD and SRNV invading the foveal avascular zone (FAZ) by pure green argon laser photocoagulation. There were 7 first eyes and 16 fellow eyes of patients who previously lost central vision due to SRNV. The SRNV lesions were treated by confluent moderate to strong intensity applications of 50μ - 300μ spots, 0.1-0.3 seconds. The membranes were completely covered by the treatment according to a careful identification by fluorescein angiography. The evaluation of the results was done by VA, visual fields, and semetimes contrast-sensitivity, as well as by fluorecein angiography (FA). The follow up period was at least two years.

R E S U L T S

In 8 eyes VA declined, in 12 it remained the same, and in 3 it improved. This means that in 60% of treated eye VA remained the same and improved. Where there was a decline, it was no more than to 6/60 if the VA at time of treatment was not less than 6/24.

Among the treated eyes, the SRNV regressed completely after the first treatment in 13 eyes; in 7 eyes it regressed after we continued to treat the membrane once or twice more during the following 6 weeks, as the membrane seemed in FA not to disappear completely; and in 3 eyes there was a recurrence which progressed beneath the fovea crossing it to the other side of the macula.

C O M M E N T S

In the 16 eyes which were the fellow eyes, if we compare the VA of the treated eye to the VA of the first untreated eye, we see that in all the patients the treated eye had a better VA than the non treated eye, and most of the treated eyes could benefit from low vision aids. (graph No. 1).

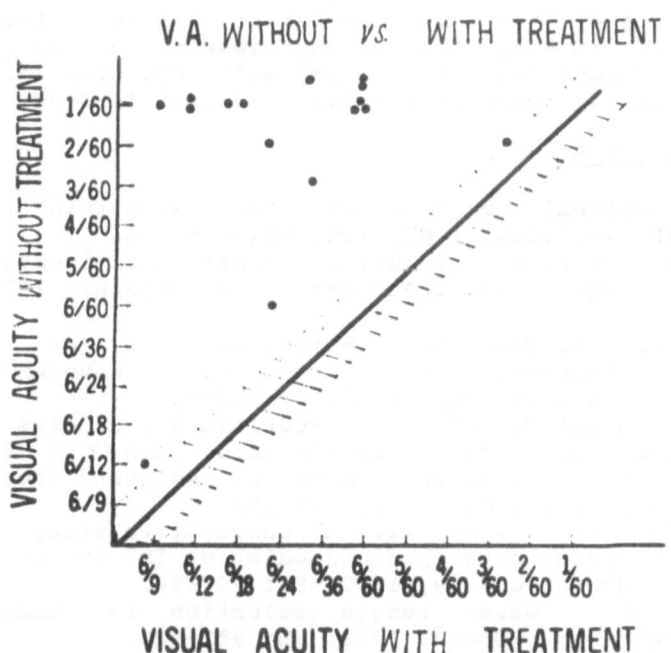

It is also interesting that quite often there was a big discrapance between the atrophic appearance of the treated macula and the relatively good VA, sometimes between 6/12 - 6/24.

It seems that sometimes the disciform scar in the eye which is treated has a completely different quality than the disciform scar of the natural history of the disease, which look thicker and with more gliosis.

Sometimes there is quite a discrepance between the good VA and and patients' low satisfaction, which may be low. This is explained by the fact that some eyes with good VA have a considarably declined contrast-sensitivity.

The results of this treatment study are on a limited number of eyes; however they draw the attention to a probable benefit of treatment of any symptomatic SRNV at the FAZ even if VA is still good. It is worth mentioning Jalkh study in 1983 and Azzolini and Jalkh in 1986: Jalkh in 1983 (10) showed that treatment with pure green argon laser for SRNV in ARMD is beneficial if being carried out while VA is better than 20/70. Jalkh and Azzolini in 1986 showed in a mode of treatment similar to ours that there was NV closure in 90%, and VA improvement in 70% of treated eyes. Future controlled study will hopefully give an answer to the efficacy of treatment of such lesions.

R E F E R E N C E S

1. Bresler. Natural course of choroidal NV within the FAZ in SMD. Am.J.Oph. 1982, Feb. 92(2)157-63.
2. Schatz, H., Patz A. Exudative senile maculopathy: results of argon laser treatment. Arch. Ophth. 1973; 90:183.
3. Trepe CL., Mainster MA., Pomerantzeff O. et al. Macular photocoagulation: optimal wavelength selection. Ophthalmology, 1982; 89: 721-8.
4. Yassur Y., Sigal R., Cohen S., Svetliza E., Bensira I. Treatment of neovascular senile maculopathy at the foveal capillary free zone with red krypton laser. Retina, 1982; Vol 2 No. 3, p. 127-133.
5. Sabates FN, Lee KY. et al. A comparative study of argon and krypton laser photocoagulation in treatment of P.O.H. Ophthalmology, 1982; 89: 729-34.
6. Mainster NA. Wave length selection in macula photocoagulation. Ophth. 1986; 93: 952-958.
7. Boettner EA, Walter JR. Transmission of the ocular media. Invest. Ophthalmology 1962; 1:776.
8. Geerates WJ., Berry ER. Ocular spectral characteristics as related to the hazards from lasers and other light sources. Ophthalmology, 1968; 66:15.
9. Yassur Y. Schlaen ND, Sigal R. The treatment of exudative senile maculopathy by red krypton laser. In: Azuberman H. et al, Docum Ophthal. Proc. Series, Vol. 25. The Hague: Dr. W. Junk 1981, 149-150. Presented at the subretinal space, Jerusalem, Sept. 1979.
10. Jalkh AE, Avila MP, Trempe CL, Schepens CL. Choroidal neovascularization in the fellow eyes of patients with advanced senile macular degeneration. Role of laser photocoagulation. Arc. Ophthal. 1983 Aug. 101(8), 1194.

LASER TREATMENT OF OCCULT SUBRETINAL NEW VESSELS IN AGE-RELATED MACULAR DEGENERATION : Feasability study and comparison with natural history.

G.SOUBRANE, G. COSCAS, C. FRANCAIS - CRETEIL (France)

In age-related macular degeneration, subretinal new-vessels are not always clearly outlined on fluorescein angiography. Often, they are so-called "occult" subretinal new-vessels which are clinically recognizable although the angiographic features are multiple : the presence of the new-vessels is established but their precise extent and location remain however extremely difficult to assess even when asociated to extensive pigmentary changes or pigment epithelium detachment (2, 3, 6).

Natural history of occult subretinal new-vessels appears to be less dramatic than clearly visible subretinal new-vessels which progress rapidly to hemorrhages, fibrous proliferations and therefore to severe loss of central vision . "Occult" subretinal new-vessels also lead to deterioration of central vision but in a slow and progressive rate : major impairment of vision occurs, in our study, only 3 years after onset of symtoms.

Three randomized trials (1, 4, 5) have demonstrated the therapeutic value of argon blue-green photocoagulation on visual outcome but only for visible subretinal new vessels. In order to assess the possible benefit of early laser treatment of occult subretinal new-vessels in age-related macular degeneration, this retrospective study was conducted about a group of 50 eyes presenting with a functional and ophtalmoscopic macular syndrome.

PATIENTS AND METHOD
Inclusion criteria of patients in the study were the following :
- ages of 55 years or more ;
- presenting with age-related macular degeneration (drusen, pigment epithelium disturbances and/or subretinal new-vessels in the other eye) whithout any other macular lesion ;
- followed-up over a six months period at least ;
- complaining of visual symptoms but still with a visual acuity of 20/200 or better ;
- biomicroscopically showing a macular retinal serous detachment associated to hemorrhages and/or exudates.
- angiographically presenting a late leakage of dye, being the essential charateristic of subretinal new-vessels, although the uneven, irregular, deep hyperfluorescence was either early or delayed.

RESULTS
Out of the 50 patients included in this study, 15 were males and 35

females with 27 right eyes and 23 left eyes involved ; in 14 cases the eye concerned was the first one and in 36 cases the second ; the latter were affected 2 to 60 months after the first eye. Symptoms duration ranged from 2 weeks to 3 years (average : 15 weeks); in 36 of 59 cases, there was a decrease of visual acuity and a third of them had metamorphopsia.

The predominance of female patients correlates to the percentage of women in the age group over 55. In the group studied, the mean age of onset of symptoms was 71.74 years.

The period of follow-up ranged from 6 to 60 months (average : 25.5 months). Half of the patients were followed-up for 2 years or more. Initial visual acuity was quite fair and 80% of the patients had still a visual acuity better than 20/70.

Biomicroscopically, the macular serous detachment was associated in all cases to hemorrhages, exudates and, in one third of the eyes, to a cystoïd degeneration of the retina. The classical precursors of age-related macular degeneration (drusen and pigment epithelial disturbances) were visible in 74% of the eyes. Moreover, pigmentary clumping was observed in the posterior pole of one third of the eyes.

On fluorescein angiography, 34% of the neovascular lesions extended into the avascular zone. Only 26% of the membranes were located at more than 400 microns of the center of the avascular zone. However, the exact location of the neovascular lesion was always difficult to ascertain and especially its peripheral limits.

The patients included in this retrospective study were treated with the different laser available at that time : blue-green argon laser (7 eyes), red krypton laser (41 eyes), green argon laser (2 eyes). The laser burns were applied on the entire lesion surpassing largely the suspected area.

In general, the destruction of subretinal new-vessels was obtained only in 18 eyes out of 50 (36%) at the end of the follow-up period. Destruction of the neovascular lesion was defined as an atrophic scar without residual serous detachment and without leakage of dye on the angiogram.

An anatomical failure, defined as the involvement of the foveola, has been observed in 64% (32 eyes) ; in most cases, the failure was due to reccurrences with rapid growth of visible new vessels ; in a few cases, failure was associated with a progressive enlargement of the disciform lesion with persistent exudation.

Recurrences, defined as the regrowth of subretinal new-vessels after a period of 4 weeks at least without any symptoms of neovascularisation, were particularly frequent : only 23 eyes were treated once (13 of them successfully but 10 with irreversible failure). Additional laser sessions enabled to obtain a small number of anatomical successes (four after two sessions ; one after three sessions ; no anatomical success was obtained after the third laser session).

Recurrences appeared mostly on the foveal side of the photocoagulation scar (26 cases or 56.5%). In one third of them, the recurrences were juxta-foveal, located at less than 200 microns from the foveola. Laser treated occult subretinal new-vessels showed more frequently central recurrences (11 cases or 23.9%) than visible subretinal new-vessels (10%) (8).

All cases of anatomical success (18 of 50 cases) but two, maintained a visual acuity of 20/100 or better (table 1). Only 6 of 18 eyes experienced a moderate decrease in visual acuity.

On the contrary, all cases in which the laser treatment could not destroy the subretinal new-vessels experienced a severe visual loss, and 26 of 32 eyes were legally blind (table 2).

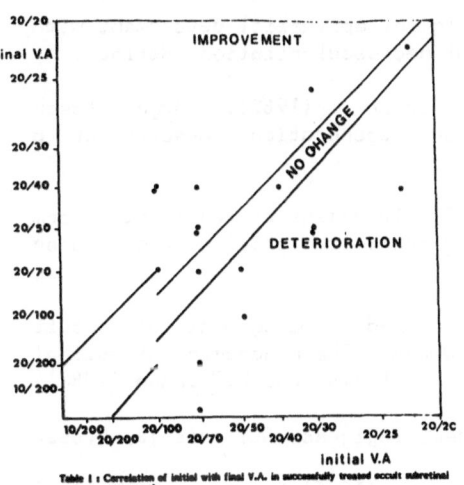

Table 1 : Correlation of initial with final V.A. in successfully treated occult subretinal new vessels

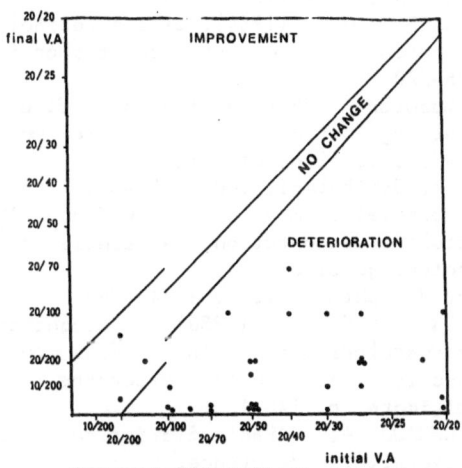

Table 2 : Correlation of initial and final V.A. in failures of photocoagulation of occult subretinal new vessels.

DISCUSSION

In the natural history 80% of the eyes retained a visual acuity of 20/200 or better three years after the onset of symptoms. The comparison between the natural history and the anatomical successes after laser treatment brought evidence that the efficient destruction of subretinal new-vessels has a beneficial effect on visual outcome even 4 years after treatment.

However, the small number of anatomical successes clearly shows the difficulty of laser treatment in occult subretinal new-vessels.

Our results suggested that "early" laser photocoagulation of subretinal new-vessels should not be recommended if it was not possible to clearly identify and precisely locate the new-vessels on the fluorescein angiography.

However, as natural history of occult subretinal new-vessels in age-related macular degeneration has shown that a severe decrease of vision occurs mainly after the third year following the onset of symptoms, it could be suggested that laser treatment should be "delayed" or that different technique should be used especially the "perifoveolar technique" of Creteil (9).

REFERENCES

1.COSCAS G., SOUBRANE G. (1983). Photocoagulation des néovaisseaux sous rétiniens dans la dégénérescence maculaire sénile par le laser à argon. Résultats de l'étude randomisée de 60 cas - Bull. Soc. Ophtalmol. Fr. 88 : 102- 106.
2.COSCAS G., SOUBRANE G., RAMAHEFASOLO C. (1986). Perifoveolar laser treatment for subretinal new-vessels in age-related macular degeneration (Preliminary results). Presented at "RETINA WORKSHOP" (Florence, May 1986).
3.GASS J.D.M. (1984). Serous retinal pigment epithelial detachment with a notch. A sign of occult choroidal neovascularization. Retina : 4,· 205-220.
4.Macular Photocoagulation Study Group (1982). Argon laser photocoagulation for senile macular degeneration. Results of a randomized clinical trial.
Arch. Ophthalmol. 100 : 912-918
5.Moorfields macular Study Group (1982). Treatment of senile disciform macular degeneration. A single blind randomized trial by argon laser photocoagulation.
Br. J. Ophthalmol. 60 : 745-753
6.ORTH P.M. (1983) Recognition and management of occult neovascularization. In : Fine and Owens : The management of retinal vascular and macular disorders. ed. Williams and Wilkinson (1983), Baltimore, p. 140-150.
7.RENAUD A. (1986) Statistiques épidémiologiques. Que sais-je, Presse universitaire de France.
8.SORENSEN J., YANNUZZI L.A., SHAKIN J.L. (1985) Recurrent subretinal neovascularization. Ophthalmology 92 : 1059-1074.
9.SOUBRANE G., COSCAS G., FRANCAIS C. (1980) Natural history of occult subretinal neovascularization. Submitted to Am. J. Ophthalmol.

SUMMARY
Occult Subretinal New Vessels in age-related macular degeneration are now recognized but their precise extent and location is critical even on fluorescein angiography.
In order to evaluate the possible results of early laser treatment on Occult subretinal new-vessels in age-related macular degeneration, 50 eyes with visual symptoms and a macular serous detachment were included in this study. A 6 months post-treatment follow-up had to be achieved. The main judgement criteria was visual acuity ; flat retina and absence of metamorphopsia were also required to define success of laser treatment.
At the end of follow-up (6 months to 6 years), 32 eyes had a visual acuity of 20/200 or better but only 13 had 20/80 or better. A severe visual loss with 20/400 or less at the end of follow-up was observed for 18 eyes despite iterative laser treatment.
These results seem to suggest that "early" photocoagulation treatment of Occult subretinal new-vessels is not beneficial on visual outcome.
As natural history of occult subretinal new-vessels in age-related macular degeneration has shown that the decrease of visual acuity became severe only in the third year after onset of symptoms, a study is actually in progress to assess the benefit of "delayed" laser treatment.

ARGON LASER TREATMENT: SHORT AND LONG TERM RESULTS OF RANDOMIZED CLINICAL TRIALS

SUSAN B. BRESSLER, M.D., NEIL M. BRESSLER, M.D. AND
ROBERT P. MURPHY, M.D.

From the Retinal Vascular Center, Wilmer Ophthalmological
Institute, Johns Hopkins University School of Medicine,
Baltimore, MD

The Macular Photocoagulation Study (MPS) is conducting three multicenter randomized controlled clinical trials designed to determine whether laser photocoagulation is effective for preventing or delaying severe visual loss in eyes with a choroidal neovascular membrane (CNVM) associated with age-related macular degeneration (AMD). Patients with an extrafoveal CNVM (outside of the foveal avascular zone), juxtafoveal CNVM (within, but not through the anatomic center of the foveal avascular zone) or subfoveal CNVM (extending into or through the anatomic center of the fovea) are randomized in separate portions of the study.

The first published report by the MPS described the treatment effect found for extrafoveal choroidal neovascularization. Eligible patients in the extrafoveal group were assigned randomly to a "treatment" group or to a "no treatment" group until recruitment was terminated in 1982. As of August 31, 1985, three or more years of scheduled follow-up examinations had been completed for 88% of the 236 eyes in the extrafoveal study. The relative risk of experiencing visual loss after three years in eyes initially assigned to the no treatment group in comparison with eyes assigned to the argon laser photocoagulation group in the extrafoveal study was 1.4. Life-table analysis curves reveal that at three years 62% of untreated eyes developed severe visual loss compared with 47% of treated eyes at this time. Consequently, treatment is recommended for eyes with extrafoveal CNVMs.

Eyes with juxtafoveal and subfoveal CNVMs currently are being assigned randomly to treatment with krypton red laser photocoagulation or no treatment. There are no differences in visual outcome in the juxtafoveal and subfoveal studies at this time to warrant a change in the protocol. Follow-up of all patients by the MPS continues so that treatment effect over a five year period can be assessed.

INTRODUCTION

Choroidal neovascularization associated with age-related macular degeneration (AMD) is a major cause of loss of central vision. In the United States, the National Eye

Institute estimates that 14% of all new cases of blindness in persons over the age of 65 or 16,000 cases of new blindness per year are from AMD. (1) Complications of the exudative stage of the maculopathy are responsible for 88% of the eyes which are legally blind from macular degeneration. (2) The majority of eyes which may ultimately be blinded from disciform scarring go through a stage of the disease, choroidal neovascularization, which is potentially treatable. Argon laser photocoagulation has been used since the 1970's to treat choroidal neovascular membranes (CNVMs) associated with AMD; however, conclusive proof as to its efficacy and ability to limit severe visual loss from choroidal neovascularization was lacking until the 1980's.

In 1979, the National Eye Institute funded the Macular Photocoagulation Study (MPS), a national collaborative clinical trial of laser photocoagulation in the treatment of choroidal neovascularization. The Senile Macular Degeneration Study, a subgroup of the MPS, was designed to answer the question, "Is argon laser photocoagulation useful in preventing severe visual loss in eyes with choroidal neovascular membranes outside the fovea?" The patients enrolled in this study had angiographic evidence of a CNVM 200 to 2500 microns (um) from the center of the foveal avascular zone (FAZ). These membranes are considered "extrafoveal" and were eligible for randomization to treatment with argon blue-green laser photocoagulation or no treatment.

Photocoagulation treatment within the FAZ was not considered at the time of the initial MPS because many investigators felt that photocoagulation in this area would be very destructive to central vision and because the argon blue-green laser was not felt to be suitable for treatment in this region. Within the macular region, xanthophyll pigment directly absorbs the blue light of the argon blue-green laser, inducing thermal damage to receptors and Henle's fiber layer. (3) Also, absorption of blue light in the inner retina blocks transmission of the thermal energy to the deeper retina and the CNVM, defeating the objectives of photocoagulation.

In 1981, krypton red photocoagulators became clinically available. Krypton red laser photocoagulation has several theoretical advantages over argon laser for macular treatments; namely, its lack of absorption by macular xanthophyll and its decreased absorption by hemoglobin. Theoretically, krypton could produce less inner retinal damage than argon within the fovea. (3) With the availability of the krypton red photocoagulator, and with reports that the natural course of CNVMs within the FAZ was very poor, (4) the MPS was expanded in 1981 to evaluate krypton red laser photocoagulation treatment of juxtafoveal CNVMs, new vessel membranes located 1 tc 200 um from the center of the FAZ. By 1986, with reports that the natural course of CNVMs extending under the center of the FAZ was very poor, (5,6) and with early successful results of photocoagulation in extrafoveal CNVMs, (7) the MPS began evaluating krypton red laser photocoagulation treatment for subfoveal CNVMs, new vessel membranes located under the center of the FAZ.

The study populations for each of these studies have been recruited from patients referred to ophthalmologists at the MPS's participating clinical centers. An MPS-certified visual acuity examiner performs a refraction according to a standard protocol on all potential subjects. Each patient receives a complete ophthalmic examination, stereoscopic color fundus photographs of the disc and macula of each eye and a fluorescein angiogram with the transit phase of the macula of the study eye. Eligibility criteria for the studies include: 1) the presence of drusen in one or both eyes; 2) an angiogram of a CNVM within 72 hours of entry in which the location, with respect to the FAZ, can be discerned; diffuse oozes (where multiple spots of hyperfluorescence can be noted in the late phases of the angiogram that do not correspond to areas of retinal pigment epithelial atrophy or drusen) are also eligible for the extrafoveal or juxtafoveal studies as long as the ooze does not extend through the center of the FAZ; 3) best corrected visual acuity of 20/100 or better for the extrafoveal study, 20/400 or better for the juxtafoveal study, and 20/100-20/320 for the subfoveal study; 4) symptoms related to the CNVM, e.g. decreased acuity, Amsler grid distortion, metamorphopsia or uniocular diplopia; 5) no prior photocoagulation in the study eye in the extrafoveal and juxtafoveal study; 6) no other ocular disease that could independently significantly affect visual acuity; 7) age 50 or older; and 8) the ability to give informed consent. In the subfoveal study, CNVMs could also be included that had documentation of prior successful photocoagulation treatment with subsequent recurrence into the center of the FAZ if all other criteria are met. In addition, CNVMs in the subfoveal study have to be less than 3.5 disc areas in size and well-defined; diffuse oozes which are subfoveal are excluded. Patients who agree to participate in a study are randomized to either immediate photocoagulation or to no treatment. The stratification to argon or krypton laser is determined by the location of the CNVM. Extrafoveal CNVMs are treated with argon while juxtafoveal and subfoveal CNVMs are treated with krypton.

Photocoagulation is performed in all centers according to a standard treatment protocol. Retrobulbar anesthesia is used to ensure akinesia and anesthesia of the globe during thetreatment. Treatment is performed using 200 um spots of 0.5 seconds duration at a sufficient intensity to produce a uniformly white lesion that extended beyond the neovascular complex by 100 to 125 um on all sides in the extrafoveal study and up to the edge of the complex in the juxtafoveal and subfoveal studies. For lesions within 350 um of the foveal center, 100 um spots of 0.2 second duration are used to treat the foveal perimeter of the neovascularization. The goal of treatment is to obliterate the neovascular complex completely with confluent photocoagulation.

Treatment is initiated by determining the threshold of a therapeutic burn. Initial "test spots" are placed on nonfoveal margins of the lesion. Once the therapeutic threshold is determined, 200 um spots are placed on the foveal side of the lesion, slightly overlapping the edge of the choroidal neovascularization. These laser burns create a curvilinear treatment line on the foveal side which overlaps the edge of the neovascularization with a margin of at least 50 to 100 um. The remainder of the perimeter of the lesion is treated in a similar manner with overlapping photocoagulation applications. Treatment of the "neovascularization complex" requires extending the treatment 100 to 125 um beyond any adjacent blood, pigmentation or blocked fluorescence in the extrafoveal study. This maneuver hopefully will treat occult neovascularization associated with the angiographically defined membrane. After the perimeter of the lesion is treated, slightly larger burns are used to create confluent treatment within the central portion of the lesion. The treatment endpoint is a confluent and uniformly white photocoagulation effect which entirely covers the extent of the CNVM. In most cases, this effect could be accomplished while keeping the photocoagulation effect limited to the outer retina, sparing the inner retina, by following the guidelines outlined above.

The Fundus Photograph Reading Center in Baltimore monitors compliance with the treatment protocol. If fluorescein leakage is observed at the margins of the treatment scars at any time during follow-up, retreatment is performed. For the argon study, retreatment has to remain outside 200 um from the foveal center. However, in the krypton study, patients may be entered into the subfoveal study if retreatment demands photocoagulation within the FAZ. (Retreatments within, but not through the center of the FAZ, are not eligible for the juxtafoveal study.)

Follow-up protocol visits are arranged for all patients at six weeks, three and six months after enrollment, and at six month intervals thereafter. Treated patients are instructed to monitor their scotomas and areas of metamorphopsia on an Amsler grid, and they are encouraged to report immediately if they develop any changes on their grids. Additional visits are obtained on patients reporting visual changes or if the treating ophthalmologist deemed it necessary to detect any possible recurrences. At each scheduled follow-up visit, the visual acuity examiner determines the best corrected acuity, an ophthalmologist performs a complete examination and photographic and/or angiographic documentation is provided.

The Coordinating Center of the study in Baltimore, Maryland receives all information, fundus photographs and angiograms from all the clinics. Coordinating center statisticians perform scheduled analysis of study data and present these to the Data and Safety Monitoring Committee on a regular basis.

The argon portion of the MPS was expected to continue

recruitment until mid-1982, with follow-up extended another three years. However, in the spring of 1982, the Data and Safety Monitoring Committee recommended terminating recruitment in the argon portion of the study because a treatment effect became apparent. (7) The Committee recommended informing all enrolled patients of the results thus far attained, and that argon laser be offered to any patients assigned to the no treatment group who currently met the eligibility criteria. The results of the argon portion of the MPS appeared as an expedited publication in the Archives of Ophthalmology in June 1982. (7)

MPS RESULTS

After only 18 months of follow-up, the MPS demonstrated that treated eyes with extrafoveal choroidal neovascular membranes fared better than untreated eyes. (7) Each of the 224 patients enrolled prior to that data were included in the statistical analysis. One year follow-up information was available on 105 patients, and 41 patients were followed for 18 months or longer. No patients were lost to follow-up. The treatment and non-treatment groups had a similar distribution of initial visual acuities. In patients who were followed for six months or longer (166 patients), twice as many treated eyes (57%) compared to untreated eyes (27%) maintained their initial acuity or showed improvement, and three times as many untreated eyes (45%) compared to treated eyes (15%) experienced a loss of at least six lines. All patients with at least six months follow-up were included in life-table analysis of cumulative events. An event was defined as a six or more line decrease from initial baseline visual acuity. At six months, and even more so at twelve months after treatment, the treated eyes appeared to have fewer events. However, this tendency did not become statistically significant until 18 months after treatment. Eighteen months after entry into the study, 60% of untreated eyes had lost six or more lines of vision compared to 25% of treated eyes (P<0.001) (Fig 1). Twice as many treated eyes (42%) as compared to untreated eyes (20%) had a visual acuity better than 20/40. Conversely, one-half as many treated eyes (14%) as compared to untreated eyes (34%) had visual acuity of worse than 20/200 (7). The treatment benefit was consistently seen when patients were evaluated by age, sex, distance of the neovascularization from the foveal center or initial visual acuity. In addition, consistency of the treatment effect was seen in eleven of the twelve clinics. The MPS had finally established the short-term effectiveness of argon blue-green laser photocoagulation in preventing severe visual loss in eyes with extrafoveal choroidal neovascularization from age-related macular degeneration.

Complications of treatment included retrobulbar hemorrhages (3 eyes), post-treatment new blood (31 eyes), a perforation of Bruch's membrane (1 eye) and a closure of a retinal arteriole (1 eye).

Although recruitment of patients into the argon study

had been terminated, follow-up of all patients continues in order to determine if the treatment benefits will persist over longer periods of time. All patients enrolled in this trial will be followed for five years. In May 1986 the three year visual acuity findings were published. (7) Three or more years of scheduled follow-up examinations had been completed for 208 (88%) of the 236 eyes in the study. At three years, the treated group was still more likely to maintain or improve their visual acuity (42%) as compared to untreated eyes (26%); and more untreated eyes (62%) lost six or more lines as compared to treated eyes (47%) (Fig 1). The relative risk of losing six or more lines of visual acuity in eyes assigned to the no treatment group in comparison with those assigned to the argon treatment group was 1.4 (95% confidence intervals were 1.1 to 1.9). Although there was a greater percentage of legally blind eyes in both groups with longer follow-up, 52% of untreated eyes versus 31% of treated eyes had an acuity of worse than 20/200. Of note, 20 of the 117 eyes initially assigned to no treatment received photocoagulation. The majority of these patients were treated after the change in protocol as recommended by the Data and Safety Monitoring Committee. The treatment benefit has persisted despite the fact that these patients continue to be analyzed as "non-treated" eyes.

The krypton portions of the MPS continue to enroll patients in the juxtafoveal and subfoveal categories. At this time there are no differences in visual outcome in either of these subcategories to warrant a change in protocol.

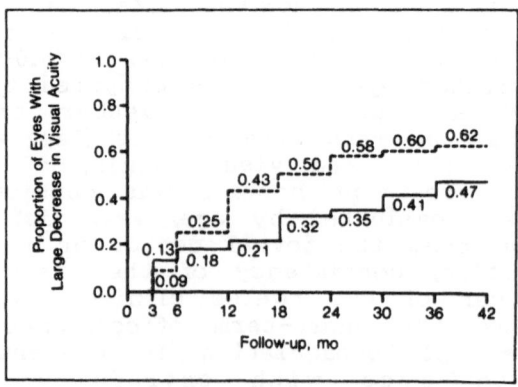

FIGURE 1. Proportion of eyes with a visual acuity loss of six or more lines from baseline in the Senile Macular Degeneration Study. Dashed line indicates no treatment group; solid line indicates treatment group. (Reprinted with permission from the American Medical Association, copyright 1986: Macular Photocoagulation Study Group: Argon laser photocoagulation for neovascular maculopathy: Three year results from randomized clinical trials. Arch Ophthalmol 104:694-701, May 1986.)

SUMMARY
When the MPS terminated its recruitment in the argon
portion of the study in 1982, the major question was whether
the reduced rate of vision loss observed during the first 18
months after treatment would persist over longer periods of
time.   Therefore, follow-up of all patients continues so
that treatment effects over a five year period can be
assessed.

In eyes with age-related macular degeneration, the
benefit of argon laser treatment for extrafoveal
neovascularization was greatest one year after treatment.
At one year, 43% of untreated eyes and 21% of treated eyes
had lost six or more lines of vision; therefore, laser
photocoagulation reduced the risk of severe loss of vision
by 51%.   At three years after treatment, the reduction in
risk of vision loss attributable to laser photocoagulation
fell to 24% (from 62% in untreated eyes to 47% in treated
eyes), predominantly because successfully treated CNVMs
developed recurrent CNVMs on the foveal side of the scar
resulting in visual loss, (see chapter on Recurrences).   In
general, argon laser photocoagulation of extrafoveal
membranes in AMD postpones, rather than prevents, severe
visual loss.   The average delay in severe loss of vision is
18 months.

The MPS has demonstrated that argon blue-green laser is
effective in reducing the risk of severe visual loss for
eyes with AMD and a symptomatic CNVM at least 200 microns
from the center of the FAZ.   At 18 months and/or three
years, untreated eyes were more likely to develop severe
visual loss than treated eyes.   The beneficial treatment
effect prevailed in all subgroups and at every point in
follow-up time.   Treatment should be considered for all eyes
that meet the MPS's eligibility criteria.   However, for this
study's results to have any significant impact on reducing
the frequency of severe visual loss from choroidal
neovascularization in AMD, patients must be identified,
evaluated and treated soon after the onset of visual
symptoms.   Unfortunately, most patients with CNVMs
associated with AMD are identified after the
neovascularization has involved the fovea (9) or has
cicatrized.   Patients with bilateral drusen, and in
particular, patients who have already experienced unilateral
exudative disease, should be followed at regular intervals
and instructed in the use of an Amsler grid or other means
of testing central acuity.   These patients should be
evaluated promptly with fluorescein angiography if new
visual symptoms arise.

It is tempting to extrapolate from the argon portion MPS
that laser photocoagulation may be beneficial in cases with
involvement within the fovea.   However, treatment of
extrafoveal CNVMs in AMD turned out to be effective, in
part, because it delayed or permanently prevented extension
of these membranes into the center of the fovea. (7)   Thus,
a paracentral scotoma from the laser scar was of greater
benefit than a subsequent central scotoma from the disciform

scar that extended into the fovea in 75% of untreated extrafoveal CNVMs. (7) Evaluating treatment of CNVMs within the FAZ, though, would compare the effects of a central scotoma from a laser scar to the effects of a central scotoma from a disciform scar. The krypton portion of the MPS is continuing to evaluate whether krypton laser photocoagulation treatment of juxtafoveal or subfoveal membranes is beneficial. As of August 1985, 328 patients have been enrolled in the juxtafoveal study. Two hundred one of these patients have been observed for at least one year, and 109 have been observed two or more years. As recently as August 1986, the Data and Safety Monitoring Committee has not yet made any recommendations that would indicate that laser photocoagulation was beneficial or harmful in such eyes. Enrollment and randomization continues in both the juxtafoveal and subfoveal controlled clinical trials of krypton red laser photocoagulation.

We look forward to the five year report on argon laser photocoagulation of extrafoveal neovascularization in eyes with age-related macular degeneration and to the results of the krypton laser trials for juxtafoveal and subfoveal choroidal neovascularization.

REFERENCES

1. Vision Problems in the United States, National Society to Prevent Blindness, Statistical Analysis prepared by Operational Research Department, New York, 1980.
2. Ferris FL III: Senile macular degeneration: review of epidemiologic features. Am J Epidemiol 1983;118:132-151.
3. Marshall J, Bird AC: A comparative histopathological study of argon and krypton laser irradiations of the human retina. Br J Ophthalmol 1979;63:657-668.
4. Bressler SB, Bressler NB, Fine SL, et al: Natural course of choroidal neovascular membranes within the foveal avascular zone in senile macular degeneration. Am J Ophthalmol 1982;93:157-163.
5. Bressler NB, Bressler SB, Fine SL, et al: Subfoveal neovascular membranes in senile macular degeneration: relationship between membrane size and visual prognosis. Retina 1983;3:7-11.
6. Guyer DR, Fine SL, Maguire MG, et al: Subfoveal choroidal neovascular membranes in age-related macular degeneration: visual prognosis in eyes with relatively good initial visual acuity. Arch Ophthalmol 1986;104:702-705.
7. Macular Photocoagulation Study Group: Argon laser photocoagulation for senile macular degeneration: results of a randomized clinical trial. Arch Ophthalmol 1982;100:912-918.
8. Macular Photocoagulation Study Group: Argon laser photocoagulation for neovascular maculopathy: three year results from randomized clinical trials. Arch Ophthalmol 1986;104:694-701.

9. Bressler NB, Bressler SB, Gragoudas ES: Clinical characteristics of choroidal neovascular membranes. Arch Ophthalmol 1986;in press.
10. Macular Photocoagulation Study Group: Recurrent choroidal neovascularization after argon laser photocoagulation for neovascular maculopathy. Arch Ophthalmol 1986;104:503-512.

PERIFOVEOLAR LASER TREATMENT FOR SUBRETINAL NEW VESSELS IN AGE-RELATED MACULAR DEGENERATION

G. COSCAS, G. SOUBRANE, C. RAMAHEFASOLO - CRETEIL (France)

The previous randomized trials have proven that argon laser photocoagulation reduces the visual loss in eyes with subretinal new vessels outside the fovea in age-related macular degeneration (1-3).

Eyes with new vessels that lie beneath the center of the fovea carry a poor visual prognosis (4, 5) and are usually considered not amenable to laser treatment. Direct treatment of the entire surface of the subfoveal membrane (6, 7) could destroy immediately the central vision and could be self defeating.
The rationale of this study was to destroy the entire neovascular membrane, sparing only the central part of the foveal avascular zone. It was intended that this "perifovealar" photocoagulation treatment would result in a stable dry scar, and that the remaining central visual function would allow an efficient use of low vision aids.

PATIENTS AND METHODS
This retrospective study included patients with subretinal new vessels growth associated with age-related macular degeneration whose eyes met the following criteria : (1) first eye with a large cicatricial subretinal membrane that involved the center of the foveal avascular zone. (2) opposite eye, included in the study with a single subretinal membrane evidenced on fluorescein angiography, involving the foveola (subfoveal membrane), and a peripheral neovascular arcade that extended more than 200 microns from the foveola but less than 2.5 disc diameters wide, without fibrous tissue. This membrane could be either primary, or secondary to a subfovealar recurrence. (3) The pretreatment visual acuity ranged from 20/100 to 20/400, in the second eye. (4) The minimum postoperative follow-up was 12 months for each patient. (5) The patient had no other ocular disease that could account for the decrease in visual acuity in the second eye.

Pretreatment and follow-up examinations included best corrected visual acuity of both eyes, measured by an optometrist, with the use of available low vision aids. The type and the power of the low vision aid was recorded.
Eyes were treated with a monochromatic krypton red laser (Coherent 900 K*). A 200-micron spot size was used for a duration of 0.5 to 1 second. The power intensity was adjusted to achieve adequate gray-white burns. Confluent overlapping spots were applied to the active peripheral neovascular arcade. The central foveal avascular zone (300

microns in diameter) was avoided to spare any possibly still functional cones.

All patients were reevaluated 3 months after treatment and at 6-month intervals thereafter. If the neovascular membrane persisted or recurred after previously documented closure, further photocoagulation, still sparing the central part of the foveal avascular zone, was repeated.

Closure of the neovascular membrane was defined as a resolution of the exudative response, a clinically flat retina, and an absence of fluorescein leakage from the membrane (Fig 1 and 2).

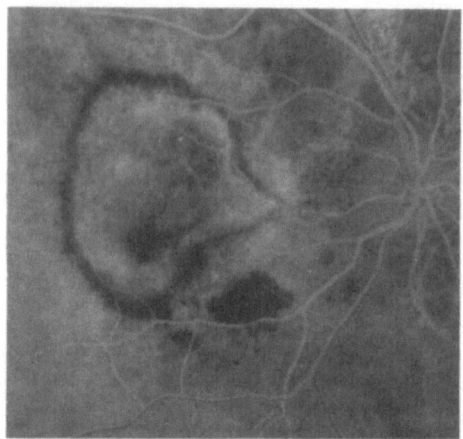 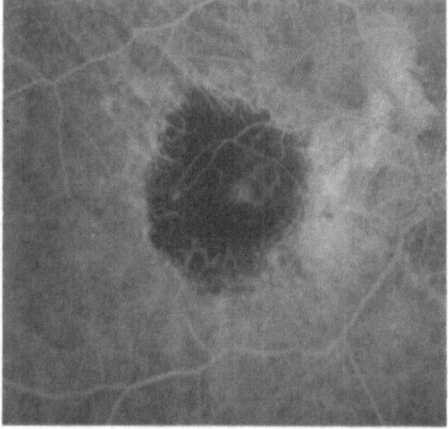

Figure 1 : Second eye of a patient with subretinal new vessels in age-related macular degeneration included in Perifoveolar Laser Photocoagulation Study (PLPS). The active neovascular membrane involves the center of the avascular zone. The neovascular anastomotic arcade is distant from the fovea.

Figure 2 : Same eye as shown in figure 1, three months after "perifoveolar" photocoagulation. In this late frame the neovascular anastomotic arcade is no longer visible. Moreover, there is no leakage of dye, even in the Foveal Avascular zone which was not treated. Visual acuity was 20/200, and normal reading (near) acuity was achieved with low-vision aids.

RESULTS

66 patients met the inclusion criteria. Of these, 10 patients were lost to follow-up soon after the initial treatment. The remaining 56 patients were 38 mens and 18 women who ranged in age from 64 to 87 years (mean age : 76.3 years).

The natural progession of macular degeneration in the patients first eye showed severe visual loss : 50 eyes (89%) had a visual acuity of 20/400 or less ; only 6 eyes (11%) retained a visual acuity of 20/200. Most of the eyes presented with a fibrovascular scar (50) ; 6 eyes had a large macular retinal detachment with exudation.

Our study was concerned with the second involved eye of each patient. Fluorescein angiography allowed accurate analysis of the initial pattern of the eyes included in the study and showed that most of the eyes (38) exhibited the typical early, lacy neovascularization with late leakage, although some (14 eyes) had an atypical occult membrane characterized by an area of gradual leakage or oozing of dye.

The subretinal new vessels were subfoveal at presentation in 22 eyes, extending beyond the foveal avascular zone. In 34 eyes, they involved the center of the fovea after multiple recurrences from a previously treated membrane that initially spared the foveola.

At the end of the follow-up period, 44 eyes had a completely obliterated subretinal membrane and a flat retina. The remaining central feeder vessels, when visible, did not leak fluorescein. A localized central retinal detachment could persist. Laser sessions were repeated in 24 eyes, for neovascular recurrences on the peripheral border of the scar but not for new visual symptoms. In 12 eyes, the serous retinal disciform detachment was unresolved due to a persistent neovascular network.

The visual results included not only distance visual acuity, but also subjective reports of visual comfort, and reading vision with low vision aids.

Distance visual acuity was initially 20/100 or worse in all cases : only 6 eyes, presented with a visual acuity better than 20/200, while 36 had a visual acuity of 20/200.

At the end of the follow-up period (12 to 44 months), distance acuity was equal to or better than 20/200 in half of the eyes (better than 20/200 in 8 eyes, and equal to 20/200 in 20 eyes) (Table I). The visual acuity remained the same or improved in 30 eyes, but worsened in 26.

TABLE I : FINAL FUNCTIONAL RESULTS

	Non treated eyes	Treated eyes
DISTANCE VISUAL ACUITY		
> 20/200	0	8
= 20/200	6	20
< 20/200	50	28
READING VISUAL ACUITY (better than Jaeger 4)	2	40

Near visual acuity was initially better than Jaeger 4 in all eyes but one. Three months after treatment, 40 eyes (71%) had recovered a normal reading acuity with low vision aids (magnification from 5 to 12X), which was retained during the follow-up period. The reading vision remained the same or improved in 42 eyes and worsened in 14 eyes (due to a tear in the retinal pigment epithelium, 2 eyes ; central pigmentary clumping, 2 eyes ; or persistent serous detachment, 8 eyes).

Only 2 patients had better reading vision, with the help of low vision aids, in the fellow non-treated eye compared with the treated eye.

DISCUSSION

Eyes with new vessel growth that lies beneath the fovea present a difficult clinical problem. Any scheme of treatment for disciform degeneration of the macula could be of no benefit to the patient if the visual potential of the fovea has been destroyed by the disease process. The preservation of macular function for a substancial period of time is not uncommon as the retina is not primarily involved in the disease process but only secondarily affected by prolonged detachment and fibrous tissue growth. Therefore neovascular tissue beneath the retina in the macular region can be expected to retain limited macular function, at least for a short period of time.

In a retrospective non randomized study of natural history, Bressler and co-workers (4) described a poor visual outcome in subfoveal membranes. In 31% of the eyes, visual acuity remained the same or improved. Visual acuity may also increase spontaneously, but very slowly, if the retina flattens. However this event is very rare (3% in our study). Singerman (8) observed spontaneous improvement in 31% of eyes after a follow-up of 33 months, which decreased to 19% after 50 months, in the first affected eye.

Many studies have suggested a poor visual outcome in subfoveal membranes (4, 5). In the "subfoveal study", it was proposed that the obliteration of a small subfoveal lesion (5) could theoretically facilitate the use of low vision aids by preserving more parafoveal retina and allowing excentric fixation. Photocoagulation delivered to the center of the fovea, even with a krypton or dye laser, might produce a dramatic decrease in vision. Thus, Decker (7) showed that even when the neovascular membrane was successfully obliterated (17 of 25 eyes), vision stabilized or improved in only 5 eyes.

Likewise, the feeder vessel technique will be rarely possible and could provide irregular and probably inefficient results.

Many reports have shown that the incomplete treatment of a neovascular network is unsatisfactory ; however, laser treatment limited to the anastomotic arcade may account for the resorption of serous and/or hemorrhagic subretinal fluid and therefore provide visual improvement or stabilization.

With the described "perifoveolar" laser treatment, anatomic results were often incomplete but (1) recurrences were mostly peripheral and therefore easily amenable to laser treatment, and (2) in the central region, the radially oriented feeder vessels become gradually competent to fluorescein and non leaking. In most cases, the foveal retina flattened and the new vessels appeared obliterated or became non leaking on fluorescein angiography. Low vision rehabilitation proved to be extremely useful.

In our study, only 11% of the nontreated eyes retained 20/200 visual acuity compared with 50% of the eyes treated with the "perifoveolar" technique. Reading (near) vision with the use of low-vision aids was possible for only 3% of the nontreated eyes compared with 71% of the treated eyes. Even though ours was not a randomized controlled study, we believed the comparison of visual outcome between the laser-treated eye and the first involved eye afforded useful information, as the follow-up period was at least one year and long enough.

REFERENCES
1.COSCAS G., SOUBRANE G. Photocoagulation des néo-vaisseaux sous rétiniens dans la dégénérescence maculaire sénile par laser à argon : résultats de l'étude randomisée de 60 cas. Bull. Mem. Soc. Fr. Ophtalmol., 1983, 94, 149-154.
2.Macular Photocoagulation Study Group : Argon laser photocoagulation for senile macular degeneration : Results of a randomized clinical trial. Arch. Ophthalmol., 1982, 100, 912-918.
3.Moorfields Macular Study Group : Argon laser photocoagulation for senile macular degeneration : results of a randomized clinical trial. Arch. Ophthalmol., 1982, 100, 912-918.
4.BRESSLER S.B., BRESSLER N.M., FINE S.L. et al. : Natural course of choroidal neovascular membranes within the foveal avascular zone in senile macular degeneration. Am. J. Ophthalmol., 1982, 93, 157-163.
5.GUYER D.R., FINE S.L., MAGUIRE M.G., HAWKINS B.S., OWENS S.L., MURPHY R.P. : Subfoveal choroidal neovascular membranes in age-related macular degeneration. Visual prognosis in eyes with relatively good initial visual acuity. Arch. Ophthalmol., 1986, 104, 702-705.
6.JALKH A.E., AVILA M.P., TREMPE C.L. et al. : Choroidal neovascularization in fellow eyes of patients with advanced senile macular degeneration. Arch. Ophthalmol., 1983, 101, 1194-1197.
7.DECKER W.L., GRABOWSKI W.M., ANNESLEY W.H. : Krypton red laser photocoagulation of subretinal neovascular membranes located within the foveal avascular zone. Ophthalmology, 1984, 91, 1582-1586.
8.SINGERMAN L.J., WONG B., EVERET A.I., SMITH S. : Spontaneous visual improvement in the first affected eye of patients with bilateral disciform scars. Retina, 1985, 5, 135-143.

246

SUMMARY

Macular subretinal new vessels extending into the center of the subfoveolar area are considered not amenable to photocoagulation treatment. Their extension associated with hemorrhages and fibrous tissue will produce a complete destruction of the central vision. During natural history, the size of the disciform lesion will usually enlarge with extensive central scotoma.

In order to assess the possible benefit of laser treatment in these most severe cases, we undertook a feasability study of a "perifoveolar" laser treatment.

Following inclusion criteria had to be met : (1) second eye involvement ; (2) visual acuity less than 20/100 ; (3) subretinal new vessels clearly defined on the angiogram involving the center of the fovea without detectable fibrous tissue ; and (4) peripheral neovascular arcade extending more than 200 microns from the foveola. 56 patients were included and the follow-up period was 12 to 44 months. Laser treatment was performed with krypton red laser directed to the perifoveal neovascular arcade. No burns were applied to the foveal avascular zone. Visual acuity of both eyes was measured (with and without low-vision aids) at 6-month intervals during follow-up.

In 54 patients, final visual acuity was better in the treated eye : in 28 eyes it was better or equal to 20/200; with low-vision aids, 40 of 56 eyes achieved fairly normal reading acuity (better than Jaeger 4). Fluorescein angiography showed a complete oblitered neovascular network in 44 eyes, with the presence of an atrophic scar.

In this study, only 11% of the nontreated eyes retained visual acuity of 20/200 compared with 50% of the treated eyes. These preliminary results suggested that useful central vision could be preserved by this "perifoveal" laser photocoagulation technique and be a benefit to patients together with low vision aids.

KRYPTON RED LASER AND ARGON GREEN LASER PHOTOCOAGULATION IN THE TREATMENT OF SICK RPE DUE TO AGE-RELATED MACULAR DEGENERATION

I. Hundert M.D., Y. Yassur M.D., L. Shani M.D., D. Ucenick M.D.

Soroka-Ben Gurion University Medical Center, Beer-Sheva and Maccabi Laser Institute, Tel-Aviv, Israel

A B S T R A C T

Krypton red laser or argon green laser photocoagulation was carried out on 15 fellow eyes suffering from sick retinal pigment epithelium (RPE) due to age-related macular degeneration (AMD). All the eyes had an initial good visual acuity (no less than 6/24), but complained of declined visual acuity or visual quality. Patients were followed-up for 6-36 months. Visual acuity test, fundoscopy and fluorescein angiography were performed before treatment and periodically during the follow-up visits. Visual acuity remained unchanged in 10 eyes, improved in 1 eye and deteriorated in 4 eyes. In all the treated eyes visual acuity was better than in the nontreated first eye.

Age-related macular degeneration (AMD) is the leading cause of new blindness in patients over 60 years old in the United States and other western countries (1,2,3), as well as in Israel. Today, there is a concept to treat AMD with laser photocoagulation only whenever there is a clear pathology such as elevation of the sensory retina due to focal leakage, detachment of the retinal pigment epithelium (RPED), or subretinal neovascularisation (SRNV) (4,5,6,7,8). Elderly patients who have lost central vision in one eye due to AMD may start to complain of visual decline in the fellow eye before a distinct lesion like RPED, central serous retinopathy-like or SRNV develops. This occurs in the presence of drusen and a typical fluorescein angiogram, which shows just a late diffuse staining of the posterior pole due to a late mild leakage through diseased RPE. This stage may be called "decompensated RPE" or "sick RPE". There are no data concerning the rate of development of distinct AMD lesions from the sick RPE stage. However, most of sick RPE eyes later develope one or all of the above mentioned lesions, which ultimately lead to low vision or blindness also in that fellow eye. The incidence of developing a disciform lesion in the second eye in patients who had it in the first eye is quite high: Teeters and Bird in 1973 reported of 12% per year (9); Gass in 1973 reported of a 33% incidence in 4 years (2); Gragudas et al. reported an incidence of 30% during a follow up period of one to four years (10); Gregor and Bird's results (11) suggested a constant risk of 12% per year of developing disciform lesion in the second eye during the first 5 years; Bressler et al. demonstated that exudative maculopathy developed in the second eye in 13% after one year, in 22% after 2 years and in 29% after 3 years (12). A lower incidence was presented by Strahlman et al., who showed a 3%-7% risk per year of exudative maculopathy developing in the second eye during the first three years (13).

We present here 15 eyes that underwent laser photocoagulation for sick RPE when they were not yet harboring the previously mentioned distinct lesion of AMD.

PATIENTS AND METHODS

In our treatment group, 15 fellow eyes of patients who had lost vision in their first eye due to disciform lesion were included. All these patients complained of decline in visual acuity and/or blurred vision in the fellow eye. Only eyes with visual acuity not worse than 6/24 were included in this treatment group. Fundus examination revealed drusen in the macula and diffuse retinal thickening of the retina at the posterior pole. The flourescein-angiogram showed diffuse late staining at the macular area and around it and no typical lesions of CSR-like, RPE detachment or SRNV. After an apropriate explanation to the patient and a concent form approval, all the 15 eyes underwent photocoagulation with Krypton red laser (11 eyes) or with pure argon green laser (4 eyes). Krypton laser was our preference in such cases, but sometimes it was not technically available.

The pattern of treatment was a grid or horseshoe starting at 500-1500µ from the center of the foveal avascular zone (FAZ) up to the temporal arcades; 0.1 sec, and 50-300µ spot size. The intensity of burns was mild to moderate. The treatment was performed in one session.

The follow-up period was at 2 and 6 weeks, and at 3, 6 and 12 months after treatment, and than every 6 months. It included a full ophthalmological examination, as well as fluorescein angiogram, color photography and sometimes contrast sensitivity. The longest follow-up period was 36 months and the average period was 1 year.

R E S U L T S

Variations in visual acuity of two lines or more were considered as "changes". In 10 eyes VA remained stable; in one eye it showed improvement and in four eyes it declined to 6/60.

Table 1

Table 1: Va before and after treatment in the 15 eyes and VA in the untreated eye.

	V.A (fellow eye) before treatment	V.A (fellow eye) after treatment	V.A first eye	Reason to V.A decline in treated eye
1)	6/18	6/24	3m	
2)	6/24	6/18	1m	
3)	6/24	6/36	3m	
4)	6/12	6/12	1.5m	
5)	6/9	6/9	1m	
6)	6/9	6/9	1m	
7)	6/12	6/12	2m	
8)	6/24	6/24	3m	
9)	6/12	6/12	1m	
10)	6/9	6/60	Hm	gliosis
11)	6/12	6/60	Hm	CME
12)	6/9	6/9	Hm	
13)	6/12	6/36	6/60	gliosis
14)	6/24	6/9	1m	
15)	6/24	6/60	2.5m	SRNV

250

Fig 1 presents these results graphically.

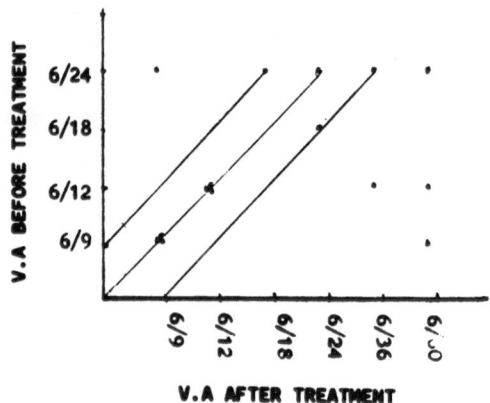

Fig. 1. V.A before VS after treatment

As to the anatomical results: In the 11 eyes in which VA stabilized or improved, and in three eyes in which it declined to 6/60, there was flattaning of the macula, and a complete regression of the late flourescein diffuse leakage, with scar staining and window defects staining only. This means that the typical fundus and flourescein angiographic appearance of sick RPE regressed.

In one eye in which VA declined from 6/12 to 6/60 cystoid macular edema occurred. In this eye there was a sever 360° peripheral SRNV with retinal elevation, which was treated later on with laser photocoagulation.

C O M M E N T S

If we compare the VA in the fellow treated eye to the VA in the first untreated eye of the same patient (tab.1), it is obvious that in all of the treated eyes VA was better than in the non-treated eyes during the follow-up period. This is true even for those four eyes in which V.A. declined after treatment.

It is worth mentioning that all the treated eyes could obtain reading ability by magnification or low vision aids, compared to the first non-treated eye which either could not get it at all, or could get it to a lower reading VA level.

We have to emphasize that it is impossible to draw any solid conclusion as to the efficacy and need of treatment in such eyes, because of lack of information as to the natural course concerning the amount, rate and time of decline of V.A. in untreated eyes with sick RPE.

It is also worth noting that sometimes there is a discrepance between the VA measured by the Snellen chart and the patient's satisfaction: This phenomen concerns the quality of vision, which is often reflected by declined contrast sensitivity.

What was the rational of treating sick RPE in patients with AMD? The statistics concerning the risk of developing disciform lesion in the second eye in patients with AMD has been already mentioned before; however there are no data as to the natural course of the fellow eye (and also of the first eye) as to the extent, time and rate of loss of macular vision after the destructive process of the sick RPE has already begun. The natural history of these eyes is not statistically recorded in the literature, although it is well clinically appreciated that once these eyes start the "sick" process they always continue to go downhill, and it is difficult to decide when is the time to start treatment so that it will not be too early or too late. Sarks in 1973 (14), and lately Miller and Miller (15), demonstrated that 20%-80% of eyes which show no signes of SRNV actually contain it. Duvall in 1985 (16) in an experiment on a Rhesus monkey reported of resolution of drusen after mild pure argon laser photocoagulation, and demonstrated that this happened by phagocytic cells derived from pericytes of the choriocapillaries. It is also worth recalling the works of Glaser (17) and Ryan (18) on the role of scars and of RPE cells in inhibiting NV formation and enhancement of gliosis or fibrosis.

Jalkh in 1985 (19) reported of beneficial results of argon laser in human eyes with what he called "decompensation of the RPE", although he particularly stressed that they were not eyes with AMD.

It may be very likely that the krypton and argon laser photocoagulation in the eyes in our treatment group stimulates the RPE cells and choriocappilaries pericytes to start a circle of inhibition of NV formation and of regression of existing occult SRNV.

It is of course impossible to get any solid conclusion out of such a small number of eyes and short follow-up period. Further data on the NH of sick RPE in age-related macular degeneration is needed, as well as controlled studies, to compare the NH to the described laser treatment.

R E F F E R E N C E S

1) Leibowitz M.M, Krueger D.E, Mander L.R et al. The Franingham Eye Study Monograph. Surv. Ophtalmol. 1980; 24(suppl.): 335-610.
2) Gass J.D.M. Drusen and disciform macular detachment and degeneration. Arch. Ophthalmol. 1973; 90: 206-217.
3) Ferris F.L, Fine S.L, Hyman L. Age-related macular degeneration and blindness due to neovascular maculopathy. Arch. Ophthalmol. 1984; 102: 1640-1642.
4) Macular Photocoagulation Study Group. Argon laser photocoagulation for senile macular degeneration; results of a randomized clinical trial. Arch. Ophthalmol. 1982; 100: 912-918.
5) Schatz H, Patz A. Exudative senile maculopathy. I. Results of argon laser treatment. Arch. Opthalmol. 1973; 90: 183-196.
6) Green W.R, McDonnel P.J, Yeo J.H. Pathologic features of senile macular degeneration. Ophthalmol. 1985; 92: 615-627.
7) Singerman L.J. Important points in management of patients with choroidal neovascularization. Ophthalmol. 1985; 92: 610-614.
8) James C, Folk B. Aging macular degeneration. Clinical features of treatable disease. Ophthalmol. 1985; 92: 594-602.

9)   Teeters V.W, Bird A.C.   A clinical study of the
      vascularity of senile disciform macular degeneration.
      Am. J. Ophthalmol. 1973; 75: 53-65.
10)   Gragudas E.S, Chandra S.R, Friedman E, Klein M.L,
      Van Buskirk M. Disciform degeneration of the macula.
      Arch. Ophthalmol. 1976; 94: 755-757.
11)   Gregor Z, Bird A.C, Chisholm I.H. Senile disciform
      macular degeneration in the second eye. Brit. J.
      Ophthalmol. 1977; 61: 141-147.
12)   Bressler L.B, Bressler N.M, Fine S.L, Hillis A,
      Murphy R.P, Olk R.J, Patz A.   Natural course of
      choroidal neovascular membranes within the foveal
      avascular zone in senile macular degeneration. Am. J.
      Ophthalmol. 1982; 93: 157-163.
13)   Strahlman E.R, Fine S.L, Hillis A. The second eye of
      patients with senile macular degeneration. Arch.
      Ophthalmol. 1983; 101: 1191-1193.
14)   Sarks S.H. New vessel formation beneath the retinal
      pigment epithelium in senile eye. Br. J. Ophthalmol.
      1973; 57: 951-965.
15)   Miller H, Miller B, Ryan S.J.   Correlation of
      choroidal subretinal neovascularization with
      fluorescein angiography. Am. J. Ophthalmol. 1985; 99:
      263-271.
16)   Duvall J, FRCS(E), Tso M.O. Cellular mechanisms of
      dursen after laser coagulation: an experimental
      atusy. Arch. Ophthalmol. 1985; 103: 694-703.
17)   Campochiaro P.A, Glaser B.M. Mechanisms involved in
      retinal pigment epithelial cell chemotaxis. Arch.
      Ophthalmol. 1986; 104: 277-280.
18)   Ohkuma H, Ryan S.J.   Experimental subretinal
      neovascularization in the monkey. Arch. Ophthalmol.
      1983; 101: 1102-1110.
19)   Jalkh A.E, Jabbour N, Avila M.P, Trempe C.L, Schepens
      C.L. Retinal pigment epithelium decompensation. II
      laser treatment. Ophthalmol. 1984; 91: 1549-1553.

SENILE SEROUS DETACHMENT OF R.P.E.-LASERTREATMENT: CONTROVERSIAL ASPECTS

A. GIOVANNINI, G.P. AMATO, G. COSTANTINI and A. PAZZAGLIA
Eye Department - University of Bologna (Italy)

Although everybody agrees with the lasertreatment of Sub-Retinal Neo-Va_
scularisations (S.R.N.V.) in course of Senile Macular Degeneration (S.M.D.),
still controversial is the approach to the Serous Detachment of R.P.E.

In respect to the size, the serous detachment could be divided in two
patterns:

a) SMALL PATTERN   b) LARGE PATTERN

$\emptyset \leqslant 1/3$ Papillary $\emptyset$ $\emptyset \geqslant 1/2$ Papillary $\emptyset$

a) Small Pattern.

In case of a small one, it usually presents itself like an "Hot-Spot" adja_
cent to a drusen. We know that "Hot-Spot" is the synonym of a S.R.N.V., but
also an early stage - serous detachment could present the same characteri_
stics. In such cases only the presence of a little deep haemorrhage led us
to a sure differential diagnosis.

In such a way, a part from the dilemma concerning the serous detachment as
constantly or not caused by a S.R.N.V. (even if an hidden one), it is
beyond doubt that lasertreatment is the only rational approach.

In such cases, of course, the lasertreatment is quite similar to the one
in course of S.R.N.V., and the whole area of the serous detachment must be
treated.

b) Large Pattern.

On the contrary there are many questions about the lasertreatment in case
of a large serous detachment.

We can distinguish schematically two types:

Type 1: Round serous detachment, the F.A.Z. is often in its centre;
great dimension (with a diameter more than or equal to one
and half papillary diameter). -(Fig. n. 1)-

Type 2: Not round serous detachment, more often quite triangular
-(Fig. n. 2)-, often involving the F.A.Z. only in part;
usually smaller than Type 1.

256

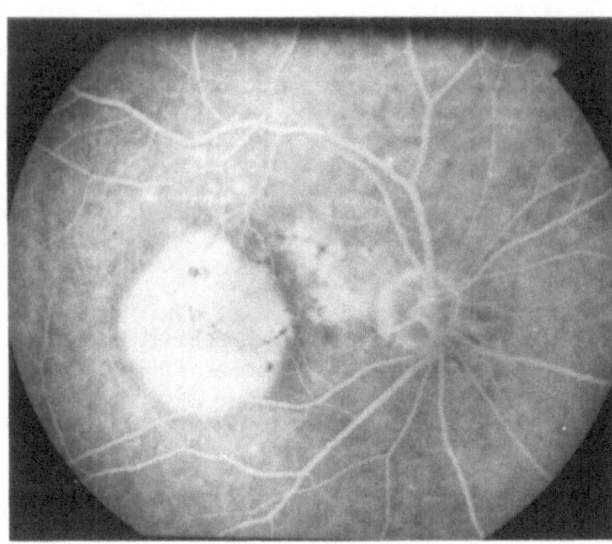

-(Fig. n. 1)-

Senile Serous Detachment
of R.P.E.:

- Large Pattern

- Type 1

(V.A. = 20/50)

As well known in type 1 - Serous Detachment, a circular or hemi-circular
lasertreatment contiguous to its rim is enough to realize a "flattening"
of the detachment -(Fig. n. 3)- with a complete recovery of Visual
Acuity (V.A.).

More over, a spontaneous "flattening" has also been described, and with a
complete recovery of V.A.

Therefore, the common approach consists in following-up these patients,
and in treating them only in case of complications: neovascularisations

-(Fig. n. 2)-

Senile Serous Detachment
of R.P.E.:

- Large Pattern

- Type 2

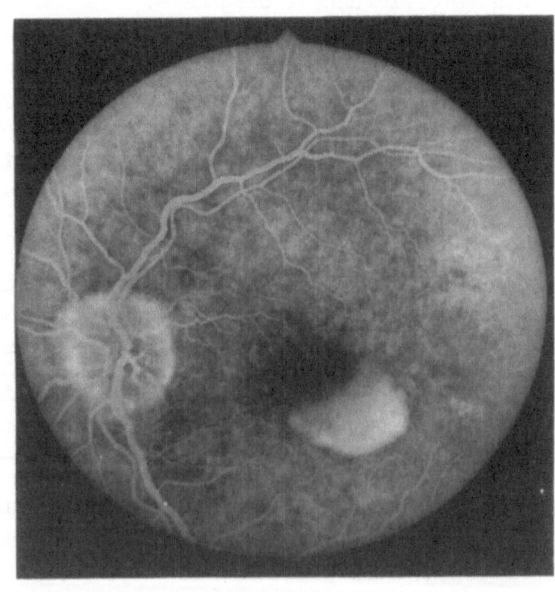

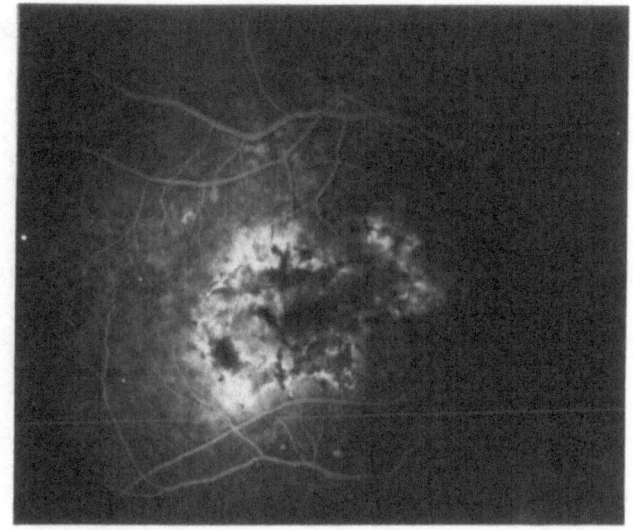

-(Fig. n. 3)-

(Same case of Fig. n. 1)

Four months after the
treatment (hemi-circular
pattern) with Dye Laser
(605 nm.- wavelength).
   V.A. = 20/20. !

(characterized by a change of pattern: often presents itself with a typical
"packman - like" aspect) (1); or deep haemorrhage in its context.

More over, a long-term detachment could produce microcystic - cystoid
alterations of F.A.Z., other lasertreatment criteria.

From our experience, a spontaneous flattening (with a good recovery of
V.A.) has been observed only in   60 years old patients presenting minimal
changes of R.P.E.

On the contrary, almost constantly in older patients and with serious

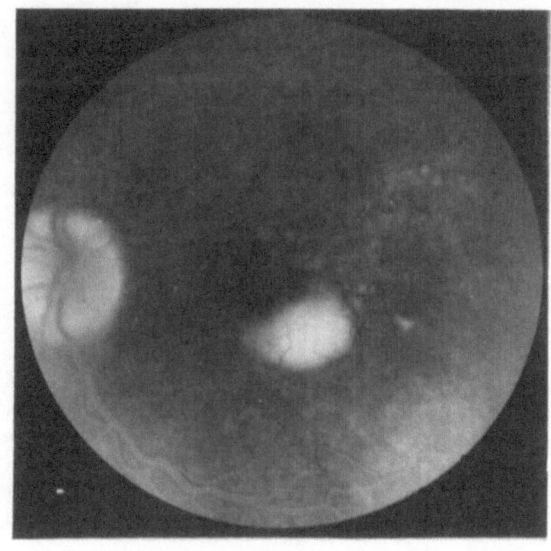

-(Fig. n. 4)-

Before treatment

258

-(Fig. n. 5)-

After Krypton Laser

V.A. = 20/20. !

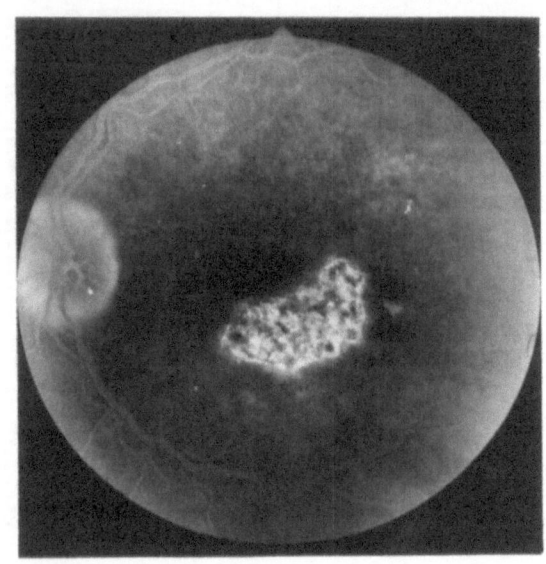

changes of R.PE., the serous detachment develops either microcystic -
cystoid alterations of F.A.Z. (that in our experience reptresents its more
frequent natural history) causing a progressive and irreversible V.A. -
impairment, or a S.R.N.V. (that is its frequent complication).

   Therefore, we emphasize that lasertreatment criteria of serous detachment
must be wider than usually considered, and in this way in case of an older
patient with serious R.P.E.- alterations we have to treat before the
complications (S.R.N.V. / microcystic - cystoid alterations) set up.

-(Fig. n. 6)-

Fellow Eye: Natural History

V.A. = 20/200.

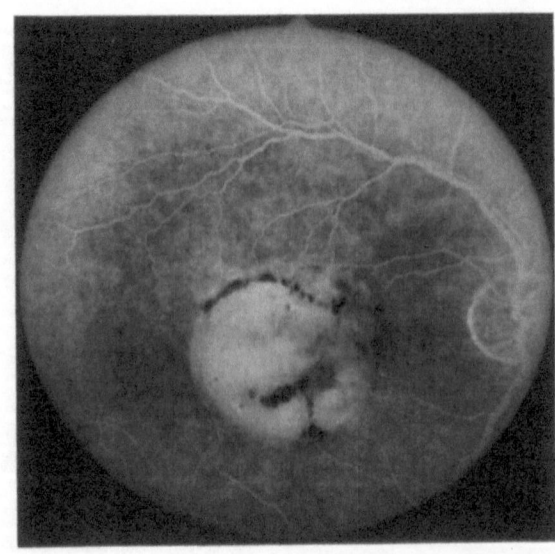

Of course, we are waiting for randomised studies to confirm our clinical opinion.

In case of young patients with minimal changes of R.P.E. we usually prefer checking and following them up.

On the other hand, in presence of Type 2 Large serous detachment, the rational approach consists in the lasertreatment of great part of its area, with saving of foveal area -(Fig. n. 4 - 5 - 6)-.

This lasertreatment, in our experience, induces a flattening of the serous detachment more frequently than the circular or hemi - circular one of Type 1.

REFERENCES

1. Gass D.M.: Present Indications and Future Promises of the Krypton Laser. in Ophthalmic Laser, March W.M. ed., 1984; 97-134.

RECURRENT CHOROIDAL NEOVASCULARIZATION FOLLOWING SUCCESSFUL PHOTOCOAGULATION IN AGE-RELATED MACULAR DEGENERATION

NEIL M. BRESSLER, M.D., SUSAN B. BRESSLER, M.D., ROBERT P. MURPHY, M.D. AND STUART L. FINE, M.D.

From the Retinal Vascular Center, Wilmer Ophthalmological Institute, Johns Hopkins University School of Medicine, Baltimore, MD

Over 50% of successfully treated choroidal neovascular membranes (CNVMs) associated with age-related macular degeneration (AMD) develop recurrences within 2 years of treatment. Most of these recurrences will have occurred 6 to 12 months following initial treatment. Unfortunately, almost all recurrences occur contiguous with the foveal side of the treatment scar, invariably resulting in further visual loss. Possible risk factors felt to be related to an increased rate of recurrence are cigarette smoking, CNVMs located closer to the center of the fovea on initial presentation and CNVMs with very light pigmentation. Additional risk factors need to be identified that may predict which eyes are likely to develop recurrences. Closer follow-up of this high risk group may allow ophthalmologists to identify recurrences earlier, before they have extended through the foveal avascular zone and destroyed central vision. Possible early clinical features which may indicate a recurrence include: (a) a further decrease in visual acuity or central visual performance; (b) subretinal fluid adjacent to the photocoagulation scar (not necessarily associated with subretinal blood or lipid early in a recurrence); (c) a change in the pigment epithelium at the edge of the scar in which focal areas of irregular hypopigmentation are seen; (d) a change in the angiographic pattern of the scar compared to previous post-treatment angiograms in which late hyperfluorescence at the edge of the scar is seen; (e) a shallow pigment epithelial detachment at the edge of the scar; (f) persistent subretinal fluid at least two weeks following treatment; and, (g) new chorioretinal folds. Careful follow-up of all successfully treated CNVMs is necessary until future studies help identify ways in which to more accurately identify and minimize recurrences.

INTRODUCTION

Argon laser photocoagulation can reduce the risk of severe visual loss in patients with extrafoveal choroidal neovascular membranes (CNVMs) associated with age-related macular degeneration (AMD). (1-4) Despite these major breakthroughs, the benefits of argon laser photocoagulation appear to be greatest at one year. (2) At that time, the risk of severe visual loss is reduced 51% by treatment, from 43% in untreated eyes to 21% in treated eyes. By three years, the risk of severe visual loss is reduced 24% by treatment, from 62% in untreated eyes to 47% in treated eyes. (2) This deterioration in treatment effect is predominantly due to recurrent CNVMs in eyes that had been successfully photocoagulated. (5) Recurrences are most apt to occur on the foveal side of previous treatments and subsequently grow toward the center of the foveal avascular zone (FAZ). (5) Thus, recurrent CNVMs account for a large majority of patients who develop severe visual loss subsequent to successful treatment of choroidal neovascularization.

Since the long term effectiveness of laser photocoagulation in reducing severe visual loss is compromised by the recurrence of CNVMs, several recent studies (5,6) have described this phenomenon in detail in an attempt to gain a better understanding of its frequency, associated risk factors and appropriate management. This paper will review these findings as well as describe our current approach to this complication.

DEFINITION OF RECURRENCES

Before discussing the frequency of recurrences, the definition of recurrences will be clarified.

Residual choroidal neovascularization. Residual choroidal neovascularization is defined as neovascularization that remains immediately after treatment, usually as a result of inadequate treatment to the neovascular complex. Inadequate treatment, in other words, failure to completely obliterate the membrane, can be minimized if a 35 mm Polaroid transparency is taken immediately after treatment to compare the treated area to the area of the membrane outlined on the initial angiogram. This is best accomplished by projecting the initial angiogram on an apparatus that permits tracing projected frames of the angiogram onto paper. The membrane as well as key landmarks around the membrane such as subretinal blood, retinal vessels and the FAZ are traced onto plain white paper. The Polaroid transparency is then projected and the area of treatment as well as some key landmarks are traced onto a separate piece of paper. The original drawing is placed over the treatment drawing on a lightbox so that the treated area can be traced onto the original drawing. Any areas not adequately treated can be "touched up" while the patient is still in the office.

Contiguous recurrent choroidal neovascularization. Usually within two weeks following adequate treatment, there should be no clinical or angiographic evidence of surviving CNVM or associated subretinal fluid. Thus, any subsequently documented fluorescein leakage contiguous with the perimeter of the treatment scar is considered a recurrent CNVM.

Some eyes identified as a recurrence actually may have had persistent or residual choroidal neovascularization that was not detected, clinically or angiographically, after treatment. However, in the current literature, a recurrence is the occurrence of neovascular activity after presumed destruction of the original CNVM has been documented clinically and angiographically, even though some overlap with residual CNVMs probably exists.

Independent recurrent choroidal neovascularization. Since AMD represents a diffuse dysfunction of the retinal pigment epithelium/Bruch's membrane/choriocapillaris complex, (7) patients with adequately treated CNVMs are also at risk for new areas of neovascularization, independent of the original treatment scar. These recurrences have been classified as independent recurrences by previous investigators. (5,6)

Central recurrent choroidal neovascularization. A third type of recurrence has been described by Sorenson and others (6) in which previously photocoagulated new vessels reopen and proliferate beyond the margins of the original membrane and treated area. In the opinion of one of the authors (RPM), this recurrence is most apt to occur when treatment is too light, as was done in initial clinical studies employing krypton red laser photocoagulation in the early 1980's.

RELIABILITY IN DETECTING RECURRENCES

Although many clinicians feel that identifying recurrent neovascularization, as defined above, can be difficult, the Macular Photocoagulation Study (MPS) showed that identification of recurrences is fairly reliable. When the MPS Reading Center's gradings were compared with three experienced ophthalmologists' gradings, agreement to the presence or absence of a recurrent membrane was 92%, (5) much higher than agreement expected by chance alone. (The chance agreement [8] that the Reading Center's gradings would agree with an ophthalmologist's gradings calculates to 51% using the data reported by the MPS. [5])

FREQUENCY OF RECURRENCES

According to the MPS, the cumulative risk of a recurrence following successful treatment of an extrafoveal CNVM among 119 patients was 10% by six weeks, 21% by three months, 24% by six months and 43% by twelve months (Fig 1). At the end of follow-up (54 months), the cumulative risk of recurrence reached 57% (Fig 1). Thus, most recurrences will occur within the first year. Nearly one-quarter of all successfully treated CNVMs developed a recurrence by three months. Subsequently, the cumulative risk of a recurrence doubled by one year.

Similar high rates of recurrence have been noted by Sorenson and coworkers. (6) Their study design, though, differed from the MPS in that patients were treated with krypton red laser photocoagulation; CNVMs were eligible for

treatment even if they came within, although not directly
under the anatomic center, of the FAZ; and, follow-up was
only for six months following treatment. Nevertheless, the
recurrence rate in their series was 54%. (6)

The frequency of recurrences following treatment of
CNVMs appears to be related, in part, to the pathologic
entity associated with the CNVM. In the MPS's most recent
report of August 31, 1985, recurrent neovascularization had
been observed following successful treatment in 59% of eyes
with AMD, 30% of eyes with presumed ocular histoplasmosis
and 33% of eyes with idiopathic CNVMs. However, the average
age of patients in the AMD group was significantly greater
than in the presumed ocular histoplasmosis or idiopathic
group. (5)   It is unclear whether the pathologic entity or
the patient's age, or both, contributes to the greater
recurrence rate in patients with age-related macular
degeneration.

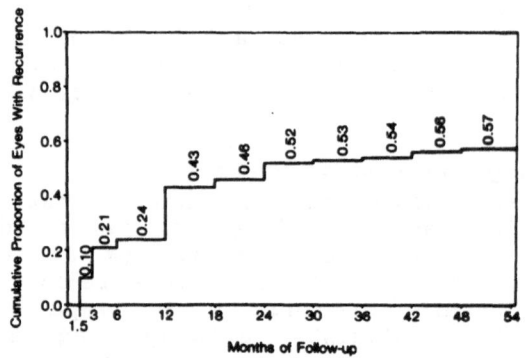

FIGURE 1.   Cumulative proportion of eyes with recurrence
following successful treatment of choroidal
neovascularization associated with macular degeneration.
(Reprinted with permission from the American Medical
Association, copyright 1986: Macular Photocoagulation Study
Group: Recurrent choroidal neovascularization after argon
laser photocoagulation for neovascular maculopathy. Arch
Ophthalmol 104:503-512, April 1986.)

IMPLICATION OF RECURRENCE ON VISUAL ACUITY

Because 97% of all contiguous recurrences in AMD involve
the foveal side of the treatment scar, recurrences are
almost invariably associated with further visual loss. (5)
In the MPS, treated eyes without recurrence had an average
visual acuity at one year of 20/40 and at three years of
20/50.   In contrast, treated eyes with recurrence had an
average visual acuity at one year of 20/125 and at three
years of 20/250.   Furthermore, at one year after treatment,
only 6% of eyes without recurrence compared to 41% of eyes
with recurrence lost more than 5.5 lines of acuity.   At
three years after treatment, 10% of eyes without recurrence
compared to 80% of eyes with recurrence lost more than 5.5
lines of acuity. (5)

RISK FACTORS ASSOCIATED WITH RECURRENCE

As noted in the chapter on Clinical Trials, the benefit of argon laser photocoagulation in the MPS was greatest one year after treatment. (2) The subsequent deterioration in treatment effect was predominantly due to the high frequency of recurrences on the foveal side of the scar. The high risk of recurrence and its effect on final visual outcome behooves us to identify risk factors that may predict which eyes are likely to develop recurrences following successful treatment. By following more closely the subset of successfully treated CNVMs who are at greatest risk for recurrence, ophthalmologists may identify recurrences earlier, before they have extended through the FAZ and destroyed central vision.

At present, risk factors felt to be related to an increased rate of recurrence are cigarette smoking, (5) CNVMs located closer to the center of the fovea on initial presentation (6) and CNVMs with very light pigmentation. (6) Predictions of which eyes will suffer recurrences, however, cannot be made accurately (5) based on this limited information.

There are several clinical and angiographic features among successfully treated CNVMs which may precede a recurrence. Identification of such factors may alert the clinician to more aggressive follow-up and may lead to retreatment of a recurrence before central vision is compromised. Possible features which need further investigation include: (a) a further decrease in visual acuity or central visual performance; (b) subretinal fluid adjacent to the photocoagulation scar (not necessarily associated with subretinal blood or lipid early in a recurrence); (c) a change in the pigment epithelium at the edge of the scar in which focal areas of irregular hypopigmentation are seen; (d) a change in the angiographic pattern of the scar compared to previous post-treatment angiograms in which late hyperfluorescence at the edge of the scar is seen; (e) a shallow pigment epithelial detachment at the edge of the scar; (f) persistent subretinal fluid at least two weeks following treatment; and, (g) new chorioretinal folds.

Given the current information and our suspected clinical and angiographic features felt to be associated with recurrences, our current approach to minimize the visual loss associated with recurrences is outlined below. Following documentation on the day of treatment that the membrane has been adequately treated, patients are re-evaluated with a fluorescein angiogram at two weeks after treatment. Any persistent subretinal fluid noted at this time should make the clinician highly suspicious that residual or recurrent neovascularization is present, and even more frequent return visits and angiograms may be necessary until the fluid is documented to resolve or a recurrence is noted. If after two weeks no persistent fluid is noted, patients return at four and six weeks for fluorescein angiography, since 10% of successfully treated patients will have a recurrence by this time. (5)   If any of the seven features noted above are seen, careful scrutiny for recurrent neovascularization is necessary.   If the clinician cannot find any definite evidence of recurrence, but one of the above features is noted, continued frequent follow-up (every seven to fourteen days) is necessary until a definite recurrence is documented or until the clinician is convinced that no recurrence is present.   If no recurrence is noted by six weeks, the patient should return for re-examination at three and six months.   Even if no recurrence is noted at six months, a fluorescein angiogram should be obtained at this time.   Areas of hypo- and hyper-fluorescence as a result of retinal pigment epithelial changes from the initial CNVM and photocoagulation treatment ("run off" [9]) can be used as a baseline for comparison to future angiograms.   By six months, most of the retinal pigment epithelial changes will have stabilized (9) so that any future areas of irregular hypopigmentation or late hyperfluorescence can be recognized as possible early harbingers of recurrence.   Of special note, careful evaluation of any further decrease in visual acuity or central visual performance on Amsler grid testing must be examined to determine if these changes are a result of atrophy of the retinal pigment epithelium and overlying photoreceptors (9) or from changes to these structures from subretinal fluid associated with a recurrence.   Since areas of atrophy will often show hyperfluorescence in the late phases of the angiogram, simultaneous projection of the fluorescein angiogram during contact lens biomicroscopy can aid in differentiating areas of atrophy from areas of new fluid.

SUMMARY AND FUTURE RESEARCH
     Over 50% of successfully treated CNVMs associated with AMD develop recurrent CNVMs within two years following treatment.   These recurrences almost invariably account for further visual loss so that severe visual loss from extrafoveal CNVMs associated with AMD is postponed by successful argon laser photocoagulation treatment for only about 18 months.   At present, we are unable to accurately predict which eyes will develop recurrences.   Careful follow-up of all successfully treated CNVMs is necessary while we await the results of future studies that will help to identify ways in which to minimize recurrences.

REFERENCES

1. Macular Photocoagulation Study Group: Argon laser photocoagulation for senile macular degeneration: Results of a randomized clinical trial. Arch Ophthalmol 100:912-918, 1982.
2. Macular Photocoagulation Study Group: Argon laser photocoagulation for neovascular maculopathy: three year results from randomized clinical trials. Arch Ophthalmol 104:694-701, 1986.

3. Coscas G, Soubrane G: Photcoagulation des neovaisseaux sous-retiniens dans la degenerescence maculaire senile par laser a argon. Resultats de l'etude randomisee de 60 cas. Bull Mem Soc Fr Ophthalmol 94:149-154, 1982.
4. Moorfields Macular Study Group: Treatment of senile disciform macular degeneration: a single-blind randomised trial by argon laser photocoagulation. Br J Ophthalmol 66:745-753, 1982.
5. Macular Photocoagulation Study Group: Recurrent choroidal neovascularization after argon laser photocoagulation for neovascular maculopathy. Arch Ophthalmol 104:503-512, 1986.
6. Sorenson JA, Yannuzzi LA, Shakin JL: Recurrent subretinal neovascularization. Ophthalmology 92:1059-1072, 1985.
7. Sarks SH: New vessel formation beneath the retinal pigment epithelium in senile eyes. Aust J Ophthalmol 8:117-130, 1980.
8. Fleiss JL: Statistical Methods for Rates and Proportions, 2nd ed. New York: John Wiley & Sons, 1981.
9. Rice TA, Murphy RP, Fine SL et al: Stability of size of argon laser photocoagulation scars in ocular histoplasmosis, in Fine SL, Owens SL (eds): Management of Retinal Vascular and Macular Disorders. Baltimore: Williams and Wilkins Co, 1983, pp 187-190.

EVALUATION OF CONVENTIONAL THERAPY VERSUS CYCLOSPORIN A IN
BEHCET'S DISEASE

David BenEzra, Evelyne Cohen, Tova Chajek, Gideon Friedman,
Sarah Pizanti, Nelson Matamoros, ImmunoOphthalmology,
Departments of Ophthalmology, Internal Medicine and Oral
Medicine, Hadassah University Hospital, Jerusalem, Israel

INTRODUCTION
    Originally identified as a disease whose main
manifestations consist of aphthous stomatitis, genital
ulcers and visual disturbances (1), Behcet disease affects
many organs (2-4). A great variability in intensity of
affection of the different organs is observed and is
responsible for the admission of Behcet's patients at the
various disciplines' departments (5-7). A high percentage
of these patients suffer from ocular involvement. When
present, it is one of the most detrimental affections that
lead to inexorable blindness early during the course of the
disease (8). Characteristically, exacerbations and
remission periods are unpredictable, making treatment
evaluation very difficult (3). Clinical as well as
laboratory observations support the concept of possible
involvement of the immune system in Behcet disease (3,9,10).
With the emergence of Cyclosporin A (CsA) as a non cytotoxic
modulator of the immune response (11), a preliminary
evaluation of its effect on Behcet disease has been carried
out (12).

MATERIALS AND METHODS
    Diagnosis of ocular Behcet's disease (8) was solely
based on the findings of involvement of the triad: Eyes,
mucous membranes and genitalia. Ocular inflammation
included iridocyclitis with or without hypopyon and/or
vasculitis retinae with or without pipe-stem sheathing,
retinal and vitreous neovascularization. The affection of
the three organs was a sine qua non for the diagnosis of
ocular Behcet and inclusion in the study protocol. However,
not all patients had to present all three symptoms at time
of examination. Diagnosis was made if active ocular
inflammation with either aphthous stomatitis or genital
ulcers was detected and evidence of the missing third
symptom was obtained from the treating physician, patient's
account of his past history or from patient's hospital
records. In most cases, other signs of the generalized
vasculitis were observed and recorded. These, however, were
not taken into consideration as diagnostic criteria.
    Selection of patients: When the clinical diagnosis of
ocular Behcet was ascertained, patients underwent chest X-
ray and thorough hematological, biochemical and

immunological tests. The decision whether a patient was compatible for inclusion in the study protocol was made during a meeting of our multidisciplinary group including ophthalmologists, internists, neurologist, dermatologist and dentist. If diagnostic criteria were met and laboratory data did not show any abnormalities of kidney or liver functions or gross hematological or immunological impairment, the patient was admitted to the study protocol.

Treatment: After a patient fulfilled all criteria for inclusion, the coordinator and/or one of the physicians explain the study to the patient who, if he agrees to the terms of the study, signs the consent form. The coordinator then draws a sealed envelope for treatment assignment prepared by Sandoz. Thus, at random, patients are assigned either to treatment with CsA or to the treatment under conventional therapy. The patient with the sealed envelope is referred to the internist who explains the treatment to the patient. The internist is responsible for the modulation of the drug regimen according to clinical response, side effects and laboratory data.

Follow-up: Each patient is scheduled for reexamination one, two and four weeks after initiation of therapy and every month thereafter for a total of six months. After this period the visits are scheduled for three-month intervals. During reexamination visits, ophthalmologists record their findings in a masked manner in "ophthalmologist file" and the internists record theirs openly in "internist file". While the internists have free access to the "ophthalmologist file", the ophthalmologists remain masked regarding the type of treatment during the whole period of follow-up. If, however, the ophthalmologist records a steady worsening of the ocular condition, he can suggest to open the protocol. In this instance, the patient is switched openly to the other mode of treatment.

During the period beginning September 1984 and ending September 1986, 29 patients have fulfilled all criteria and were included in this study. Eleven of the patients are female and 18 are males with a total number of 56 eyes for evaluation (two eyes were phthisic and could not be evaluated). The average age of these patients was 30 years with a range between 18 and 46. Sixteen of the patients are Jews and 13 Arabs. Among the Jews, 15 are of Sephardic extraction and only one is of Ashkenazi origin.

RESULTS

Of the 29 patients, 15 have been randomly assigned to conventional therapy (steroids - 12 patients, leukeran - 3 patients) and 14 to treatment with Cyclosporin A. Three of the 15 patients on conventional therapy dropped out: one patient did not return after the first visit, one patient did not keep his third-month visit appointment and another one, his visit of the fourth month. Eight of the patients from this group had to be crossed over to Cyclosporin therapy because of steady worsening of their symptoms. Among the patients who were assigned to Cyclosporin therapy, two

out of the 14 dropped out of the study: one patient failed
the visit of one month and the second, the fourth month
visit... Only one patient had to be crossed over because of
worsening of her ocular condition. It is interesting to
note that on unmasking of the treatment we found out that
the blood Cyclosporin level of this patient fluctuated
markedly and were most probably due to the patient's
inconsistency in taking the drug according to treatment
protocol. The ocular condition of this patient showed
marked variations which correlated well with her varying
levels of Cyclosporin. Patients under conventional therapy
showed either a stabilization of their condition (5
patients) within 3 to 6 months of therapy or a marked
worsening (8 patients). Those under Cyclosporin A showed a
stabilization or improvement (13 patients) or worsening (1
patient). Figure 1 illustrates the visual acuity and
inflammatory ocular reaction of a patient assigned to the
conventional therapy. Her ocular condition worsened and
therefore she was crossed over openly to Cyclosporin
therapy. Shortly after CsA was started, a marked and steady
improvement in visual acuity and ocular inflammation was
observed.

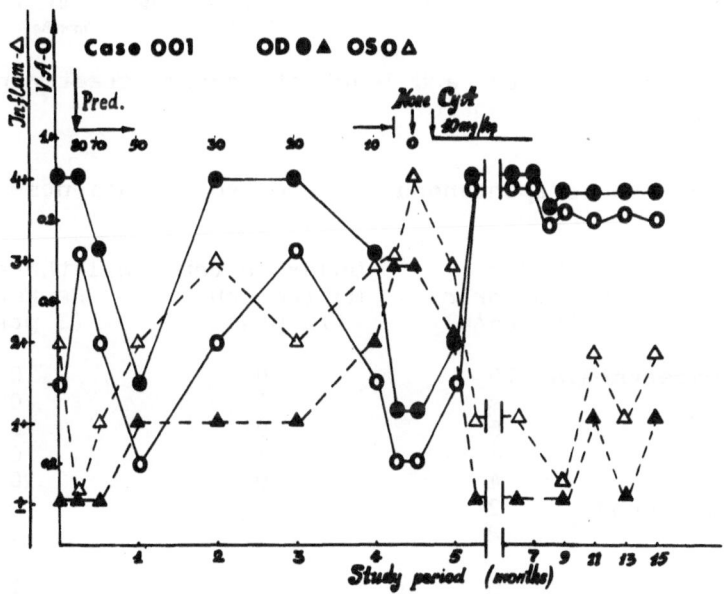

Figure 1. Ocular inflammation and visual acuity during
conventional and Cyclosporin treatment periods in one of the
patients.

Figure 2 illustrates a representative case who was
assigned to Cyclosporin therapy and followed for a period of
21 months. In this case an improvement of visual acuity and
a decrease in the inflammatory signs are observed shortly

after initiation of therapy. These improvements remained unchanged during the period of follow-up.

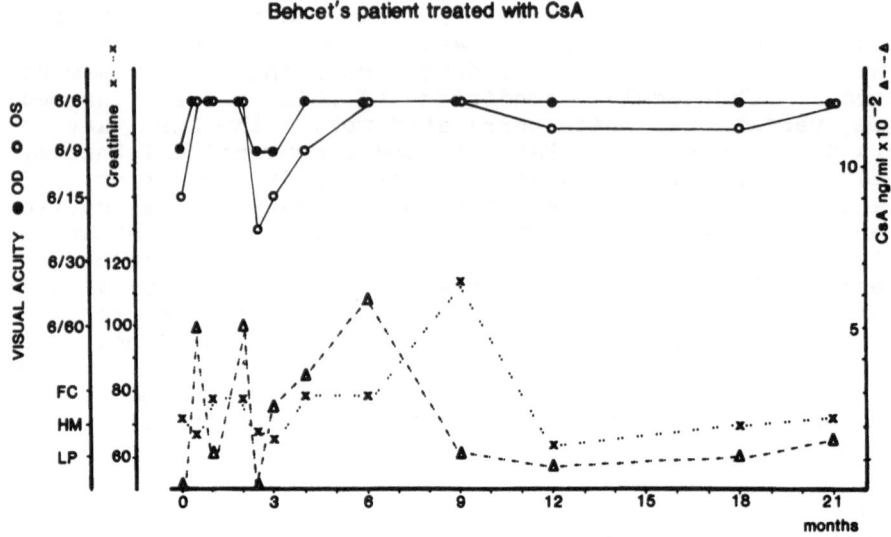

Figure 2. Visual acuity and level of serum creatinine during therapy with Cyclosporin.

Table 1: Side effects spontaneously reported by patients*

Side effect	Under Cyclosporin (19 pts**)	Under conventional therapy Meticorten (12 pts)	Leukeran (3 pts)
Paresthesia/Hypesthesia	19	0	0
Fatigue	8	1	0
Hirsutism	6	0	0
G.I. distress	4	1	0
Nausea/Vomiting	4	0	0
Gingival hypertrophy	2	0	0
Headaches	8	1	1
Muscle pain	5	1	1
Arthralgia	5	1	0
Acne	0	4	0
Moon face	0	3	0

*   In most cases, side effects were transient.
**   Number of patients included in the various groups. Under Cyclosporin are listed five additional patients crossed over from conventional therapy.

Table 1 represents the spontaneous side effects as reported by the patients on the study. The group under Cyclosporin shows a higher incidence of side effects. Most of these were tolerated without additional medications. Table 2 summarizes the more serious side effects observed during the follow-up. These necessitated modulation of the treatment regimen.

Table 2: Major side effects of therapy*

Side effect	CsA (19 pts)	Meticorten (12 pts)	Leukeran (3 pts)
Nephrotoxicity**			
Moderate	3	1	0
Severe	2	0	0
Hepatotoxicity***			
Slight	6	2	0
Severe	6	2	1

* Most patients treated with CsA showed transient marked increase in sedimentation rate. Hypertension was not observed among this group of patients. It was recorded, however, in two out of two patients treated with CsA in our open protocol.

** Nephrotoxicity was arbitrarily classified as moderate if an increase of 50 to 99% in creatinine levels were recorded at any time during therapy. Severe toxicity was considered when an increase of 100% or more was recorded.

*** Hepatotoxicity was arbitrarily classified as moderate if an increase of 50 to 99% of total bilirubin was recorded at any time during therapy. Severe toxicity was considered when an increase of 100% or more was observed.

DISCUSSION

A chronic and relentless disease manifested in various organs, Behcet ocular affections are among the most prevalent and dramatic effects of this phenomenon. Patients suffering from the ocular type of Behcet's disease demonstrate both anterior and posterior segment involvement. Manifestations at the posterior pole may lead to total loss of visual abililty in 74% of the affected eyes within 6 to 10 years (13). Moreover, the effectiveness of conventional therapy to influence the visual outcome has been at best limited (3,8,13-15). Therefore, the possible theoretical advantages of the use of Cyclosporin in Behcet's disease has been suggested (16). Early encouraging results have already been observed (12,17-19). However, because of the chronicity of the disease process, the unpredictability of remissions and exacerbations and the unavoidable bias of the treating physician, a need for masked studies, larger groups of patients and longer follow-up periods has been stressed (12). In the present report we have evaluated 29 patients in a masked manner and carefully followed them for a period of two years. The comparison between the group of patients under conventional therapy and those receiving CsA is in favor of the latter. Eight of the patients assigned to the conventional therapy showed a continuous worsening of their ocular symptoms. All have shown rapid improvement when switched (openly) to CsA therapy. On the other hand, only one out of the 14 patients randomly assigned to CsA showed deterioration of her ocular condition. Analysis of this case revealed the fact that this patient was not taking the medication regularly. The CsA blood level fluctuated markedly, demonstrating minimal (50 to 100 ug/ml) to undetectable levels in a few instances. It is interesting that these periods correlated with the exacerbations of the ocular condition observed clinically.

Although these results are very promising, the relatively large number of early drop-outs (5 out of 29) and the still short period of follow-up of many of the patients prevent any further optimism. Nonetheless, while the systemic therapeutic effects of CsA in Behcet's disease are doubtful (manuscript in preparation), its beneficial influence on the ocular manifestations of Behcet's disease is, so far, very encouraging. From our observations as reported here and our additional data from an ongoing open study with intractable bilateral uveitis, our surmise is that Cyclosporin A will be an important adjunct to our therapeutic modalities in severe non-infectious intraocular inflammations that do not respond to conventional therapy. When using Cyclosporin A, its potential side effects (especially its nephrotoxic and hepatoxic influence) have to be carefully monitored in order to avoid any irreversible damage.

REFERENCES
1. Behcet H: Uber rezidivierende Aphthose, durch ein virus verursachte Geschwure am Munde, am Auge am Genitalien. Dermatol Monatschr 105:112, 1937.
2. Chajek T, Fainaru M: Behcet's disease. Report of 41 cases and a review of the literature. Medicine (Baltimore) 54:179, 1975.
3. BenEzra D, Nussenblatt RB: Ocular manifestations of Behcet's disease. J Oral Pathol 17:431, 1978.
4. Michelson J, Chisari FV: Behcet's disease. Surv Ophthalmol 26:190, 1982.
5. Mason RM, Barnes CG: Behcet's syndrome with arthritis. Ann Rheum Dis 28:95, 1969.
6. Haim S, Barzilai D, Hazani E: Involvement of veins in Behcet's syndrome. Br J Dermatol 84:238, 1971.
7. Lehner T: Progress report. Oral ulcerations and Behcet's syndrome. Gut 18:491, 1977.

8. BenEzra D: Diseases of the choroid and anterior uvea. In: Michaelson IC: Textbook of the Fundus of the Eye. 3rd ed., Longman, Edinburgh and London, p. 703, 1980.
9. Lehner T: Behcet's syndrome and autoimmunity. Br Med J 1:465, 1967.
10. Chan CC, Palestine AG, Nussenblatt RB, Roberge FG, BenEzra D: Anti retinal auto-antibodies in Vogt-Koyanagi-Harada syndrome, Behcet's disease and sympathetic ophthalmia. Ophthalmology 92:1025, 1985.
11. Borel JF, Lafferty KJ: Cyclosporine: Speculation about its mechanism of action. Transplant Proc 15:1881, 1983.
12. BenEzra D, Brodsky M, Pe'er J, Chajek T, Pizanti S, Vertman E, Sachs U: Ciclosporin versus conventional therapy in Behcet's disease. Preliminary observations of a masked study. In: Ciclosporin in Autoimmune Diseases. Springler-Verlag, p. 58, 1985.
13. BenEzra D, Cohen E: Treatment and visual prognosis in Behcet's disease. Br J Ophthalmol 70:589, 1986.
14. Tricoulis D: Treatment of Behcet's disease with chlorambucil. Br J Ophthalmol 60:55, 1976.
15. Mamo JG: Treatment of Behcet's disease with chlorambucil. Arch Ophthalmol 94:580, 1976.
16. BenEzra D: Cyclosporin A in Behcet's disease - an overview. In: Recent Advances in Behcet's Disease. Lehner and Barnes (ed). Royal Society of Medicine Services, International Congress and Symposium Series 103:319, 1986.
17. Nussenblatt RB, Palestine AG, Chan CC: Cyclosporin A therapy in the treatment of intraocular inflammatory disease resistant to systemic corticosteroids and cytotoxic agents. Am J Ophthalmol 96:275, 1983.
18. Graham EM, Sanders MD, James DG, Hamblin A, Dumonde D: Cyclosporin A in the treatment of posterior uveitis. Trans Ophthalmol Soc UK 104:146, 1985.
19. Massuda K, Nakajima A: A double masked study of Cyclosporin treatment in Behcet's disease. In: Ciclosporin in Autoimmune Diseases, Springer-Verlag, p. 162, 1985.

THE EFFECTS OF THE CYCLOSPORINES ON OCULAR INFLAMMATORY DISEASE

ROBERT B. NUSSENBLATT, M.D.
ALAN G. PALESTINE, M.D.
LABORATORY OF IMMUNOLOGY, NATIONAL EYE INSTITUTE,
NATIONAL INSTITUTES OF HEALTH, BETHESDA, MD, U.S.A.

The search for newer immunosuppressive therapies remains an important goal in the treatment of intra-ocular inflammatory disease. With this goal in mind, we have had the opportunity to evaluate several animal models for intra-ocular inflammatory disease, in particular the retinal S-Ag induced experimental autoimmune uveitis model (1). This disorder can be transferred to naive recipients by T-cell lines specific to the S-antigen that have been maintained in vitro for extended periods of time (2). The demonstration of the strong T-cell role in this animal model that has many aspects strikingly similar to the human condition supported strongly the concept that specific anti-T-cell medications could be effective in some types of human disease. This report deals with several aspects of our work concerning the cyclosporines, a group of medications with specific anti-T-cell qualities, both in the animal model, and in patients with ocular inflammatory disease.

Cyclosporin-A is a lipid soluble cyclic peptide which is unchanged at physiologic pH, and has a molecular weight of 1202. It has been the most extensively tested of all the cyclosporines for its capacity to immunomodulate. The mechanism of action of cyclosporine is via an inhibition of the production of interleukin-2 by T-lymphocytes and the expression of IL-2 receptors (3). Cyclosporine was initially described as having an effect on the afferent limb of the immune system as well. Further studies, however, have demonstrated that this drug was also effective in inhibiting an immune response in a previously immunized animal, indicating an effect on the efferent limb of the immune system. These observations supported strongly its use in the retinal S-antigen model. Cyclosporine was noted to be very effective in this model. We have reported that the administration of CsA at the time of S-antigen immunization effectively prevented the expression of this disease (4). Perhaps more importantly, therapy initiated one week after immunization also resulted in a positive therapeutic result (4,5). These findings permitted us to embark on a long-term evaluation of this compound in the treatment of human uveitis. Our initial entry criteria required patients to have severe posterior or intermediate endogenous disease not well controlled on either systemic corticosteroid or cytotoxic agent therapy. These patients initially began on cyclosporine as the sole therapeutic agent. This therapeutic approach has been changed and will be detailed later on in this discussion. We have reported our results concerning these patients, demonstrating a positive therapeutic response in the majority of the patients treated (6,7). Long-term follow-up of these patients demonstrated that at three months after the initiation of cyclosporine therapy, over 78% of the patients were considered therapeutic successes, and at one year's time, the figure was at greater than 62% (7). The vast majority of these individuals developed visual disturbances due to the inflammation's effect on the integrity of the ocular vasculature, particularly that of the retina and choroid. Of particular note was the profound effect this drug had on the ocular course of Behcet's disease (8), with the number of ocular attacks diminishing dramatically, and sometimes being stopped completely. These observations have been corroborated in a recently completed randomized, double masked trial in Japan (9), and results of the Israel study under the guidance of Prof. BenEzra are anxiously being awaited. Further, the non-Behcet patients involved in our study invariably had decompensation of the blood/ocular barrier, leading either to cystoid macular edema, or to serous detachments, as in the case of the patients with Vogt-Koyanagi Harada's syndrome. Such an example is the following: This 35 year old white female with American Indian heritage developed bilateral posterior uveitis with serous retinal detachments with a subsequent fall in visual acuity to 20/400 in both eyes. She also developed severe headaches, and two months later experienced a significant hearing loss. Therapy with 120 mg of prednisone daily did not lead to an improvement of her symptoms. An evaluation at the NIH revealed a severe vitritis, a 50Db hearing loss, and 20-30 mononuclear cells were noted in her cerebral spinal fluid (Fig. 1). The patient began cyclosporine as the sole immunosuppressive agent. A relatively rapid decrease in inflammatory activity was noted, and gradual improvement in visual acuity ensued. However, over the first 6-8 months, the patient suffered two vitreal hemorrhages, both of which cleared. After approximately one year of cyclosporine therapy, and excellent control of her inflammatory disease, the vitreal hemorrhages ceased to be a problem, and the patient has maintained good visual acuity with maintenance low dose cyclosporine (Fig. 2). Additionally, it was noted that her central auditory disturbance improved as well.

However, we have seen that some patients with well established retinal vascular problems due to uveitis will continue to manifest these problems even after the initiation of CsA therapy. Young patients with pars planitis, obtaining good inflammatory control with the medication, will at times continue to have vitreal hemorrhages due to neovascularization. Additionally, patients with Behcet do not seem to have regression of neovascularization with cyclosporine therapy, as has been seen in sarcoid patients.

We have noted cyclosporine induced renal toxicity in our patients treated long term (10). Because of these observations, we have attempted to develop newer therapeutic approaches using CsA. In addition to lowering the dosage of CsA and combining it with low dose systemic prednisone, we have explored the immunosuppressive characteristics of Cyclosporine G (CsG) in the EAU model (11), finding it a potentially useful compound. We evaluated the concentration of CsG needed for an immunosuppressive effect if the medication was placed intravitreally in S-antigen immunized rats. Placing varying concentrations of CsG

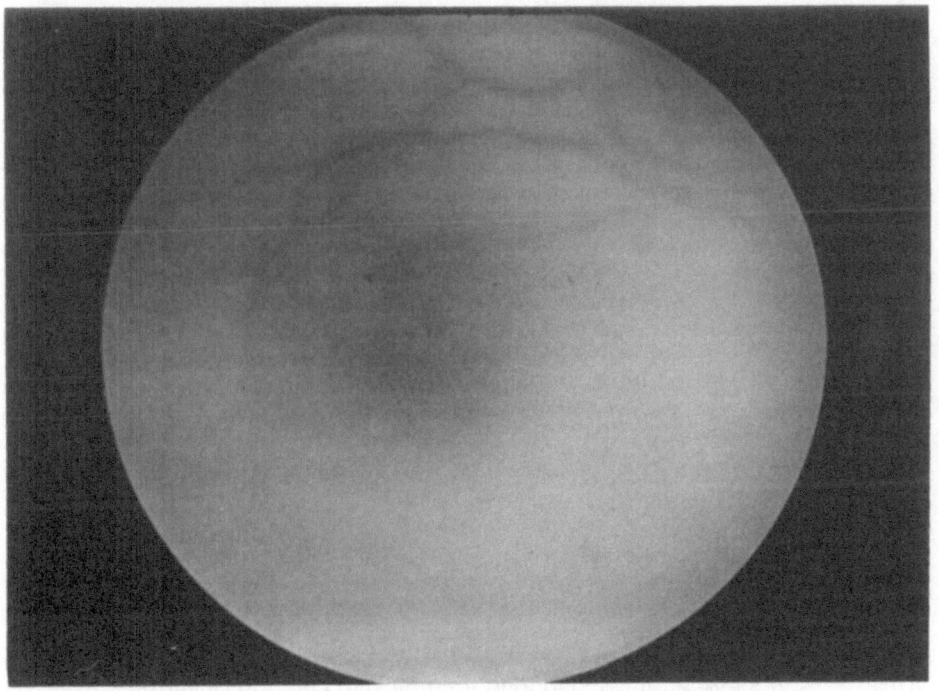

FIGURE 1. Patient with Vogt-Koyanagi-Harada's disease, before cyclosporine therapy. Very hazy detail is due to severe inflammatory response.

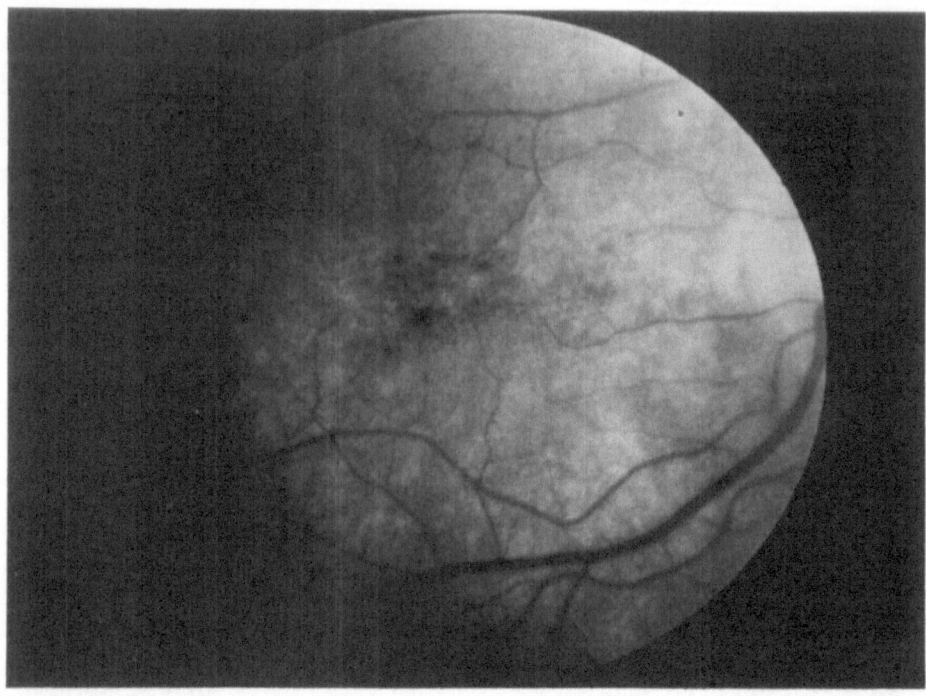

FIGURE 2. Same eye after cyclosporine therapy with clearing of vitreal inflammation and marked improvement in visual acuity.

intravitreally on day 11 following S-Ag immunization provided information as to whether end organ protection could be obtained. The results are shown in Table 1:

The Local Effect of Intravitreal CsG on EAU

Amount of Drug	Treated Eyes # Eyes Normal/Total	Untreated (olive oil injection) # Eyes Normal/Total
500 ng CsG	4/7	1/7
100 ng CsG	0/6	0/6
50 ng CsG	0/6	0/6

Thus protection could be elicited locally using this medication. Grisolano et al (12) have recently reported that intra-ocular CsA was not toxic at amounts 10 fold higher than were used in this study. Therefore, we feel that systemical cyclosporine appears to be a significant therapeutic modality in the treatment of ocular inflammatory disorders with significant retinal vascular complications. Further, it appears that local immunosuppression can be achieved with the cyclosporines, paving the way for newer therapeutic approaches to these most difficult collection of diseases.

REFERENCES

1. Nussenblatt RB, Kuwabara T, deMonasterio FM, Wacker WB: S-antigen uveitis in primates: A new model for human disease. Arch Ophthalmol 99:1090-1092, 1981.
2. Caspi RR, Roberge FG, McAllister CG, El-Saied M, Kuwabara T, Gery I, Hanna E, Nussenblatt RB: T-cell lines mediating experimental autoimmune uveoretinitis (EAU) in the rat. J Immunol 136:928-933, 1986.
3. Nussenblatt RB, Palestine AG: Cyclosporine: Immunology, pharmacology, and therapeutic usages. Survey of Ophthalmology (in press).
4. Nussenblatt RB, Rodrigues MM, Wacker WB, Cevario SJ, Salinas-Carmona MC, Gery I: Cyclosporin A: Inhibition of experimental autoimmune uveitis in Lewis rats. J Clin Invest 67:1228-1231, 1981.
5. Nussenblatt RB, Rodrigues MM, Salinas-Carmona MC, Gery I, Cevario SJ, Wacker WB: Modulation of experimental autoimmune uveitis with Cyclosporin A. Arch Ophthalmol 100:1146-1149, 1982.
6. Nussenblatt RB, Palestine AG, Chan CC: Cyclosporine therapy in the treatment of intra-ocular disease resistant to systemic corticosteroids or cytotoxic agents. Amer J Ophthal 96:275-282, 1983.
7. Nussenblatt RB, Palestine AG, Chan CC: Cyclosporine therapy for uveitis: long term followup. J of Ocular Pharmacology 1:369-382, 1985.

8.   Nussenblatt RB, Palestine AG, Chan CC, Mochizuki M, Yancey K: Effectiveness of cyclosporin therapy for Behcet's disease. Arthritis Rheumatism 28:671-679, 1985.

9.   Masuda K, Nakajima A: A double masked study of ciclosporin treatment in Behcet's disease. In: Ciclosporin in Autoimmune Diseases. Schindler,Rosemarie (Ed), Springer-Verlag, Berlin, pp 162-164, 1985.

10. Palestine AG, Austin III HA, Balow JE, Antonovych TT, Sabnis SG, Preuss HG, Nussenblatt RB: Renal histopathologic alterations in patients treated with cyclosporine for uveitis. New Engl J Med 314:1293-1298, 1986.

11. Nussenblatt RB, Caspi RR, Dinning WJ, Palestine AG, Hiestand P, Borel J: A comparison of the effectiveness of cyclosporine A,D, and G in the treatment of experimental autoimmune uveitis in rats. J of Immunopharmacol 8:427-435, 1986.

12. Grisolano Jr J, Peyman GA: Retinal toxicity study of intravitreal cyclosporin. Ophthal Surg 17:155-156, 1986.

LYMPHOCYTE ACTIVITY AND THE ROLE OF HUMORAL FACTORS IN PATIENTS WITH CHRONIC OCULAR INFLAMMATION

David BenEzra and Genia Maftzir, Immuno-Ophthalmology, Hadassah University Hospital, Jerusalem, Israel

INTRODUCTION

Chronic ocular inflammation is one of the important causes leading to vascularization (1-3). Humoral factors derived from activated leukocytes have been found to be angiogenic in the rabbit cornea (1). The possible relationship between substances released during chronic inflammatory processes and neovascularization could explain the neovascularization of ocular tissues observed in chronic uveitis and Behcet's disease (4). With the emergence of Cyclosporin A as a potent immunomodulator that influences mainly the release of interleukins (5), its use in ophthalmology is being investigated (6,7). We report herein the effect of Cyclosporin A and steroid treatment on the lymphocyte activity and the release of humoral factors of patients with chronic uveitis and Behcet's disease treated with these drugs.

MATERIALS AND METHODS

Subjects: Patients suffering from intractable chronic bilateral uveitis not responding to conventional therapy, were treated with Cyclosporin A under an open protocol. Patients fulfilling the criteria for the ocular type of Behcet's disease were included in a masked protocol and randomly assigned to conventional therapy (steroids or Leukeran) or Cyclosporin A (7). Before starting the protocol treatment and at various intervals thereafter, blood was withdrawn for biochemical and immunological studies.

Serum: Blood withdrawn into non heparinized tubes was incubated for 30 minutes at 37°C and transferred to 4°C overnight. Separation of the serum from the blood clot was performed by two times centrifugation of the supernatants at 2500 g for 15 minutes under aseptic conditions. The sterile serum was then transferred to plastic tubes and stored at -20°C until assayed.

Leukocytes: Lymphocytes (mononuclear) cells were separated using ficoll hypaque as previously described (8). After the harvest of mononuclear cells, the polymorphonuclears were isloated using Dextran. Residual red blood cells were eliminated after short incubations in hypotonic solutions (9).

Lymphocyte cultures: Blast transformation to S-Ag and Concanavalin A (Con A) was evaluated in microcultures as reported (8,10). The level of interleukin-1 (IL-1)

production was assessed by stimulating murine thymocytes as described by Gery et al (11).

Chemotaxis: Boyden blind-chambers and cellulose nitrate filters with a pore size of 8 um and a thickness of 15 um (Sartorious) were used (12).

RESULTS

As illustrated in figure 1, little changes in the capacity of the patients' lymphocytes to undergo blood transformation when stimulated with Con A are observed. Repeated examination at various intervals from time zero (before treatment) to one year after the initiation of treatment demonstrate a level of response comparable to the mean of response shown by a panel of 60 control volunteers. The response to S-Ag was unassessable as no specific blast transformation to this antigen was observed among any of the patients or controls.

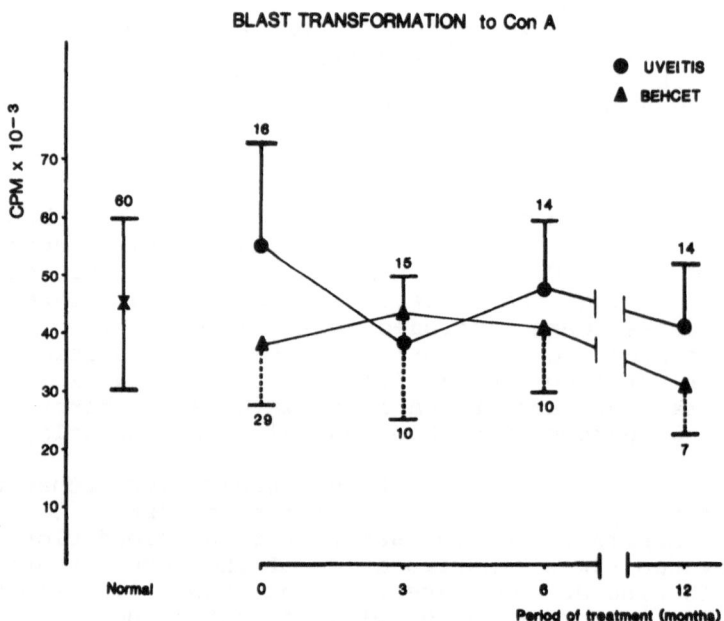

Figure 1. Extent of non-specific blast transformation to Con A during the period of follow-up. The numbers on each bar represent the number of patients tested at this point.

The level of IL-1 production varied markedly among individual patients with a tendency of a lower average 6 and 12 months after the start of therapy (figure 2).

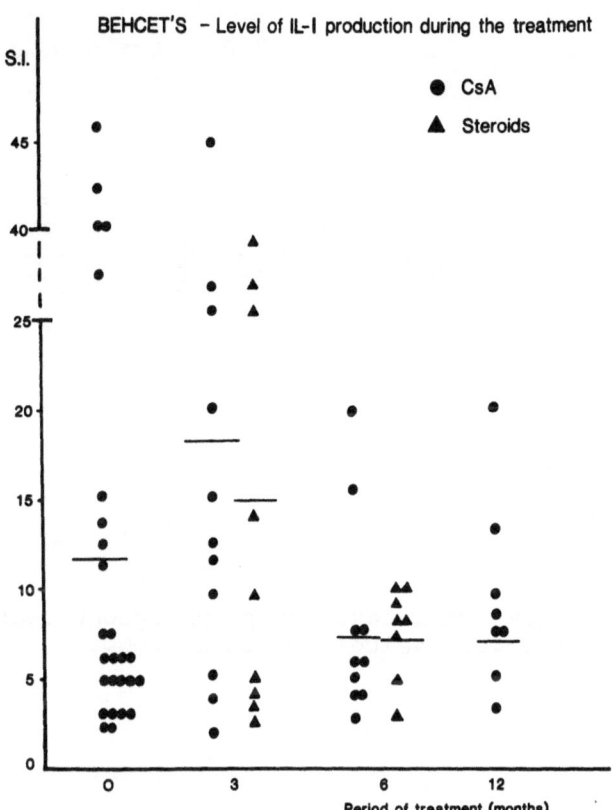

Figure 2. Levels of IL-1 production of individual patients at various intervals of follow-up. Bars represent the mean level for all patients at that point.

The random (figure 3) as well as the directional (figure 4) chemotactic potential of the polymorphonuclear cells did not differ significantly during the period of follow-up. The chemotactic ability shown by the patients' leukocytes remained within the normal range demonstrated by a large panel of control volunteers.

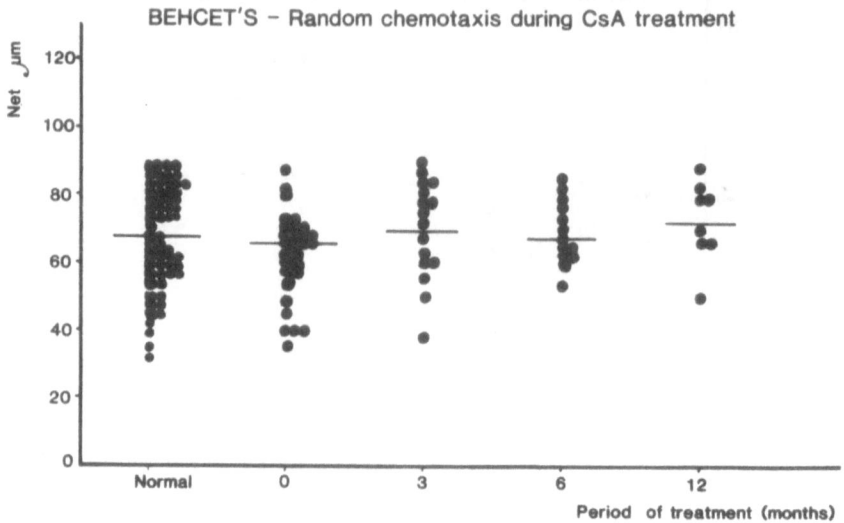

Figure 3. Random chemotaxis of polymorphonuclear cells. Bars represent the mean values for each group.

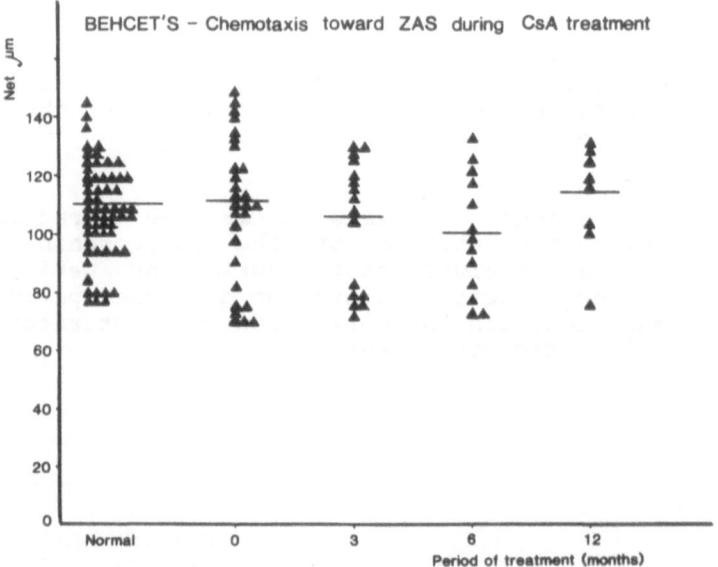

Figure 4. Directional chemotaxis of polymorphonuclear cells to zymozan activated serum (ZAS). Bars represent the mean values for each group.

Thus, no indications for any significant affection at the cellular level has been observed during therapy with Cyclosporin A or steroids. On the other hand, when the serum of patients under Cyclosporin A therapy was tested, a marked inhibition of the blast transformation ability to Con A stimulation was observed (figure 5).

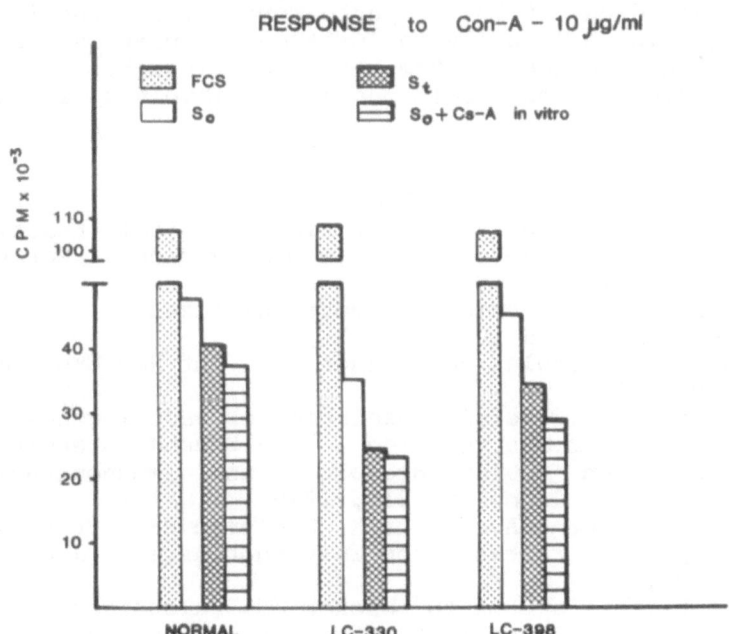

Figure 5. Effect of various sera on the extent of non specific blast transformation to Con A.

As one can see, in the presence of fetal calf serum (FCS) the patients' lymphocytes undergo blast transformation at a level comparable to control. However, the extent of blast transformation is markedly inhibited when the lymphocytes are cultured in the presence of patient's serum (St) withdrawn during the period of treatment with CsA. This effect is observed when both normal and patients' lymphocytes are tested. The level of inhibition is similar to that obtained when similar concentrations of CsA are added to the culture (figure 5).

DISCUSSION
The data presented in this study clearly demonstrate that Cyclosporin A (and steroids) at dosages used during the study period, do not have any striking effect on the activity of lymphocytes and polymorphonuclear cells of the treated patients. These tests were carried out after the isolation of these cells from the blood and then thorough washings. Therefore, the treatment had no longstanding

effect on the tested activities of the lymphoid cells. Patients' ɹera with detectable levels of CsA, however, showed a marked influence on the lymphocytes' capacity to proliferate. This effect was identical whether cells from normal volunteers or those from patients under treatment were tested. Thus, a direct inhibition of proliferation is only observed in the presence of CsA. These findings may have implications on the understanding of the mode of action of this novel drug (10,13). Furthermore, the potential use of Cyclosporin A locally in external ocular affections involving the immune system may add insight into the possible immunopathological mechanism involved in these diseases (14).

REFERENCES
1. BenEzra D: Mediators of immunological reactions. Function as inducers of neovascularization. Metabolic Ophthalmol 2:339, 1978.
2. Archer D: Retinal neovascularization. Trans Ophthalmol Soc UK 103:2, 1983.
3. Garner A: Ocular angiogenesis. Int Rev Exp Pathol 28:249, 1986.
4. BenEzra D: Possible mediation of vasculogenesis by products of immune reaction. The Second International Symposium on Ocular Immunology and Immunopathology. Paris, Masson & Co., p. 315, 1979.
5. Granelli-Piperno A, Inaba K, Steinman RM: Stimulation of lymphokine release from T-lymphoblasts. J Exp Med 160:1792, 1984.
6. Nussenblatt RB, Rook AH, Wacker WB, Palestine AG, Scher I, Gery I: Treatment of intraocular inflammatory disease with Cyclosporin A. Lancet 2:235, 1983.
7. BenEzra D, Brodsky M, Pe'er J, Chajek T, Pizanti S, Vertman E, Sachs U: Ciclosporin A versus conventional therapy in Behcet's disease. Preliminary observations of a masked study. In: Ciclosporin in Autoimmune Diseases. Springer-Verlag, p. 158, 1985.
8. BenEzra D, Gery I, Chan CC, Nussenblatt RB, Palestine AG, Kaiser-Kupfer M, Maftzir G, Pe'er J: Cellular and humoral immune parameters among patients with retinitis pigmentosa and other retinal disorders. Ophthal Ped Gen 4:193, 1984.
9. Ramsey WS: Locomotion of human polymorphonuclear leukocytes. Exp Cell Res 72:489, 1972.
10. BenEzra D: Cyclosporin A in Behcet's disease - an overview, in Recent Advances in Behcet's Disase, Lehner and Barnes (ed). Royal Society of Medicine Services, International Congress and Symposium Series 103:319, 1986.
11. Gery I, Gershon RK, Waksman BH: Potentiation of the T-lymphocyte response to mitogens. I. The responding cell. J Exp Med 136:128, 1972.

12. Snyderman R, Pike MC: Methodology for monocyte and macrophage chemotaxis. In: Leukocyte Chemotaxis, Gallin and Quie (ed). Raven Press, New York, p. 73, 1978.
13. Borel JF, Lafferty *J: Cyclosporine: Speculation about its mechanism of action. Transplant Proc 15:1881, 1983.
14. BenEzra D, Pe'er J, Brodsky M, Cohen E: Cyclosporin A for the treatment of severe vernal kerato-conjunctivitis. Am J Ophthalmol 101:278, 1986.

ANTIBODIES TO ORAL MUCOSA IN PATIENTS WITH OCULAR BEHCET'S DISEASE

Joseph B. Michelson, M.D., and Francis V. Chisari, M.D.

This is publication number 3064-BCR from the Research Institute of Scripps Clinic. This work was supported in part by a grant from the Eye Bank, San Diego County Medical Society.

1. SUMMARY

A method is reported for the identification of cytoplasmic antibodies in patients with Behcet's disease with uveitis. The assay appears positive in at least 80% of patients with definite or probable Behcet's disease, with a false-positive rate of 6.5% among non-Behcet's ocular inflammatory disorders with vasculitis. This test may prove useful to the ophthalmologist in selecting those patients with Behcet's disease from the larger group of patients with uveitis for whom no systemic etiology is identified.

2. INTRODUCTION

Behcet's disease is characterized by three primary components: iridocyclitis with hypopyon, aphthous ulceration in the mouth, and ulceration of the genitalia. Erythema nodosum, arthropathy, thrombophlebitis and nervous system involvement often accompany these manifestations, but the ocular symptoms may be the most important manifestations of the disease. The burden of diagnostic recognition of Behcet's disease often lies with the ophthalmologist since he/she may be the first physician to encounter the patient or put the patient's random systemic complaints into meaningful order.

The hallmark of Behcet's disease is an obliterative, necrotizing vasculitis affecting both arteries and veins characterized microscopically by fibrinoid degeneration, endothelial cell swelling and proliferation and a mononuclear cell infiltrate (1,2). These findings are characteristic of several immunologically induced vasculitides, especially those associated with circulating immune complexes (3). Indeed, it has been reported that approximately 40% of patients with Behcet's disease have circulating immune complexes detectable by the Raji cell assay (3). Others have reported the presence of autoantibodies reactive with oral mucosal antigens in Behcet's disease, especially during relapse (4). The antigenic specificity and diagnostic sensitivity of assays for these autoantibodies has not been determined. The importance of mucosal antigen stimulation in these patients is emphasized by the reported evidence of macrophage migration inhibitory factor production by mucosal antigen-stimulated T-cells from these patients (5). Additionally, peripheral blood lymphocytes from Behcet's patients have been reported to be cytotoxic for cultured oral epithelial cells in vitro (6). The immunologic basis of Behcet's disease is strengthened by the favorable therapeutic effect of corticosteroids (7) and isolated reports of improvement following transfer factor (8,9) or levamisole therapy (9,10).

Clearly, ancillary diagnostic assistance is required in the identification of patients with Behcet's disease because of the absence of strictly pathognomonic clinical findings. Because of the potential importance of additional diagnostic criteria for Behcet's disease we have developed an indirect immunofluorescence assay for the detection of serum antibodies to oral mucosal cytoplasmic antigens. An exhaustive evaluation of the organ and species specificity of these antibodies has been performed and the potential cross-reactivity of other known anti-tissue autoantibodies with oral mucosal epithelium has been assessed. We have applied this assay in a survey of patients with Behcet's disease and other vasculitides with uveitis in order to evaluate the sensitivity and specificity of the test. The results of these studies are reported herein. A clinical summary of the patients with definite Behcet's disease is given in Table 4. The three patients with false-positive assays were each diagnosed as juvenile rheumatoid arthritis, Toxocara canis, and toxoplasmosis, respectively.

3. MATERIALS AND METHODS
3.1. Subjects
Eight patients with clinically definite, 4 patients with probable, and 2 patients with possible Behcet's disease, and 60 patients with non-Behcet's vasculitis and uveitis from Scripps Clinic and Research Foundation were studied. Additionally, the serum of 16 patients with known Behcet's disease from Haceteppe University School of Medicine, Ankara, Turkey, were studied.

3.2. Assays
Antibodies to cytoplasmic antigens in the stratified squamous epithelium of guinea pig lip were identified by indirect immunofluorescence. Cryostat secretions were incubated for 45 minutes at 20°C with serial dilutions of patient and control serum in 0.01 M NaH_2PO4, 0.15 MNaCl, pH 7.2 (phosphate buffered saline, PBS). They were then washed three times for five minutes in PBS, dried and incubated with an optimal dilution of goat antiserum to human immunoglobulines previously conjugated with fluorescein isothiocyanate (0.1 mg/ml fluorescein/protein ratio equal 3:1), according to the method of Clark and Shapard (11). After 45 minutes of incubation at 20°C, the slides were washed as previously described and the stained sections were examined for fluorescence with a Zeiss RA microscope equipped with an HB-200 mercury arc lamp, a 490 nm interference filter, a NA 1.2:1.4 dark field condenser and a 530 nm barrier filter. Positive staining was interpreted as apple green fluorescence restricted to the squamous epithelial cytoplasm of the lip characterized with sparing of epithelial cell nuclei and intercellular bridges (Figure 1).

The species and organ specificity of the antibodies present in reactive sera was assessed by their ability to stain a wide variety of other tissues from the guinea pig and numerous other species (Table 1).

The possibility that reactivity with cytoplasmic antigens in guinea pig lip might be due to the presence of other, potentially crossreactive, autoantibodies that ordinarily react with other tissues was also assessed. The autoantibodies that were studied and their usual tissue substrate and disease association are listed in Table 2.

Finally, all of the Behcet's sera from Turkey were evaluated on appropriate substrates for the presence of several anti-tissue antibodies of the specificity listed in Table 2.

Table 1. Indirect Immunofluorescence Reactivity of Behcet's Sera with Various Tissue Substrates

Species	Tissue	Result
Guinea pig	Lip, Squamous	4+
"	Lip, Mucosal	0
"	Facial Skin	2+
"	Tongue	1+
"	Abdominal Skin	Trace
"	Dorsal Skin	Trace
Human	Lip	2+
Rat	Lip	1+
Mouse	Lip	1+
Rabbit	Lip	1+
All Species	Esophagus	Negative
"	Heart	"
"	Lung	"
"	Kidney	"
"	Liver	"
"	Pancreas	"
"	Adrenal	"
"	Stomach	"
"	Thyroid	"

Sera were assayed at a 1:2 dilution on fresh, snap-frozen cryostat sections prepared from each tissue.

Table 2. Reactivity of Other Human Autoantibodies with Guinea Pig Lip.

Autoantibody	Disease Association	Usual Substrate	G.P. Lip Cytoplasm Reactivity
Epidermis	Bullous	G.P. Esophagus	Negative
Epidermis	Pemphigus Vulgaris	G.P. Esophagus	Negative
Native DNA	Systemic Lupus Erythematosus	Mouse Kidney	Negative
Sm	Systemic Lupus Erythematosus	Mouse Kidney	Negative
Ribonucleopro-tein	Mixed Connective Tissue Disease	Mouse Kidney	Negative
Histone	Drug Induced Lupus	Mouse Kidney	Negative
SSA, SSB	Sjogren's Syndrome	Mouse Kidney	Negative
Mitochondrial	Primary Biliary Cirrhosis	Mouse Kidney	Negative
Liver Kidney Microsomal	Chronic Liver Disease	Mouse Kidney	Negative
Smooth Muscle	Chronic Active Hepatitis	Mouse Stomach	Negative
Parietal Cell	Pernicious Anemia	Mouse Stomach	Negative
Adrenal	Idiopathic Addison's Disease	G.P. Adrenal	Negative
Thyroid Microsomal	Hashimoto's Thyroiditis	Human Thyroid	Negative
Thyroglobulin	Hypothyroidism	Human Thyroid	Negative
Skeletal Muscle	Myasthenia Gravis	G.P. Muscle	Negative

Sera were assayed at a 1:2 dilution on fresh snap-frozen cryostat sections of usual substrate (see above) and guinea pig lip.

Table 3. Occurrence of Behcet's Antibody in SCRF and Turkish Sera.

	Guinea Pig Lip Antibody	
	Positive	Negative
Behcet's Disease		
Definite	8	0
Probable	2	2
Possible	0	2
Non-Behcet's Disease		
Turkish Sample	3	60
Definite	10	6

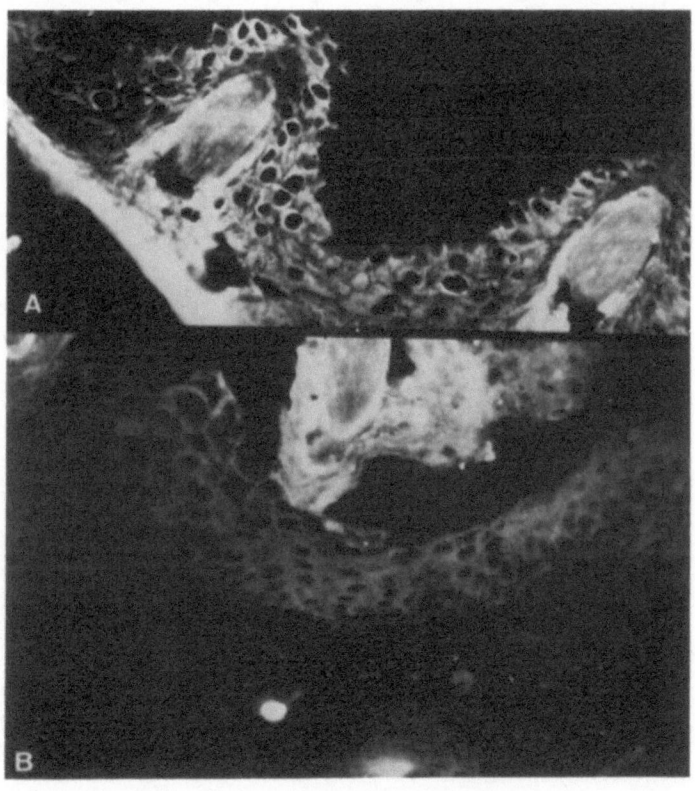

LEGEND
Figure 1.: (Michelson and Chisari) Indirect immunofluorescence analysis of
serum of Behcet's antibody (substrate, guinea pig lip X125). A. Serum
from patient with Behcet's disease. Note brighter fluorescent staining of
cytoplasms of epidermis. Nuclei and intercellular bridge areas are
negative. B. Serum from normal control. Note absence of epidermal
fluorescence.

Table 4. Patients with Definite Behcet's Disease.

Patient	Irido-cyclitis	Retinal vasculitis	Oral ulcers	Genital ulcers	Erythema nodosum	Other	GPL Titer
#1-LM	+	+	+	+	+	CNS disease Renal disease	1:30
#2-SM	+	+	+	+	+	s	1:10
#3-MM	+	-	+	+	+	s	1:10
#4-TH	+	+	+	+	-	Thrombo-phlebitis	1:10
#5-M(N)M	+	+	+	-	+	-	1:10
#6-SF	+	+	+	-	+	-	1:3
#7-IS	+	-	+	+	-	-	1:10
#8-LS	+	-	+	+	-	-	1:4

4. RESULTS

Antibody to guinea pig lip cytoplasmic antigens was present in all eight patients with definite Behcet's disease and in two of four patients with a probable diagnosis of Behcet's disease (Table 3). Antibody titer was low, varying from 1:2 to 1:8, and did not appear to be related to disease activity. The antibody was present in only three of 60 patients without Behcet's disease, and was negative in both patients in whom a diagnosis of Behcet's disease was possible, but far from definite, on clinical grounds. To date, sera from several patients with non-Behcet's mucosal ulceration (including bullous pemphigoig and pemphigus vulgaris) have been negative in our assay. Thus, the assay is positive in at least 80% of patients with definite or probable Behcet's disease from the SCRF study and has a false positive rate of only 6.5% among non-Behcet's disease ocular diseases, suggestive that this may be a diagnostically helpful test in these disorders.

Ten of the 16 Behcet's patients from Turkey were positive in our assay. It is interesting that 5 of these patients from Turkey also have coexisting basal cell antibodies, 4 had antibodies reactive with basement membrane antigens at the dermoepidermal junction (as in bullous pemphigoid) and four had low titer antinuclear antibodies of nondiagnostic specificity.

The nature of the antigen in the cytoplasm of guinea pig lip epidermis with which Behcet's sera react is not known. Interestingly, the antigen is present only in the squamous epithelium but is not present in the mucosal epithelium of the lip. Reactivity is seen to a lesser degree with the epithelial cytoplasm of the tongue, facial skin, and to a much lesser degree with abdominal and dorsal skin of the guinea pig. Human, rat, mouse and rabbit lip squamous epithelial cytoplasm is also positive but to a lesser degree than guinea pig lip. Positive sera do not stain the cytoplasm of any cells within the esophagus, heart, lung, kidney, liver, pancreas, adrenal, stomach or thyroid of numberous species. The specificity of the Behcet's antibody for guinea pig lip epithelial cytoplasm is further strengthened by the failure of these sera to react with other tissue substrates in a pattern compatible with a presence of autoantibodies such as those listed in Table 2. Conversely, sera known to contain autoantibodies of those diverse specificities fail to stain guinea pig epithelial cytoplasm in a Behcet's specific fashion. Therefore, this antibody represents a new and distinct specificity and does not represent a cross-reactivity of other previously identified autoantibodies that are associated with an assortment of more common diseases.

5. DISCUSSION

It is important to state that although hypothetical schemes can be devised in which these antibodies play an important pathogenetic role in Behcet's disease, there is no definite evidence to support this hypothesis presently. The etiology and pathogenesis of this disease must, therefore, be currently designated as still unknown.

All antibody titer measurements were low, varying from 1:2 to 1:8, and the degree of disease activity is reflected either by clinical severity of involvement or by Raji cell assay for circulating immune complexes did not influence the low amount of antibody seen. Patient L.M., who died of central nervous system vasculitis, and demonstrated a Raji cell titer in the 2×10^3 range, showed a maximal titer of only 1:30, while 3 other patients, demonstrating a titer of 1:10 had only the mild, fleeting symptoms of aphtha with intermittent iridocyclitis and retinal vasculitis. While this tendency toward uniformity shows that eye disease may be the

most common and disabling feature of Behcet's disease, the antibody titer
to guinea pig lip cannot select out those patients who have the profound
and unrelenting form of the disease. Conversely, patients I.S. (titer 1:4;
trace positive) and S.F. (1:3), have severe, disabling aphthi and permanent
visual loss, underscoring that those patients with the most severe eye and
mucosal disease may have the lowest titers. An amplification and clarification of the present findings may be achieved when the specificity and
selectivity of this test are refined. Perhaps with improved specificity
antibody titer might reflect disease activity in much the way that immune
complex deposition does, and shed some light upon pathogenesis of disease.
Or, equally feasible, antibody recognition may play no role in the disease
process. But at the very least, prompt recognition of those patients with
propensity to develop Behcet's disease, with all of its disease and
potentially lethal manifestations, will be an asset to the clinician faced
with the puzzling uveitis patients whose systemic evaluation may be
neglected at worst and incomplete at best.

REFERENCES
1. Ehrlich GE: Intermittent and Periodic Arthritic Syndromes. In:
   Arthritis 8th Edition, Hollander JL and McCarty D (eds). Philadelphia:
   Lea & Febiger, 1972.
2. Enoch BA, Castillo-Olivares J, Khou TCL, et al: Major vascular
   complications in Behcet's syndrome. Postgrad. Med. J. 44:453-9, 1968.
3. Gupta RG, O'Duffey JD, McGuffie FC: Circulating immune complexes in
   active Behcet's disease. Surv. Ophthalmol. 12:324-34, 1967.
4. Lehner T: Characterization of mucosal antibodies in recurrent aphthous
   ulceration and Behcet's syndrome. Arch. Oral Biol. 14:843-53, 1969.
5. Lehner T: Pathology of recurrent oral ulceration and oral ulceration
   in Behcet's syndrome: Light, electron, and fluorescein microscopy.
   H. Pathol. 97:481-94, 1969.
6. Rogers RS, Sams WM, Shorter RG: Lymphocytotoxicity in recurrent
   aphthous stomatitis: Lymphocytotoxicity for oral epithelial cells in
   recurrent aphthous stomatitis and Behcet's syndrome. Arch. Dermatol.
   109:361-3, 1974.
7. Michelson JB, Chisari FV: Behcet's disease. Surv. Ophthalmol.
   (Review) 26:190-203, 1982.
8. Bernhard GC, Heim LR: Transfer factor treatment of Behcet's syndrome.
   J. Rheumatol. 1:34-7, 1974.
9. Inaba G, Aoyama J, Shimizu T. Transfer factor therapy of fifteen
   patients with Behcet's disease (in press).
10. Oson JA, Nelms D, Silverman S, Spitler LE: Levamisole: A new treat-
    ment for recurrent aphthous stomatitis. Oral Surg. 41:588-600, 1976.
11. Clark HF, Shepard CC: A dialysis technique for preparing fluorescent
    antibody. Urology 20:642-4, 1963.

BEST'S VITELLIFORM MACULAR DYSTROPHY
SUBRETINAL NEOVASCULARIZATION

VICTOR GODEL,[1] LUCIAN REGENBOGEN,[1,2] GILLES CHAINE[2] AND
GABRIEL COSCAS.[2]
Eye Departments, Tel Aviv University Medical School[1] and
Paris-Val de Marne University Medical School.[2]

INTRODUCTION

Best's Vitelliform Macular Dystrophy (BVMD) is one of the
most pleomorphic of the hereditary macular degenerations
with respect to its manifestation in the ocular fundus(1).
The presence of the disease is heralded by the awareness of
the typical egg-yolk abnormality in the macula and the pathog
nomonic electrooculogram. This macular dystrophy with its
autosomal dominant inheritance is characterized by a progressive temporal course that may have an awkwardly broad
spectrum of appearances in various morphologic stages.

We wish to describe our retrospective analysis of 47 cases
diagnosed as BVMD, to portray its various stages and to
provide some ideas about its pathogenesis and sequence of
events.

MATERIAL AND METHODS

A retrospective review was made of 47 patients diagnosed
as BVMD between the years 1973-1984. The criteria for
inclusion in this study were the characteristic macular
findings associated with impaired EOG or decreased light/
dark ratio in EOG in those autosomal dominant families
where at least one member had a typical vitelliform lesion.

In addition to having their best corrected visual acuity
determined, all patients were examined by a high intensity
red free light ophthalmoscopy, photograohy of the maculas,
visual fields, color vision testing, ERG and EOG.

The classification of the lesions was made accòrding to
the stages proposed by Deutman(2) and modified by Mohler &
Fine(3). In stage 0 the macula is normal without any pigment
epithelial disturbances at angiography, but the EOG is altered
In stage 1 pigment epithelial granularity of the macular
region is seen. It appears as window defect at fluorescein
angiography. Stage 2 is characterized by the typical vitelliform changes that ressembles egg-yolk lesions-sunny-side up.
A scrambled egg appearance in the macula defines stage 2 when
the contents of the lesion becomes less homogenous and more
fragmented. Stage 3 is delineated by the organisation of the
pseudohypopion phase with the development of a fluid level
of a yellow-colored material. In stage 4a the macula develops
an orange-red color with peripheric dispersion of the vitellin deposit associated with increased visibility of the
choroid through the atrophic pigment epithelium. Due to these
atrophic changes the choroidal blood flow could be more

brightly visualized on the transit phase of the fluorescein angiogram. In stage 4b typical fibrous scar tissue in the macula appears, which stains and increases in the late phase of the angiogram. This lesion evolves into a non-specific, often pigmented atrophic scar. Stage 4c was characterized by the presence of definite neovascularisation, as evidenced by vessels visible on a fibrous scar or subretinal haemorrhages adjacent to fibrous proliferation. In rare instances the disease appears with multiple vitelliform cysts scattered outside the foveal region. The lesions are usually round or oval, and situated at the level of retinal pigment epithelium Fig.1 illustrates examples of the macular lesions according to the above mentioned classification.

RESULTS

The 47 patients with BVMD who were examined and tested for this study ranged in age from 13 to 68 years(means 36 years). Twentyone were males and 26 were females. Of 94 eyes of the 47 patients with BVMD, 31 eyes (33%) had stage 0 lesions, 19 eyes (20%) had stage 1 lesions, 9 eyes (10%) had stage 2 lesions, 2 eyes (2%) had stage 3 lesions, and 33 eyes (35%) had stage 4 lesions.

Nineteen of our examined patients were familial occurrences with autosomal dominant pattern of inheritance. Eight additional cases informed us about familial incidences of similar ocular complaints in relatives of their families, however, these probably affected individuals could not be examined by us. Twenty of our patients seemed to be sporadic occurrences.

The spectrum of the retinal manifestation and the encountered frequency of their various stages showed that the progression of the lesion moved from a quiet and quite stable stage 0 and 1, through a transient stage 2 and 3, towards a more stable and destructive stage 4. This transient nature of stages 2 and 3 explains their relatively lower incidence.

The lesions do not significantly alter visual functions in its early stage. The visual acuity was surprisingly good in view of the ophthalmoscopic picture of macular involvement. Individuals with stage 0,1,or 2 had normal or nearly normal vision. Seventy-four percent of our patients had a best corrected vision of 20/40 or better. During the rupture of the egg-yolk the visual acuity remained good, however, during the pseudohypopion stage there was transient loss of vision. When acute haemorrhage or edema accompanied the progression of the lesion a sudden visual acuity drop occurred. After such exacerbations the visual acuity improved again in some cases, and its range was wide, varying from pretty good acuity to lower vision, depending on the severity of the macular findings. Prolonged visual loss was seen only in the eyes of elderly patients with atrophic macular stages. Metamorphopsia and central or paracentral scotomas were variable depending on the severity of the involvement.

From the 47 cases investigated 16 presented anomalous color discrimination. The most commonly encountered acquired color vision defect appeared in the red-green range and was

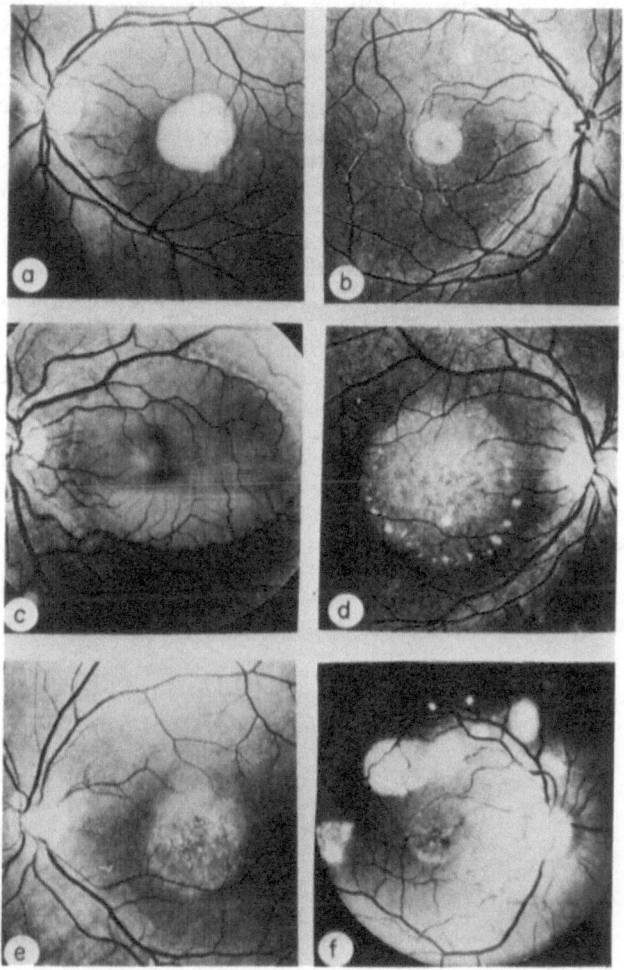

Fig.1. Stages of the macular lesion in BVMD. a) Typical
vitelliform or egg-yolk lesion. b) Scrambled egg phase with
fragmentation of the vitellin material. c) Pseudohypopion
with a fluid level in the vitelliform cyst. d) Atrophy of
pigment epithelium producing an orange-red macular lesion
with peripheral dispersion of the vitellin deposit.
e) Hypertrophic macular scar with fibrous tissue. f) Multiple
vitelliform cysts outside the fovea.

was diagnosed in 12 patients. In 4 cases tritanomaly was observed. It appears that in the later stages of the disease there is an acquired reduction of hue discrimination in some cases.

Little or no electroretinographic abnormalities were found in our series. Almost all of the 47 BVMD patients showed normal b-wave amplitudes at all stimulus values. Only 4 cases of stage 4 with atrophic macular scars showed reduced amplitudes, but responses were all considered to be within the normal range of values of our laboratory.

Flicker fusion threshold intensities were measured as a function of flicker frequency for 22 patients with BVMD having normal or nearly normal visual acuities. An abnormal elevation of the foveal cone threshold and a loss of cone temporal resolution were observed in 16 cases.

All the 47 patients with BVMD included in this study had abnormally low light/dark ratio on the EOG. Ophthalmoscopically normal eyes presented abnormal EOGs which were transmitted in familial cases in an autosomal dominant pattern. Re-evaluation of the EOG in some cases showed progressive decrease of the light/dark ratio.

Subretinal neovascularisation and subretinal haemorrhages have rarely been observed (Fig.2). In our only case with subretinal haemorrhage an early staining of the lesion was followed by late leakage into the surrounding retina. Following the reabsorbtion of the haemorrhage the neovascular frond remained visible until it later contracted into a small fibrotic subretinal scar.

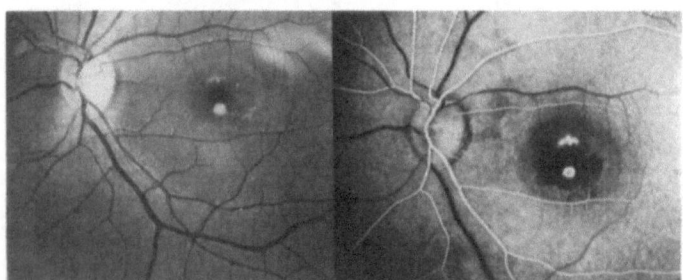

Fig.2. An uplifting of the sensory retina due to a serous detachment of the pigment epithelium (left). A deep retinal haemorrhage was visualized at fluorescein angiography (right). The serous detachment covered the neovascular network.

DISCUSSION

Knowledge concerning the pathogenesis and the nature of the primary defect in BVMD is incomplete. Traditional modes of thinking, in general, perpetuated the notion that BVMD might be a condition that has the potential to affect the retinal pigment epithelium. Such assumptions were built on the result of abnormally low light/dark ratio on the EOG of every BVMD patient(4-6). Moreover, the finding of relatives, in familial cases, with only EOG abnormalities as intense as those of the cases with severe macular destructions substantiates the possibility that the degenerative process is more widespread than in just the macula. Further support to the pathologic localization of the retinal lesion in the pigment epithelium is provided by fluorescein angiography which is quite sterotyped in most of the typical cases to permit accurate diagnosis (7,8).

Primarily on the basis of visual acuity measurements it was generally accepted that BVMD does not involve the neurosensory retina in most stages. However, the lack of visual acuity loss is not indicative of the lack of photo-receptor damage. Visual acuity is at least a gross assessment of the behaviour of mechanism underlying spatial resolution. Subtle abnormalities of retinal function that do not interfere with lateral interactions are not likely to be detected by measurements of visual acuity. The flicker ERG findings gave some hints that BVMD affects the neuro-sensory retina even when visual acuity was normal (9).

In the presence of a negative family history the typical cases of BVMD are generally labeled as sporadic and thought to be fresh mutations of a dominant gene. However, the amount of the so-called "sporadic" cases seem to be far too large for them all to be due to fresh mutations. It is more reasonable to believe that the gene having no complete penetrance and causing sometimes skipping of generations may add to this apparent sporadicity.

On the other hand in an adult patient, one may wonder if the so called "sporadic" case do not correspond to one of the so-called pseudovitelliform varieties. It is currently apparent that a wide range of macular disorders of varied etiologies masquerade as BVMD(10). Descriptions of various vitelliform-like lesions which are unassociated with genetic alterations are continuously growing (11-14). It is worth-wile to point out that,unfortunately, these vitelliform-like diseases are encumbered by an abundance of eponyms, tending to obfuscate rather than clarify their real origin.

The exact sequence of events in BVMD remains uncertain. The most actual, and by far the most impressive and exhaustive works trying to correlate knowledge concerning the histopathology of this disorder were offered quite recently(15,16). Weingeist et al.(1982) had labored long and well to clarify the central issue of the primary site of involvement in BVMD. Their histopathologic results in a young patients with well documented BVMD are logically compelling to warrant the postulation that the primary site of involvment is the retinal pigment epithelium. But one should not lose sight of the contradictory histologic and ultrastructural evidence of Frangieh et al.(1982) who examined the eyes of an elderly woman with BVMD. Because the photoreceptor cell layer was found to be severely affected, whereas the retinal pigment epithelium was nondisrupted and because the photoreceptor cell degeneration was found to extend beyond the boundaries of the involved retinal pigment epithelium within the macula, the authors concluded that the sensory retina may be the primary site of the disease process.

What both of these studies had in common was the description of an electron dense granular material believed to be lipofuscein found within the retinal pigment epithelium by both groups (15,16), and within the photoreceptor cells by Frangieh et al.(16).

Subretinal neovascularisation as an integral part of BVMD has several times been suggested(17-19). Subretinal neovascular membranes with clearly demonstrable feeder vessels and leakage of fluorescein into the subretinal space have also been reported(18). In rare instances it is probable that the break down and resorption of this yellow granular deposit in the pigment epithelium lead to a disruption or atrophy of pigment epithelial cells which may weaken the underlying Bruch's membrane enabling breaks in it. The hypothesis is appealing that the damaged tissue have an intrinsic ability to regenerate. This adaptive healing mechanism once established, the break in Bruch's membrane permits neovascular proliferation from the choriocapilaris into the subretinal pigment epithelial space with the resulting choroidal neovascularisation.

The question of the primary defect in BVMD continues to be thought provoking. As the sensory retina-pigment epithelium complex forms an integrated whole of inseparable functional unity it is very probable that the interruption of the mutual interplay of these tissues may induce either the predominance of retinal pigment epithelial alteration in some cases or the predominance of photoreceptor cell damage in others.

SUMMARY

We evaluated retrospectively the ophthalmological and electrophysiological findings of 47 patients with Best's Vitelliform Macular Dystrophy (BVMD). Our sample re-confirm that BVMD is a progressive disease which may have several appearances from the egg-yolk, scrambled egg and pseudo-hypopion stages to atrophic macular scars and subretinal neovascularization. The heredity of this disorder is autosomal dominant with reduced penetrance and variable expressivity. Some contradictions exist regarding the nature of the primary defect in this entity. Electrooculographic and angiographic investigations lend support to the belief that the basic pathological changes are located in the retinal pigment epithelium. However, recent histopathological findings and flicker electroretinographic results indicate the possibility that the photoreceptor cells are equally involved, even before the pigment epithelium. In view of the

existing disagreements about the pathogenesis of this
disorder, certain considerations are advanced which
suggest that the basic pathologic process in this entity
produces a disorganisation in the structural and functional
interdependance of both the photoreceptor cells and pigment
epithelium.

REFERENCES
1. Best F: Ueber eine hereditare Maculaaffektion:Beitrage
zur Vererbungslehre. Z Augenheilkd 13:199–212,1905.
2. Deutman AF: The Hereditary Dystrophies of the Posterior
Pole of the Eye. Royal van Gorlum, Assen, The Netherlands
1971
3. Mohler CW & Fine SL: Long term evaluation of patients
with Best's vitelliform dystrophy. Ophthalmology
88:688–691,1981.
4. Krill AE: The electroretinographic and electrooculographic
findings in patients with macular lesions. Trans Am Acad
Ophthalmol Otolaryngol 70:1063–1071,1966.
5. Francois J, DeRouk A & Fernandez-Sasso D: Electrooculography in vitelliform macular degeneration. Arch Ophthal
77:726–733,1967.
6. Deutman AF: Electrooculography in families with vitelliform dystrophy of the fovea. Arch Ophthalmol 81:3o5–316,
1969.
7. Curry HF & Moorman LT: Fluorescein photography of vitelliform macular degeneration. Arch Ophthalmol 77:7o5–709,
1968.
8. Morse PH &McLean AL: Fluorescein fundus studies in
hereditary vitelliruptive macular degeneration. Am J
Ophthalmol 66:485–494,1968.
9. Massof RW, Fleischman JA, Fine SL & Yoder F: Flicker
fusion threshold in Best macular dystrophy. Arch Ophthal
95:991–994, 1977.
10. Gass JDM, Jallow S &Dawis B: Adult vitelliform macular
detachment occuring in patients with basal laminar
drusen. Am J Ophthalmol 99:445–459, 1985.
11. Birndorf LA & Dawson WW: A normal EOG in a patient with
a typical vitelliform macular lesion. Invest Ophthalmol
12:830–833, 1973.
12. Gass JDM: A clinicopathologic study of a peculiar
foveo-macular dystrophy. Trans Am Ophthalmol Soc 72: 139–
156, 1974.
13. Fishman GA, Trimble S, Raab MF & Fishman M: Pseudovitelliform macular degeneration. Arch Ophthalmol 95: 73–76,
1977.
14. Kingham JD & Lochen GP: Vitelliform macular degeneration.
Am J Ophthalmol 84:526–531, 1977.
15. Weingeist TA, Kobrin JL,& Watzke RC: Histopathology of
Best's macular dystrophy. Arch Ophthalmol 100:1108–1114,
1982.
16. Frangieh GT, Green R & Fine SL: A histopathologic study
of Best's Macular Dystrophy. Arch Ohthalmol 100:1115–
1121, 1982.

17. Benson WE, Kolker AE, Enoch JM, van Loo JA & Honda Y:
    Best's vitelliform macular dystrophy. Am J Ophthalmol
    79:59-60,1975.
18. Miller SA, Bresnick GH & Chandra SR: Choroidal neovascular membrane in Best's vitelliform macular dystrophy.
    Am J Ophthalmol 82:252-255,1976.
19. Noble KG, Scher BM, Carr RE: Polymorphous presentations
    in vitelliform macular dystrophy. Subretinal neovascu-
    larisation and central choroidal atrophy. Br J Ophthalmol
    62:561-570,1978

PIGMENT EPITHELIOPATHIES-CLINICAL AND HAEMATOLOGICAL CHANGES

P.Souza-Ramalho,PA.Jorge,Carlota Saldanha and J Martins-Silva

Departments of Ophthalmology and Biochemistry,University of Lisbon, Hospital de Santa Maria, Lisbon, Portugal

There are a variety of clinical conditions which are characterized by discret grey,white or yellow-white lesions or focal infiltrates at the level of outer retina,often situated at the posterior pole,in macular or peripapillary areas. These patchy lesions can resolve or progress to the periphery leaving areas of chorioretinal atrophy with depigmentation. Such patients can show signs of intraocular inflammation and evidence of choriocapillary involvement.

Abnormal choroidal haemodynamics with delayed perfusion of the dye in the choriocapillaris have been reported in acute posterior multifocal placoid epitheliopathy (APMPE) and other similar conditions (1,2,3).

In our preliminary studies presented at OSUK meeting in Harrogate (1984) and later at Baden-Baden (1985) we reported,besides circulatory changes in choriocapillaris,some haemorheological abnormalities in geographic,serpiginous,helicoidal chorioretinopathy and in acute posterior multifocal placoid epitheliopathy.

In a group of five patients known to have pigment epitheliopathy (APMPE and geographic chorioretinopathy) we further investigated haemorheological parameters and chorioretinal circulatory changes using fluorescein angiography.

Material and Methods

In two male patients,32 and 37 years old,with geographic chorioretinopathy and in two females,45 and 31 years old,and in one young boy of 20 years of age with APMPE,repeated and periodic,serial clinical,laboratory routine tests and ophthalmological investigations were carried out during 8 to 37 months period. Chorioretinal circulation was studied with fluorescein angiography using standart technique. Blood rheology parameters were investigated:red cell filterability index using modified method of Reid at all (4),plasma viscosity determined with Leonard's method (5). These parameters and other tests such as haematocrit,red cell aggregation (6),acetylcholinesterase (7) and buterylcholinesterase(8) were also accessed after diagnosis and repeated periodically during follow up period. Results were analysed and compared to normal healthy controls. Routine periodic ophthalmological examination with visual acuity,still lamp microscopy,fundus photography,fluorescein angiography,ERG,EOG and PEV was carried out initially and later during the progress of the pathological process. Colour photographs and fluorescein negatives were carefully examined

by projection in order to evoluate the extend of changes of
lesions and their progression. These clinical and circulatory
changes were compared and tried to correlate with laboratory
findings.

Results

JMB 37 years old male with geographic chorioretinopathy presented with floaters and metamorphopsia in both eyes and reduction of vision in the right eye (RE = 3/10;LE = 9/10). His
vitreous showed moving opacities and his fundii had typical
yellow-white patches in the posterior pole (fig.1-RE) not involving the macular area in left eye. Later these lesions extended to the equator alternating with pigmented spots. On
fluorescein angiography small lobular areas of non perfusion
(arrows) others of delayed filling,with hyperfluorescent edges
and staining were seen (figs 2 and 3). There were also other
larger areas of non perfusion,probably of early atrophy.

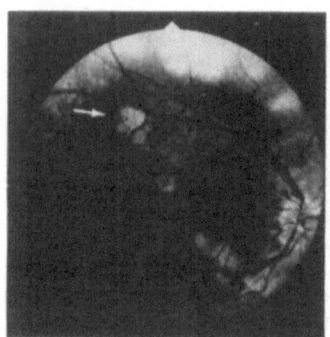 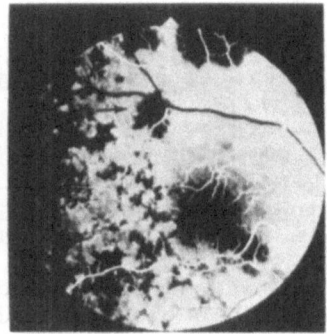 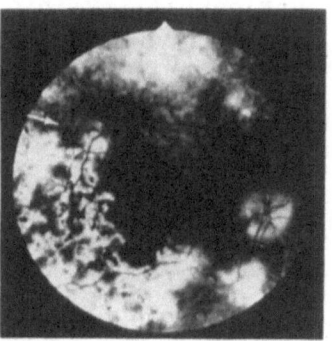

Fig.1   Fig.2   Fig.3

All the clinical and laboratory investigations were negative except white cell count of 16.800,haematocrit (52%),red
cell filterability reduced (24.4) and plasma viscosity high
(1.35cP). He developed phlebitis of superior temporal vein the
papillitis in the right eye. EOG and ERG were abnormal since
the beginning and they remained so during the period of follow
up (37 months) in spite of improvement,of both his vision
(10/10) and haemorheological parameters(table 1).

At present his retinal lesions are not active although
there are large areas of chorioretinal atrophy in both eyes.

The second case of geographic chorioretinopathy (32 years
old man) presented with sudden lowering of vision in his left
eye. The right eye was atrophic since childhood.
On fluorescein angiography at the time of lowering the vision
there was abcence of choriocapillary filling around the disc
area even in the later stages of dye transit(Fig.4).
Later he developed yellow-white atrophic lesions alternating
with pigmented spots. His vision was finger counting and all
laboratory and clinical investigations (blood,urine,neurologi-
cal,dermatological)were negative. EOG was abnormal (Arden In-

dex 120%) and ERG showed depression of a and b waves.

Table I

Haemorheology (JMB)

Red cell filterability (initial values)	Plasma Viscosity (initial values)	Vision	
		RE	LE
17.2	1.35		
24.4	1.28	3/10	9/10
23.1	1.29		
(later values)	(later values)		
14.0	1.30	9/10	10/10
14.8	1.25	10/10	10/10
Normal 13.94 ± 2.24	1.25 - 1.27		

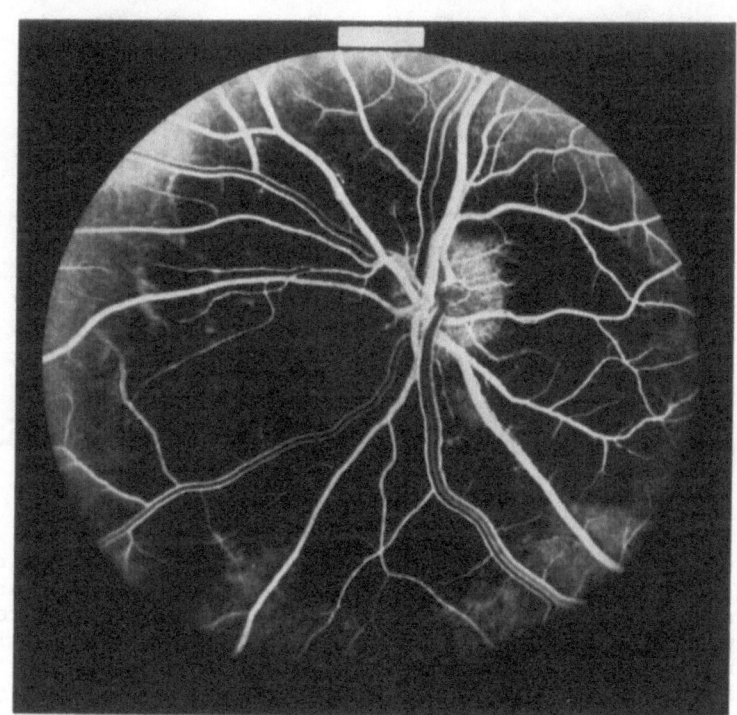

Fig.4

Red cell filterability was abnormal (21.9) so was the plasma viscosity (1.36cP). As he presented new and fresh active lesions he was administered steroids (prednisolone 100 mg/day) and later a combination of therapy to reduce blood viscosity. Fundus lesions ceased activity after 2 months of intensive therapy as blood viscosity parameters gradually normalized:

Red Cell Filterability Index (normal 13.94 $\pm$ 2.24)	Plasma Viscosity (normal 1.25 - 1.27cP)
21.9	1.36
17.5	1.21
14.8	1.21
14.8	1.22
12.8	

Visual acuity stabilized with litlle improvement because macular area was damage (LE = 1/10 with full peripheral field)
and the fudus presented many areas of chorioretinal atrophy
(fig.5 and 6).Active lesions were not seen during last twelve
months in spite of not having steroids or any other treatment.

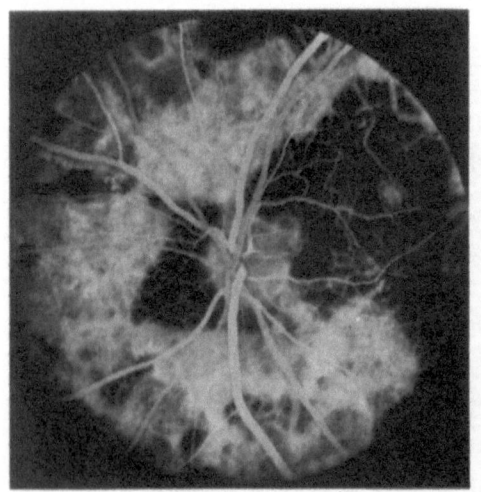
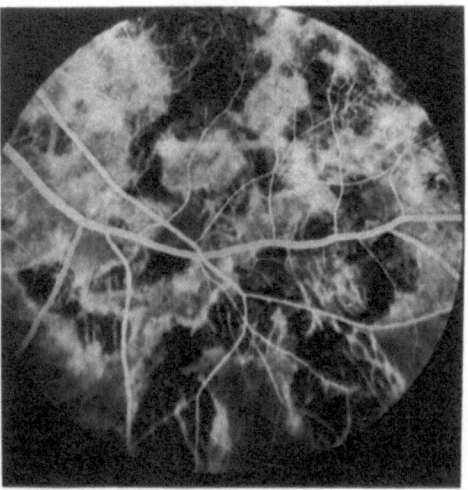

Fig.5   Fig.6

Three cases of acute posterior multifocal placoid epithe-
liopathies have been investigated recently. In all cases clinical features and fundus changes were typical with yellow/
white spots in the posterior pole showing delayed filling
areas and later hyperfluorescence and low vision. All routine
clinical and laboratory investigations were negative in all
three cases and haemohreological parameters normal in 2 cases.
   LBDR,45 years old female presented with haedaches and mental depression followed by sudden reduction of vision RE=4/10
and LE = FC. General and neurological examination was normal
including EEG. Blood and urine test were negative (ESR = 12mm.
Typical yellow-white patches in the posterior pole in both
eyes were present. Early choriocapillary filling defects and
late hyperfluorescence and staining of these lesions were
seen. Blood viscosity parameters:
   Red cell filterability index was very high(125.5-normal =
13.9 $\pm$ 2.22),haemoglobin 16.2, WBC = 9.800.

On high doses of steroids within a week,red cell deformability index normalized (14.00) and acetylcholinesterase increased (from 254 to 537). A focus of chorioretinitis was seen
in the left superior temporal area.
Her vision improved dramatically:

RE = 4/10 week later   RE = 6/10 2 weeks later   RE = 10/10
LE = FC   LE = 5/10   LE = 10/10

Considerable improvement of fundus and angiography features
were noticed 4 weeks after the initial obsrvation (almost
normal). Haemorheological parameters were normal.

AHM,20 years old male presented with sudden and severe reduction of vision in the left eye (FC) with typical yellow-
white patches in the posterior pole without any other signs
of ocular inflammation or general clinical or laboratory abnormalities. Haemorheological parameters studied only after
recovery of vision 2 months after first signs,were normal.
Fluorescein angiography showed hyperfluorescent spots 3 months later.

ZB,31 years old female patient presented with sudden reduction of vision in both eyes (more in left eye) coinciding
with tonsilitis and dermatological complaints. General and laboratory tests were normal. On fundus photography and fluorescein angiography showed typical yellow-white spots in posteri-
or pole of placoid epitheliopathy with choriocapillary filling
defects. Without any treatment her vision improved to almost
normal within 8 weeks. Haemorheological parameters studied in
the recovery stage (AchE,BuchE,red cell filterability index,
plasma viscosity,red cell aggregation index,haematocrit),were
within normal limits.

Discussion and Comments

In two cases of geographic serpiginous chorioretinopathy choriocapillary filling defects were recorded when subjective
reduction of vision was noticed and when deep retinal lesions
or focal infiltrates were seen in the posterior pole and around the disc. In the early stages some areas of delayed filling
and others of non perfusion were seen in the choriocapillaris.
Later these patches were hyperfluorescent and some presented
stainning. After weeks of evolution some of these areas were
normally perfusing and others were atrophic with hyperfluorescent edges. Most of these patches still presented hyperfluorescence after 2/4 months of evolution.   Almost all clinical
and laboratory investigations which were carried out on these
two cases were normal except haemorheological parameters.Hae-
matocrit,white cell count,red cell deformability,plasma viscosity were abnormal and they gradually improved as the vision
and the fundus changes normalized with steroid treatment in
the second case.

In three cases of acute posterior multifocal placoid epitheliopathy studied also typical fundus changes with lobular
choriocapillary filling defects and later hyperfluorescence
and staining of retina were seen. In these 3 cases all clinical and laboratory tests were negative including haemorheological parameters in two out of 3 cases.

In all five cases of pigment epitheliopathy investigated

312

flow changes in the choriocapillaris were confirmed - absence
and delayed lobular filling and later hyperfluorescence,stai-
ning and chorioretinal atrophy. These flow changes were related to the typical grey,white-yellow spots which could be recovered or transformed in to atrophic areas in spite of steroid therapy. In two cases total recovery was obtained without
any therapy
   Although all the clinical and laboratory tests investigated
were negative (in 2 cases WBC 16.800 and 9.800) some parameters of blood rheology more abnormal suggesting high blood
viscosity in the beguinning of the process.Later,after 8 to
12 weeks,these abnormal haemorheological parameters improved
or normalized even without any therapy. Normal haemorheological parameters recorded in two cases of placoid,were investigated only 8 and 10 weeks after beguinning of pathological
process.
   We think that haemorheological abnormalities recorded,for
the first time to our knowledge,in this type of disorders,
could be accidental or secondary to inflammatory or immunologic process. They could certaily interfere with normal flow
in the affected areas, specially at the capillary level and
in already damaged blood vessels and at low shear rates,thus
inducing ischaemic changes.
Further work is needed to support our hypothesis and to clarify the pathophysiology of these disorders.

References

1 - Gass,JDM: Acute multifocal posterior placoid pigment epi-
    theliopathy.Arch.Ophthalmol.80,173 1968
2 - Hamilton,AM and Bird,AC:Geographical choroidopaty.
    Br.J.Ophthalmol.-58.784,1974
3 - Deutman,FD and Lion,F:Choriocapillaris non perfusion in
    acute multifocal placoid pigment epitheliopathy.Amer. J.
    Ophthalmol. 84,652, 1977.
4 - Reid,HL.Barnes,A.,Lock,PJ and Dormandy,JA: Simple method
    of measuring erythrocyte deformability.J.Clin.Pathol.
    29,855, 1976.
5 - Leonard,RCF:Simple technique for measuring serum or plas-
    ma viscosity with disposable apparatus.Brit.Med.J. 283,
    1154. 1981.
6 - Kiesewetter.H.,Radtker,M.,Schneider,R.,Mussker,K.Scheffler
    A. and Schimid-Schonbein,H: Erythrocyten aggregometer:Ein
    neues Gerät zur schnellen quantifizierung des ausmaBas der
    erythrozytenaggregation, Biomed.Technik. 27.219, 1982.
7 - Kaplan,E.,Tildon,JT: Changes in red cell enzyme activity
    in relation to red cell survivae in infancy.Pediatrics,32,
    371,1963.
8 - Kutty,KM.,Redheendran,R. and Murphy,D: Serum cholynestera-
    se: function in lipoprtein metabolism. Experientia,4,420,
    1977.

SUB-RETINAL NEO-VASCULARISATIONS OF UNCOMMON ORIGIN

A. GIOVANNINI, G.P. AMATO., A. PAZZAGLIA, P. CHILLEMI and S. VOLANTI
Eye Department - University of Bologna (Italy)

Since its first angiographic description by Gass in 1967, (1), Sub-Reti_
nal Neo-Vascularisations (S.R.N.V.) have been described more and more fre_
quently as complications of several ocular diseases (2).
   Since then, more and more associations of S.R.N.V. and ocular diseases
have been reported (Congenital, Hereditary, Inflammatory, Degenerative,
Tumoral, Traumatic, Systemic and Idiopathic), and in the present paper we
report new and uncommon ones.
- Our first case is represented by a S.R.N.V. associated to Gyrate Atrophy
of choroid and retina -(Fig. n. 1)-.
   A 73 years old female complained night blindness since childhood and
reduced Visual Acuity (V.A.) in the Right Eye for the last twenty days. Her
best corrected V.A. was 20/20 in R.E. and 20/200 in L.E. The anterior seg_
ment was unremarkable except for a nuclear sclerosis of both lenses; the
fundus of both eyes presented round, sharply defined, atrophic areas some

-(Fig. n. 1)-

S.R.N.V. appeared in
course of Gyrate Atrophy
of choroid and retina.

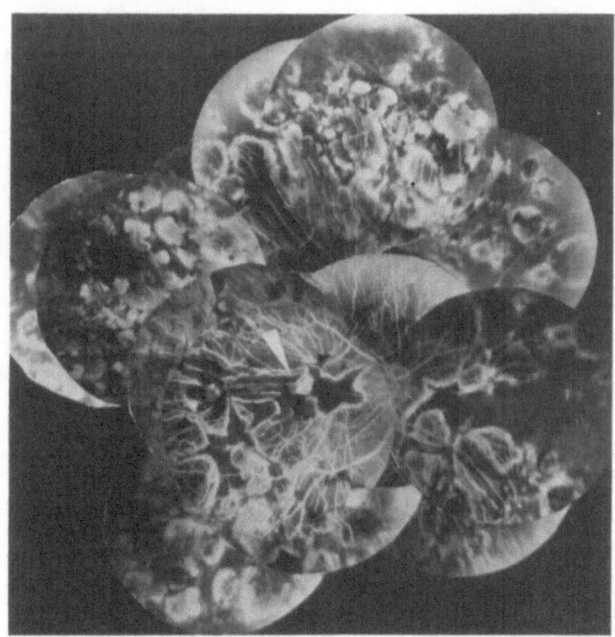

314

of them showing tendency towards confluence. In R.E. an islet of normal
retina was present in the macular region, and its temporal border showed a
deep haemorrhage. Fluorescein angiography was performed; besides the atro_
phy of R.P.E., choriocapillaris and large choroidal vessels in the atrophic
areas, it showed the presence of a serous haemorrhagic detachment of R.P.E.
with a S.R.N.V. at the temporal border of the islet of normal retina, just
underneath the fovea, while in the fellow eye no S.R.N.V. was detected.

In our knowledge, this association has never been reported in Literature.
- The second case is a S.R.N.V. observed in the follow-up of a sub-intra-
retinal haemorrhage caused by a Retinal Macroaneurysm -(Fig. n. 2 a-b)-.

A 66 years old female, with a reduced V.A. in the R.E. (3/50) presented
the Fundus a great haemorrhage in macular region, that seemed to be origina_
ted from a branch of inferior temporal arteria; because of its possible
origin from a Retinal Macroaneurysm, the patient underwent to many Fluore_
scein Angiography-controls, and at about 60 days after, a S.R.N.V. presen_
ted itself with a typical hyper-fluorescence with a late diffusion and the
R.M. in the early phases with a "mouse-tail" - like aspect.

The disruption of the R.P.E.- Bruch membrane complex due to haemorrhage
might induce a S.R.N.V.. We know that S.R.N.V. caused by sub-retinal
haemorrhages have been observed in course of Sickle Cell-Anemia, but never
in macular area.

In our knowledge, this one seem to be the first case of S.R.N.V. due to a
Retinal Macroaneurysm.
- The third case of our material of study is represented by a S.R.N.V. that
appeared in course of a Diffuse Retinal Pigment Epitheliopathy (D.R.P.E.),
-(Fig. n. 3 a-b-c)-. Fluorescein angiography showed a typical hyper-fluore_

-(Fig. n. 2)- a ; b - A S.R.N.V. complicates (after 10 months) a R.M.-indu_
ced pre- intra and sub-retinal haemorrhage.

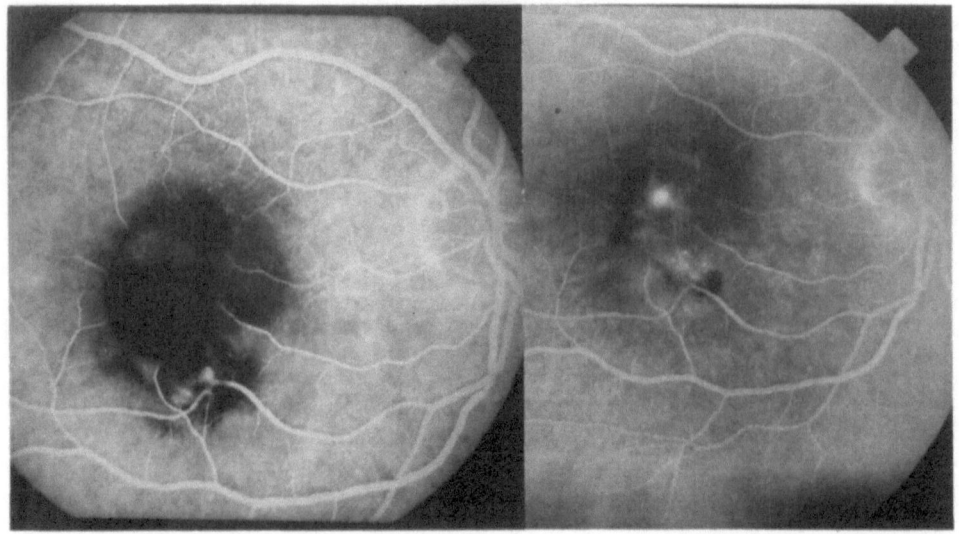

scence with late diffusion in the R.E.; V.A. was 20/30 with metamorphopsia.

This S.R.N.V. has been treated with Dye Laser (Orange wavelength: 610nm), and V.A. is actually 20/20 .

The S.R.N.V. origin must be related to the chronic decompensation of the R.P.E.- Bruch membrane complex in course of Diffuse Retinal Pigment Epithe_ liopathy.

- Our fourth report concerns a S.R.N.V. observed in course of a Giant Coloboma of the optic disk -(Fig. n. 4)-.

A 31 years old female came to us complaining blurried vision in the L.E. Her best corrected V.A. was 20/20 in R.E. and 20/40 in L.E. Biomicroscopy of the anterior segment was unremarkable. The R.E.- Fundus was normal, while in the L.E. both a Giant Coloboma of the optic disk and inferiorly a Coloboma involving the retina and choroid was present. On the temporal

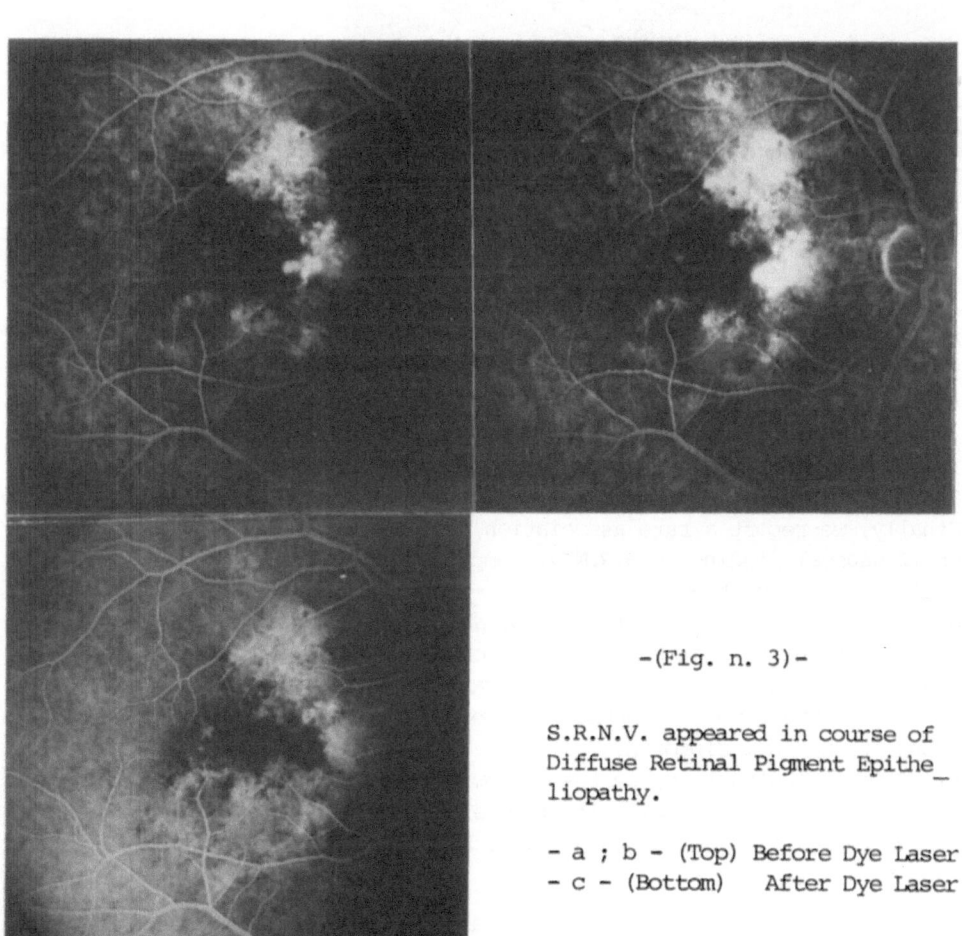

-(Fig. n. 3)-

S.R.N.V. appeared in course of Diffuse Retinal Pigment Epithe_ liopathy.

- a ; b - (Top) Before Dye Laser
- c - (Bottom)   After Dye Laser

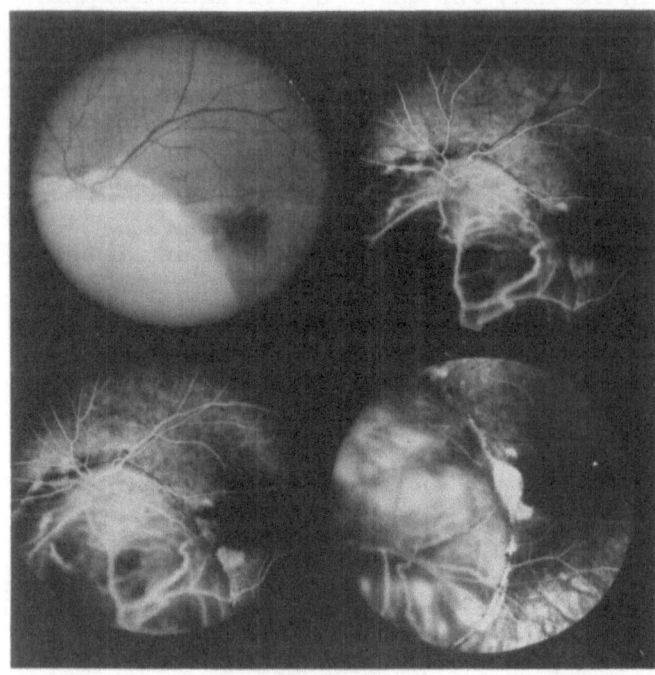

-(Fig. n. 4)-

S.R.N.V. in course of
Giant Coloboma of.the
Optic disk.

border of the optic disk coloboma a deep haemorrhage was present.

A Fluorescein Angiography was performed, and showed the presence of a
Serous Haemorrhagic Detachment of Retinal Pigment Epithelium (S.H.D.R.P.E.)
due to a Sub-Retinal Neo-Vascularisation located just at the temporal rim
of the optic disk coloboma.

·This association has been previously reported in a "Letter to the Journal"
(1984),(3).

- Finally, we report a rare association, previously reported in Literature,
even if unusual finding: a S.R.N.V. complicating a case of Toxocara canis
granuloma -(Fig. n. 5)-.

A 5 years old childgirl, affected by a macular Toxocariasis in both eyes:
more in particular, in the Right Eye a choroidal Toxocara Granuloma, while
in the Left Eye a typical retinal Toxocara Granuloma were present.

The latter one showed a marked involvement of the inner retina and an
evident pre-retinal fibrosis.

Fluorescein Angiography, in the follow-up (two years after), showed in
the Left Eye a S.R.N.V., with its typical hyperfluorescence, located at the
superior-temporal border of the retinal Toxocara canis granuloma .
-(Fig. n. 5)-

In conclusion, more and more numerous are the reports in Literature of new
associations between Sub-Retinal Neo-Vascularisations and ocular diseases,
and we think that the list is bound to grow longer.

-(Fig. n. 5)-

S.R.N.V. complicating a
retinal Toxocara canis
granuloma.

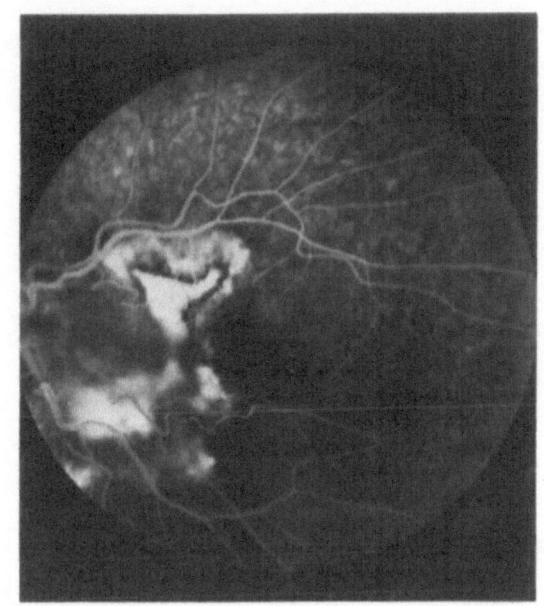

REFERENCES

1. Gass J.M.: Pathogenesis of disciform detachment of the neuroepithelium.
   Am. J. Ophthalmol. 63: 563-571 (1967).
2. Shatz H., Laser treatment of fundus diseases. S. Anselmo Pacific Medical
   Press (1981).
3. Jay W.M. and Coll.: Juxtapapillary sub-retinal neovascularisation asso_
   ciated with congenital pit of the optic nerve. in Letters to the Journal
   Am. J. Ophthalmol. 97: 655-657 (1984).

VASCULITIS AND MORPHOLOGY OF MICROVILLI OF THE CONJUNCTIVA IN SJOGREN SYNDROME

Ewy Meyer+, Judith Scharf+, Rina Schechner+, Shlomo Zonis+, Yehuda Scharf*, Menachem Nahir*
Department of Ophthalmology+ and B. Shine Department of Rheumatology, Rambam Medical Center, Faculty of Medicine, Technion-Israel Institute of Technology, Haifa, Israel.

The conjunctiva plays an important role in external ocular physiology by contributing to maintenance of the tear film. Light and electron microscopical studies of the conjunctiva in Sjogren syndrome have been studied and changes such as stratification of the epithelium, elongation of the epithelial cells, widening of the intercellular spaces and reduction of the number of microvilli and number of goblet cells have been described(1,2).

Material and Methods

Conjunctival biopsies of 14 patients with Sjogren syndrome as well as from 8 patients without apparent conjunctival disease of the same age group, were examined under light and transmission electron microscopy. Of the 14 patients with Sjogren syndrome, 11 presented with secondary Sjogren syndrome due to the presence of a well documented inflammatory connective tissue disease and 3 had primary Sjogren syndrome.

The biopsies were removed from the lower bulbar conjunctiva with topical anesthetic drops at the same site which was 6 mm. from the limbus.

Results

The common feature on light microscopy was superficial flattening and irregularity in thickness of the epithelium of the conjunctiva. In 4 cases chronic inflammatory cells were found surrounding blood vessels in the conjunctival stroma (Fig. 1). These findings were consistent with

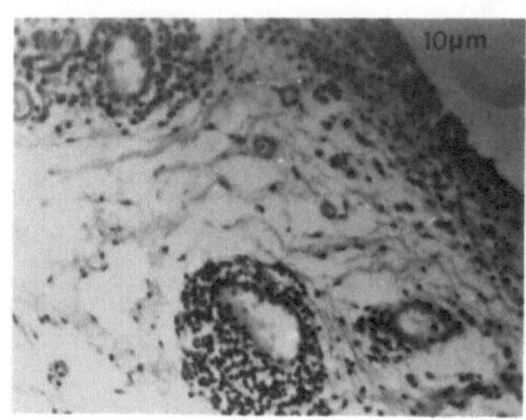

Fig. 1. Chronic inflammatory cells surrounding a conjunctival blood vessel.

vasculitis. Two of those had clinically inactive rheumatoid arthiritis and two had Sjogren syndrome without inflammatory connective tissue disease. Under electron microscopy we found marked changes in the microvilli namely loss of microvilli, decrease in height, the microvilli being only 1000-2000 A high, almost no branching of microvilli and no presence of secretory vesicles (Fig. 2). The control conjunctiva revealed high microvilli

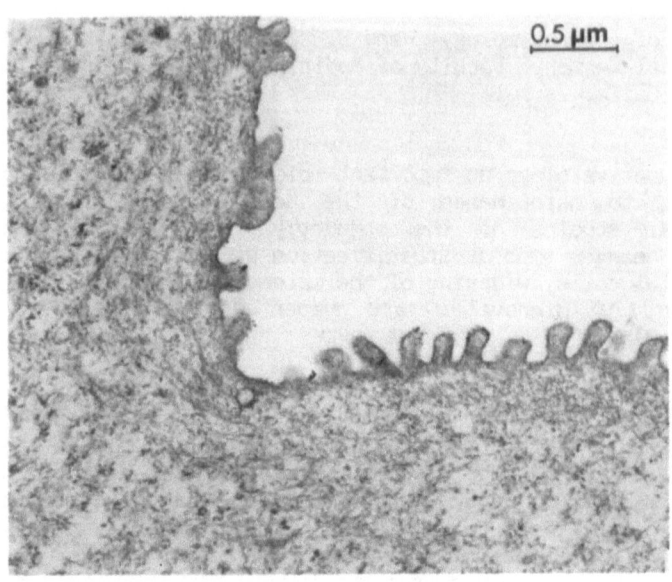

Fig. 2. Transmission electron micrograph showing attenuation in height, loss of branching and fusion of microvilli of the superficial cell.

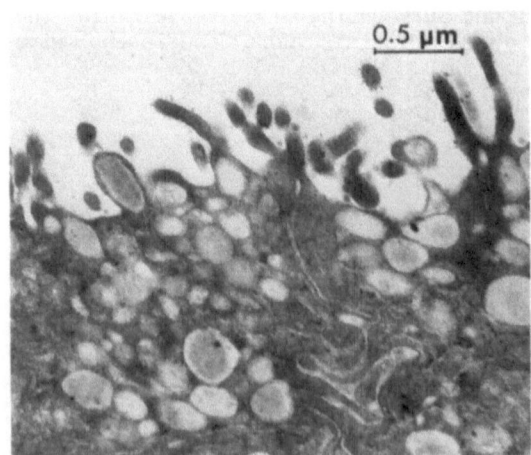

Fig. 3. Transmission electron micrograph of control conjunctiva showing high microvilli and many secretory vesicles.

measuring 4000 A in height with many secretory vesicles (Fig. 3). Two
cases with rheumatoid arthritis were of special interest because of
aggravation of the rheumatoid arthritis the patients were treated with
immunosuppressive drugs. Conjunctival biopsies were taken before and
following this treatment. Before the treatment the microvilli were
decreased in height and there was loss of microvilli (Fig. 4). Following

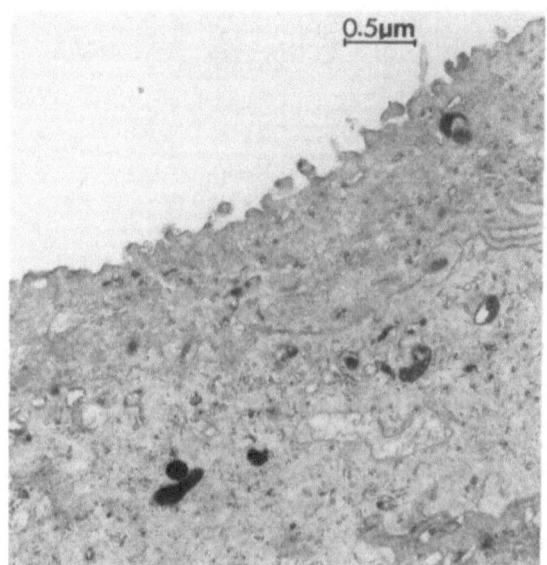

Fig. 4. Transmission electron micrograph showing loss and decrease in height of microvilli.

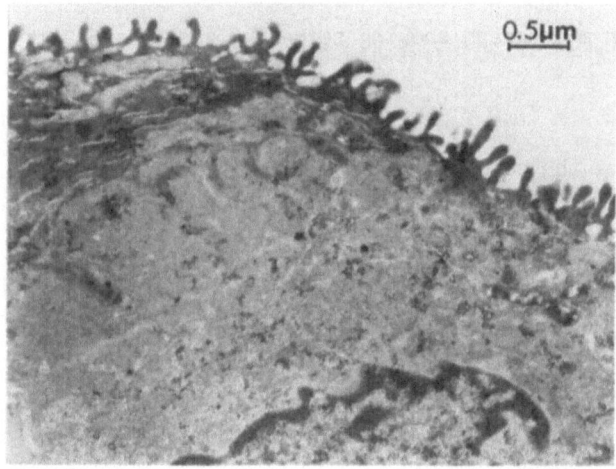

Fig. 5. Transmission electron micrograph showing increase in height and number of microvilli.

the treatment there was an increase in height, number and branching of microvilli and secretory vesicles appeared beneath the microvilli (Fig.5,6). Another very common feature in all cases was widening of the intercellular spaces between the superficial and the subjacent cells (Fig. 7).

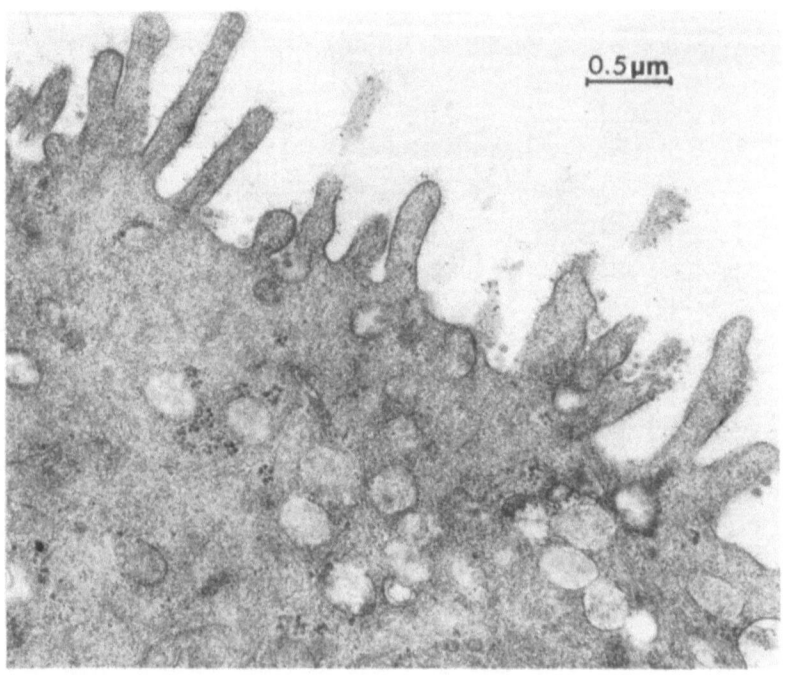

Fig. 6. Transmission electron micrograph showing secretory vesicles beneath the microvilli.

There was a separation of the superficial layer with stunting of the cell processes in the intercellular space (Fig. 8). The goblet cells seemed normal and filled with secretory granules (Fig. 9).

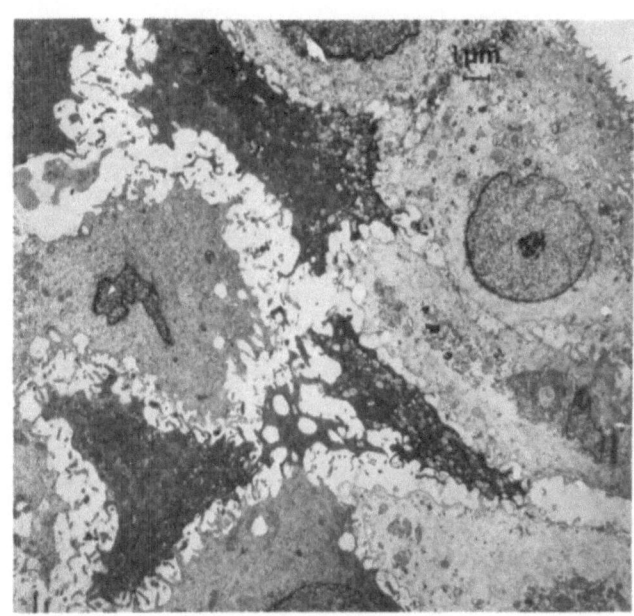

Fig. 7. Transmission electron micrograph showing widening of the intercellular spaces between the cells in the deeper layers.

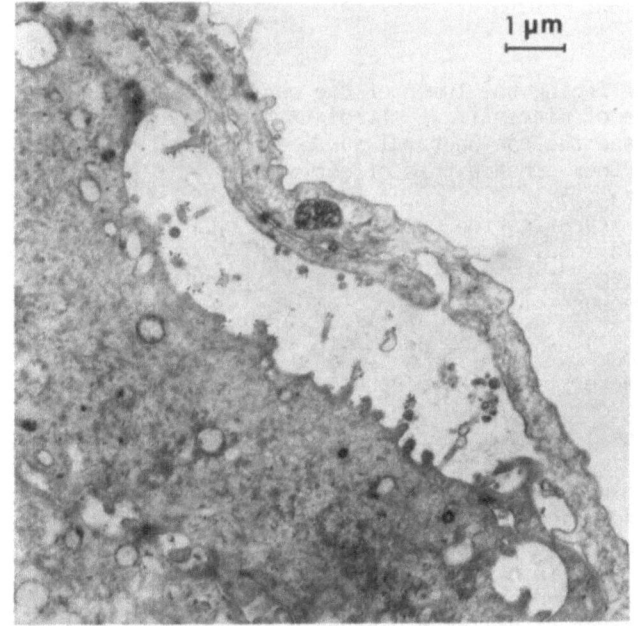

Fig. 8. Transmission electron micrograph showing severe loss of microvilli and separation of the superficial cell layer and stunting of the cell processes in the intercellular space.

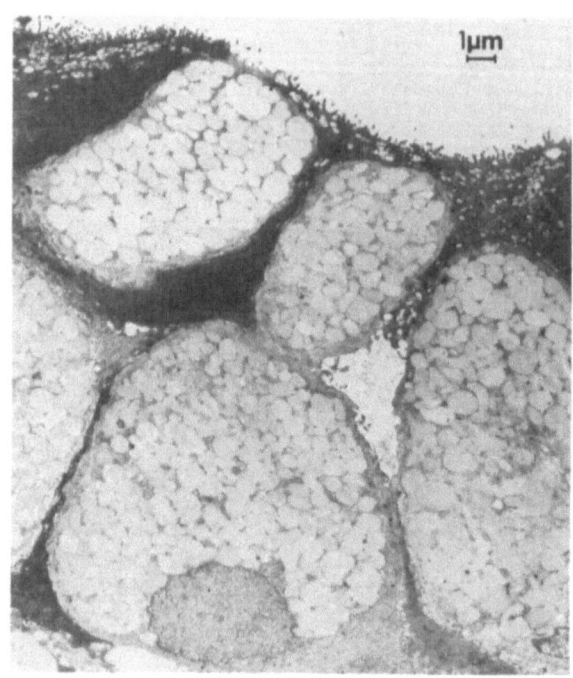

Fig. 9. Transmission electron micrograph showing a group of goblet cells filled with secretory granules.

Discussion

The conjunctival surface facing the lumen of the conjunctival sac is characterized by the presence of microvilli. Straight tubular microvilli have been estimated to increase the conjunctival surface area several folds and branched microvilli further enhance this effect and thereby increase the cells' absorbtive capacity (3).

A constant feature in our investigation were the severe changes found in the microvilli namely dramatic loss, decrease in height, no branching and fusion in comparison with aged matched conjunctiva from patients with normal tear secretion. Because of these morphological changes in the microvilli the stability of the tear film cannot be maintained even if aqueous tear production is normal. Another constant finding were the wide intercellular spaces. The severity of the morphological changes found in the microvilli, the widening of the intercellular spaces and separation of sheets of the superficial cells in our patients were proportional to the severity of the clinical findings in the sicca syndrome.

Another interesting finding in our cases was the vasculitis of the conjunctiva not previously described to our knowledge in cases of Sjogren syndrome. In the two cases of rheumatoid arthritis it appeared in an inactive stage of the disease without systemic manifestations and with negative tests for rheumatoid factor. The finding of vasculitis in Sjogren syndrome without clinical signs of collagen disease does not exclude an autoimmune mechanism as well. Recently two cases of retinal vasculitis caused by systemic lupus erythematosus and Sjogren syndrome were described by Farmer (4).

There seemed to be no difference in the morphological changes of the conjunctiva between patients with primary Sjogren syndrome and secondary Sjogren syndrome. The morphological changes in the microvilli following the treatment with immunosuppressive drugs has to the best of our knowledge not been described before. The association of these structural changes with clinical improvement suggests the relationship between the tear film stability and conjunctival structure. Most probably the irregular surface of microvilli with an absorbed layer of mucin contributes to a prolonged effect of artificial tears.

The finding of other authors of secretory vesicles in normal human conjunctiva suggests that the conjunctival epithelium secretes mucus from two sources: one the goblet cells and the second the secretory vesicles which are non goblet epithelial mucus producing cells (5,6). We have found secretory vesicles in the normal conjunctiva and in the two cases after immunosuppressive treatment. They were also found in an increased number by Greiner and Allansmith in soft and hard contact lens wearers (5).

The morphological findings in the two cases after immunosuppressive treatment must by necessity be considered a preliminary study and should be followed by more extensive investigation.

REFERENCES

1. Abdel-Khalak, L.M.R.: Morphological changes in the human conjunctival epithelium. II. In Keratoconjunctivitis sicca. Br. J. Ophthal. 62:800, 1978.
2. Torok, N., Suveges, I.: Morphological changes in dry eye syndrome. Grafes Arch. Klin. Exp. Opthal. 219:24, 1982.
3. Greiner, J.V., Gladstone, L., Corington, H.J., Korb, D.K., Weidman, T.A., Allansmith, M.R.: Branching of microvilli in the human conjunctival epithelium. Arch. Ophthalmol. 98:1253, 1980.
4. Farmer, S.G., Kinyoun, J.L., Nelson, J.L., Wener, M.H.: Retinal vasculitis with autoantibodies to Sjogren's Syndrome. An Antigen. Am. J. Ophthalmol. 100:814, 1985.
5. Greiner, J.V., Allansmith, M.R.: Effect of contact lens wear on the conjunctival mucous system. Ophthalmology 88:821, 1981.
6. Greiner, J.V., Weidman, T.A., Korb, D.R., Allansmith, M.R.: Histochemical analysis of secretory vesicles in non goblet conjunctival epithelial cells. Acta Ophthalmol. 63:98, 1985.

CORNEAL NEOVASCULARIZATION: AN OVERVIEW

GORDON K. KLINTWORTH

Three months after the first elections in the new state of Israel in which Dr. Chaim Weizmann was elected first President of Israel with David Ben-Gurion as Prime Minister a classic paper appeared in the ophthalmic literature. In this paper, Campbell and Michaelson (2) drew attention to the clinical and experimental observation that a localized corneal lesion usually elicited a vascular ingrowth from the corneoscleral limbus nearest to the lesion and that the neovascularization typically filled an isoceles triangle. They also pointed out that the distance between the lesion and the limbus influenced the angiogenic response. Based on these observations Campbell and Michaelson proposed that blood vessels invade the normally avascular cornea in response to locally generated diffusible vasostimulatory factor(s). Michaelson appreciated the importance of testing this hypothesis and stimulated others to collaborate with him in thoughtful experiments. The results of these additional studies (8-10) remained consistent with this "vasostimulatory theory" and recent studies are still compatible with it.

This report provides an overview of our current knowledge about the cause and pathogenesis of corneal neovascularization. Because of space restrictions most statements are not referenced. Sources from the older literature are cited in several reviews (4,5,7). More recent studies are cited in a comprehensive critical review on corneal neovascularization (6).

1. CAUSES OF CORNEAL NEOVASCULARIZATION

In numerous diverse natural and experimental situations, blood vessels extend into the normally avascular cornea from the pericorneal vascular plexus (4). In all situations in which corneal vascularization has been thoroughly studied it has occurred in association with inflammation. Immunological reactions are particularly potent stimulators of corneal neovascularization as in graft rejection and after the intracorneal instillation of an antigen into presensitized animals.

2. PATHOGENESIS OF CORNEAL VASCULARIZATION

2.1. Inflammation

Numerous studies emphasize the association of corneal vascularization with the inflammatory response. Within the complex cellular and humoral events of inflammation exist many potential sources for the initiation and potentiation of neovascularization.

During the past decade many of the participants in the drama of corneal neovascularization have been identified, but innocent bystanders have not been distinguished from active participants with certainty. Indeed progress is only now beginning in the assessment of the relative roles of putative factors. From the many studies on corneal vascularization it has become apparent that its pathogenesis involves a complex cascade of events. While the fundamental events that lead to corneal vascularization remain unknown, it seems likely that different stimuli initiate corneal neovascularization by several pathways.

2.1.1. Cellular Components. A considerable amount of data supports the hypothesis that leukocytes, which liberate a wide variety of biologically active substances, produce one or more factors which either stimulate directional vascular growth directly or by way of intermediaries. The relative importance of these different types of leukocytes in corneal neovascularization undoubtedly varies with the vascularizing corneal conditions, but how they facilitate corneal angiogenesis remains uncertain.

Capillaries invade the cornea after leukocytes in a wide variety of situations, including corneal injuries produced by chemicals (silver nitrate, sodium hydroxide, colchicine, or alloxan), antigens (intracorneal antigens in sensitized animals), and metabolic disorders (hypertyrosinemia, as well as riboflavin and vitamin A deficiency). Moreover, in these models new vessels grow into the cornea only in areas in which leukocytes are present.

Several studies in a variety of experimental models have demonstrated a reduction in the degree of induced corneal neovascularization in leukopenic animals. The extent of the vascular ingrowth is also decreased in experimental situations in which the number of leukocytes in the corneal stroma is diminished. The intensity of new vessel formation is directly related to the degree of leukocytic infiltration and is enhanced by conditions that promote leukocytes to infiltrate the corneal tissue. Leukocytes do not appear to be essential for the initiation of corneal neovascularization, at least in some experimental models, but they seem to facilitate or augment the process by incompletely understood mechanisms.

Polymorphonuclear Leukocytes (PMNs). PMNs, common companions of newly formed blood vessels in many tissues, including the cornea have been suspected of playing a role in angiogenesis. While PMNs do not seem to be essential for the initiation of corneal vascularization they may play a facilitatory role. Not only do PMNs accompany the growth of blood vessels into the cornea in most experimental models that have been studied extensively to date, but they emigrate from the pericorneal blood vessels and enter the cornea prior to corneal neovascularization. It is also noteworthy that corticosteroids, as well as non-steroidal inflammatory drugs (fluriprofen and indomethacin) that suppress corneal vascularization also inhibit PMN migration following corneal injury. Factors that lead to the corneal infiltration of PMNs varies with the experimental situation and local prostaglandin synthesis may be important following at least certain injuries.

PMNs (as well as other leukocytes and other cells) are a source of cyclooxygenase and lipoxygenase products of arachidonic acid. Extracts of PMNs are also reported to be weakly mitotic for umbilical vein endothelial cells. However, some investigators have been unable to induce neovascularization in the cornea by injecting PMNs into the cornea of rabbits and guinea pigs.

Lymphocytes. A vast body of evidence supports the hypothesis that activated lymphocytes can induce angiogenesis (1). Corneal vascularization has been induced by the intrastromal injection of mitogen stimulated lymphocytes into rabbits and mice. Strain-related differences in reactivity and host recognition of histocompatibility differences have been shown to both be important in this response. How lymphocytes induce angiogenesis remains to be determined, but following their stimulation by mitogens lymphocytes undergo blastogenesis and secrete a variety of mediators including prostaglandins and lymphokines which have been implicated in angiogenesis.

Macrophages. Several studies implicate monocytes (macrophages) in angiogenesis. Lactate, but not pyruvate, have been found to cause macrophages to secrete angiogenic factors that cause corneal vascularization in the rabbit cornea. Antigenically stimulated macrophages produce increased amounts of mitogens, while hypoxic macrophages do not.

Platelets. During the early hours of the inflammatory response, as after chemical injuries to the cornea, platelets are prominent in the dilated stagnant blood vessels. These cellular elements release substances that stimulate deoxyribonucleic acid (DNA) synthesis and cell migration in vascular endothelium. Platelets are rich in ADP and 5-hydroxytryptamine both of which induce endothelial cell growth in vitro and in vivo.

Mast Cell. For a long time the mast cell has been suspected of having more than a passive role in angiogenesis and this cell type has been identified in association with new vessel formation in the cornea and other tissues. Recent studies have implicated two products of these cells in angiogenesis: heparin and histamine. Heparin promotes endothelial cell migration and that this activity can be blocked by protamine sulfate. Heparin has also been found to bind several growth factors that have angiogenic activity. Heparin is stated to not promote endothelial cell proliferation in some systems, but it has been found to enhance the growth of some strains of vascular endothelial cells.

Histamine, a potent component of the inflammatory response, and the suspected angiogenic factor of Campbell & Michaelson (2) may contribute to angiogenesis. Some investigators have not been able to produce vascular labeling of the pericorneal vasculature with H^3-thymidine either with or without a corneal lesion with this constituent of mast cell granules. Other investigators have found histamine to be mitogenic to human microvascular endothelial cells in culture, and with the use of specific agonists and antagonists this effect has been shown to be mediated through an H_1 receptor. Histamine may also conceivably enhance angiogenesis through the resultant increased vascular permeability that it causes in the inflammatory response.

2.1.2. <u>Humoral Aspects of Inflammation</u>. During the inflammatory response the cornea not only becomes infiltrated by leukocytes, but inflammatory mediators are liberated within the injured tissue, and constituents of plasma enter the cornea as a result of the increased permeability of the pericorneal blood vessels. Potential mediators of neovascularization include fibrin, biogenic amines, serotonin, constituents of plasma, plasminogen activator, and eicosanoids.

Fibrin. The complex web of reactions during inflammation include the activation of the coagulation pathway via tissue thromboplastic activity leading to fibrin deposition. In many tissues, fibrin has been implicated as a proinflammatory mediator following its activation by other systems, such as complement, and as a primary trigger of such a reaction. That fibrin may play a role in corneal vascularization is suggested by its presence within the inflammatory exudate of vascularizing tissue and an apparent enhancement of corneal vascularization in the presence of antifibrinolysins (epsilon-aminocaproic acid and BP 961).

Biogenic Amines (Histamine, Bradykinin and Acetylcholine). Zauberman et al. (9) found that blood vessels from the corneoscleral limbus grew into the lumen of a plastic tube in one third of the rabbits into whose corneas they perfused acetylcholine, histamine, serotonin or bradykinin. However, other investigators have been unable to produce or stimulate the vascular labelling of the pericorneal microvasculature with bradykinin.

At least in the rat cornea acetylcholine stimulates the formation of phosphatidic acid from ^{14}C arachidonate labelled phospholipids. Since phosphatidic acid is an obligatory intermediate in the inositol phospholipids pathway, the enzymes involved in that cycle of reactions are also presumably present.

Potentially important in corneal neovascularization are the phosphoinositol pathway and protein kinase-C. Several biological systems have pointed to the importance of protein phosphorylation in the regulation of normal cellular functions including proliferation. Various kinases and phosphatases govern such phosphorylations and they are targets for the action of growth factors. The multifunctional protein kinase C appears to play a critical role in this activity and this depends on physiological concentrations of calcium and diacylglycerol. Phosphatyl inositol hydrolysis forms diacetylglycerol which is subsequently phosphorylated to produce phosphatidic acid. Phospholipase C generates 2 important second messengers from inositol phospholipids: inositol 1,4,5-triphosphate which releases calcium from intracellular stores, and diacylglycerol, which activates protein kinase C, a potential regulator of cell proliferation and differentiation. That this pathway may be involved in corneal neovascularization finds support in the following observations: (i) phorbol esters activate protein kinase C in a manner analogous to diacylglycerol; (ii) phorbol esters induce corneal angiogenesis after their instillation into the cornea; (iii) phorbol esters stimulate angiogenesis in the chick chorioallantoic membrane; and (iv) when added to vascular endothelial cells cultured on a collagenous matrix these biologically active substances stimulate capillary formation. Phorbol esters appear to initiate this response by binding to a receptor, identified as protein kinase C, in the responding cells.

Serotonin (see platelets).

Constituents of Plasma. Edema of the corneal stroma not only accompanies corneal neovascularization, but precedes and apparently facilitates the growth of blood vessels into it. The stromal edema that antecedes corneal neovascularization is of the inflammatory type caused by an increased permeability of the pericorneal vasculature, rather than edema due to corneal endothelial cell dysfunction or destruction. Corneal neovascularization is usually not a feature of some settings in which corneal edema secondary to endothelial dysfunction is prominent, such as Fuchs' dystrophy, congenital endothelial corneal dystrophy, and bullous keratopathy.

The increased vascular permeability associated with the inflammatory response occurs primarily at the postcapillary venular endothelial cells and can be created by a wide variety of inflammatory mediators including histamine, 5-hydroxytryptamine, bradykinin, substance P, ADP, adenosine, inosine, prostaglandins (E_1, E_2, $F_{2\alpha}$), leukotrienes (C_4, D_4, E_4, B_4), components of complement cascade (C3a, C5a), platelet-activating factor, fibrin-derived peptides, free radicals, ischemia, and immune aggregates.

As a consequence of the increased permeability of the pericorneal vasculature during acute inflammation, many constituents of plasma including a wide variety of growth factors (mesodermal growth factor, insulin, platelet derived growth factor, epidermal growth factor, fibroblast growth factor) capable of enhancing the proliferation of various cell types including vascular endothelium gain access to the cornea.

Plasminogen Activator (Urokinase) and other Proteases. Plasminogen activator has also been implicated in corneal neovascularization. Blood vessels grow into the cornea following the intracorneal instillation of plasminogen activator and, as with intracorneal injections of other substances, this reaction, is accompanied by a leukocytic infiltration. However, the reaction is diminished if the urokinase is inactivated by heat or by an inhibitor of a specific active site of plasminogen activator (Phe-ala-arg-chloro-methylketone).

Eicosanoids (Prostaglandins and other Metabolites of Arachidonic Acid). Soon after cell injury from any cause, phospholipids within various cells are degraded by phospholipase A to liberate nonesterified fatty acids, including arachidonic acid. The latter is metabolized further by cyclooxygenase to prostaglandins and by lipoxygenase to leukotrienes.

Following injury, prostaglandins (PG) form within the cornea and conjunctiva. While this can occur in the absence of exogenous cells, prostaglandins can also arise from other sources in situations in which corneal neovascularization occurs. These include platelets (that aggregate) in the pericorneal vasculature, activated lymphocytes and macrophages. Angiogenic activity has been attributed to the prostaglandins (most notably PGE_1) because of several observations: (i) corneal vascularization follows the intracorneal instillation of several prostaglandins (PGE_1 > PGE_2 and $PGF_{2\alpha}$ inconsistent); (ii) corneal neovascularization is suppressed by drugs that inhibit the metabolism of arachidonic acid, including corticosteroids, flurbiprofen, indomethacin, Kerorolac, and Phenidone; (iii) corneas exposed to prostaglandins (especially PGE_1) induce endothelial cell migration whereas PGE_2 has a very much smaller effect.

The angiogenic effect of prostaglandins may be mediated via polymorphonuclear leukocytes, which are attracted chemotactically to metabolites of arachidonic acid. Also, the marked neovascularization of corneas with implants sequestering PGE_1 are infiltrated by polymorphonuclear leukocytes.

2.2. Hypoxia

A low oxygen tension appears to be important in angiogenesis in several settings and there is reason to suspect a similar situation in the cornea, especially when corneal vascularization is induced by corneal contact lenses. The possibility of lactate, a product of anerobic metabolism, playing a role in corneal neovascularization has been considered and this view finds support in the observations that the lactate levels at the corneal margins are increased prior to corneal neovascularization, and that lactate stimulates macrophages to secrete factors with angiogenic activity. However, in several experimental models, including some performed by Michaelson, Herz & Kertecz (9), oxygen has not influenced corneal angiogenesis.

2.3. Reactive Corneal Epithelium

Since the non-pathologic cornea is avascular its epithelium clearly does not normally induce angiogenesis. Also, it is apparent that the corneal epithelium is not essential for the induction of corneal neovascularization, because blood vessels can grow into corneas devoid of it. Nevertheless, several observations suggest that a reactive epithelium may contribute to neovascularization: (i) corneal epithelial injury and vascularization frequently coexist; (ii) the vascular endothelium in thermally injured skin has a higher labeling index (^{3}H-thymidine) beneath foci of incomplete reepithelialization compared to nonepithelialized injured sites; (iii) homogenates of excised or cultured corneal epithelial cells induce neovascularization when infused into the cornea; and (iv) the growth of cultured vascular endothelium is stimulated by corneal epithelial cells; and (v) a substance that elicits the growth of vessels in the hamster cheek pouch has been extracted from skin epidermis.

3. SUPPRESSION OF ANGIOGENESIS

Valuable insights into the pathogenesis of corneal neovascularization are gained by an understanding of circumstances that suppress the phenomenon. Support for the hypothesis that corneal vascularization is a component of inflammation and that leukocytes play a cardinal role comes from experiments that show that corneal angiogenesis and the accompanying leukocytic infiltration into the cornea following corneal injury are suppressed by total body x-irradiation, and by antiinflammatory agents such as corticosteroids, indomethacin, and flurbiprofen.

3.1. Irradiation

Corneal vascularization is suppressed in animals exposed to total body irradiation (TBI), total lymphoid irradiation (TLI) and total body irradiation followed by bone marrow transplantation. The suppression of corneal vascularization by TBI appears to be due in part to the effect of irradiation on the peripheral leukocyte count, as it can be reversed to some extent if a bone marrow transplant is performed immediately after the irradiation. However, the extent of the corneal neovascularization in these reconstituted mice is not equivalent to comparable mice that only receive head irradiation. This suggests that TBI may inhibit corneal neovascularization not only by the effect of irradiation on the pericorneal vasculature and the bone marrow, but also by some yet to be defined additional effect. While corneal vascularization does follow irradiation of the head the amount is less than in non-irradiated animals, presumably because the blood vessels that invade the cornea in such cases are formed only from endothelial cell migration rather than by migration and mitosis in the usual manner.

The degree of corneal vascularization is dependent upon the timing of the irradiation in respect to the corneal cauterization. Corneas vascularize more extensively if they are cauterized immediately after total body x-irradation prior to the onset of leukopenia.

While beta irradiation has not been shown to prevent the onset of experimentally induced corneal vascularization it is reported to be effective in enhancing the regression of experimentally induced corneal neovascularization.

3.2 Steroids

Corticosteroids suppress new vessel formation in the cornea in a variety of clinical and experimental circumstances. This suppression of corneal neovascularization has been noted with cortisone, methylprednisolone, dexamethasone, prednisolone, and ticabesone propionate. The timing of the drug administration seems to effect the degree of resultant angiogenesis. It has a greater effect if provided prior to, or immediately after, corneal injury rather than 1 day later. Corticosteroids have not been effective in the treatment of neovascularization induced in the cornea by alkali-burns. How corticosteroids suppress corneal neovascularization remains incompletely understood, but this presumably relates to its anti-inflammatory action and part of the effect could be due to the suppressive effect of corticosteroids on the leukocytic infiltrate that occurs in injured corneas as pointed out more than a decade ago by Fromer & Klintworth (3) and confirmed by others. The combination of heparin with cortisone has been shown to enhance the anti-angiogenic effect of cortisone in post-traumatic corneal vascularization.

Medroxyprogesterone has been reported to decrease substantially the polymorphonuclear leukocytic and vascular infiltration into rabbit corneas with experimental herpes simplex keratitis and to moderately decrease corneal neovascularization following thermal burns.

3.3 Non-steroidal anti-inflammatory drugs

At least in some experimental models corneal neovascularization is suppressed, but not abolished, by non-steroidal anti-inflammatory drugs (including flurbiprofen, indomethacin, Keroralac, and Phenidone) that inhibit the metabolism of arachidonic acid. As with corticosteroids non-steroidal anti-inflammatory drugs suppress the leukocytic infiltrate.

3.4. Antimitotics

Triethylene thiophosporamide (Thio TEPA) has been noted to be effective in suppressing corneal vascularization, but it has toxic side effects.

3.5. Protamine

Protamine, an arginine-rich basic protein that binds heparin, suppresses the rate of corneal angiogenesis in rabbits after the intracorneal implantation of silica particles or rabbit lymph nodes. Polymer pellets of ethylene vinyl acetate (EVA) containing protamine positioned between a tumor (V2 carcinoma) implanted in the rabbit cornea and the corneoscleral limbus have also suppressed corneal angiogenesis, and under such circumstances removal of the protamine has been followed by a resumption of capillary growth into the cornea.

3.6. Tissue Extracts

Extracts of cartilage, vitreous and aorta have been shown to contain anti-angiogenic material. Intracorneal implants of cartilage have retarded and sometimes completely inhibited tumor induced capillary proliferation in the rabbit cornea. An extract of cartilage containing antiprotease activity has also been found to inhibit tumor induced angiogenesis in the rabbit cornea.

Vitreal extracts from several species (rabbit, human, bovine) inhibit angiogenesis in a variety of bioassays, including neovascularization induced by tumor implants in rabbit cornea.

When administered either subconjunctivally or topically a low molecular weight extract of bovine aorta has been reported to inhibit corneal vascularization in rabbits and also to enhance the regression of newly formed corneal vessels.

4. ENHANCEMENT OF CORNEAL VASCULARIZATION

Experimental models that enhance corneal neovascularization also provide valuable information relevant to the pathogenesis of corneal vascularization even though some of these observations are difficult to interpret at present. The degree of corneal vascularization following a focal lesion is influenced by the distance of the focal lesion to the corneoscleral limbus, as shown years ago by Campbell & Michaelson (2). This finding strongly supports the concept that a diffusible angiogenic factor plays a role in corneal neovascularization. In our laboratory we have observed an enhanced corneal angiogenic response to chemical cautery with silver nitrate/potassium nitrate in several situations for reasons that are incompletely understood. These include corneal cauterization of the nude mouse (which lacks T lymphocytes), mice immunized with rabbit anti-mouse-platelet serum, and in mice with retrobulbar injections and sutured eyelids.

5. QUANTITATION OF CORNEAL VASCULARIZATION

Since the degree of corneal vascularization following various corneal injuries or intracorneal innoculations varies considerably, corneal neovascularization needs to be quantitated in studies that evaluate the angiogenic effect of different variables on experimentally induced corneal angiogenesis. Many methods of variable sensitivity and reproducibility have been used by different investigators. Computerized planimetry and a morphometric technique have been valuable but tedious. Our laboratory has recently refined a rapid, reproducible technique for measuring neovascularization in corneal flat preparations of rodents after India Ink perfusion using computerized image analysis. Particularly important in such analyses has been the capability to quantitate objectively the size of burns created by silver nitrate/potassium nitrate. We have found a positive correlation between the burn size and the angiogenic response. This observation has clearly demonstrated that relatively subtle differences in size need to be taken into account in the analysis of different experimental groups after chemical cauterization.

REFERENCES

1. Auerbach R: Angiogenesis inducing factors: a review. In Pick, E. and Landy, M. editors. Lymphokines: A forum for immunoregulatory cell products. New York, 1981, Academic Press, pp. 69-88.
2. Campbell FW and Michaelson IC: Blood vessel formation in the cornea. Br. J. Ophthalmol. 33:248, 1949.
3. Fromer CH and Klintworth GK: An evaluation of the role of leukocytes in the pathogenesis of experimentally induced corneal vascularization: II. Studies on the effect of leukocyte elimination on corneal vascularization. Am. J. Pathol. 81:531, 1975.
4. Garner A: Ocular angiogenesis. Internat. Rev. Exp. Pathol. 28:249, 1986.
5. Klintworth GK: The cornea: structure and macromolecules in health and disease. Am. J. Pathol. 89:719, 1977.
6. Klintworth GK: Corneal neovascularization: a critical review. In preparation.
7. Klintworth GK and Burger PC: Neovascularization of the cornea: current concepts of its pathogenesis. Int. Ophthalmol. Clin. 23:27, 1983.
8. Maurice DM, Zauberman H. and Michaelson IC: The stimulus to neovascularization in the cornea. Exp. Eye Res. 5:168, 1966.
9. Michaelson IC, Herz N and Kertecz D: Effect of increased oxygen concentration on new vessel growth in the adult cornea. Brit. J. Ophthalmol. 38:588, 1954.
10. Zauberman H, Michaelson IC, Bergman F and Maurice DM: Stimulation of neovascularization of the cornea by biogenic amines. Exp. Eye Res. 8:77, 1969.

THE RABBIT CORNEA - A MODEL FOR THE STUDY OF ANGIOGENIC FACTORS

David BenEzra, Itzhak Hemo and Genia Maftzir, Immuno-Ophthalmology and Laboratory of Ocular Angiogenesis, Department of Ophthalmology, Hadassah University Hospital, Jerusalem, Israel

INTRODUCTION

The avascular cornea has ideal organ characteristics for the study of angiogenic stimuli. Indeed, early on, Michaelson and colleagues used the rabbit cornea to study the effect of heat injury (1,2) and to analyze the basic histological and possible chemical phenomena involved in neovascularization (3,4). Later, a more meticulous approach to the study of neovascular stimuli was devised by Zauberman and colleagues (5) and used also by Folkman's group (6) studying the "Tumor Angiogenic Factor" (TAF). Although the corneal model had many advantages, it became evident that the variability among experiments was very large. Furthermore, the possibility that cornea vascularization could be induced by "nearly everything" (7, Zauberman - personal communication) prompted us to look for a reliable and reproducible methodology for the study of neovascular factors.

We report herein our experience using a slow-release device implanted within the rabbit corneal stroma as a model for the study of angiogenic factors. Special emphasis is made regarding the most important aspects that have to be carefully considered during the evaluation of corneal angiogenesis.

MATERIALS AND METHODS

Preparation of implants: The tested compounds are sequestered into ethylene-vinyl-acetate copolymer made by 40% vinyl acetate (Elvax-40). Under a laminar flow hood, 100 ul of a 10% casting solution of Elvax-40 in methylene chloride is mixed with the substance to be tested. The methylene evaporates quickly and a thin film of polymer is formed (8). Pieces of 1 mm^2 of the film are prepared with a blade and used as implants. Ten to 12 implants are obtained from each preparation using the central part of the film and discarding the edges. This step increases homogeneity and decreases the variability of response among individual implants of the same set experiments. Thorough washings of Elvax-40 preparations in absolute alcohol decrease to a minimum the incidence of non specific corneal reactions to the slow-release device.

Implantation: In all experiments, male or female albino mongrel rabbits weighing 2 to 3 kg were used. Under aseptic conditions using the operating microscope, an

incision of half the depth of the corneal thickness and 4 mm
wide is made at the apex of the cornea (Fig. 1). Two
midstromal tunnels toward the corneoscleral limbus are
formed with a thin cyclodialysis spatula at 6 and 12 o'clock
(Fig. 2).

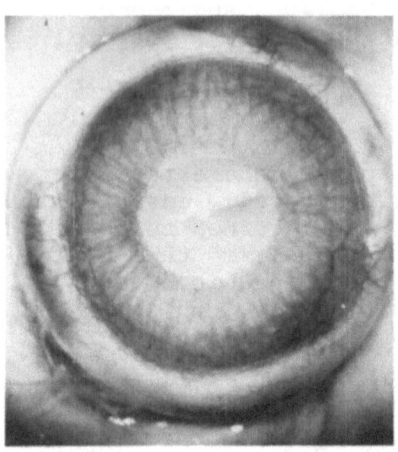
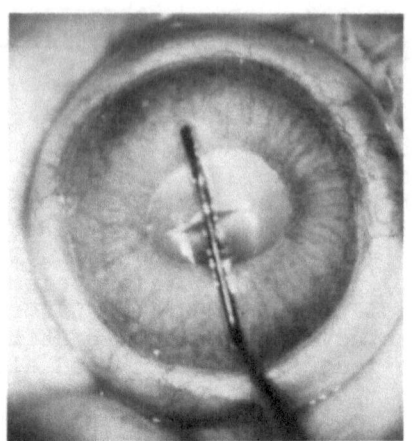

Figure 1 (L). Central incision.
Figure 2 (R). Formation of tunnels.

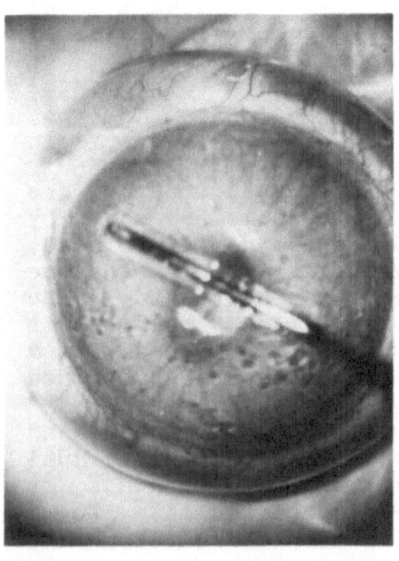
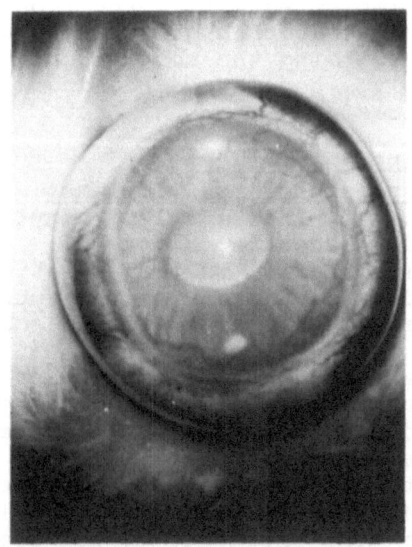

Figure 3 (L). Enlarging the tunnels.
Figure 4 (R). Cornea with implants.

These tunnels are enlarged by introducing a larger cyclodialysis spatula (Fig. 3). The implants are introduced within the tunnels and positioned exactly at the desired distance from the limbus (Fig. 4). "Empty" implants of Elvax-40 are used as controls and inserted at random opposite implants sequestering material to be tested.

Assessment of angiogenic stimulus: The corneas are examined daily under the microscope. Corneal edema and engorgement of vessels at the limbus are noted if present. Neovascularization is recorded as the length of the leading vessel from the limbus toward the implant and the length of the active base of new vessel sprouting at the limbus. Although daily records are made, for practical evaluations the findings on day 6 after implantation are reported. At different intervals, representative eyes were removed and subjected to histological studies.

RESULTS

When implants are positioned at the same distance from the corneoscleral limbus, the extent of neovascularization is closely dependent on the concentration of the stimulating substance as demonstrated in figures 5 and 6.

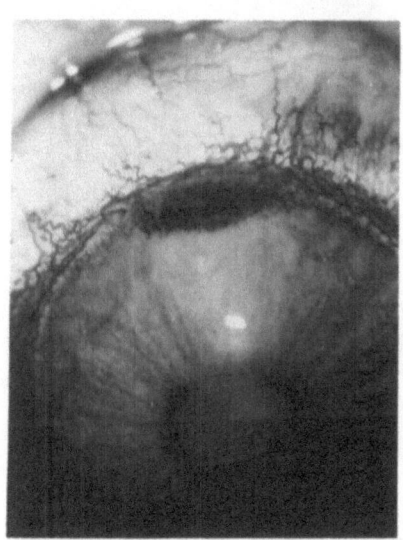 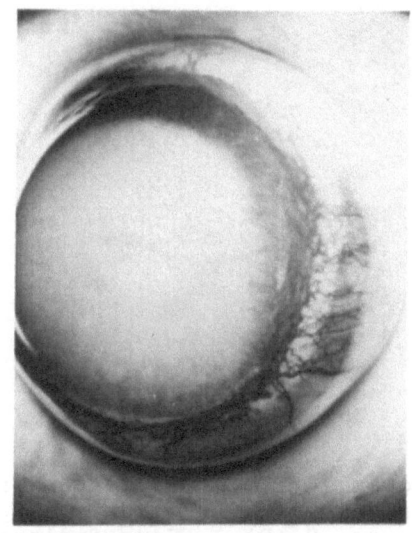

Figure 5 (L). Implant sequestering 1 ug of prostaglandin El.
Figure 6 (R). Implant sequestering 10 ug of prostaglandin El

Table 1 illustrates the crucial role of the distance from the limbus at which the implant is positioned. Two similar implants positioned at a slightly different distance will give variable results. Furthermore, a much higher concentration of the same stimulating substance is needed if an implant is positioned at a distance of 2.0 or 3.0 mm from the limbus. This tendency is enhanced if the implant is positioned at a distance of 4 mm from the limbus (Table 1).

Table 1.   Changes in the minimal effective neovascular
concentration at various distances from the limbus

| Distance* | Minimal effective concentration** | | ug/implant |
(mm)	FGF	EGF	PGE2
2	5	5	<1
3	15	10	3
4	>50	25	10

*   Earlier studies showed that at a distance of 1.5 mm or
     less, a non specific stimulus is obtained also with
     "empty" Elvax-40 implants. No non specific stimuli are
     obtained at a distance of 2.0 mm from the limbus.
**   Concentration that induces significant   neovascular
     budding in at least 50% of the tested implants (EC_{50}).

     Specificity of the stimulus can be demonstrated by the
regression of blood vessels on "emptying" of the implant
(figures 7 and 8).

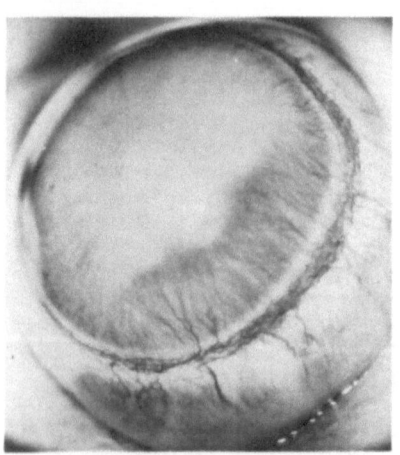 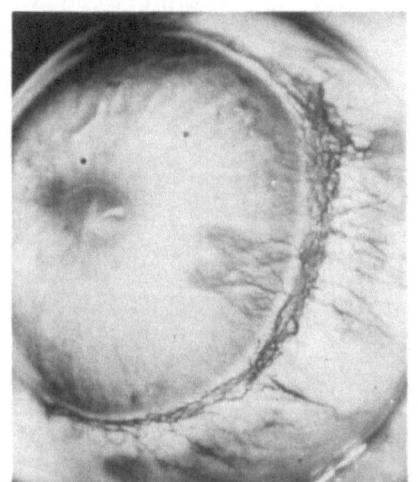

Figure 7 (L). A very strong stimulus is observed early after
implantation.
Figure 8 (R).   Same implant as in Figure 6, fourteen days
later.

     When active implants (as in figure 6) are removed and
reimplanted in new corneas, a strong angiogenic activity
(similar to the original) is observed. Reimplantation of an
inactive implant, on the other hand, does not induce
angiogenic activity.

DISCUSSION
     Numerous models for the evaluation of neovascular
stimuli have been investigated (7,9-11).   In all, variation

among individual experiments and adequate assessment of the extent of neovascular budding is problematic. The rabbit cornea seems an ideal tissue for this purpose (1). However, the high sensitivity of the cornea to neovascular stimuli enhanced the incidence of non specific reactions. In this report, we reexamined the crucial steps of the rabbit corneal model of angiogenesis. An outline of the practical measures that have to be considered in order to increase specificity and reliability of this model are described. The use of thoroughly washed Elvax-40 for the preparation of slow-release devices, careful preparation of individual implants and their insertion within tunnels of the rabbit corneal mid-stroma are very crucial steps. However, as shown in this study and in previously reported data (12,13), the positioning of the implant and its distance from the limbus are factors of the utmost importance. We have shown that a carefully designed rabbit corneal model can be most reliable and reproducible. The question that still remains open is whether the processes that are activated in corneal neovascularization are similar or identical to the ones taking place in other tissues. From clinical and experimental observations, it is clear that various stimuli can trigger neovascularization in different organs. Our surmise has been that although different stimuli are responsible for the trigger of the observed neovascular processes, the final steps leading to the sprouting of neovascular buds are probably identical (12,13). Recently, other investigators are rallying to this very appealing postulation (11).

REFERENCES
1. Campbell FW, Michaelson IC: Blood vessel formation in the cornea. Br J Ophthalmol 33:248, 1949.
2. Michaelson IC: Effect of cortisone upon cornea vascularization produced experimentally. Arch Ophthalmol 47:459, 1952.
3. Michaelson IC: Proliferation of limbal melanoblasts into the cornea in response to a corneal lesion. Br J Ophthalmol 36:657, 1952.
4. Maurice DM, Zauberman H, Michaelson IC: The stimulus to neovascularization of the cornea. Exptl Eye Res 5:168, 1966.
5. Zauberman H, Michaelson IC, Bergmann F, Maurice DM: Stimulation of neovascularization of the cornea by biogenic amines. Exptl Eye Res 8:77, 1969.
6. Folkman J, Merler E, Abernathy C, Williams G: Isolation of a tumor factor responsible for angiogenesis. J Exp Med 133:275, 1971.
7. Klintworth GK: The cornea - structure and macromolecules in health and disease. Am J Pathol 89:719, 1977.
8. BenEzra D: Neovasculogenic ability of prostaglandins, growth factors and synthetic chemoattractants. Am J Ophthalmol 86:455, 1978.

9. Sidky YA, Auerbach R: Lymphocyte-induced angiogenesis in tumor-bearing mice. Science 192:1237, 1976.
10. Auerbach R, Kubai L, Sidky Y: Angiogenesis induction by tumors, embryonic tissues and lymphocytes. Cancer Res 36:3435, 1976.
11. Garner A: Ocular angiogenesis. Int Rev Exp Pathol 28:249, 1986.
12. BenEzra D: Neovasculogenesis. Triggering factors and possible mechanisms. Surv Ophthalmol 24:167, 1979.
13. BenEzra D: Neovascularization. A unitarian phenomenon. Docum Ophthalmol Proc Series 25:125, 1981.

IMMUNOLOGICALLY MEDIATED CORNEAL NEOVASCULARIZATION IN INBRED MICE

Randy J. Epstein, M.D.* and R. Doyle Stulting, M.D. Ph.D.**

* Cornea Service, Department of Ophthalmology, Rush-Presbyterian-St. Luke's Medical Center, Chicago, and University of Illinois, Chicago IL 60612 USA
** Department of Ophthalmology, Emory University, Atlanta GA 30322 USA

SUMMARY

The rabbit cornea has previously been utilized as a model for the study of corneal neovascularization (CNV) induced by the intrastromal injection of stimulated lymphocytes. In order to determine the relative importance of host-related variables in the pathogenesis of immunologically mediated CNV, we studied this response in inbred mice.

A/J, C3H/He, C57BL/6, and BALB/6 mice, and F_1 hybrids derived from these strains were used as donors of Con A stimulated splenic mononuclear cells (SMC) injected into the corneas of allogeneic recipients. Controls included non-stimulated and stimulated-irradiated allogeneic SMC, stimulated-syngeneic SMC, and unfractionated, concentrated supernates from cultures of stimulated SMC.

A marked, strain-related variability in the intensity of CNV induced by allogeneic-stimulated SMC was noted, with A/J > BALB/c > C57BL/6 > C3H/He. Syngeneic SMC and supernates induced CNV only in A/J mice and in F_1 hybrids derived from this strain, suggesting that the gene(s) involved in this response are dominantly inherited. Variability in the intensity of CNV is similar to the pattern of susceptibility to HSV stromal keratitis previously demonstrated in these same strains, and may share a similar pathogenetic mechanism.

INTRODUCTION

Lymphocyte induced angiogenesis (LIA) was first described by Auerbach and associates (1), who used this system to study neovascularization in an intradermal model and, subsequently, in the cornea (2). Because of the clinical importance of corneal neovascularization (CNV), both with regard to worsening the prognosis for a successful penetrating keratoplasty (3), as well as the direct visual loss associated with CNV (4), this model has been important to ophthalmic researchers. BenEzra first described LIA in the rabbit cornea (5), and showed that CNV can be induced by prostaglandins, which are among the mediators elaborated by these stimulated cells (6, 7). Epstein and Hughes noted a significant host related variability in CNV induced by allogeneic, Con-A stimulated lymphocytes (8). In order to better characterize the variables which are important in the host's response, we performed a series of experiments using inbred mice.

MATERIALS AND METHODS

8 week old female BALB/c, C57BL/6, C3H/He, A/J mice were purchased from the Jackson Laboratory (Bar Harbor, ME, USA) and maintained in our colony. B6AF$_1$ hybrids were bred from C57BL/6 and A/J parents. Splenic mononuclear cells (SMC) were obtained using minor modifications of previously described techniques (9, 10). Spleens were pressed through fine nylon mesh, and crudely purified by hypotonic lysis of erythrocytes and density gradient centrifugation. 2×10^6 viable lymphocytes/ml were suspended in 75 cm^2 tissue culture flasks in medium consisting of RPMI 1640 with glutamine, Hepes buffer, penicillin-streptomycin and 10% heat-inactivated fetal calf serum. The cells were incubated for 66 hours with 5.0 ug/ml of concanavalin A (Con A). Dose-response curves were previously plotted in order to determine the optimal parameters for mitogen concentration and culture duration, as assessed by ^{3}H-thymidine incorporation. At the conclusion of the culture period, cells were gently pipetted from the culture flasks, in order to avoid dislodging adherent macrophages. The cells were washed in plain medium and alpha-methyl-mannoside to remove bound Con A, and concentrated to 5×10^8 cells/ml. Viability was assessed by trypan blue dye exclusion, and always exceeded 55% of the cells.

Donor-recipient combinations utilized in these studies are described in Tables I and II. Control injections included syngeneic-stimulated SMC, allogeneic-stimulated irradiated SMC, and allogeneic non-stimulated SMC. Supernatants from stimulated SMC were concentrated 40X in Minicon gradients (15,000 m.w. exclusion) and injected into syngeneic recipients. Intrastromal injections were performed in the following manner: Mice were anesthetized with intramuscular ketamine and acepromazine. Following proptosis of the globe, a 30g disposable hypodermic needle was used to enter the superficial corneal stroma. A 10 ul syringe with a 33g removable needle and 30 degree bevel (Hamilton Corp., Reno, NV), was used to inject 0.2 ul of cells or supernatant (Fig. 1).

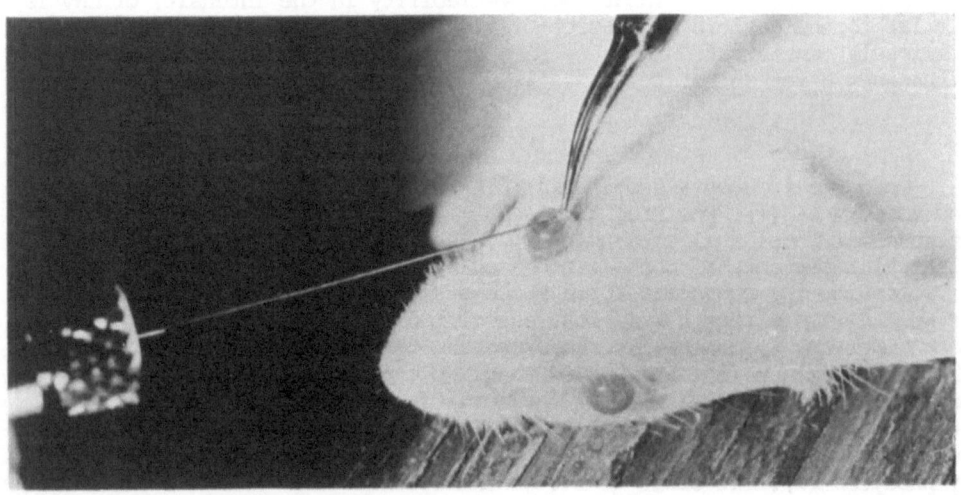

Fig. 1   Technique for performing intrastromal injections

Care was taken not to allow the injected material to enter the
anterior chamber or to spread to the limbus. In cases where this occurred
(less than 5%), the animals were excluded from the study. A positive
response was defined as the induction of new corneal vessels which
persisted for at least two weeks following the injection. Light microscopy
was performed on eyes enucleated from 1-30 days following the injections.

RESULTS

As illustrated in Table I, 50% of BALB/c mice underwent CNV in response
to the injection of allogeneic stimulated lymphocytes from C57BL/6 donors.
Conversely, only 38% of C57BL/6 mice underwent CNV in response to a similar
injection from BALB/c donors. C3H/He mice did not undergo CNV in response
to the injection of donor SMC from either C57BL/6 or BALB/c mice. 100% of
A/J mice underwent CNV in response to the injection of SMC from BALB/c and
C57BL/6 donors. A typical example of the variability seen in the response
of C57BL/6 mice is illustrated in Fig. 2.

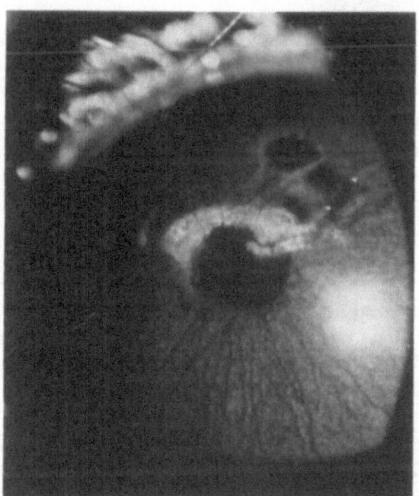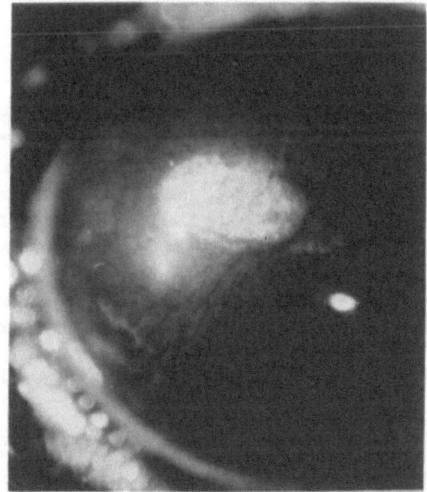

Fig. 2. C57BL/6 mouse one week post-injection of nonstimulated-allogeneic
         splenic mononuclear cells (left). This control injection failed
         to elicit any inflammatory or neovascular response. Contralateral
         eye, (right) injected with allogeneic stimulated lymphocytes, has
         marked acute inflammation, as evidenced by whitening of the
         injection site.

344

The response seen in the more intensely reactive A/J strain is
illustrated in Figs. 3 and 4, below.

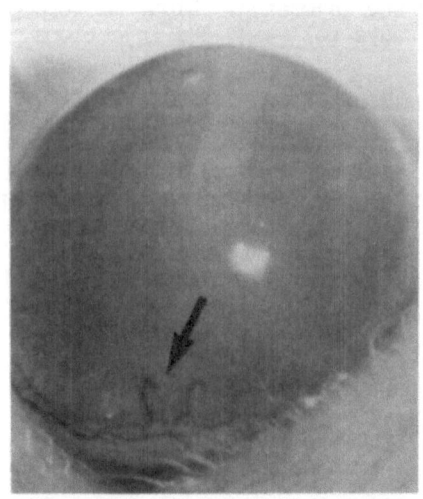 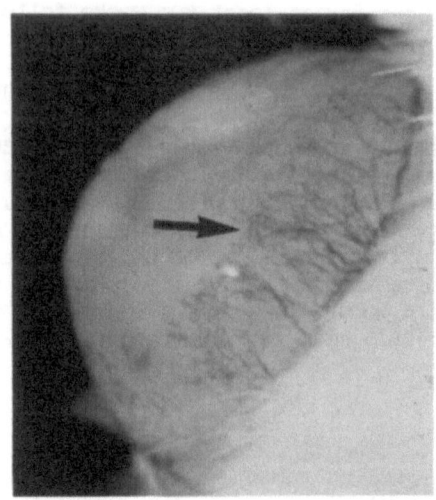

Fig. 3 (Left): A/J mouse at one week post-injection. The cornea is
                beginning to undergo neovascularization (arrow) even at
                this early stage. Vessels measure 0.5 mm in length.
Fig. 4 (Right): A/J mouse two weeks post-injection. Diffuse corneal
                stromal inflammation is associated with 1.5 mm neovascula
                fronds (arrow) growing toward the injection site.

There were marked strain-related differences in the intensity of
inflammation induced by the injected cells, with the corneas of A/J mice
experiencing far more infiltration of PMN both acutely, and at the later
stages, in association with neovascularization, (Fig 5.).

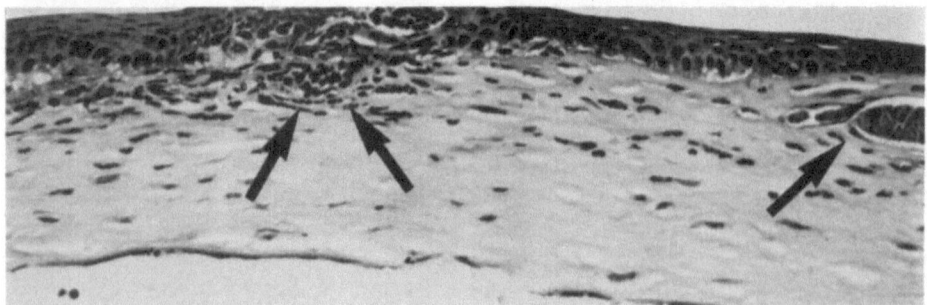

Fig 5. Histologic section of cornea four weeks post-injection. Diffuse
       lymphocytic and PMN infiltration of the injection site (double
       arrows) is noted. Neovascularization (single arrow) is proceeding
       from the limbus toward the center of the cornea.
       (Hematoxylin-eosin, 20x)

There was a marked difference in the percentage of positive responses to allogeneic-stimulated lymphocytes among the four strains, with A/J > BALB/c > C57BL/6 > C3H/He. Quantitative analysis of the area of neovascularization, compared with the Student's t-test, has shown that these differences are significant at the P<.05 level (Epstein, RJ and Stulting, RD, Invest. Ophthalmol. Vis. Sci., 1987, in press.)

TABLE I. Corneal Neovascularization Induced by Allogeneic-Stimulated Lymphocytes.

Recipient	Donor	Number of eyes	Percentage of positive responses
A/J	C57BL/6	15	100%
A/J	BALB/C	15	100
BALB/c	C57BL/6	14	57
C57BL/6	BALB/c	16	38
C3H/He	C57BL/6	7	0
C3H/He	BALB/6	7	0

*A positive response was defined as new corneal vessels persisting for at least two weeks following the intrastromal injection of 10^5 Con A stimulated lymphocytes. BALB/c > C57BL/6 (p <.05), BALB/c > C3H/He (p <.001), and C57BL/6 > C3H/He (p <.001, one-tailed Student's t-test).

The results of control injections were as follows: Allogeneic-nonstimulated, allogeneic-stimulated-irradiated, and syngeneic-stimulated SMC failed to induce CNV in C57BL/6, BALB/c or C3H/He recipients. However, A/J mice and B6AF$_1$ hybrids (A/J x C57BL/6) underwent CNV in response to the injection of allogeneic-nonstimulated, allogeneic-stimulated-irradiated and syngeneic-stimulated cells (Table II). Conditioned medium did not induce CNV, except in the A/J strain, and, to a lesser extent in B6AF$_1$.

TABLE II. Corneal Neovascularization Induced by Syngeneic-Stimulated Lymphocytes.

Recipient	Number of eyes	Percentage of positive responses
A/J	14	93%
B6AF$_1$	15	40
BALB/c	14	0
C57BL/6	16	0
C3H/He	7	0

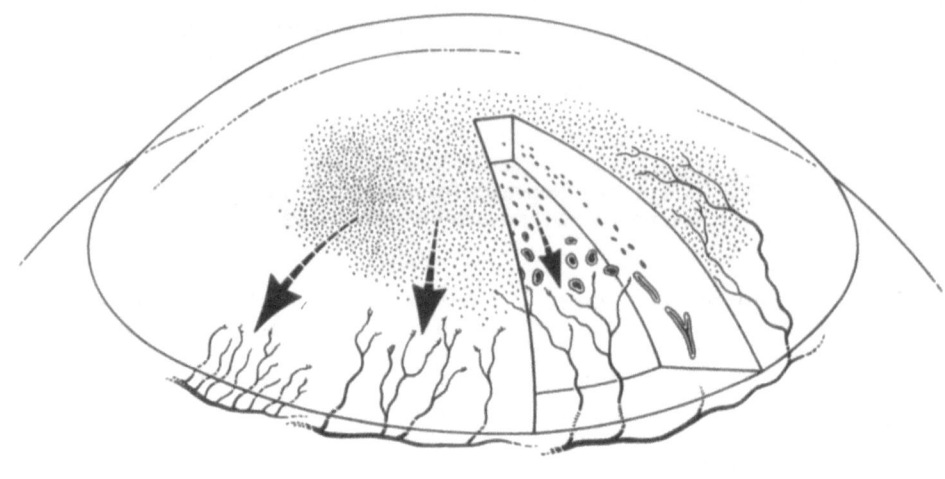

Fig 6. Proposed mechanism of corneal neovascularization.

DISCUSSION

This study demonstrates that corneal neovascularization (CNV) can be effectively studied in inbred mice, and provides some insights into various host-related variables which may have a bearing on this response. Although our experiments in rabbits suggested that host-related variables were important in determining the intensity of CNV (8), we were unable to prove this hypothesis due to limitations inherent in the outbred rabbit model, as previously emphasized by Auerbach (2). Inbred mice have been useful in the study of lymphocyte-induced neovascularization intradermally (1, 11), and are also the model of choice for the study of immunologically mediated corneal neovascularization (2).

We noted significant strain-related differences in the intensity of CNV, as manifested by the percentage of positive responders, with A/J > BALB/c > C57BL/6 > C3H/He. We selected these strains based on their differing H-2 haplotypes, spectrum of variability in immune responses (12, 13), and variable susceptibility to herpes simplex virus (HSV) stromal keratitis (14). A/J mice, which are the most susceptible to HSV stromal keratitis, also seem to be most prone to develop CNV in response to the injection of allogeneic stimulated lymphocytes. A/J mice also have an enhanced blastogenic response to HSV antigen in vitro (15). This "hyper-reactivity" may account for their unique propensity to undergo CNV in response to the injection of allogeneic-nonstimulated and syngeneic-stimulated control lymphocytes. The response to syngeneic cells has not previously been noted by us in outbred rabbits (8) or in any of the other strains tested in the present study. This hyper-reactivity is dominantly transmitted to the F_1 offspring of "CNV-resistant" C57BL/6 crossed with "CNV-susceptible" A/J mice. We have also recently reported that CNV in response to the intrastromal injection of stimulated lymphocytes is a host-versus-graft response, controlled by genes which are non-H-2 (16).

It is likely that variability in the recipients' response to the injected cells (which is presumably related to differences in their immunogenetic makeup), as well as angiogenic activity present in the soluble mediators elaborated by the donor cells are important in the pathogenesis of this response. It has been demonstrated that T-cell mediators, including prostaglandins (6, 7) and lymphokines (17) are angiogenic in the cornea. However, these substances have only been shown to induce neovascularization when complexed to slow-release polymers. In the present study, unfractionated conditioned medium from syngeneic-stimulated lymphocyte cultures was angiogenic after direct intrastromal injection into the corneas of A/J and B6AF$_1$ mice. Experiments currently in progress, utilizing this strain and related congenics have indicated that one of the vasoactive components of these supernatants is interleukin 2 (IL-2), as the direct intrastromal injection of IL-2 will also induce CNV in these strains. IL-2 may stimulate T-helper cells to proliferate (18) and produce additional lymphokines or other factors (19) which act on endothelial cells. Soluble mediators, continuously elaborated by viable, proliferating donor cells likely play a central role in the pathogenesis of this response, (Fig. 6) as it is abrogated, to a significant extent, by irradiation of donor SMC prior to injection (16).

The importance of PMN in the pathogenesis of CNV has been previously demonstrated by Klintworth and associates (20, 21). PMN are also important in this model, as demonstrated by their infiltration following the injection of both stimulated lymphocytes and controls. The degree of PMN infiltration appears to be quantitatively related to the amount of CNV which is induced, as it is most marked in the A/J strain and minimal in non-vascularizing corneas. Therefore, while PMN infiltration is involved in CNV induced by stimulated lymphocytes, it is not the sole mechanism.

Immunologically mediated CNV is important clinically, and it can be a source of significant visual morbidity (4). In addition to its association with stromal scarring and opacification, a vascularized cornea leaves the patient at poor risk for success in penetrating keratoplasty (3). Further investigations, currently underway, will attempt to characterize the mediators responsible for inducing CNV, in order to develop therapies to inhibit it.

ACKNOWLEDGEMENTS

The authors wish to express their appreciation to J. Clifford Waldrep, Ph.D., for essential assistance with immunologic rationale and methodology, and Janice C. Kindle, M.S., who provided extraordinary technical support.

This study was funded by United States Public Health Service Research Service Award EY-05765-01 (Dr. Epstein), and the Seymour R. Marco Foundation.

REFERENCES

1. Sidky YA and Auerbach R: Lymphocyte-induced angiogenesis: A quantitative and sensitive assay of the graft-versus-host reaction. J Exp Med 141:1084, 1975.
2. Muthukkaruppan VR and Auerbach R: Angiogenesis in the mouse cornea. Science 205:1416, 1979.

3. Khodadoust AA: The allograft reaction: The leading cause of late failure in clinical corneal grafts. In Corneal Graft Failure, Ciba Foundation Symposium, Jones BR, ed. Amsterdam, 1973, Elsevier, p. 151.
4. Cogan D: Corneal vascularization. Invest Ophthalmol 1:253, 1962.
5. BenEzra D: Mediators of immunological reactions: Function as inducers of neovascularization. Metab Ophthalmol 2:339, 1978.
6. BenEzra D: Possible mediation of vasculogenesis by products of the immune reaction. In Immunology and Immunopathology of the Eye. Silverstein AM and O'Connor RG, editors. New York, 1978, Masson Publishing USA, Inc., p. 315.
7. BenEzra D: Neovascularization ability of prostaglandins, growth factors and synthetic chemoattractants. Am J Ophthalmol 86:455, 1978.
8. Epstein RJ and Hughes WF: Lymphocyte-induced corneal neovascularization: A morphologic assessment. Invest Ophthalmol Vis Sci 21:87, 1981.
9. Mishell B, and Shiigi SM, editors: In vitro immune responses. IN: Selected methods in cellular immunology, 1980, San Francisco, W.H. Freeman, pp. 3-156.
10. Meo T: The MLR test in the mouse. In Immunological methods, Lefkovits I, and Pernis B, editors. New York, 1979, Academic Press, p. 234.
11. Auerbach R: Angiogenesis inducing factors: A review. In Pick E and Landy M, editors, Lymphokines: A forum for immunoregulatory cell products. New York, 1981, Academic Press, pp. 69-88.
12. Festing MFW: Inbred strains in biomedical research. New York, 1979, Oxford University Press, pp. 137-266.
13. Hume DA and Weidemann MJ: Mitogenic lymphocyte transformation. Amsterdam, 1980, Elsevier, pp. 46-50.
14. Stulting RD, Kindle JC, and Nahmias AJ: Patterns of herpes simplex keratitis in inbred mice. Invest Ophthalmol Vis Sci 26:1360, 1985.
15. Kindle JC, Epstein RJ, and Stulting RD: Cell-mediated immunity to herpes simplex virus (HSV) in inbred mice. Invest Ophthalmol Vis Sci 27 (Suppl.): 116, 1986.
16. Epstein RJ and Stulting RD: Genetic control of corneal neovascularization (CNV) in inbred mice is dominantly inherited and non-H-2. Invest Ophthalmol Vis Sci 27 (Suppl.):46, 1986.
17. Lutty GA, Liu SH, and Prendergast RA: Angiogeneic lymphokines of activated T-cell origin. Invest Ophthalmol Vis Sci 24:1595, 1983.
18. Niederkorn NJ and Streilen JW: Lymphoma allografts abrogate immune privilege within the anterior chamber of the eye. Invest Ophthalmol Vis Sci 27:1235, 1986.
19. Watt SL and Auerbach R: A mitogenic factor for endothelial cells obtained from mouse secondary mixed leukocyte cultures. J Immunol 136(1):197, 1986.
20. Fromer CH, and Klintworth GK: An evaluation of the role of leukocytes in the pathogenesis of experimentally induced neovascularization. I. Comparison of experimental models of corneal neovascularization. Am J Pathol 79:537, 1975.
21. Fromer CH and Klintworth GK: An evaluation of the role of leukocytes in the pathogenesis of experimentally induced neovascularization. III. Studies related to the vasoproliferative capability of PMNs and lymphocytes. Am J Pathol 82:157, 1976.

VASOFORMATIVE FACTORS IN THE CORNEAL EPITHELIUM

J.A. Eliason

INTRODUCTION

The classic work of Campbell and Michaelson[1] first demonstrated a spatial relationship between stimulus and response in corneal vascularization. Their work implied the presence of a diffusible, vasogenic substance. Maurice, Zauberman and Michaelson[2] utilizing both open and blind ending tubes in the stroma further proved that vascularization is accompanied by the movement of a substance from the site of stimulus through the stroma to the limbal vessels. The other indispensible requirement for vessel growth in the cornea is the presence of edema. Cogan and others[3,4] have provided evidence that the normally compact stroma is too tightly apposed to allow the incursion of vascular structures unless it is separated by fluid. A bewildering array of growth promotors, specific agents and circumstances capable of initiating corneal vascularization have made it difficult to determine the true mediators in a given clinical or experimental situation.

In a series of articles by Fromer and Klintworth[5,6] and the work of others[7,8] convincing evidence has been generated that leukocytes are the source of a vasostimulating substance. Histologic information and the results of injected leukocyte extracts have implicated white blood cells. There has been some conflict among these reports comparing the roles of different leukocytes (lymphocytes, basophils, macrophages and polymorphonuclear cells) in this process. It seems likely that this role is not limited to one cell type. Despite the evidence gathered, no specific angiogenic agent has yet been purified from leukocytes.

Sholley et al[9] were the first to report an animal model (rat) in which eliminating leukocytes did not prevent vascularization. Eliason[10] reported the same results in another animal model (rabbit). Sholley used both whole body X-irradiation as well as antineutrophil serum while Eliason utilized only the former to depress the white blood cell population. Eyes were shielded to prevent local effects from the irradiation. Histology documented the absence of leukocytes in the stroma and vascularization was observed in response to a cauterization of the cornea. In both reports the growth was less vigorous in leukopenic than in normal animals (Table 1). Glatt et al[11] examined the effect of irradiation by transplanting injured and irradiated rat corneas to chorioallantoic membranes where they observed a depressed vascular response compared to non-irradiated ones. This correlated with the degree of leukocytic infiltration. However, they did not rule out the possibilities that the irradiation damaged local corneal elements which may have limited their ability to produce angiogenic substances or that it may have caused the release of antiangiogenic materials.

TABLE 1.

Days After Cauterization

	1	2	3	4	5
Control	0.34±0.03	0.32±0.03	0.57±0.04	0.97±0.06	1.28±0.06
Leukopenic	0.33±0.02	0.38±0.03	0.51±0.04	0.68±0.03	0.98±0.04

Vascular invasion from the limbus after cauterization of the cornea. Expressed as the mean invasion in mm±1 S.E. (n = 5 to 14 for controls and 12 to 31 for leukopenic). The indicated difference on day 5 is significant at $p < 0.001$.

In the above irradiated rabbit model the corneal epithelium was the only viable cell population present in the wound area which could act as the source of an angiogenic substance. Neither leukocytes nor corneal endothelium were present in the injured area and the keratocytes did not take up stain thus appearing nonviable. To pursue the theory presented by this model the corneal epithelium has been examined for activities that one might associate with angiogenesis.

IN VIVO ANGIOGENIC ACTIVITY

An aqueous extract of both fresh and cultured rabbit corneal epithelium was prepared by homogenizing the cells in isotonic saline followed by centrifugation and filtration. In most circumstances, except where indicated, the extract was also heat precipitated at 80° C for 10 minutes. This became the standard practice when it was determined that such heating did not destroy the angiogenic activity. In order to examine this extract for activity in vivo it was perfused by way of an osmotic pump into the corneal stroma of rabbits at a point 3 mm from the limbus at a constant rate of 1 μl/hr[12]. The vascular reaction from the adjacent vessels was observed and recorded. A vigorous growth of vessels directed toward the tube tip resulted and was accompanied by an inflammatory infiltrate in the stroma[13]. Both fresh and cultured epithelial extract evoked vessels when the perfusion system provided a solution containing as little as 50 μg/ml total protein. With lesser amounts of extract the vascular response became inconsistent.

Vessel growth still occurred when the perfusion system was implanted after the white blood cell population had been depleted by irradiation. The extent of vascularization was not statistically different between normal and leukopenic animals (Table 2). Histology confirmed the absence of leukocytes in the stroma in this situation as with the corneas that were injured by cautery in the previous study. Different here was the presence of the endothelial and epithelial layers of cells as well as the keratocyte population which were absent or nonviable in the cauterized model. Obviously the quantitative comparison of the angiogenic signals in these two models are not comparable and it is possible that the native corneal cells may have played a contributing role.

TABLE 2.

Area of Vascularization

Normals	2.08±0.93 (n = 11)
Leukopenics	1.28±0.19 (n = 4)

Area of vascularization calculated from photographs in normal and leukopenic rabbits. Expressed as the mean in mm±1 S.D.. The observed difference of the means is not statistically significant.

IN VITRO ANGIOGENIC ACTIVITY

In vivo studies generally bear many uncontrolled parameters. Depleting the leukocytes is one step to simplify the model. In order to provide further controls, the epithelial extract was tested for its ability to stimulate growth of vascular endothelial cells in tissue culture[14].

Cutaneous vessel endothelial cells were obtained from rabbit ears by perfusion with a trypsin solution[15]. Extract was added to the media of replicate cultures and cell counts were used to measure the response. Culture medium was selected which supported less than optimal growth to allow a further stimulating effect to be manifest (Eagle's Minimal Essential Medium with 5% - 10% rabbit serum or 10% human serum). When an optimal medium was used (i.e. 15% fetal bovine serum) the cells grew at a maximum rate in the control cultures without extract added and no further stimulation of growth could be appreciated. When heated extract was added to cells in medium with 5% rabbit serum to achieve a concentration of 34 µg/ml total protein, growth was stimulated by slightly less than five times (4.89 ± 0.33, S.E., n = 5). Medium conditioned by the growth of epithelial cells was also able to stimulate growth. When endothelial cells were obtained from the aorta, stimulation did not occur (1.05 ± 0.22, not statistically significant). This is consistent with the results of Keegan et al[16] who found a similar distinction between these cell types. An extract was prepared from cultured keratocytes in the same fashion as for epithelial cells. When this was applied to the endothelial cells, significant stimulation of growth did not occur (1.16 ± 0.21, S.E., not statistically significant).

Directed migration of vascular endothelial cells towards a stimulus along with mitotic activity are the most obvious components of the response of these cells in vascularization. Boyden chambers were used to examine for chemotactic activity in the epithelial extract[17]. They were prepared using millipore filters to separate the two chambers. With cells plated on the upper surface of the membrane, the extract was added to the medium in the inferior chamber. For these slow moving cells incubation was carried out for 14-16 hours. Cells were counted on both surfaces of the membrane and the fraction migrating through was calculated. Vascular endothelial cell migration was increased by eighteen times over control in the presence of the epithelial extract (Table 3). Migration increased with higher concentrations of the extract. In comparison, significant migration was not observed when keratocytes were placed into the chamber instead of endothelial cells.

A further marker that may reflect vascular endothelial cell activity is plasminogen activator production. This is not a function unique to these cells but is generally felt to be an important aspect of their function. Activator was measured using a specific chromogen substrate in a modification of the spectrophotometric method described by Verheijen et al[18]. Cells were extracted at a low pH (2.8) and then neutralized to maximize the recovery. Results were standardized with urokinase. We have found that plasminogen activator is present in all three corneal cell types and their conditioned medium in the rabbit in addition to cutaneous vascular endothelial cells[19] (Table 4). The highest levels were recovered from epithelial cells. When confluent vascular endothelial cells were exposed to the epithelial extract then subsequently extracted themselves, their content of plasminogen activator was increased by a fraction of 2.31 over baseline levels (Table 5). Epithelial conditioned medium was also able to stimulate this production of activator. The cells were generously washed prior to extraction to remove activator present in the epithelial extract added to the medium. This did not control for possible internalization of the activator which might then be included in the assay.

TABLE 3.

	Epithelial Extract (mg/ml)			
	0	0.88	1.75	3.5
Vascular Endothelium	0.24±0.08	0.28±0.05	1.29±0.68	4.36±0.81
Keratocytes	0.30±0.1	0.29±0.1	0.28±0.1	0.49±0.06

Migration of vascular endothelial cells through a membrane exposed to a gradient of epithelial cell extract expressed as a fraction of the plated cells (±1 S.D., n = 3).

TABLE 4.

	Activator
Vascular Endothelial Extract	7.14 ± 1.53
Vascular Endothelial Medium	8.33 ± 2.35
Epithelial Extract	48.0 ± 8.6
Epithelial Medium	309.0 ± 22
Keratocyte Extract	11.6 ± 4.3
Keratocyte Medium	9.3 ± 1.2
Corneal Endothelial Extract	11.2 ± 2.0
Corneal Endothelial Medium	33.0 ± 0.9

Plasminogen activator activity present in cellular extracts and conditioned medium in corneal cells and vascular endothelium expressed as mean urokinase standard milliunits/mg total protein (±1 S.D., n = 4 to 6).

Several angiogenic related activities have thus been demonstrated in the corneal epithelium. Vessel growth can be provoked in the intact animal. Vascular endothelium in culture can be stimulated both in growth and chemotactic migration by an extract of epithelium, and synthetic activity in the form of plasminogen activator production is also stimulated by the extract. These may be related to one or several species in the epithelial extract. They all do share the common features of being aqueous soluble and stable to heating.

TABLE 5.

	Activator	Fraction of Control	
Control	7.14 ± 1.53	1.00	
Epithelial Extract	16.51 ± 0.99	2.31	p < 0.001
Epith. Cond. Medium	10.50 ± 0.73	1.47	p < 0.01

Stimulation of plasminogen activator production (expressed as milliunits/mg total protein ± S.D., n = 4 to 6) in vascular endothelial cells when exposed to an extract of corneal epithelial cells and medium conditioned by epithelial cells.

CHARACTERIZATION OF ACTIVITY

Characterization of the growth stimulating activity and in vivo vascularization activity has resulted in several findings. As already mentioned, these activities share a polar character being soluble in aqueous medium and are stable to heating. They are also not destroyed by extremes of pH when the extract is titrated to values of 2 or 12 then neutralized. Stimulation remains comparable to nontitrated extract. Extraction of the extract with chloroform depressed the activity by 15% suggesting that it has some non-polar character.

Interesting results were encountered when the extract stability was examined. Heated material was stable; retaining activity up to 14 days at temperatures varying from 20° C to -20° C. Extract which had not been heated lost its activity within a matter of days throughout this temperature range. This was evaluated using in vivo perfusion into the cornea to create vascularization.

Incubation of the extract with insoluble trypsin completely destroyed the activity. This was true for both the in vitro stimulation of vascular endothelial cells as well as stimulation of vascularization in vivo.

The extract has been separated into several fractions using ultrafiltration. Using filters having nominal cutoff values of 500, 10,000 and 30,000 the activity of the extract to stimulate endothelial cell growth in culture has been examined (Table 6). The results suggest that the angiogenic activity is largely excluded by the 500 filter and passed by the 10,000 one. There further seems to be activity retained by the 30,000 membrane. If the angiogenic activity is less than 10,000 in size this would place it in the same range as many other growth factors[20-22]. The higher molecular weight material may represent a complexed form of the activity. Further steps to purify these activities may prove them to be related and may find correlations with other known factors.

TABLE 6.

Nominal Cutoff	% of Protein	Stimulation
500	0.19	1.31 ± 0.24
10,000	0.74	2.11 ± 0.47
30,000	0.81	2.12 ± 0.41
Whole Extract	1.00	3.03 ± 0.9

Ultrafiltration separation of epithelial extract using membranes as indicated in the first column. Protein content is expressed as a fraction of the whole extract and stimulation is expressed as a fraction of control cultures (± S.D., n = 6).

REFERENCES
1. Campbell FN and Michaelson IC (1949) Blood vessel formation in the cornea. Brit. J. Ophthal. 33:248
2. Maurice DM, Zauberman H and Michaelson IC (1966) The stimulus to neovascularization in the cornea. Exp. Eye Res. 5:168
3. Cogan DG (1949) Vascularization of the cornea. Arch. Ophthal. 41:406
4. Dohlman CH (1965) Corneal edema and vascularization. in The Cornea - World Congress. Butterworths p. 80
5. Fromer CH and Klintworth GK (1975) An evaluation of the role of leukocytes in the pathogenesis of experimentally induced corneal vascularization: II Studies on the effect of leukocyte elimination on corneal vascularization. Am. J. Pathol. 81:531
6. Fromer CH and Klintworth GK (1976) An evaluation of the role of leukocytes in the pathogenesis of experimentally induced corneal vascularization: III Studies related to the vasoproliferative capability of polymorphonuclear leukocytes and lymphocytes. Am. J. Pathol. 82:157

354

7. Polverini PJ, Cotran RS, Gimbrone MA Jr. and Unanue ER (1977) Activated macrophages induce vascular proliferation. Nature 269:804
8. Epstein RJ and Hughes WF (1981) Lymphocytes-induced corneal neovascularization: a morphologic assessment. Invest. Ophthal. & Vis. Sci. 21:87
9. Sholley MM, Gimbrone MA and Cotran RS (1978) The effects of leukocyte depletion on corneal neovascularization. Lab. Invest. 38:32
10. Eliason JA (1978) Leukocytes and experimental corneal vascularization. Invest. Ophthal. & Vis. Sci. 17:1087
11. Glatt HJ, Vu MT, Burger PC and Klintworth GK (1985) Effect of irradiation on vascularization of corneas grafted onto chorioallantoic membranes. Invest. Ophthal. & Vis. Sci. 26:1533
12. Eliason JA and Maurice DM (1980) An ocular perfusion system. Invest. Ophthal. & Vis. Sci. 19:102
13. Eliason JA (1985) Angiogenic activity of the corneal epithelium. Exp. Eye Res. 41:721
14. Eliason JA (1979) Stimulation of vascular endothelium by an epithelial homogenate. Invest. Ophthal. & Vis. Sci. 18(Suppl):75
15. Davison PM, Bensch K and Karasek MA (1980) Growth and morphology of rabbit marginal vessel endothelium in cell culture. J. Cell Biol. 85: 187
16. Keegan A, Hill C, Kumar S, Phillips P, Schor A and Weiss J (1982) Purified tumour angiogenesis factor enhances proliferation of capillary but not aortic, endothelial cells in vitro. J. Cell Sci. 55:261
17. Eliason JA, Deshmukh A and Elliott JP (1984) Chemotactic activity from the corneal epithelium. Invest. Ophthal. & Vis. Sci. 25(Suppl):323
18. Verheijen JH, Mullaart E, Chang GTG, Kluft C and Wijngaards G (1982) A simple, sensitive spectrophotometric assay for extrinsic (tissue-type) plasminogen activator applicable to measurements in plasma. Thromb. Haemostas. 48:266
19. Eliason JA and Schwietz E (1985) Plasminogen activation by corneal cell and vascular endothelium. Invest. Ophthal. & Vis. Sci. 26(Suppl):319
20. Taylor JM, Mitchell WM and Cohen S (1972) Epidermal growth factor: physical and chemical properties. J. Biol. Chem. 247:5928
21. Gospodarowicz D (1975) Purification of a fibroblast growth factor from bovine pituitary. J. Biol. Chem. 250:2515
22. Gospodarowicz D and Moran JS (1976) Growth factors in mammalian cell culture. Ann. Rev. Biochem. 45:531

ACKNOWLEDGMENTS
This work was supported in part by NIH grants EY00431 and EY00051, and by The Pemberton Fund. I express my gratitude to Dr. David M. Maurice for his invaluable criticism and timely encouragement.

MACROPHAGE-INDUCED NEOVASCULARIZATION IN THE MOUSE EYE: CORRELATION WITH
OTHER IN VIVO AND IN VITRO TESTS OF ANGIOGENESIS

M. KAMINSKI, Y. HAYARI, G. KAMINSKA, VR. MUTHUKKARUPPAN, L. KUBAI and R.
AUERBACH
Laboratory of Developmental Biology, Department of Zoology, University of
Wisconsin, Madison WI 53706 USA

1. INTRODUCTION

Macrophages play an important role in the neovascular process. A clear
demonstration of an angiogenic response to macrophages was shown when
macrophages introduced into the guinea pig cornea were found to elicit a
vascular response from the limbus (1). Interleukin-1 (IL-1), tumor necrosis factor (TNF), prostaglandin E2 and/or other factors produced by activated macrophages have been directly implicated both in the corneal
vascular response and in tissue culture models assessing endothelial cell
proliferation and migration (2,3,4,5). Moreover, while the relationship
of macrophage function to immune-mediated lymphocyte-induced angiogenesis
(LIA) has not yet been defined, it may be assumed that stimulation of the
T-lymphocytes mediating LIA leads not only to a direct production of
angiogenic factors (e.g. proliferation-inducing endothelial cell lymphokine (ECL-1); see ref.6) but also to the activation of resident macrophages. Our experiments were designed to examine the role of macrophage and
macrophage-derived cell products on angiogenesis in the mouse. We report
on the effects of resident macrophages, activated macrophages, a macrophage cell line and macrophage-derived factors on angiogenesis in the cornea, on angiogenesis in the skin, and on mouse microvascular and lymphatic
endothelial cell proliferation in vitro.

2. MATERIALS AND METHODS

2.1 Mice
BALB/cAu, 129/J, and (BALB/cAu x 129/J)F_1 animals were bred in our own
colony.
2.2 Cells and cell lines
P388D$_1$ cells, an IL-1 producing macrophage line (7), were obtained from
the American Type Culture Collection. Mouse brain microvascular endothelial cells and mouse thoracic duct lymphatic endothelial cells were isolated following collagenase digestion and characterized by flow cytometry
on the basis of cell-surface associated angiotensin-converting enzyme and
a receptor for acetylated low density lipoprotein, as described in detail
previously (8,9). Resident macrophages were obtained from BALB/c mice by
peritoneal lavage with Dulbecco's modification of Eagle's Minimum
Essential Medium (DMEM). Activated macrophages were generated by injection of thioglycolate solution (Difco) 3 days prior to peritoneal lavage.

2.3 Intradermal angiogenesis assay

Macrophages suspended in DMEM were injected intradermally into syngeneic mice, at a dose of 1×10^6 cells per inoculation, in a volume of 0.1ml.
DMEM medium alone served as a control to establish vessel background.
Recipient mice were exposed to 700 rad gamma irradiation (cesium source)
2 hours prior to injection of cells. Animals were killed and assessed for
vascular response after 72 hours as described in detail previously (10).

2.4 Corneal neovascularization assay

Initial experiments were carried out using the corneal pocket protocol
described previously by us (11,12) as modified by R.Epstein (this volume).
BALB/c or (BALB/c x 129/J)F_1 mice were anesthetized with avertin, a transverse incision was made into the corneal stroma, and a narrow pocket was
made using a finely ground iris spatula. The pocket terminated within 1mm
of the limbus. The opening of the pocket was kept as narrow as possible.
0.3-0.5 µl of a concentrated cell suspension was then introduced using a
Hamilton syringe terminating in a 33-gauge needle.

2.5 Proliferation assay

The assay was performed in 96 well flat bottom plates (Costar, Cambridge
MA) using 10^4 endothelial cells/well (cf.6). Differing numbers of resident
or activated macrophages were then added. After 48 hours of incubation at
37°C, cells were labelled overnight with ^{3}H-thymidine (.2 µCi/well).
Subsequently cells were cultured in medium containing unlabelled thymidine,
then rinsed, detached with trypsin and EDTA, processed by harvesting on
filter paper, and assessed for radioactivity using liquid scintillation
measurements.

3. RESULTS

3.1 Angiogenesis in the cornea

We compared the angiogenesis-inducing capacity of unstimulated macrophages, stimulated macrophages and a macrophage cell line, by introducing test
cells into the cornea of adult, syngeneic mice. Normal, syngeneic spleno-
cytes served as a negative control. The results are shown in Table I.

TABLE I

Angiogenesis-inducing capacity of macrophages: Intracorneal assay

Cells Tested	# exp.	# cases	# pos.	# neg.	P value
splenocytes (control)	4	17	13	4	
resident macrophages	5	17	12	5	NS
activated macrophages	6	25	23	2	<.005
P388D$_1$ cells	2	12	12	0	<.005

The experiments indicate that syngeneic macrophages obtained from the peritoneal cavity are at best weak inducers of angiogenesis. However, if the macrophages are stimulated with thioglycolate they rapidly acquire the ability to induce angiogenesis in the corneal assay. The P388D$_1$ macrophage cell line is also highly angiogenic.

3.2 Angiogenesis in the skin

Verification of the angiogenic properties of activated mouse macrophages was carried out using the intradermal angiogenesis assay developed for LIA measurements. In this assay injection of medium was used as a control. The results are shown in Table II.

TABLE II

Angiogenesis-inducing capacity of macrophages: Intradermal assay

Cells tested	Number of assays	New blood vessels (Mean ± S.E.)	P value
medium alone (control)	24	6.1 ± 0.8	
syngeneic thymocytes	10	7.5 ± 1.4	NS
resident macrophages	9	6.2 ± 0.5	NS
activated macrophages	42	17.3 ± 1.0	<.005

An additional experiment, involving a different set of strain combinations and controls, was carried out with the P388D$_1$ cell line. As expected, the macrophage cell line was also found to be angiogenic.

3.3 Effect on endothelial cell proliferation

We next examined the effect of macrophages on endothelial cell proliferation. We prepared cell cultures with a fixed number of mouse thoracic duct (MLE) or brain (MBE) endothelial cells, and added variable numbers of resident or activated macrophages to these cultures. Control groups included endothelial cells alone and macrophages alone. After two days in vitro, cell proliferation was assessed by thymidine incorporation. The results are shown in Figure 1. It can be seen that both unstimulated and stimulated macrophages have a moderate effect on thymidine incorporation, leading to a stimulation index of about 1.6-2.2. An inhibitory effect of activated macrophages at high density was seen for both MLE and MBE cells.

358

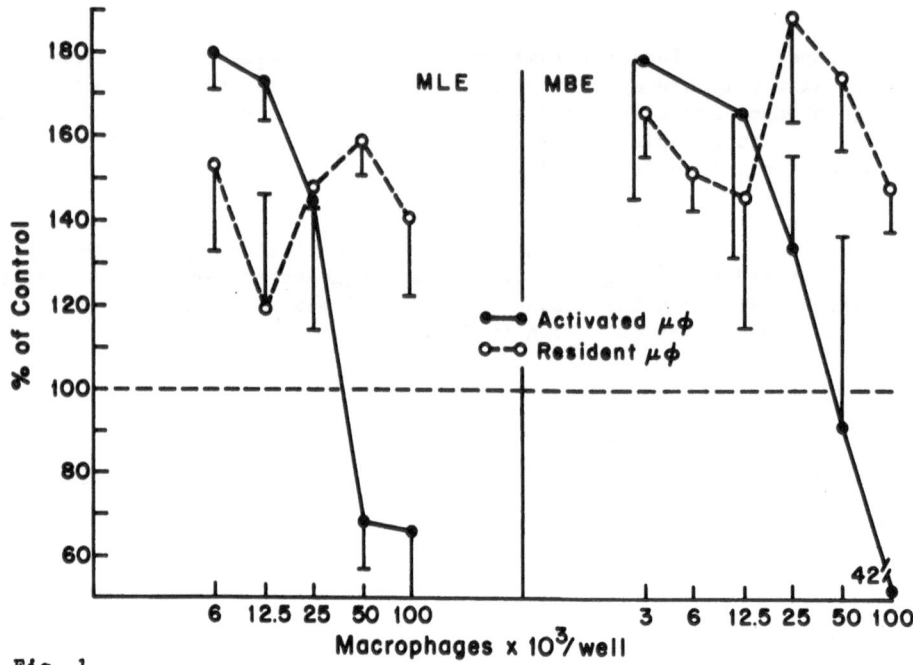

Fig. 1

The effect of syngeneic macrophage cocultivation on proliferation of syngeneic mouse lymphatic (MLE) or brain (MBE) endothelial cells

4. DISCUSSION

Our experiments extend to the mouse the earlier observations of Polverini, Gimbrone and their colleagues that activated but not unstimulated macrophages can elicit a neovascular reaction (1,13). Moreover, they demonstrate that the intradermal assay originally developed for immune-mediated lymphocyte-induced angiogenesis can be used to provide quantitation of the angiogenic reaction evoked by these macrophages.

That both activated and resident macrophages can elicit a proliferative response from lymphatic as well as microvascular endothelial cells is not necessarily contradictory, since it has been shown that macrophages become activated by overnight incubation in tissue culture (14). On the other hand, this leaves unanswered the question of why thioglycolate-induced macrophages are inhibitory to endothelial cell proliferation when added at high density.

Our studies show that the P388D$_1$ cell line also is an effective inducer of angiogenesis. Similar observations were made with two other macrophage cell lines by Polverini and Leibovich (15). Although it was likely that the IL-1 and other cytokines produced by P388D$_1$ cells were responsible for the observed effects, we nevertheless considered the possibility that this cell line may be transformed and therefore active because of its tumor properties rather than because of its macrophage phenotype. The line, however, is contact inhibited in vitro and did not produce tumors on transplantation into syngeneic mildly irradiated host animals (data not shown). Thus we believe it will serve as a useful model in further studies directed at characterizing the nature of macrophage-induced angiogenesis.

Our studies do not address the question of mechanism. Macrophages are known to produce a variety of cytokines with effects on endothelial cells, including prostaglandins, IL-1, and TNF. In addition, a separate population of macrophages has been shown to be cytostatic for tumor cells in vitro (16). Moreover, indirect effects have also been demonstrated since macrophages or their products stimulate production of additional cytokines by both lymphocytes and endothelial cells (17). It is likely, moreover, that the angiogenic effects that we have reported represent the net effect of mediators that enhance and mediators that inhibit neovascularization.

REFERENCES

1. Polverini PJ; Cotran PS; Gimbrone MA Jr; Unanue ER: Activated macrophages induce vascular proliferation. Nature 269, 804-6, 1977.
2. Stolpen AH; Guinan EC; Fiers W; Pober JS: Recombinant tumor necrosis factor and immune interferon act singly and in combination to reorganize human vascular endothelial cell monolayers. Am.J.Pathol. 123, 16-24, 1986.
3. Sato N; Goto T; Haranaka K; Satomi N; Nariuchi H; Mano-Hirano Y; Sawasaki Y: Actions of tumor necrosis factor on cultured vascular endothelial cells: morphological modulation, growth inhibition and cytotoxicity. J.Natl.Cancer Inst. 76, 1113-1121, 1986.
4. Nawroth PP; Bank I; Handley D; Cassimeris J; Chess L; Stern D: Tumor necrosis factor/cachectin interacts wih endothelial cell receptors to induce release of interleukin 1. J.Exp.Med. 163, 1363-1375, 1986.
5. Form DM; Auerbach R: PGE$_2$ and angiogenesis. Proc.Soc.Exp.Biol.Med. 172, 214-218, 1983.
6. Watt SL; Auerbach R: A mitogenic factor for endothelial cells obtained from mouse secondary mixed leukocyte cultures. J.Immunol. 136, 197-200 1986.
7. Mizel SB; Mizel D: Purification to apparent homogeneity of murine interleukin 1. J.Immunol. 126, 834-837, 1981.
8. Auerbach R; Alby L; Grieves J; Joseph C; Lindgren C; Morrissey LW; Sidky YA; Tu M; Watt SL: A monoclonal antibody against angiotensin-converting enzyme: Its use as a marker for murine, bovine and human endothelial cells. Proc.Natl.Acad.Sci.(USA) 79, 7891-7895, 1982.
9. Gumkowski F; Kaminska G; Kaminski M; Morrissey LW; Auerbach R: Heterogeneity of mouse vascular endothelium: in vitro studies of lymphatic, large blood vessel and microvascular endothelial cells. Blood Vessels (in press).
10. Sidky YA; Auerbach R: Lymphocyte-induced angiogenesis: A quantitative and sensitive assay of the graft-vs.-host reaction. J.Exp.Med. 141, 1084-1100, 1975.
11. Muthukkaruppan VR; Auerbach R: Angiogenesis in the mouse cornea. Science 205, 1416-1418, 1979.
12. Muthukkaruppan VR; Kubai L; Auerbach R: Tumor-induced neovascularization in the mouse eye. J.Natl.Cancer Inst. 69, 699-708, 1982.

Supported by grants EY 3243 and CA 28656 from the National Institutes of Health

HETEROGENEITY OF VASCULAR ENDOTHELIAL CELLS: ITS POSSIBLE ROLE IN SELECTIVE
NEOVASCULARIZATION IN THE EYE

ROBERT AUERBACH, G. KAMINSKA, J. WEBER, F. GUMKOWSKI, M. KAMINSKI, L.W.
MORRISSEY, J. BIELICH, V. WOODS, W.C. LU, and L. KUBAI
Laboratory of Developmental Biology, Department of Zoology, University of
Wisconsin, Madison WI 53706 USA

1. INTRODUCTION

The central hypothesis of our laboratory is that vascular endothelial
cells are not all alike, and that their differences reflect in large part
their developmental origins (1-4). In order to document these differences
between endothelial cells of different organs we have used monoclonal and
polyclonal antibodies to delineate organ-specific determinants (1-3). We
have used a variety of plant lectins to characterize cell surface-
associated lectin-binding sites (5). Further, we have demonstrated that
differences exist in the adhesion of different tumor cells to various
endothelial cell monolayers (6,7).

In this report I will review this work briefly, and then describe our
initial research on vascular endothelial cells obtained from various parts
of the mouse eye. These studies led to the hypothesis that selective ocular
neovascularization reflects at least in part the differential responsiveness
of endothelial cells obtained from different tissue sites within the eye.

2. MATERIALS AND METHODS

2.1 Mice
All of our studies have been carried out with BALB/cAu mice. Mouse
embryos staged by the vaginal plug method were used to obtain trophoblast
tissue.

2.2 Endothelial cell cultures
Endothelial cells were obtained using collagenase treatment of minced
tissues, followed by selective retention of microvascular fragments on 15μ
Nitex mesh. Fragments were then placed in dishes coated with gelatin, or
20% Matrigel and permitted to grow to confluence. Culture medium in
general included endothelial cell growth factor as well as tumor-
conditioned medium. Details were modified for endothelial cells from different sources (2,5).

2.3 Cell identification
Characterization of endothelial cells included binding of acetyl-LDL and
of a monoclonal antibody to angiotensin-converting enzyme (4). Cell sorting
to enrich for endothelial cells in mixed cultures was carried out on the
basis of these two markers. An antibody to a macrophage antigen not shared
by endothelial cells (Ly 5) was used to assure absence of macrophage

contamination. Endothelial cell identification was confirmed by electron microscopy and by the gross morphological appearance of cells in vitro. Formation of tubes resembling microvessels in vitro served as further confirmation of the endothelial nature of these cells.

2.4 Transplantation protocols

Preliminary experiments have now been carried out in which anterior eye chamber grafts (cf.9) or intracorneal grafts (10,11) were used to elicit intraocular hemorrhage and neovascular reactions. A detailed report of these procedures is in preparation.

3. RESULTS

The fact that organ-specific antigens are expressed on endothelial cells is shown in Figure 1. Endothelial cells from the mouse brain express brain-specific anti-MBE 1, they express allele-specific Thy 1.2, and they lack Ia antigens. This contrasts to ovary-derived endothelial cells which do not express MBE-1 or Thy 1.2, but do express Ia antigens as well as an ovary-specific antigen detected by antibody RO-15.

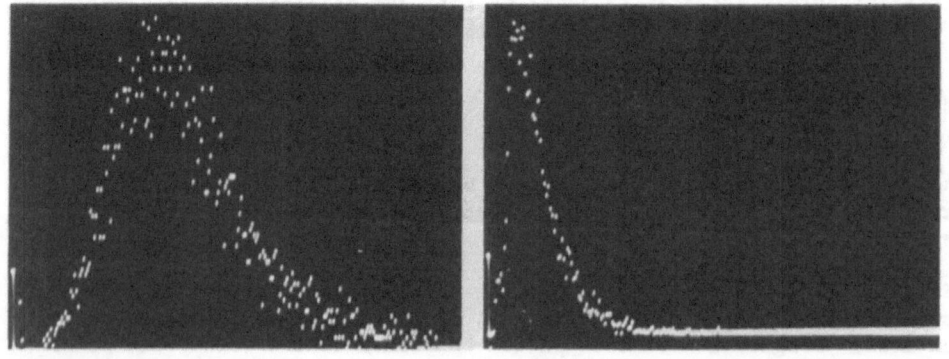

Fig. 1 Fluorescence profile of mouse brain (left) or ovary (right) endothelium stained with anti-MBE antibody. (from ref. 3)

Organ-associated differences are also seen in adhesion experiments involving different tumor cell lines (Figure 2). Thus glioma cells show greater adhesion to mouse brain endothelial cells than to ovary-derived endothelium, while ovary-seeking teratoma cells show the reverse specificity.

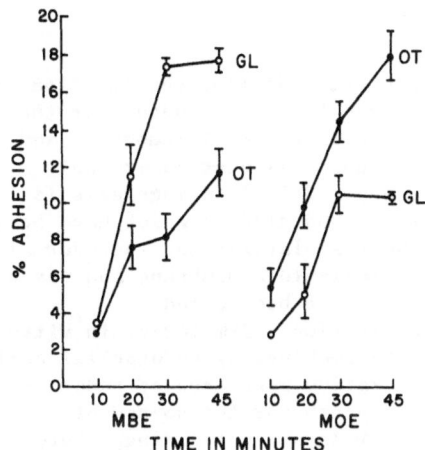

Fig. 2 Adhesion of glioma (GL)
and ovary seeking teratoma (OT)
cells to mouse brain (MBE) or
ovary (MOE) endothelial cell
monolayers. (from ref. 7)

The diversity of endothelial cells from different sources has been further
documented. For example, using 4 different tumor types and 5 different
target monolayers, we have documented that each tumor differs in its adhesion pattern (6). Hepatomas adhere preferentially to liver endothelial
cells; mammary tumor cells show preferential adhesion to lymphatic endothelium. Similarly, using a panel of 8 plant lectins we have been able to show
that each endothelial cell type has a unique profile of lectin binding properties (5).

Recently in our laboratory (unpublished observations) we have extended our
analysis to include vascular endothelial cells derived from different portions of the mouse eye. Our first isolates were from normal adult mouse
retina. Retinas were dissected and subjected to standard collagenase
digestion. Following isolation of microvascular fragments a second collagenase treatment was used to generate retinal endothelial cell cultures. These
cultures could be passaged provided tumor-conditioned medium was used.

To obtain vascular endothelial cells we have used intracorneal grafts of
murine, syngeneic, activated macrophages to elicit corneal neovascularization (cf.12). At the height of the reaction the region containing vessels
was isolated, corneal endothelium was removed by scraping, and the remaining
tissue was placed in culture to permit cell outgrowth. Cells were then
removed from the dishes, dissociated using collagenase, labelled with a
monoclonal antibody to angiotensin-converting enzyme, and sorted using a
FACS-IV cell sorter to generate corneal vascular endothelial cell cultures.
As a second approach we have introduced Elvax pellets into the cornea to act
as an inflammatory stimulus for vascularization. Corneas were then processed for cell culture in similar manner.

To obtain iris-derived endothelial cells we have implanted mouse
embryonic trophoblasts into the anterior eye chamber to elicit a hemorrhagic
reaction. Subsequently massive iris neovascularization was observed, and
the reactive irises were fragmented and placed in vitro to permit outgrowth
of cells. Cultures containing a preponderance of endothelial cells were
obtained, and cell sorting protocols are now being applied to permit
establishment of pure endothelial cell lines from the iris.

4. DISCUSSION

Studies of experimental angiogenesis have not addressed the question of selective neovascularization (13). It has been tacitly assumed that the sequence of reactions that include dissolution of basement membranes and the induction of endothelial cell migration and proliferation are uniformly involved and that, for this reason, any model of angiogenesis is equally useful in providing analytical data. Thus studies which have been carried out using the corneal model, iris neovascularization, intradermal angiogenesis, vessel formation in the chorio-allantoic membrane and vascular responses in the explanted chick yolk sac have been cited interchangeably to document the angiogenic reaction. Similarly, in vitro models of directed (chemotactic) or random (chemokinetic) endothelial cell movement or of enhanced or inhibited proliferative responses of endothelial cells in vitro have been used without concern for the source of endothelial cells used in these bioassays. It is not surprising, therefore, that angiogenesis inducers as well as angiogenesis inhibitors have not appeared to be selective in their actions.

We have proposed one method for obtaining selective neovascularization. We have suggested that endothelial cell lymphokines, i.e. lymphocyte-produced factors that act on endothelial cells, may lead to site-specific neovascularization if the release of those factors is locally restricted. Thus we have argued that if such lymphokines are released only on antigenic stimulation, then the organ-specific presentation of antigens by endothelial cells may lead to localized release of these angiogenic lymphokines (14). In local sites of immune reactions and inflammation the corresponding selectivity could be mediated by cytokines released from macrophages and other leukocytic effector cells.

A second possible means of obtaining selective neovascularization, however, takes advantage of the fact that endothelial cells are not a uniform cell population. Examples that we have already demonstrated include variation in lectin-binding sites indicating marked differences in terminal sugar moieties, and differences in cell adhesion molecules that may lead to selective adhesion of migrating tumor cells.

Given these striking differences it appears reasonable to propose that there will be a wide spectrum of responses of different vascular endothelial beds to the bewildering array of angiogenesis-inducing factors. The hypothesis leads to the prediction that such diverse factors as heparin binding growth factors (ECGF, FGF, RDGF), non-heparin binding factors (ECL-1, angiogenin), proteases (tissue plasminogen activator, urokinase), and prostaglandins (PGE_1, PGE_2) do not all act equally on all endothelial cells. Similarly, the hypothesis predicts that different inhibitors of angiogenesis such as heparin, corticosteroids, aortic inhibitor, cartilage-derived inhibitor, platelet factor IV, protamine or interferon or specific antibodies may also act selectively in influencing neovascular reactions evoked in different sites.

The concept of differential neovascular reactions seems particularly relevant to the problem of ocular neovascularization where corneal, iris, choroidal and retinal vascular reactions have different etiologies and different outcomes (15). While this concept may appear to complicate the design of experiments and the interpretation of results, it supports the belief that selective methods can be developed that will be effective in regulating specific neovascular reactions associated with ocular disease.

REFERENCES

1. Auerbach R; Joseph J: Cell surface markers on endothelial cells: A developmental perspective. In: "The Biology of Endothelial Cells," Jaffe EA, ed. Martinus Nijhoff, The Hague, 393-400, 1983.
2. Joseph J; Tu M; Alby L; Grieves J; Houser B; Kubai L; Morrissey L; Sidky Y; Watt SL; Auerbach R: Immunological probes for the study of endothelial cell diversity. In: "The Endothelial Cell - A Pluripotent Control Cell of the Vessel Wall," Thilo-Korner DGS; Freshney RI, eds. Karger, Basel, 55-66, 1983.
3. Auerbach R; Alby L; Morrissey LW; Tu M; Joseph J: Organ-specificity of capillary endothelial cells. Microvasc.Res. 29, 401-411, 1985.
4. Auerbach R; Alby L; Grieves J; Joseph J; Lindgren C; Morrissey LW; Sidky YA; Tu M; Watt SL: A monoclonal antibody against angiotensin-converting enzyme: Its use as a marker for murine, bovine and human endothelial cells. Proc.Natl.Acad.Sci. (USA) 79, 7891-7895, 1982.
5. Gumkowski F; Kaminska G; Kaminski M; Morrissey LW; Auerbach R: Heterogeneity of mouse vascular endothelium: In vitro studies of lymphatic, large blood vessel and microvascular endothelial cells. Blood Vessels (in press).
6. Auerbach R; Lu WC; Pardon E; Gumkowski F; Kaminska G; Kaminski M: Specificity of adhesion between tumor cells and capillary endothelium: an in vitro correlate of preferential metastasis in vivo. Cancer Res. (in press).
7. Alby L; Auerbach R: Differential adhesion of tumor cells to capillary endothelial cells in vitro. Proc.Natl.Acad.Sci. (USA) 81, 5739-5743, 1984.
8. Kaminski M; Auerbach R: Presence of endothelium decreases mouse NK cell activity against tumor cells. (Submitted)
9. Kubai L; Auerbach R: A new source of embryonic lymphocytes in the mouse. Nature 301, 154-156. 1983.
10. Muthukkaruppan VR; Auerbach R: Angiogenesis in the mouse cornea. Science 205, 1416-1418, 1979.
11. Muthukkaruppan VR; Kubai L; Auerbach R: Tumor-induced neovascularization in the mouse eye. J.Natl.Cancer Inst. 69, 699-708, 1982.
12. Epstein RJ: (this symposium)
13. Folkman J: Tumor angiogenesis. Adv.Canc.Res. 43, 175-230, 1985.
14. Joseph J; Cairns JS; Auerbach R: Ia antigens of murine epididymal fat pad endothelial cells. Immunohistology and mixed lymphocyte endothelial cell culture studies. Transplantation (in press).
15. Garner A: Ocular angiogenesis. Internat.Rev.Exp.Pathol. 28, 249-306, 1986.

Supported by grants EY 3243 and CA 28656 from the National Institutes of Health

CORNEAL ENDOTHELIALIZATION IN EXPERIMENTAL ANTERIOR SYNECHIAS AND RUBEOSIS
IRIDIS

Z. ZAGÓRSKI, K.W. RUPRECHT, G.O.H. NAUMANN

1. INTRODUCTION

Corneal endothelial cells respond to different kinds of trauma by migration and production of a new basement membrane. They proliferate not
only on the denuded Descemet membrane but also over suitable surfaces within the eye. Such ectopic endothelial proliferation is most commonly seen
in cases of anterior synechias of iris or vitreous, angle contusion deformities, rubeosis iridis or in the presence of abnormal endothelium,
like in posterior polymorphous dystrophy or irido-corneo-endothelial syndrome[9].

Histopathological and experimental studies suggest that factors inducing corneal endothelial proliferation are trauma to endothelium (growth
stimulus), availability of suitable substrate (extracellular matrix) and
growth factors released by chronic inflammation or trauma[5,7,10]. Our
earlier observations of endothelialization of experimental anterior synechias have shown that endothelium does not proliferate over normal iris
surface or proliferation stops soon[10]. This paper presents observations
on the corneal endothelial proliferation in experimental reactive neovascularization of iris and experimental anterior synechias.

2. MATERIAL AND METHODS

Alloplastic, autologous and homologous material was implanted into
the anterior chamber of 19 eyes of 18 pigmented rabbits weighing from 2,5
to 5 kg. All experiments were done in general anesthesia of Xylazine and
Ketanest i.m. Six rabbits received alloplastic material (silicone rubber
1 eye, silicone sponge 3 eyes and glass splitter 2 eyes), 5 autologous
material (ear cartilage 1 eye, conjunctiva 4 eyes) and 7 homologous Brown-
Pierce tumor. Fluorescein angiography was then performed periodically up
to 4 months. The animals were sacrified with an overdose of Nembutal i.v.
after a time varying from 3 days to 4 months, eyes were enucleated, fixed
in 4% paraformaldehyde-1% glutaraldehyde solution and embedded in paraffin .
8μ sections were then stained with PAS and hematoxyline and studied under
light microscope.

An additional group of 13 rabbits was used to produce anterior
synechias. In 10 eyes iris and cornea were approximated by means of transcorneal 10-0 nylon suture and in the remaining 3 eyes by introduction of
fibrine glue (Tissucol) between iris and cornea after evacuation of aqueous. The histologic studies were done as above between 3 weeks and 5 months
after surgery.

Neovascularization was found in 14 out of 18 eyes where foreign
material was implanted into the anterior chamber. Implantation of Brown-
Pierce tumor had the strongest angiogenic action, however the very fast
growing rate of tumor filling the anterior chamber after 2-3 weeks did not
allow to study its possible influence on corneal endothelial proliferation.

In another 2 groups where alloplastic or autologous material was implanted new vessel formation was found in 7 out of 11 eyes (Fig. 1, Table I).

Endothelialization was seen in 7 eyes, in 5 being simultaneous with neovascularization (Table II). Retrocorneal fibrous membranes were endothelialized in all these 7 eyes while endothelial proliferation over the iris was seen in 4 eyes where iris was in contact with cornea or retrocorneal membrane (Fig. 2).

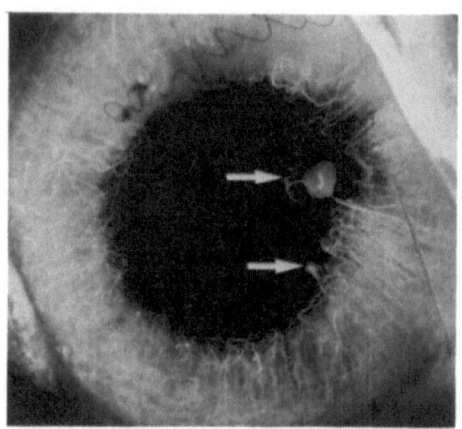

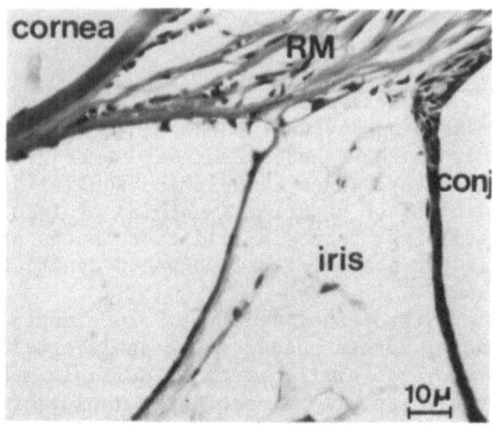

Fig. 1 Focal neovascularization of the iris 13 weeks after implantation of autologous conjunctiva into anterior chamber, rabbit

Fig. 2 Corneal endothelial proliferation over retrocorneal membrane (RM) and iris 13 weeks after implantation of autologous bulbar conjuntiva into anterior chamber. PAS-staining

TABLE 1 Experimental focal neovascularization of iris

Foreign material in A.C.: 18 eyes		Neovascularization: 14 eyes
1. Alloplastic	6	4
Silicone rubber	1	1
Silicone sponge	3	3
Glass splitter	2	–
2. Autologous	5	3
Ear cartilage	1	–
Conjunctiva	4	3
3. Homologous	7	7
(Brown-Pearce tumor)		

Experimental anterior synechias were in all eyes accompanied by a small amount of retrocorneal membrane, which was always endothelialized. Endothelial growth over the iris was found in 4 eyes (Table III), although proliferation stopped at the area where iris was not covered with fibrous tissue or basement membrane (Fig. 3). In some broad synechias a new basement membrane was produced by endothelial cells both towards cornea and iris (Fig. 4).

TABLE II   Corneal Endothelial Proliferation in Experimental Neovasculariza-
           tion of iris

Endothelialization:	7 eyes	RM	Iris
Silicone rubber	1	1	1
Silicone sponge	1	1	1
Glass splitter	1	1	–
Ear cartilage	1	1	–
Conjunctiva	3	3	2

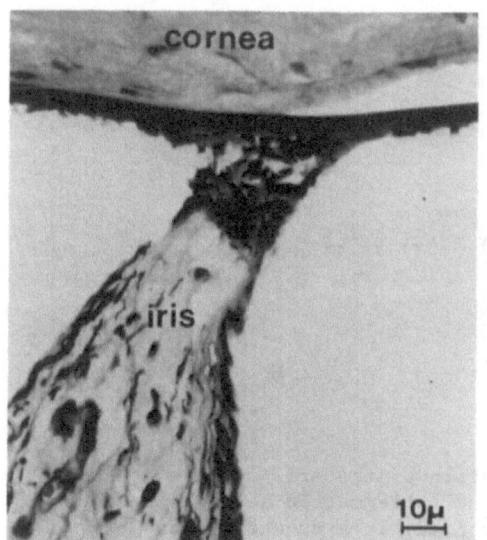 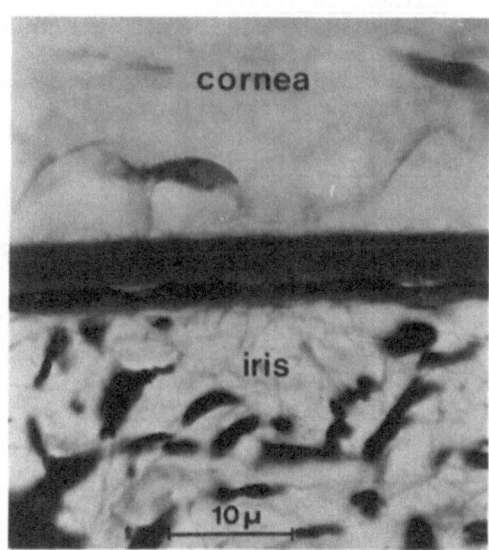

Fig. 3 Experimental anterior synchia
produced by 10-0 nylon sutures 8 weeks
postoperative. Endothelial proliferation stops at the normal iris surface.
PAS-staining

Fig. 4 "Stressed" endothelial cells
in the area of synechia produce a
new basement membrane both toward
cornea and iris. PAS-staining.

3. DISCUSSION

High coincidence of rubeosis iridis and endothelialization of anterior
chamber suggests that there are common factors promoting both symptoms[2,6,7].
This view is further supported by facts showing that some growth factors,[8]
like Fibroblast Growth Factor[4] and Retina-Derived-Growth-Factor (Crude
Retinal Extract)[3] support proliferation of both corneal and vascular endothelial cells in vitro[1].   In eyes with implanted Brown-Pierce carcinoma,
Tumor Angiogenic Factor could influence vascular neoformation. This model
however was unsuitable for studies of corneal endothelial proliferation.
In the remaining eyes new vessel formation was induced by factors released
by inflammation and trauma caused by foreign material implanted into anterior chamber. These factors stimulated also corneal endothelial proliferation. It seems probable, that inflammation and trauma not only delivered

TABLE III   Corneal Endothelium in Experimental
             Anterior Synechias

Method	Endothelialization		
		EM	Iris
10-0-nylon suture	10	10	4
Fibrin glue	3	3	-

TABLE IV   Factors Influencing Corneal Endothelial
            Proliferation

I.   Suitable substrates
     1. Basement membrane with acellular surface
     2. Retrocorneal fibrous tissue
     3. Modified iris surface (rubeosis, necrosis, scarring)
     4. Vitreous strands

II. Unsuitable substrates
     1. Normal iris surface
     2. Normal trabecular meshwork
     3. Other tissue surfaces covered by vital cells

III. Promoting factors
     1. Chron. inflamm. or trauma
     2. (defect blood-acqueous-barrier)
     3. Retinal angiog. factor
     4. Healthy endothelium

growth factors but also caused modification of the iris surface enabling
endothelial proliferation. Some amount of inflammation seems to be necessary to support endothelial growth over iris. In eyes where anterior
synechias were produced by fibrin glue and the degree of inflammation was
minimal no endothelial proliferation over iris was found. Transcorneal 10-0
nylon suture approximating iris and cornea produced much more inflammation
and more retrocorneal fibrous tissue could be found. This fibrous tissue
(retrocorneal membrane) was always covered by endothelial cells which represented a normal mechanism of corneal wound healing process. Fibrous
proliferation ceased after being covered by endothelial cells. Endothelial
growth over the iris was seen only in the areas where iris surface was
covered with fibrous tissue or basement membrane. In some eyes such a membrane was extensively produced by endothelial cells. It is possible that
endothelial cells, which began to grow over modified iris surface, may slowly continue to proliferate, laying their own extracellular matrix. Such
mechanism needs however constant delivery of growth factors and probably
more time than in our experiments. So we believe that in our cases another
mechanism could be important. Stressed endothelial cells in contact with
iris in the area of synechia produce extracellular matrix (new basement
membrane) not only on the corneal side but also toward the iris. Iris,
covered with the new basement membrane can further separate from the cornea
and, being a suitable substrate for endothelial growth, may be repopulated
with endothelial cells (Fig. 5). This mechanism is shown on Fig. 6, modified from Waring et al[9], where production of a new basement membrane by
stressed endothelial cells was proposed only on one cell side.

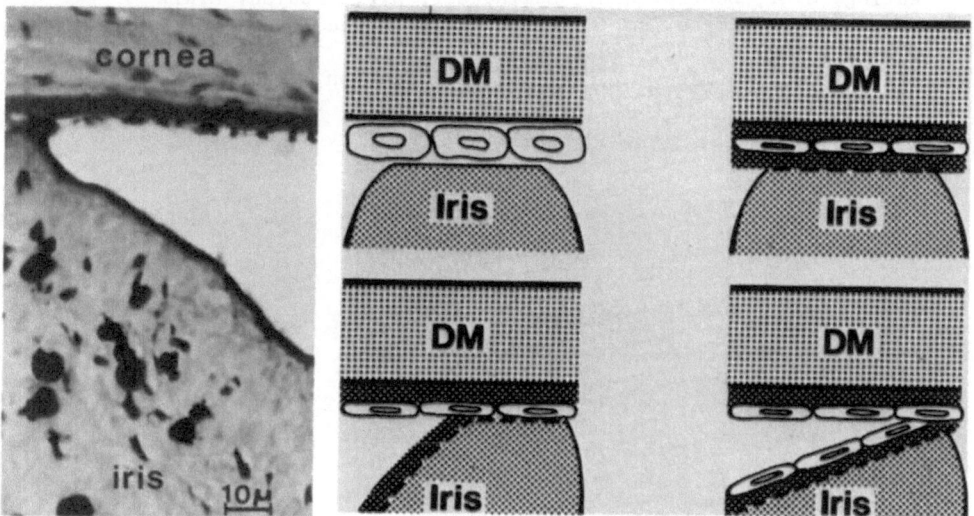

Fig. 5 Basement-membrane covered iris
after partial separation of the synechia. PAS-staining.

Fig. 6 Schematic presentation of a
possible mechanism of endothelialization of iris in anterior synechias

Acknowledgement
This work was supported in Part (Z.F. Zagórski, M.D.) by Alexander von
Humboldt Foundation, 5300 Bonn-Bad Godesberg, Federal Republic of Germany

References
1. Boulton, M. (1986): personal communication.
2. Gartner, S., Taffet, D., Friedman, A.H.: The association of rubeosis
    iridis with endothelialization of the anterior chamber. Br. J. Oph-
    thalmol. 61: 267-271 (1977)
3. Glaser, B.M., D'Amore, P.A., Michels, R.G., Patz, A., Fenselau, A.:
    Demonstration of vasoproliferative activity from mammalian retina.
    J. Cell Biol. 84: 298-304 (1980)
4. Gospodarowicz, D., Giguére, L.: Growth factors, effect on corneal
    tissue. In: McDevitt, D.S. (ed.): Cell Biology of the Eye. pp. 98-142
    (Academic Press, New York, 1982)
5. Jonas, J., Zagórski, Z., Völcker, H.E.: Corneale Endothelialisierung
    zentraler vorderer Synechien. Klin. Mbl. Augenheilk. (in preparation)
6. Naumann, G.O.H., Apple, D.J.: Pathology of the Eye (Springer Verlag,
    New York, 1986)
7. Pabst-Hofacker, M., Domarus, D.v.: Die Endothelialisierung der Vorder-
    kammer. Klinik und Histopathologie. Klin. Mbl. Augenheilk. 177: 174-179
    (1980).
8. Ruprecht, K.W., Naumann, G.O.H.: Zur Klinik und Histopathologie der
    Rubeosis Iridis. Ber. Dtsch. Ophthalmol. Ges. 76: 797-799 (1979)

9. Waring, G.O., Bourne, W.M., Edelhauser, H.F., Kenyon, K.R.:
    The Corneal Endothelium. Normal and Pathologic Structure and Function.
    Ophthalmology 89: 531-590 (1982).
10. Zagŕski, Z., Hofmann, C., Gossler, B., Naumann, G.O.H.: Corneale
    Endothelialisierung experimenteller zentraler vorderer Synechien.
    Zbl. f. Ophthalmologie (in press).

NEOVASCULAR GLAUCOMA: ETIOLOGIC FACTORS AND MANAGEMENT CONSIDERATIONS

LARRY E. MAGARGAL, M.D.
GARY C. BROWN, M.D.
JAMES J. AUGSBURGER, M.D.
LARRY A. DONOSO, M.D., PH.D.

INTRODUCTION

Neovascular glaucoma (NVG) is a devastating complication of a variety of ischemic disease processes that affect the eye.[1-17] Previous studies[1-6] have elucidated various etiologic entities associated with NVG; presented herein are the presumed etiologic factors in 208 consecutive patients with NVG referred to the senior author (LEM) for evaluation and treatment.[7] The long term result of therapeutic intervention is summarized according to the primary underlying condition and the status of the angle at the time iris neovascularization (NVI) was established.

MATERIALS AND METHODS

Included in this study were 208 consecutive cases referred to the Retina Vascular Unit (LEM) with NVG over a four year period (1978-1981). Each patient underwent a complete ophthalmologic examination and fundus-iris fluorescein angiography[8] was utilized to assess the degree of retinal ischemia and document the presence of iris neovascularization (NVI). Medical and neurovascular consultations were obtained in selected cases; carotid studies were obtained only in patients with clinical features of the ocular ischemic syndrome.[9]

RESULTS

The patients ranged in age from 19 to 89 years, with a mean age of 62 years. Females comprised 54% of the entire group; 51% had systemic arterial hypertension and 46% had diabetes mellitus. The presumed etiologic factors found in this series of 208 patients are listed in Table 1.

RETINAL VEIN OBSTRUCTION

Retinal vein obstruction (RVO) was the most common primary association accounting for 36% (75/208) of the NVG cases. Central retinal vein obstruction (CRVO) was present in 67 cases, hemispheric vein obstruction (HBRVO) occurred in 5 eyes, and temporal branch retinal vein obstruction (TBRVO) was documented in 3 eyes. No cases of bilateral NVG were encountered in this group of RVO patients. Although 20% (15/67) of the patients with an ischemic RVO pattern also had diabetes, the fellow eyes exhibited only background or no diabetic retinopathy; therefore diabetes was considered to be a secondary factor in these cases. Systemic arterial hypertension was found in 53% (40/75) of patients in the RVO group. Digital subtraction angiography found an underlying carotid stenosis in 13% of those studied (20 cases), a figure not felt to be higher than that expected in this age group.[13]

DIABETIC RETINOPATHY

Overall, 46% (96/208) of our patients had diabetes mellitus, making it the most commonly encountered primary systemic disease found in association with NVG. Preproliferative or proliferative diabetic retinopathy (PDR) was primarily associated with the development of NVG in 32% (67/208) of our cases. Women comprised 66% (44/67) of diabetics with NVG and systemic arterial hypertension was present in 60% (40/67).

Bilateral NVG was present in 12% (25/208); 24 of the 25 bilateral cases occurred secondary to bilateral PDR, the remaining non-diabetic patient had bilateral high grade carotid obstructive disease and was classified as having the ocular ischemic syndrome (OIS).

CAROTID ARTERY OBSTRUCTION

Of the 208 patients, 27 (13%) had NVG in association with a high grade ipsilateral carotid artery obstruction. Each case of the OIS had at least 90% or greater carotid artery obstruction as demonstrated by either digital subtraction or conventional carotid angiography. Men comprised 74% of this group and 30% (8/27) of the patients were diabetic.

OTHER ASSOCIATED CONDITIONS

In nine patients (4%) no unequivocal etiology was found to explain the NVG. Most of these patients presented to us with advanced disease and blind painful eyes hoping for an alternative to enucleation.

The eight patients (4%) with NVG and CRAO either refused carotid angiography or were felt to be in such poor general health that carotid surgery was not indicated. These patients may well be cases of the OIS, although the stenosis may involve the ophthalmic artery rather than the cervical vessels.[7,9]

Of the eight patients (4%) with evidence of a combined retinal arterial-venous obstruction, four had a CRAO-CRVO combination and four had a BRAO-CRVO pattern. One case of CRAO-CRVO occurred following a retrobulbar injection and NVG developed two weeks later.[7]

Rhegmatogenous retinal detachment accounted for NVG in 3 (2%) of our cases, including one case of Wagner's vitreo-retinopathy.[7]

Miscellaneous factors were present in eight patients (4%) and are included in Table 1.

LONG TERM RESULTS OF TREATMENT

Whenever possible, the posterior segment ischemia was treated with either panretinal laser photocoagulation (PRP) or pan retinal cryo ablation after being placed on our maximum tolerated medical regimen which usually included Atropine Sulfate 1%, Inflammase Forte 1%, Propine 0.1%, Timoptic 0.5% topical drops and Diamox sequels 500 mgs orally all twice daily. Those cases with angle vessels received angle photocoagulation in an attempt to prevent complete synechial angle closure. Cases with greater than 50% angle closure or cases unresponsive to medical and laser/cryo treatment, underwent various combinations of cyclocryo therapy and/or filtering surgery with or without insertion of a seton. All but 2 patients with the OIS had carotid bypass surgery in an effort to improve the ocular and cerebral circulation. Table 1 summarizes each treatment category and the long term response to treatment.

Only 18 of the 75 patients (24%) with RVO and NVG still had less than 50% synechial angle closure at the time of initiating treatment. While only 11% (2/18) lost vision completely, 4 required additional glaucoma surgery and all required topical glaucoma medication to maintain a satisfactory pressure at their last visit. No enucleations were required in this group. In contrast, of the 57 cases with extensive angle closure initially, 49 (86%) ended with complete loss of vision (NLP). Of the 49 blind eyes, all had multiple surgical procedures and 35 (70%) are either phthisical or cosmetically unacceptable but pain free on topical medication. Four eyes required enucleation for control of pain and 13 received retrobulbar alcohol injections. The remaining 8 cases (14%) have either LP or HM visual acuity and a cosmetically acceptable pain free eye on medication.

Of the 67 patients with diabetic retinopathy and NVG, 24 of whom had bilateral disease, 38 (57%) presented with less than 50% angle closure and 61% (25/38) responded to our initial treatment regimen. While only 4 patients (11%) lost vision completely, two had bilateral NVG and one eye required enucleation. Surprisingly, 80% (30/38) achieved CF or better vision with 12% at least 20/200. Nineteen (50%) patients are maintained on topical drops for pressure control. In contrast, 29 of the 67 patients had over 50% angle closure initially and 13 (44%) of these cases progressed to complete loss of vision (NLP) following multiple glaucoma surgical procedures. Of the 16 eyes with vision, only 2 are better than CF. Four blind eyes required enucleation and the other 9 are either phthisical or cosmetically unacceptable but remain pain free on topical medication.

Of the 27 cases with the ocular ischemic syndrome, 23 underwent carotid bypass surgery in conjunction with treatment to control the intraocular pressures which tended to be low preoperatively (6-28 mmHg) due to ciliary body shutdown. At presentation 20 (74%) of cases had less than 50% angle closure and all but one case (which had reocclusion of the carotid vessels postoperatively) maintained vision and satisfactory intraocular pressures during follow up.[10] Of the seven cases presenting with extensive angle closure, one refused surgery and had the eye enucleated elsewhere and 3 lost vision completely after successful carotid surgery due to an abrupt rise in intraocular pressure postoperatively. Overall, of the 23 cases that underwent carotid surgery, the vision was completely lost in 3 (13%), was maintained in 18 (78%) and improved at least 2 lines in 2 (9%).[10]

Thirty-nine eyes had a variety of ischemic diseases and the final outcome tended to parallel the intensity of the ischemic event and the extent of angle closure at the time of initiating treatment. Overall, 10 eyes presented with greater than 50% angle closure, 8 eyes ended with a final visual acuity of NLP and 2 eyes were enucleated.

DISCUSSION

Systemic arterial hypertension was found to be the most common underlying disease entity, being present in 51% of our patients as compared to an expected rate of 30% in an age matched population.[7,9] Since hypertensive retinopathy per se does not appear to be a primary cause of NVG, we believe that hypertension most likely contributes secondarily by exacerbating other ischemic vascular disease (i.e. diabetic retinopathy), or predisposes to the development of other known primary etiologic entities (i.e. RVO) that lead to NVG.

Diabetic retinopathy was the second leading primary cause of NVG in our series; likewise diabetes was second only to arterial hypertension as an associated systemic disease entity, being present in 46% of our patients.

Perhaps the most surprising finding was the high incidence of chronic ophthalmic artery insufficiency (13%) in this study. However, the actual incidence is probably even higher since we only studied those patients with strong clinical evidence of the ocular ischemic syndrome and who were in satisfactory general health to be a candidate for carotid surgery. The recent availability of non-invasive techniques, such as duplex ultrasound, will enable further clarification of this important relationship.[9]

This study strongly suggests that the presence of bilateral NVG occurs overwhelmingly in patients with underlying PDR. Since diabetic retinopathy tends to be bilateral and symmetrical[4] whereas bilateral RVO is relatively uncommon (4-6%)[11] as is bilaterality of the OIS (8%),[12] this observation serves as a distinguishing feature in the management of advanced cases.

As in other studies[6,14] we found that the age at the time of NVG was younger in patients with diabetes (55 years) than in those with RVO (69 years), or in people with the OIS (64 years). Although the differences were not statistically significant,[7] they correlate well with the onset of posterior segment neovascularization.[11,12,13]

The sex distribution appears to differ according to the primary etiology of NVG. Whereas women comprised 66% of the diabetic group with NVG and 57% of the RVO group, men were far more commonly seen in the OIS group by a 3:1 margin. Since 61% of diabetics in the United States are female[14] and 75 % of patients with severe carotid obstructive disease are male,[9,13] the observed differences are closely correlated with the prevalence of the underlying disease entities.

Of the 208 patients in our study, 97% had an associated posterior segment disease known to produce retinal ischemia. One entity not encountered as a primary factor for NVG was chronic open angle glaucoma. Although others have reported such an association[3,4,5] in from 2-6% of cases, we believe that these cases actually occur in the context of an unrecognized RVO or an unsuspected OIS.

Because of our interest in retina vascular disease, our etiologic data may be biased in this direction; however, our experience subsequent to 1981 has indicated that with the aggressive use of treatment to stabilize posterior segment ischemia, the incidence of NVG has been dramatically reduced.[15,16,17]

The result of treatment of early NVG depends on the underlying condition being best in cases of ischemic TBRVO and worst in ischemic CRVO, probably because the ischemic drive is proportionate to the location, extent and rapidity of onset of the vaso-obstructive event.[9,17] The status of the anterior chamber angle is a critical factor in the final visual outcome; once angle closure is essentially complete, many eyes lose vision completely (38% in this series overall) and many end up either phthisical, chronically hypertensive and cosmetically unacceptable, or were enucleated (5%). It is especially important to recognize the often rapid rise in intraocular pressure that occurs following successful carotid surgery in cases with the OIS; unless anticipated and treated aggressively pre and post operatively, the benefits of improved ocular circulation will be negated. With the application of early laser treatment in high risk ischemic eyes, neovascular glaucoma has almost disappeared in our practice, the failure rate being approximately 1-2%.

SUMMARY

This updated review of 208 patients with neovascular glaucoma (NVG) referred to the senior author (LEM) over a four year period was undertaken to determine associated etiologic conditions and the long term results of therapeutic intervention. The most common primary predisposing conditions were retinal venous obstructions (36%), preproliferative or proliferative diabetic retinopathy (32%), and the ocular ischemic syndrome (13%). Systemic arterial hypertension was present in 51% of all patients followed by diabetes mellitus in 46%. Females comprised 65% of the diabetics and 57% of the RVO group with NVG, whereas 74% of the NVG cases due to the ocular ischemic syndrome (OIS) were males. Of the 25 bilateral cases of NVG, 24 patients had long standing diabetes. Overall, 97% of NVG eyes exhibited extensive retinal capillary non-perfusion on fluorescein angiography. Chronic ophthalmic artery insufficiency due to severe underlying carotid obstructive disease (the OIS) should be considered in cases of NVG and central retinal artery obstruction (CRAO) or in cases where the degree of retinopathy alone does not explain the presence of iris neovascularization (NVI).

TABLE 1

Etiology of NVG	Number of Cases %	Mean Age in Years	Diabetics %	Hyper-tensives %	Angle Closure %	NLP Eyes %	Enuc-leations %
RVO	75 (36%)	69.1	15 (20%)	40 (53%)	57 (76%)	51 (68%)	4 (5%)
DR	67 (32%)	54.7	67 (100%)	40 (60%)	29 (43%)	17 (25%)	5 (7%)
CAD	27 (13%)	64.2	8 (30%)	14 (52%)	7 (26%)	3 (13%)	1 (4%)
MISC CAUSES	39 (19%)	47.1	6 (12%)	12 (24%)	10 (20%)	8 (16%)	2 (4%)
TOTALS	208 (100%)	61.5	96 (46%)	106 (51%)	103 (50%)	79 (38%)	12 (5%)

Legend: RVO-Retinal Vein Obstruction; DR-Diabetic Retinopathy; CAD-Carotid Artery Disease; MISC-Miscellaneous

REFERENCES

1. Smith JL: Unilateral Glaucoma in Carotid Occlusive Disease. JAMA 1962; 182:683-684.
2. Anderson DM, Morin JD, Hunter WS: Rubeosis Iridis. Can J Ophthalmol 1971;6:183-188.
3. Hoskins HD: Neovascular Glaucoma: Current Concepts. Trans Am Acad Ophthalmol Otolaryngol 1974;78:330-333.
4. Gartner S, Henkind P: Neovascularization of the Iris (Rubeosis Iridis). Surv Ophthalmol 1978;22:291-312.
5. Schulze RR: Rubeosis Iridis. Am J Ophthalmol 1967;63:487-95.
6. Madsen PH: Haemorrhagic Glaucoma: Comparative Study in Diabetic and Non-Diabetic Patients. Br J Ophthalmol 1971;55:444-450.
7. Brown GC, Magargal LE, Schachat A, Shah H: Neovascular Glaucoma: Etiologic Considerations. Ophthalmology 1984;91:315-320.
8. Sanborn GE, Symes DJ, Magargal LE: Fundus-iris Fluorescein Angiography: Evaluation of its use in the Diagnosis of Rubeosis Iridis. Ann Ophthalmol 1986;18:52-58.

REFERENCES

9. Sanborn GE, Magargal LE: Retinal Manifestations of Carotid Disease. Clinical Ophthalmology. T.D. Duane (ed), J.B. Lippincott Company, Philadelphia, 1985.

10. Ros M, Magargal LE: Ocular Ischemic Syndrome: Long Term Complications. Ann Ophthalmol (accepted) 1986.

11. Magargal LE, Brown GC, Augsburger JJ, Parrish RK: Neovascular Glaucoma Following Central Retinal Vein Obstruction. Ophthalmology 1981;88:1095-1101.

12. Brown GC, Magargal LE, Simeone FA, et al. Arterial Obstruction and Ocular Neovascularization. Ophthalmology 1982;89:139-146.

13. Hedges TR, Giliberti OL, Magargal LE: Intravenous Digital Subtraction Angiography and its Role in Ocular Vascular Disease. Arch Ophthalmol 1985;103:666-669.

14. West EM: Epidemiology of Diabetes and its Vascular Lesions. New York: Elsevier-Dutton 1978;138.

15. Tasman W, Magargal LE, Augsburger JJ. Effects of Argon Laser Photocoagulation on Rubeosis Iridis and Angle Neovascularization. Ophthalmology 1980;87:400-402.

16. Magargal LE, Donoso LA, Sanborn GE: Retinal Ischemia and Risk of Neovascularization Following Central Retinal Vein Obstruction. Ophthalmology 1982;89:1241-1245.

17. Sanborn GE, Magargal LE, Jaeger E: Venous Occlusive Disease of the Retina. Clinical Ophthalmology, T.D. Duane (ed), J.B. Lippincott Company, Philadelphia 1986.

ACKNOWLEDGEMENTS

From the Retina Vascular Unit (LEM,GCB), the Oncology Service (JJA) and the Research Department (LAD) Wills Eye Hospital, Thomas Jefferson University, Philadelphia, Pennsylvania.

Presented in part at the 1983 American Academy of Ophthalmology Meeting, Chicago, the 1985 Annual Wills Eye Hospital Conference, Philadelphia, and the 1986 International Symposium of Ocular Circulation and Neovascularization, Jerusalem.

Supported in part by the Retina Research and Development Foundation of Philadelphia and the Pennsylvania Lions Sight Conservation Corporation.

The authors wish to acknowledge the late Professor I.C. Michaelson and Paul Henkind, M.D., Ph.D. for their pioneering contributions to our current understanding of retina vascular disease and to P. Robb McDonald, M.D., Thomas D. Duane, M.D. and William H. Annesley, Jr., M.D. for their support of the Retina Vascular Unit of the Wills Eye Hospital over the past ten years.

NEOVASCULAR GLAUCOMA AFTER EXTRACAPSULAR CATARACT EXTRACTION IN DIABETIC PATIENTS WITH DIABETIC RETINOPATHY

E. Bessler, B.Z. Biedner, M. Badarna, R. David, Y. Yassur

Ophthalmology Department, Soroka University Hospital and Faculty of Health Sciences, Ben-Gurion University of the Negev, Beer-Sheba, Israel

It is a well accepted observation that diabetic patients who undergo intracapsular cataract extraction, particularly those with PDR, develop rubeosis iridis and neovascular glaucoma more often than non-diabetic patients (1).

We conducted a retrospective study on diabetic patients who underwent extracapsular cataract extraction in order to try to determine if the posterior capsule has any role in the prevention of neovascular glaucoma after that operation.

MATERIAL AND METHODS

We examined 117 eyes of diabetic patients who underwent extracapsular cataract extraction between January, 1984 and December, 1985. This means that the follow-up was between 8-31 months, with a mean of 14 months. In 79 eyes no diabetic retinopathy was proved immediately after the operation and in 38 eyes some degree of diabetic retinopathy was then observed. Our study investigated these 38 eyes with diabetic retinopathy.

In 18 out of the 38 eyes, the posterior capsule was left intact, and in 20 eyes it was opened during the operation, either deliberately due to posterior capsule opacity, or non-deliberately due to an intrasurgical event of capsule rupture. Of the 38 eyes, 26 remained aphakic and in 12 eyes, artificial lenses were implanted: ten posterior chamber implants and two anterior chamber implants.

RESULTS

Of the 38 eyes with diabetic retinopathy, three eyes developed neovascular glaucoma during a period of 4 to 8 months. From the 18 eyes with intact capsule, in 16 the capsule remained intact during all the follow-up period, and only one eye out of these 16 developed neovascular glaucoma. This was a patient who had background diabetic retinopathy at the time of operation who developed proliferative diabetic retinopathy two months later and neovascular glaucoma four months postoperatively.

There were two eyes whose capsule remained intact during the operation but underwent secondary capsulotomy during the follow-up period. One of these two eyes developed neovascular glaucoma five months following the posterior capsulotomy. From the 20 eyes with rupture of posterior capsule at the time of surgery, one eye developed neovascular glaucoma eight months after the extraction.

COMMENT

Neovascular glaucoma following cataract extraction in diabetic patients was until now reviewed in the literature only in two reports of results for intracapsular cataract extraction (1,2) and in only one report for eyes which underwent extracapsular cataract extraction (3). As to neovascular glaucoma after intracapsular cataract extraction, Aiello (2) stressed the importance of risk factors like the type of diabetes mellitus (type I or II) and the severity of the diabetic retinopathy. As to neovascular glaucoma after extracapsular cataract extraction, Poliner (3) reported that in the 78 eyes of diabetics which he reviewed, the neovascular glaucoma developed only in the eyes which had a primary capsule rupture during the operation.

Our study results from the 38 diabetic eyes which had extracapsular cataract extraction were somehow different from those of Poliner: one patient in each of the three operation groups - intact posterior capsule, primary ruptured posterior capsule, and secondary capsulotomy at some later time during the follow up period - developed neovascular glaucoma. This is demonstrated in Fig. 1.

TABLE 1. NEOVASCULAR GLAUCOMA AFTER EXTRACAPSULAR CATARACT EXTRACTION.

	Intact post. capsule	Second post. capsulotomy	Rupture of post. capsule
Poliner's study NV - glaucoma	0/53	0/8	2/17
Present study NV - glaucoma	1/16	1/2	1/20

It is impossible to draw any solid conclusion concerning the importance of the various risk factors from such small numbers as Poliner's or our's. However, there are no other data in the literature. It seems reasonable that the integrity of the posterior capsule has some important role in the development of neovascular glaucoma, but other factors, as well, play a role, like vasoproliferative substances, vasoproliferative inhibitors and hypoxia which are factors in the pathogenesis of neovascularization. Glaser and Associates (4) demonstrated an angiogenesis factor in an eye with active proliferative disease and conceived that after intracapsular extraction, this factor may easily reach the anterior chamber due to altered dynamics of intraocular fluids and due to destruction of the barriers between the vitreous and the anterior chamber. They suggested that from this point of view, extracapsular procedure may be less harmful and thereby more protective against anterior chamber neovascularization, particularly if the posterior capsule is intact.

There is no doubt that following our results and the fact that the reports in literature concerning this matter are so scarce, prospective controlled studies, as well as retrospective evaluations of previously operated eyes are necessary to assess if it is true that there is a protective effect of extracapsular cataract extraction from the development of neovascular glaucoma. Also the necessity of performing laser treatment with intact and ruptured posterior capsule should be assessed by such studies.

REFERENCES

1. Beasley H. Rubeosis iridis in aphakic diabetics. JAMA 1970; 213:128.
2. Aillo LM, Ward M, Liang G: Neovascular glaucoma and vitreous hemorrhage following cataract surgery in patients with diabetes mellitus. Ophthalmology 1983; 90: 814-819.
3. Poliner LS, Christianson DJ, Escoffery RF et al: Neovascular glaucoma following intracapsular and extracapsular cataract extraction in diabetic patients. Abstract. Invest Ophthalmol Vis Sci 1985; 26 (Suppl): 25.
4. Glaser BM, D'Amore PA, Michels RG: The effect of human intraocular fluid on vascular endothelial cell migration. Ophthalmology 1981; 88: 986-991.

CRYOTHERAPY FOR IRIS NEOVASCULARIZATION AND NEOVASCULAR GLAUCOMA

Moshe Lahav, Joseph Tauber, and Stephen Haug, Department of Ophthalmology, New England and Boston VA Medical Centers and Tufts University School of Medicine, Boston, Massachusetts

INTRODUCTION

Numerous and diverse clinical entities are associated with iris neovascularization, but the most frequently encountered are diabetes mellitus and central retinal vein occlusion. The prevalence of iris neovascularization is between 1 - 10% among all diabetic patients and over 40% in patients with proliferative retinopathy (1-3). The incidence of iris neovascularization among patients with central retinal vein occlusion is about 15% (4), but is only 1 to 2% in patients with central retinal artery occlusion (5). The clinical presentation, histologic pathology, and theories of pathogenesis of this disorder have been reviewed (6-14).

The management of iris neovascularization and neovascular glaucoma is difficult. In the past, most cases of neovascular glaucoma ended as blind painful eyes. Recently, it has been shown that panretinal photocoagulation (15-18) or panretinal cryotherapy (19) are beneficial.

In the present study we report a long-term follow-up of 11 eyes treated for iris neovascularization and neovascular glaucoma by panretinal cryotherapy and cyclocryotherapy.

METHODS

Seven patients (11 eyes) had diabetic retinopathy and were included in this study. They presented with decreased vision, advanced iris neovascularization, and hazy media precluding laser panretinal photocoagulation (PRP). Therefore, all were treated by panretinal cryotherapy. Seven eyes in four of these patients also had neovascular glaucoma, defined as intraocular pressure (IOP) greater than 21 mmHg, associated with iris and angle neovascularization and/or anterior synechiae. Patients with neovascular glaucoma and gonioscopic evidence of a fibrovascular membrane or peripheral anterior synechiae were treated with cyclocryotherapy in addition to panretinal cryotherapy. Preoperatively, all of the patients were evaluated with detailed slit lamp biomicroscopy, gonioscopy, visual fields and indirect ophthalmoscopy. In selected cases, fluorescein angiograms of the iris were performed.

Local akinesia and anesthesia were achieved by retrobulbar injection of a mixture consisting of xylocaine 1%, bupivacaine hydrochloride 0.5% and hyaluronidase. Perilimbal peritomy was performed for 360° and the ora serrata identified by transillumination and a 3 mm curved retinal cryoprobe was applied posterior to the ora serrata.

Cryo was applied for seven seconds from the time of ice ball formation on the sclera. Three rows of three applications each were placed between the ora serrata and the retinal vascular arcade for a total of nine applications per quadrant. Four quadrants were treated in all patients. Additional applications were placed when it was felt that the retina on both sides of the equator had not been adequately treated. This treatment was designed to create uniform retinal destruction anterior and posterior to the equator and to leave untreated retina between the applications. Cyclocryotherapy was performed by applications over 180° of the ciliary body. The duration of each application was 30 seconds. Postoperatively, all patients were treated with topical cycloplegic and steroid eye drops three times daily for two to three weeks. Postoperatively, tonometry, gonioscopic and slit lamp examinations were performed regularly to evaluate the intraocular pressure and iris neovascularization status.

RESULTS

All patients had diabetes for 10 years or more and demonstrated disc neovascularization with evidence of ischemic retinopathy and capillary drop out. All presented at a late stage of the disease with poor visual acuity. Only two eyes had a vision of 20/60 or better. In all but three eyes, the angle was totally or partially closed by peripheral anterior synechiae. All eyes had a fibrovascular membrane which extended from the iris surface to the trabecular meshwork. The IOP was elevated in all but two eyes. After panretinal cryotherapy, the rubeosis regressed in 10 of the 11 eyes. In four eyes cyclocryotherapy was performed in addition to panretinal cryotherapy. In one of these eyes, the pressure was not controlled.

The visual acuity deteriorated during the period of follow-up (14 to 73 months). In one eye, cataract and vitreous hemorrhage developed following cryotherapy. In four eyes the vision remained stable. Those eyes were treated early following the diagnosis of iris neovascularization.

DISCUSSION

Iris neovascularization presents an extremely difficult management problem. Generally, secondary angle closure glaucoma induces progressive deterioration of vision leading to a blind painful eye. In diabetes and central retinal vein occlusion, iris neovascularization is associated with diffuse retinal ischemia (6,13,17). This association is in favor of the theory regarding a diffusable angiogenic substance . This factor is produced by hypoxic retina and is probably responsible for both anterior and posterior segment neovascularization (6-9,14). The high incidence of iris neovascularization after vitrectomy and lensectomy in eyes with proliferative diabetic retinopathy lends support to this theory (22). Local iris ischemia may also play a role in the production of iris neovascularization (23).

The most widely-used treatment for iris neovascularization is panretinal photocoagulation (PRP) (9-15). This technique may be effective in maintaining IOP below 21 mmHg in up to 80% of patients with iris neovascularization. By destroying ischemic retina, one destroys the source of the presumed angiogenic factor, and eliminates the stimulus for local and distant neovascularization. In cases where PRP treatment is not possible, panretinal cryotherapy can be "the other" alternative. Moderate cryoapplication will create a chorioretinal scar which is slightly larger than the size of the probe. As in PRP, the mechanism of neovascular regression by panretinal cryotherapy remains unclear. The destruction of hypoxic angiogenic retina or increased availability of oxygen may play a role in the regression process (23).

The present study demonstrates that prompt panretinal cryotherapy, prior to closure of the chamber angle by anterior synechia, may prevent further deterioration of vision due to progressive retinal and/or optic nerve ischemia. However, once the filtration angle closes, treatment is ineffective in maintaining useful vision. Pain control of non-seeing eyes becomes the only achievable goal once this stage is reached. In this study, the incidence of complications following panretinal cryotherapy has been low. Only one eye developed a cataract directly related to the treatment.

It is our impression that, for best results, panretinal cyrotherapy should be done as soon as it is realized that adequate laser panretinal photocoagulation cannot be performed. A combination of additional cyclocryotherapy to control elevated IOP should also be considered if the filtration angle is closed by peripheral anterior synechiae.

REFERENCES
1. Ohrt V: The frequency of rubeosis iridis in diabetic patients. Acta Ophthalmol 49:301, 1971.
2. Armaly MF and Baloglou PJ: Diabetes mellitus and the eye. Arch Ophthalmol 77:485, 1967.
3. Madsen PH: Rubeosis of the iris and haemorrhagic glaucoma in patients with proliferative diabetic retinopathy. Br J Ophthalmol 55:368, 1971.
4. Hayreh SS, Rojas P, Podhajsky P, et al: Ocular neovascularization with retinal vascular occlusion. III. Incidence of ocular neovascularization with retinal vein occlusion. Ophthalmology 90:488, 1983.
5. Hayreh SS and Podhajsky P: Ocular neovascularization with retinal vascular occlusion. II. Occurrence in central and branch retinal artery occlusion. Arch Ophthalmol 100:1585, 1982.
6. Brown GC, Magargal LE, Schachat A, Shah H: Neovascular glaucoma - etiologic considerations. Ophthalmology 91:319, 1984.
7. Henkind P: Ocular neovascularization. The Krill Memorial Lecture. Am J Ophthalmol 85:287, 1978.

8. BenEzra D: Neovasculogenesis. Triggering factor and possible mechanisms. Surv Ophthalmol 24:167, 1979.

9. Gartner S and Henkind P: Neovascularization of the iris (Rubeosis iridis). Surv Ophthalmol 22:291, 1978.

10. Nomura T: Pathology of anterior chamber angle in diabetic neovascular glaucoma: Extension of corneal endothelium onto iris surface. Jap J Ophthalmol 27:193, 1983.

11. John T, Sassani JW, Eagle RC Jr: The myofibroblastic component of rubeosis iridis. Ophthalmology 90:721, 1983.

12. Jocson VL: Microvascular injection studies in rubeosis iridis and neovascular glaucoma. Am J Ophthalmol 83:508, 1977.

13. Madsen PH: Haemorrhagic glaucoma. Comparative study in diabetic and nondiabetic patients. Br J Ophthalmol 55:444, 1971.

14. Glaser BM, D'Amore PA, Michels, RG et al: The demonstration of angiogenic activity from ocular tissues. Preliminary report. Ophthalmology 87:440, 1980.

15. Laatikainen L: Preliminary report on the effect of retinal panphotocoagulation on rubeosis iridis and neovascular glaucoma. Br J Ophthalmol 61:278, 1977.

16. Little HL, Rosenthal AR, Dellaporta A, Jacobson DR: The effect of panretinal photocoagulation on rubeosis iridis. Am J Ophthalmol 81:804, 1976.

17. Magargal LE, Brown GC, Augsburger JJ, Donoso LA: Efficacy of panretinal photocoagulation in preventing neovascular glaucoma following ischemic central retinal vein obstruction. Ophthalmology 89:780, 1982.

18. Wand M, Dueker DK, Aiello LM, Grant WM: Effects of panretinal photocoagulation on rubeosis iridis, angle neovascularization, and neovascular glaucoma. Am J Ophthalmol 86:332, 1978.

19. Hilton GF: Panretinal cryotherapy for diabetic rubeosis. Arch Ophthalmol 97:776, 1979.

20. May DR, Bergstrom TJ, Parmet AJ, Schwartz JG: Treatment of neovascular glaucoma with transscleral panretinal cryotherapy. Ophthalmology 87:1106, 1980.

21. Mohan V and Eagling EM: Peripheral retinal cryotherapy as a treatment for neovascular glaucoma. Trans Ophthalmol Soc UK 98:93, 1978.

22. Rice TA, Michels RG, Maguire MG, Rice EF: The effect of lensectomy on the incidence of iris neovascularization and neovascular glaucoma after vitrectomy for diabetic retinopathy. Am J Ophthalmol 95:1, 1983.

23. Wolbarsht ML and Landers MB III: The rationale of photocoagulation therapy for proliferative diabetic retinopathy: A review and a model. Ophthalmic Surg 11:235, 1980.

MOLTENO IMPLANTS IN NEOVASCULAR GLAUCOMA

Robert David[1], George Baerveldt[2], Don Minckler[2], Jeffrey Freedman[3] and
Yuval Yassur[1], Soroka Medical Center, Beer Sheva, Israel[1], Estelle Doheny
Eye Foundation, Los Angeles[2] and Kings County Hospital, Brooklyn, New York,
U.S.A.[3]

The therapy of neovascular glaucoma constitutes one of the most
frustrating problems facing the practicing ophthalmologist. Medical
treatment has little effect, pan-retinal-photocoagulation is often not
performable due to opaque media, usually associated with the condition, and
none of the conventional surgical procedures have been found to be
particularly helpful in this specific type of glaucoma.
With the introduction of the setons in glaucoma surgery, it was the
next obvious step to try and improve the rather discouraging results
obtained so far in cases of neovascular glaucoma by using these devices.
The authors in the 3 departments have cooperated in developing and
improving techniques for the insertion of setons in severe cases of
glaucoma. The seton used was the Molteno type implant. This type of
implant was chosen as it is the one which has been in use, and constantly
improved, through the last 15 years and during which period, some of the
authors (G.B.& J.F) were keeping close contact with Dr. Molteno concerning
the accumulating experience.

CLINICAL MATERIAL AND OPERATIVE TECHNIQUES
Thirty-eight patients suffering from neovascular glaucoma from the
three participating centers were included regardless of the underlying
disease causing the neovascularization, number or type of operations
performed prior to the Molteno implantation (as long as they were not lost
for follow-up), and were followed for at least 6 months after surgery.
The Molteno implant used is the one manufactured by OPTOMAT, New
Zealand (Fig. 1); its circular plate is 13mm in diameter and is elevated
on a peripheral ring from the underlying sclera. On both sides of the
0.6mm wide polyethylene tube emerging from the plate are 2 holes through
which the plate is anchored into the sclera.

Fig. 1

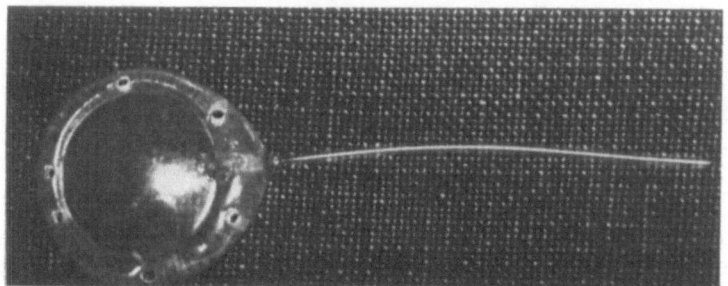

The surgical procedure is performed through a large fornix-based conjunctival flap, one quadrant in size, which is dissected as far as possible behind the equator. The two adjacent rectus muscles are fixated with bridle sutures to facilitate exposure and all bleeding points carefully cauterised. The plate is inserted under the flap, anchored firmly to the sclera with 2 dacron sutures through the anterior holes at 10 mm from the limbus. The rest of the plate floats freely under the flap.

Fig. 2

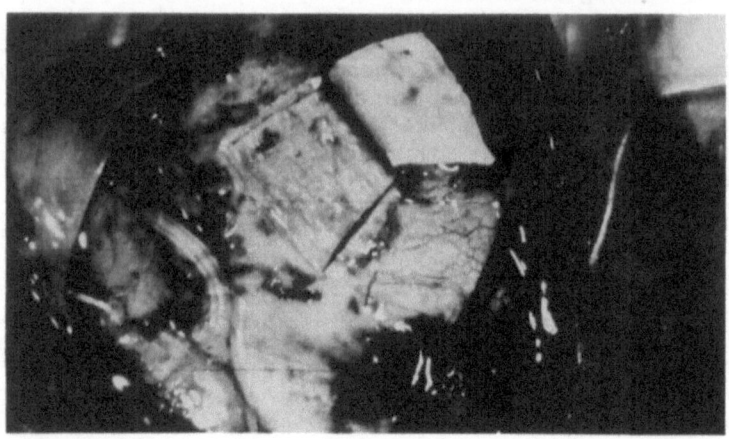

At this stage, either a 5 x 5 mm limbal based scleral pocket, 1/3 in thickness is raised (Fig. 2) before the polyethylene tube is cut to the desired size (Fig. 3), or a full thickness scleral graft 5mm wide and 8mm long is prepared to cover the tube.

Fig. 3

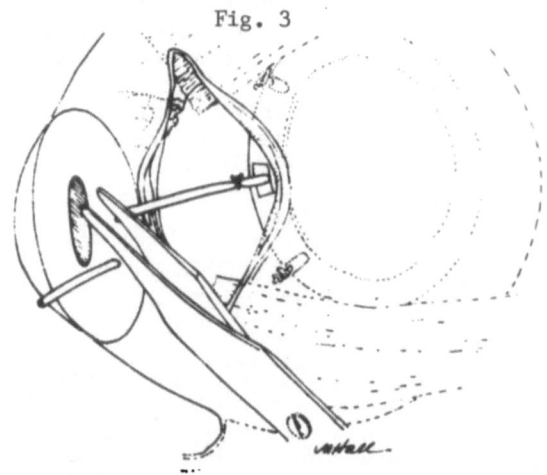

The tunnel through which the tube will be inserted into the anterior chamber is made with a 22 gauge needle to phakic eyes and a 23 gauge for aphaks (Fig. 4).

Fig. 4

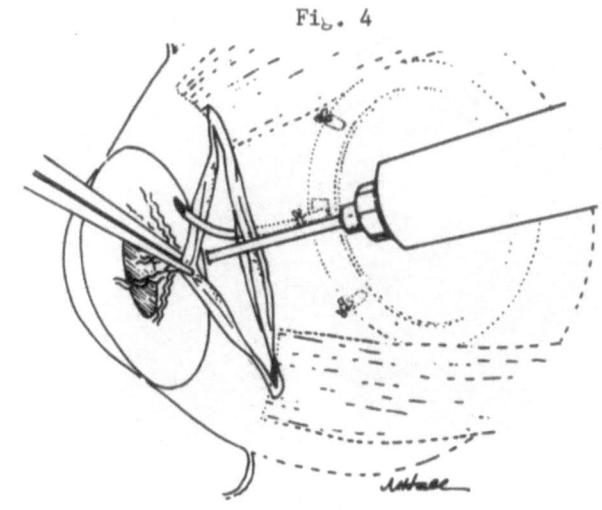

To prevent post-operative hypotony, a ligature of the tube with an absorbent suture before entrance to the tunnel has been suggested, followed by water-tight closure of the scleral flap or firm suturing of the overlay, full thickness, scleral graft (Fig. 5).

Fig. 5

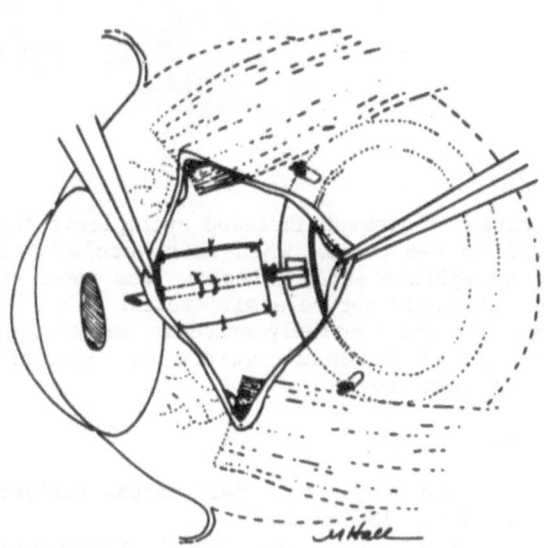

The tube protuding in the anterior chamber should ideally be away from both iris and corneal endothelium as seen in Fig. 6 or through gonioscopic view (Fig. 7).

Fig. 6

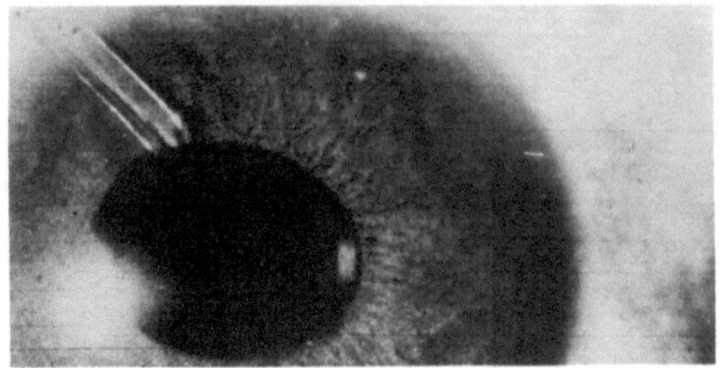

Fig. 7

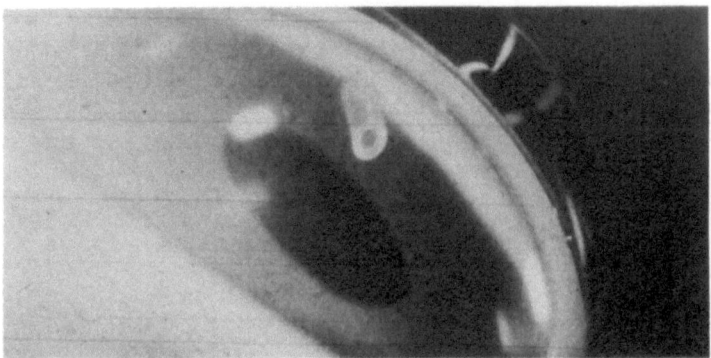

The post-operative treatment included cycloplegic drops and a steroid antibiotic compound for 6–8 weeks. When intra-ocular pressure elevation was encountered, epinephrine and/or timolol was used. Carbonic anhydrase inhibitors should preferably not be administered.

Some surgeons also use routinely systemic medications. These include steroids, colchicine and flufenamic acid. The value of such treatment, however, has not yet been proven.

RESULTS AND COMMENTS

The follow-up period ranged from 6–27 months following surgery; the average follow-up time was 13.7 months.

Surgery was considered successful when the intraocular pressure on the last follow-up visit was equal or less than 24 mmHg in 2 centers and 26 mmHg at the third. Visual acuity was not a criteria for success, as several patients suffered deterioration in sight due to complications of the underlying condition, deterioration which was not related to the neovascular glaucoma or the surgery.

Of the 38 eyes that underwent surgery, 28 or 73% were considered successful according to the criteria described above. There was however, a significant difference in the outcome when the eyes were divided into phakic and aphakic: among the phakic eyes, the success rate was as high as 90% while aphakes only 53% (see Table 1).

TABLE 1

SUCCESS RATE

	Done	Success	Failure
Phakic	21	19 (90%)	2 (10%)
Aphakic	17	9 (53%)	8 (47%)
Total	38	28 (73%)	10 (27%)

The complications encountered are listed in Table 11. Transient hypotony was the most common and unpredictable complication. Water-tight passage of the tube through a 23 gauge tunnel and/or temporary ligature of the tube neck were attempts to control this complication. In one of the corneal-touch cases, decompensation occurred and necessitated surgical reintervention, while in six others the corneal touch was intermittent with occasional localized edema.

Vitreous hemorrhage occurred in diabetic patients during the hypotony period and were probably triggered by the surgery. The case with iris touch produced a plugging of the tube with iris tissue which was consequently released by laser applications.

TABLE II

COMPLICATIONS

Transient hypotony	7 (18%)
Corneal touch	7 (18%)
Early vitreous hemorrhage	5 (13%)
Iris touch	1 (2.6%)
Phthisis bulbi	1 (2.6%)

The results are encouraging, especially if one considers the rather disappointing outcome of surgery for neovascular glaucoma in general. It should be remembered however, that this is a rather small series of cases, that there were slight differences in the surgical technique during the years and it is our impression that the outcome of the cases operated late in our series were doing better. This is an indication that experience and refining of the techniques are playing major roles in the improving results.

BASEMENT MEMBRANES AND RETINAL NEOVASCULARIZATION

ROBERT N. FRANK, M.D., The Kresge Eye Institute of
Wayne State University School of
Medicine, Detroit, MI 48201
U.S.A.

INTRODUCTION

Basement membrane abnormalities, including thickening, multilamina-
tion, vacuolization, and the inclusion of bundles of fibrillar collagen
within the normally homogeneous basement membrane structure, have been
recognized in diabetic subjects for many years (1-4). These abnormalities involve basement membranes in a variety of locations, including
both vascular and non-vascular tissues. However, the major interest in
the pathophysiology of basement membranes in diabetes to date has been
to discover their role in diabetic microangiopathy. One of the initial
hypotheses in this regard was that abnormalities of the basement membranes of the diabetic renal glomerulus led to disturbances of glomerular filtration in the early stages of diabetic nephropathy (5). More
recently, investigators in this field have placed greater emphasis on
the role of the glomerular mesangial cell in this disorder (6). Since
basement membranes appear to function normally only as rather coarse
filters, it would seem that disturbances in their filtration property
would have at best only a relatively minor effect on diabetic microangiopathy in most tissues.

What other functions might extracellular matrix in general, and basement membranes in particular, have that might be subject to disturbance
in diabetes mellitus? One such function, whose importance is receiving
increasing recognition, is to promote cellular differentiation, while at
the same time, inhibiting uncontrolled cellular proliferation. A recent
editorial emphasized this role for the glycosaminoglycans, which comprise one class of macromolecular components of basement membranes (7).
However, other basement membrane components may also serve as modulators
of cellular proliferation and differentiation. Thus, basement membrane
abnormalities in diabetic tissues could be a factor enhancing cellular
de-differentiation or at least, markedly disturbed cell function. In
tissues such as the retina, where other stimuli to vascular cell proliferation are likely to be present in certain disease states, abnormalities of vascular basement membranes may enhance the neovascular process
In this paper, I shall summarize some of the evidence for this hypothesis, including recent studies from my own laboratory.

IN VITRO STUDIES

Recently, a number of investigations using cultured cells have shown
that several types of cells demonstrate a variety of "differentiated"
characteristics when grown on matrices composed of collagens, fibronectin, and other extracellular macromolecules. For example, mammary epi-
thelia form structures resembling glandular acini when the cells are
"sandwiched" between collagen gel layers, while mammary cells grown on

plastic do not demonstrate such properties (8). Lens epithelial cells grown on type I collagen gels (9), and microvascular endothelial cells grown under similar conditions (10), form structures that resemble basal laminae. Microvascular endothelial cells grown on collagen matrices have a greater tendency to form lumen-like tubes than when they are grown in the absence of such matrices (11). In cultures of retinal microvascular endothelial cells, we have made similar observations. We also find a greater tendency of the cells to lay down basal lamina-like structures, and to form intracellular junctional complexes, when they are grown on type I collagen gels than when they are grown on plastic culture dishes alone (12). In addition, we have observed differences in the morphology of cultured microvascular pericytes grown on type I collagen gels, and on gelled substrates consisting of various proportions of type I collagen and "Matrigel"®, an extract of basement membrane macromolecules derived from the Engelbreth-Holm-Swarm (EHS) chondrosarcoma of mice (13, 14). By phase contrast microscopy, we observe that pericytes grown on such gels extend long processes that are not present when the cells are cultured on plastic dishes lacking the substrate. By electron microscopy, it is apparent that these processes extend within the substrate (13). Finally, when either cultured microvascular endothelial cells or pericytes are fixed and stained with Alcian blue to demonstrate glycosaminoglycans, it is evident that the pericellular glycocalyx is much thicker in cells cultured on a collagenous substrate, than when the substrate is lacking (13; a manuscript detailing all of these findings is in preparation).

Many investigators, including ourselves, have cultured cells on dried films or gels of extracellular matrix materials that are readily available commercially. Some of these, such as type I collagen, are not normally considered part of the native basement membrane, although our own work (15) and that of Jerdan and Glaser (16) indicates that type I collagen is present in normal retinal microvascular basement membranes. More recently, a number of workers have begun to isolate complex extracts of native basement membranes, and to use these as substrates for cultured cells. There is indication that cells grown on these may not only display more highly differentiated characteristics, but also to proliferate more slowly than when they are grown on plastic alone, or on non-native matrices of simpler composition. For example, in a study of cultured rat mammary epithelium, the cells incorporated [^{3}H]-thymidine more slowly when they were grown on an extracellular matrix extracted from rat mammary tissue than when they were cultured on plastic (17; see especially Fig. 2 of this paper). We (13) have made similar observations on retinal microvascular cells grown on substrates containing greater than 50% Matrigel by comparison with cells grown on other substrates, on plastic alone, or on substrates containing a small proportion of Matrigel.

IN VIVO STUDIES

Several years ago, Ausprunk and Folkman (18) demonstrated in a model of corneal neovascularization that digestion of the basement membrane was necessary before the vascular endothelial cells could proliferate. The suggestion was, that vascular endothelium, under conditions that favored neovascularization, could elaborate collagenase(s) and, perhaps, other enzymes capable of digesting basement membrane macromolecules. A direct demonstration of this was reported by Kalebic, et al. (19) in an in vitro study, which showed that proliferating large vessel endothelial cells could elaborate a collagenase specific for type IV collagen, the principal collagen of basement membranes.

We have seen evidence for such lysis of basement membranes in a model of retinal neovascularization in rats with varieties of hereditary dystrophy. Spontaneously hypertensive (SHR) rats develop a dystrophy with late onset (the first anatomic abnormalities are observed only after the first year of life), and which appears to originate in the photoreceptor cells. Ultimately, the entire neural retina degenerates and, as has been observed in rats with other types of hereditary retinal dystrophies as well as induced retinal degenerations, abnormal vessels extend from the retinal circulation, first outward into the retinal pigment epithelium (RPE). Evidence has been presented by Shiraki and Burns (20) that these intra-RPE vessels represent true neovascularization, rather than simply vessels that were previously present but have become anatomically altered. The intra-RPE vessels are present in nearly all rats with extensive retinal dystrophies or degenerations. Like true retinal neovascularization, they have thinned, often fenestrated cytoplasm (21, 22), and they are "leaky" to molecules like microperoxidase (mol. wt. 1,200; Fig. 1), and even to relatively large molecules like horseradish peroxidase (mol. wt. 40,000; photomicrograph not shown).

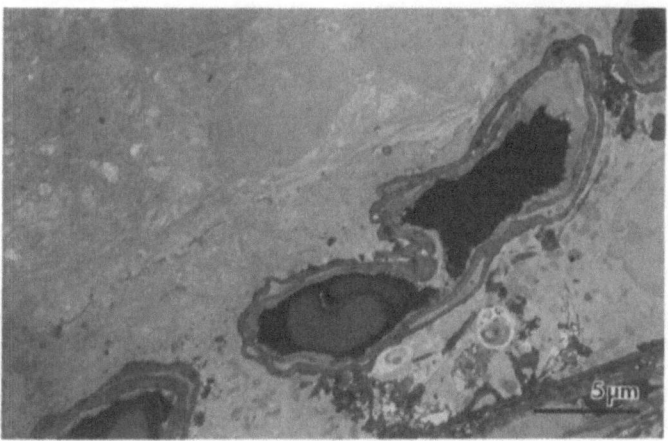

FIGURE 1. An intra-RPE (?new) vessel in a dystrophic Royal College of Surgeons (RCS) rat. The animal was first injected intraperitoneally with methysergide and diphenhydramine and then, after 5 min., received intravascular microperoxidase (Sigma Chemical Co., St. Louis, MO, USA; 75 mg/100 g body weight, in 1 ml Dulbecco's phosphate-buffered saline, pH 7.2), which was allowed to circulate for 15 min. before the animal was euthanized. Fixation of the tissue, the histochemical reaction for peroxidase, and thin sectioning were by standard methods. The reaction product is seen in the photomicrograph as a dark precipitate within the vascular lumina. It also stains the vascular basement membranes, indicating that the vessel has become "leaky," at least to this molecule.

396

We have observed, in several older, dystrophic SHR rats, that the intra-RPE vessels may change their course by 180°, and extend inward into the dystrophic neural retina again, now accompanied by RPE cells (23). Once the vessels, together with their accompanying RPE cells, reach the inner limiting membrane (ILM) of the retina, several things happen. The vascular cells burst through the ILM into the vitreous cavity, where they display features identical to that of retinovitreal neovascularization in human disease, as it has been observed by several authors using electron microscopy (24, 25): abnormalities of the vascular basement membranes, thinned and often fenestrated endothelial cytoplasm, scarce and often bizarre pericytes, and abnormal intra-endothelial junctional complexes (Figs. 2 and 3). The RPE cells, however, are never seen to enter the vitreous cavity in this model. Rather, they line up along the ILM, which appears to impart differentiated properties upon these cells. While they are growing through

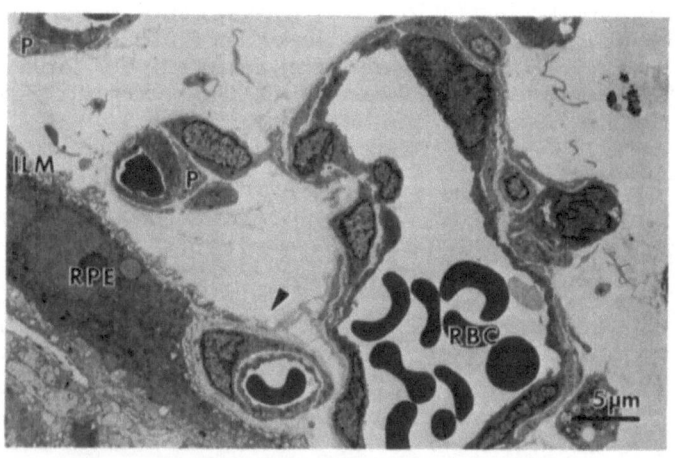

FIGURE 2. Apparent new vessels break through the inner limiting membrane (ILM) of the dystrophic retina of a spontaneously hypertensive rat. The ILM is ruptured at the arrowhead. A retinal pigment epithelial cell (RPE) does not break through the ILM. Note the basal plasma membrane infoldings of the RPE cell, adjacent to the ILM, and the parallel rows of microvilli on the apical side of the cell, facing the retina. Note that the intravitreal vessels are functional, since their lumina are filled with red blood cells (RBC), but their appearance is abnormal with thin endothelium, thin, often multilaminar basement membranes, and small, bizarre pericytes (P).

the retina, the proliferating RPE cells lack polarity. Once they reach the ILM, however, the RPE cells become polarized. The surface that abuts the ILM develops multiple invaginations of its plasma membrane, much like the basal plasma membrane invaginations of the normal RPE (Figs. 2, 4; refs. 23, 26). The cell surface that faces the now degenerated neural retina produces multiple microvilli, like the apical microvilli of normal RPE cells (Figs. 2, 4; ref. 23). In addition, glial elements (perhaps Müller cells) adjacent to these RPE cells develop junctional complexes resembling those of the "external limiting membrane" of the normal retina, except that they are in the wrong location (23)! These observations strongly suggest that the ILM exerts an influence upon the RPE cells to differentiate and polarize, but in an anatomically upside-down orientation. Because proliferating RPE cells do not produce enzymes capable of lysing basement membranes, they must remain inside the ILM, while the proliferating microvascular endothelial cells, which produce collagenase(s) and, perhaps, other enzymes that can digest basement membrane components, can rupture the ILM and enter the vitreous.

The stimulus to retinovitreal neovascularization in this dystrophic rat model remains unknown. Because the retinal neurons in these animals have almost completely degenerated, it appears unlikely that a completely identical stimulus is operating here, to that which operates, say, in proliferative diabetic retinopathy in humans, as well as in other human retinal diseases. This would seem evident from the clinical

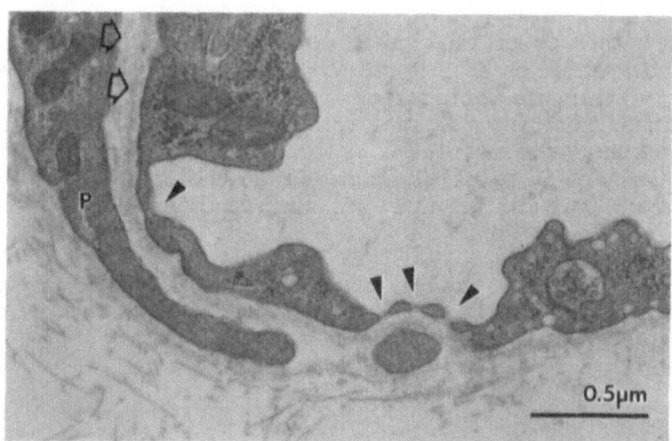

FIGURE 3. A higher power view of an intravitreal, apparent new vessel in a one year-old Royal College of Surgeons (RCS) rat with a dystrophic retina. Note the thinned endothelium with fenestrations (closed arrowheads), and the thin, multilaminar basement membrane (open arrowheads). A pericyte process is indicated by P.

behavior of retinal neovascularization in the various circumstances in which it arises. Thus, while an ischemic stimulus, perhaps leading to the production of an angiogenic factor endogenously in retinal cells, has recently been the most widely advanced hypothesis (27), it seems unlikely that this explanation accounts for all cases of retinal neovascularization (28, 29). It has been the purpose of this presentation to suggest that the chemical abnormalities of retinal vascular basement membranes in diabetes serve to modify the behavior of the adjacent

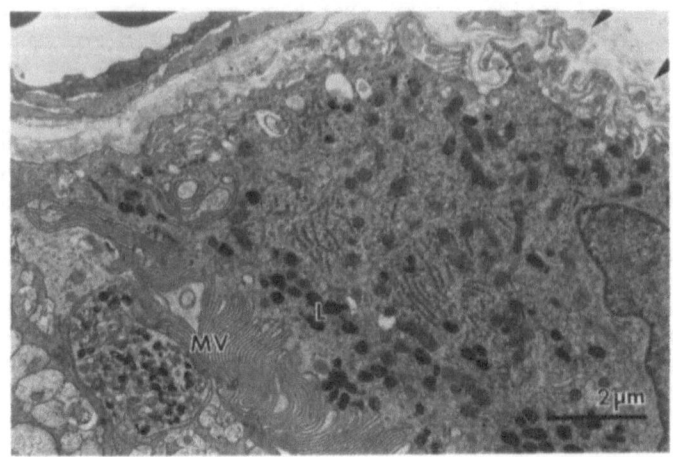

FIGURE 4. A higher power view of an ectopic RPE cell lying on the inner surface of the retina of an SHR rat with retinal dystrophy. Part of a vessel lying within the vitreous cavity is seen at the upper left. Note the intact inner limiting membrane (closed arrowheads) over the RPE cell, with extensive basal plasma membrane infoldings adjacent to it. Microvilli (MV) are in parallel alignment at the apical end of the cell, with multiple lipofuscin granules (L) just beneath them.

vascular cells, providing an additional factor leading to the physiological malfunctions of early diabetic retinopathy, and in many cases, resulting ultimately in retinal neovascularization.

REFERENCES

1. Friedenwald JS: Diabetic retinopathy. Amer. J. Ophthalmol. 33: 1187-1199, 1950.
2. Yamashita T and Becker B: The basement membrane in the human diabetic eye. Diabetes 10: 167-174, 1961.
3. Kilo C, Vogler NJ, and Williamson JR: Muscle capillary basement membrane changes related to aging and to diabetes mellitus. Diabetes 21:881-995, 1972.
4. Caird FI, Pirie A, and Ramsell TG: Diabetes and the Eye. Oxford: Blackwell, 1969, pp. 37-58.
5. Farquhar MG, Courtoy PJ, Lemkin MC, and Kanwar YS: Current Knowledge of the functional architecture of the glomerular basement membrane. In, New Trends in Basement Membrane Research, Kuehn K, Schoene, H-H, and Timpl R (eds). New York: Raven Press, 1982, pp. 9-30.
6. Mauer M and Shvil Y: The glomerular mesangium. In, Renal Disease, Black D and Jones NF (eds), 4th edition. Oxford: Blackwell, 1979, pp. 93-106.
7. Trelstad RL: Glycosaminoglycans: mortar, matrix, mentor. Lab. Invest. 53: 1-4, 1985.
8. Hall HG, Faison DA, Chin S, and Bissell MJ: Extracellular matrix and morphogenesis: collagen overlay induces lumen formation by epithelial cell lines. In, Extracellular Matrix, Hawkes S and Wang JL (eds). New York: Academic Press, 1982, pp. 233-238.
9. Heathcote JG, Bruns RR, and Orkin RW: Biosynthesis of sulphated macromolecules by rabbit lens epithelium. II. Relationship to basement membrane formation. J. Cell Biol. 99: 861-869, 1984.
10. Kramer RH, Bensch KG, Davison PM, and Karasek MA: Basal lamina formation by cultured microvascular endothelial cells. J. Cell Biol. 99: 692-698, 1984.
11. Montesano R, Orci L, and Vassalli P: In vitro rapid organization of endothelial cells into capillary-like networks is promoted by collagen matrices. J. Cell Biol. 97: 1648-1652, 1983.
12. Kennedy A, Frank RN, and Mancini MA: In vitro production of glycosaminoglycans by retinal microvessel cells and lens epithelium. Invest. Ophthalmol. Vis. Sci. 27: 746-754, 1986.
13. Kennedy A, Mancini MA, and Frank, RN: A type I collagen gel substrate stimulates cultured retinal cells to produce insoluble proteoglycan. Invest. Ophthalmol. Vis. Sci. 27 (Suppl.): 327, 1986.
14. Kleinman HK, McGarvey ML, Hassell JR, Star VL, Cannon FB, Laurie GW, and Martin GR: Basement membrane complexes with biological activity. Biochemistry 25: 312-318, 1986.
15. Kennedy A, Frank RN, Mancini MA, and Lande M: Collagens of the retinal microvascular basement membrane and of retinal microvascular cells in vitro. Exp. Eye Res. 42: 177-199, 1986.
16. Jerdan JA and Glaser BM: Retinal microvessel extracellular matrix: an immunofluorescent study. Invest. Ophthalmol. Vis. Sci. 27: 194-203, 1986.
17. Wicha MS: Growth and differentiation of rat mammary epithelium on mammary gland extracellular matrix. In, Extracellular Matrix, Hawkes S and Wang JL (eds). New York: Academic Press, 1982, pp. 309-314.
18. Ausprunk DH and Folkman J: Migration and proliferation of endothelial cells in preformed and newly formed blood vessels during tumor

angiogenesis. Microvasc. Res. 14: 53-65, 1977.

19. Kalebic T, Garbisa S, Glaser B, and Liotta LA: Basement membrane collagen: degradation by migrating endothelial cells. Science 221: 281-283, 1983.

20. Shiraki K and Burns MS: Neovascularization in urethane rat retinopathy demonstrated by thymidine labeling. Curr. Eye Res. 5: 683-696, 1986.

21. Bellhorn RW, Bellhorn M, Friedman AH, and Henkind P: Urethan-induced retinopathy in pigmented rats. Invest. Ophthalmol. 12: 65-76, 1973.

22. Mancini MA, Frank RN, Keirn RJ, Kennedy A, and Khoury JK: Does the retinal pigment epithelium polarize the choriocapillaris? Invest. Ophthalmol. Vis. Sci. 27: 336-345, 1986.

23. Frank RN and Mancini MA: Presumed retinovitreal neovascularization in dystrophic retinas of spontaneously hypertensive rats. Invest. Ophthalmol. Vis. Sci. 27: 346-355, 1986.

24. Frank KW and Weiss H: Unusual clinical and histopathological findings in ocular sarcoidosis. Brit. J. Ophthalmol. 67: 8-16, 1983.

25. Taniguchi Y: Ultrastructure of newly formed blood vessels in diabetic retinopathy. Japan. J. Ophthalmol. 20: 19-28, 1976.

26. Grimes P and Laties AM: Early morphological alteration of the pigment epithelium in streptozotocin-induced diabetes: increased surface area of the basal cell membrane. Exp. Eye Res. 30: 631-639, 1980.

27. Weiter JJ and Zuckerman R: The influence of the photoreceptor-RPE complex on the inner retina. An explanation for the beneficial effects of photocoagulation. Ophthalmology 87: 1133-1139, 1980.

28. Henkind P: Ocular neovascularization. Amer. J. Ophthalmol. 85: 287-301, 1978.

29. Patz A: Studies on retinal neovascularization. Invest. Ophthalmol. Vis. Sci. 19: 1133-1138, 1980.

LOCALIZATION OF ANGIOGENESIS MARKERS TO INNER AND OUTER RETINA

PETER A. CAMPOCHIARO AND STEVEN H. BLAYDES

Department of Ophthalmology, University of Virginia School of Medicine, Charlottesville, Virginia 22908, U.S.A.

INTRODUCTION

Ever since the pioneering observations of Dr. Michaelson (1) and others (2,3), there has been mounting evidence to suggest that there is a diffusible substance released by retina that plays a role in the development of neovascularization. Several authors have noted the association of retinal capillary nonperfusion and neovascularization (2-5), implicating ischemia in the pathogenesis. The diffusible nature of the factor is suggested by the occurrence of neovascularization remote from the area of ischemia, such as neovascularization on the disc and rubeosis. Angiogenic activity has been demonstrated in mammalian retina (6,7), and several laboratories are in the process of purifying it. Since assays for angiogenesis are difficult to perform and hard to quantitate, assays for cellular events involved in the process of neovascularization are often substituted. These include vascular endothelial cell migration (8), proliferation (8), and production of plasminogen activator by vascular endothelial cells (9). Extracts prepared from mammalian retina contain significant activity for each of these three parameters (7,9,10). However, little is known about the source of these activities within the retina, or whether they are mediated by one agent or multiple agents. In this study, we examined the retinal localization of these markers for angiogenesis by selectively ablating portions of rabbit retinas.

MATERIALS AND METHODS

Pigmented rabbits were divided into three groups. One group received two doses of iodoacetate (IA), 15 mg/kg IV, eight hours apart, which has previously been demonstrated to cause selective loss of photoreceptors (11). Another group received a 0.1 ml intravitreous injection of 200 nmol of kainic acid (KA) in one eye and a 0.1 ml intravitreous injection of saline in the other eye. Kainic acid is an analog of glutamate which at appropriate doses causes selective destruction of the inner retina (12). The third group received no treatment.

Three weeks after treatment the rabbits were sacrificed, and several eyes from each group were examined histologically. Using the remainder of the eyes in each group, retinas were carefully dissected free of contamination from other ocular structures and homogenized in balanced salt solution. Protein content was determined by the method of Lowry et al (13), and an equivalent protein concentration of 200 µg/ml was used for each assay. Homogenates were assayed for their ability to stimulate vascular endothelial cell migration, proliferation, and production of plasminogen activator.

Bovine aortic endothelial cells were cultured by the procedure of Fenselau and Mello (14). They were maintained in Eagle's minimal essential medium (MEM) supplemented with 10% fetal calf serum. Cells at passage 8 through 12 were used for all experiments.

Endothelial cell migration was measured using a modified Boyden chamber apparatus. Retinal homogenates diluted to a protein concentration of 200 µg/ml in MEM were placed in the bottom wells and covered with a collagen coated polycarbonate membrane containing 5 µm pores. Endothelial cells suspended in MEM at a concentration of 6.0×10^5 cells per ml were placed in the top wells. After four hours of incubation at $37^\circ C$, the membranes were removed, and all cells were scraped from the upper side, leaving only cells that had migrated through the pores. After fixation and staining, the number of cells in ten 400 x fields were counted for each well.

Endothelial cell proliferation was measured in cell counting assays. Cells at a concentration of 5.0×10^4 cells per ml were plated in 24-well plates. After attachment, they were transferred to serum free-media for 24 hours, and then retinal homogenates diluted to 200 µg/ml in MEM were added to each well. After 48 hours the media were harvested and stored at $-20^\circ C$ for assay of plasminogen activator activity. The cells were trypsinized and counted in a Coulter electronic cell counter.

The production of plasminogen activator by endothelial cells was measured in fibrin degredation assays (15). Media (300 µl) that had been conditioned on endothelial cells in the presence and absence of retinal homogenates (200 µg/ml) were placed in wells coated with ^{125}I-labelled fibrin. Plasminogen (4 µg) was also added to each well. After a 2 hour incubation at $37^\circ C$, the media were harvested, and radioactivity was counted by liquid scintillation spectroscopy.

Each assay was performed in triplicate to generate one experimental value and numbers reported represent the mean (± SEM) from at least three separate experiments. Statistical comparisons were made by the Student's unpaired t-test.

RESULTS

Retinas from rabbits treated with IA showed a selective loss of

photoreceptors throughout their entire extent, which at the light
microscopic level is seen as complete loss of the outer nuclear layer
with sparing of the inner nuclear, inner plexiform and ganglion cell
layers (Fig. 1a and b). This contrasts with control retinas (Fig. 1c),
which showed all of the normal retinal cell layers. Note that though the
IA-treated retina is artifactually separated from the RPE, the loss of
the outer retina is not artifactual, as the outer edge of remaining
retina is smooth with no torn or jagged edges (Fig. 1a and b). Retinas
from eyes treated with KA showed selective destruction of the inner
layers. This is demonstrated by the marked attenuation of the inner
nuclear, inner plexiform, and ganglion cell layers with preservation of
the outer nuclear and outer segment layers (Fig. 1d). Only rare inflammatory cells were noted in both IA-treated and KA-treated retinas.

Fig. 1. Histology of
iodoacetate-treated,
control, and kainate-
treated retinas. a)
Low power (150 X) of
iodoacetate-treated
retina to show rela-
tionship to artifac-
tually separated RPE.
b) High power (300 X)
of iodoacetate-treated
retina. c) High power
(300 X) of control
retina. d) High power
(300 X) of kainate-
treated retina.

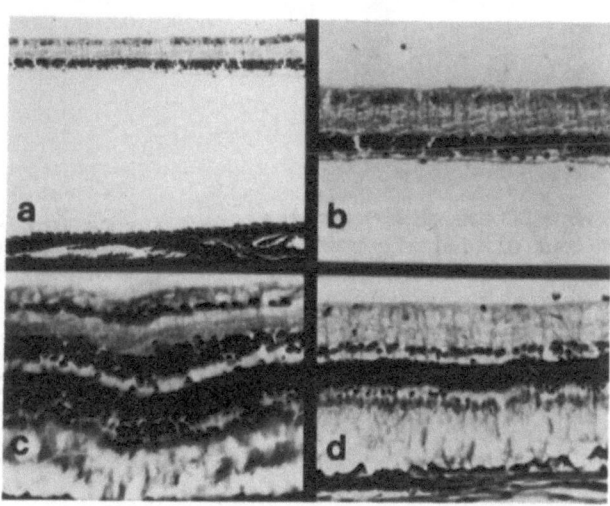

Retinal homogenates from control eyes significantly enhanced the
migration of endothelial cells above migration that occurred in the
presence of media alone (Fig. 2). Homogenates of retinas that had been
treated with KA or IA, caused an even greater enhancement. The results
in the endothelial cell proliferation assays were similar, with retinal
homogenates from KA or IA treated eyes causing even greater stimulation
than the moderate increase seen in the presence of control retinal homogenates (Fig. 3).

Media conditioned on endothelial cells caused [^{125}I]fibrin degredation that was 2-fold above background (Fig. 4). This difference
represents the baseline production of plasminogen activator. It is
significantly stimulated by the presence of control retinal homogenate

404

in the conditioning media and is even further stimulated by the presence
of homogenates of IA- or KA-treated retinas (Fig. 4).

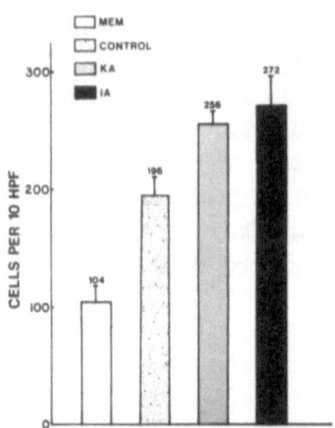

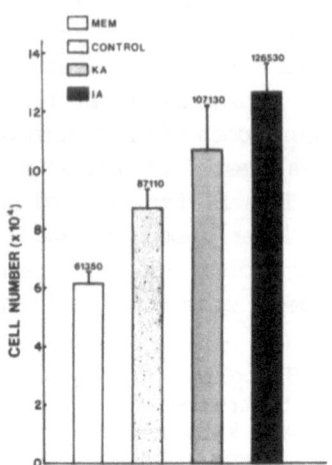

Fig. 2. Effect of homogenates
from control, kainate-treated
(KA), and iodoacetate-treated
(IA) retinas on vascular endothelial cell migration. Bars
represent the mean (± SEM)
number of migrated cells per
ten 400 X fields calculated
from at least three separate
experiments.

Fig. 3. Effect of homogenates
from control, kainate-treated
(KA), and iodoacetate-treated
(IA) retinas on vascular endothelial cell proliferation.
Bars represent the mean (± SEM)
number of proliferated cells
after 48 hr in the presence of
test media calculated from at
least three separate experiments.

Fig. 4. Effect of homogenates from control
(RF-CM), kainate-treated (KA-CM), and
iodoacetate-treated (IA-CM) retinas on
production of plasminogen activator by
vascular endothelial cells. Bars represent
the amount of [^{125}I]fibrin degraded by
media conditioned on endothelial cells for
48 hr in the presence of homogenates. The
amount of [^{125}I]fibrin degraded in the
presence of media containing retinal
homogenates (MEM) and media conditioned on
endothelial cells in the absence of homogenates (CM) is also shown. Results are
expressed as disintegrations per minute
(DPM) and represent the mean (± SEM) of at
least three experiments.

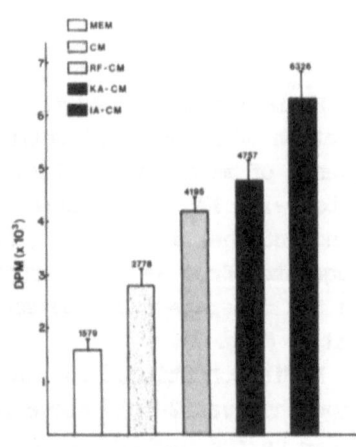

The table below summarizes the data from each of the three assays. It shows that the relative increases above control for all three markers were similar in both treatment groups, with that for the IA group being somewhat greater.

Table 1. Effect of retinal homogenates on 3 markers for angiogenesis.

| | Percent above baseline | | |
	Control	KA-treated	IA-treated
Migration	89	146	162
Proliferation	42	74	106
PA Production	51	71	128

DISCUSSION

In this study, we have demonstrated that ablation of the inner retina or outer retina does not result in a decrease in any of three markers for angiogenesis. Quite the contrary, there is an increase in all three markers when the inner retina has been destroyed and an even greater increase when the photoreceptors have been destroyed. This suggests that there is angiogenic activity in both inner and outer retina.

It is unclear why these treatments which ablate portions of retina result in enhanced activity for angiogenic markers. It may be that though the ablated portion of retina is primarily affected, the remaining viable retina is compromised in a manner similar to what occurs in the presence of ischemia, resulting in enhanced production of angiogenic activity. Regardless of the reason for the increase, it does suggest that cells of the inner and outer retina have the capacity to produce angiogenic activity.

Our original hypothesis was that we would find the greatest concentration of angiogenic activity in the outer retina, because of circumstantial evidence in the literature: 1. The photoreceptors have the highest level of metabolic activity (16) and, therefore, might be expected to be most affected by retinal ischemia regardless of whether its origin is from retinal vasculature or choroidal vascular compromise. 2. Retinal detachment which affects most the oxygenation of the outer retina is an extremely potent stimulus for neovascularization in diabetics. 3. Patients with diabetes who also have Retinitis Pigmentosa, a disease associated with a generalized loss of photoreceptors, have an extremely low incidence of proliferative diabetic retinopathy (PDR) (17). 4. Photocoagulation treatment, which has a beneficial effect on neovascularization, ablates the outer retina while leaving the

406

inner retina intact (18).

Our data do not support this hypothesis and require re-evaluation of the circumstantial evidence: 1. Though the high level of metabolic activity in photoreceptors may explain why retinal detachment is such a potent stimulus for neovascularization, our data suggest that the inner retina is capable of producing angiogenic activity and is likely to be the source in the early stages of PDR. 2. The low incidence of PDR in patients with Retinitis Pigmentosa is not likely to be due to photo-receptor cell loss, but might instead be explained by thinning of the retina allowing better oxygenation of the inner retina from the choroid in the presence of retinal capillary drop out. 3. The mechanism by which photocoagulation exerts its beneficial effect in PDR is not likely to be by ablation of ischemic retina alone. Our data suggest that other factors are likely to play a role. One possibility is that thinning of the retina associated with destruction of the outer layer by photoco-agulation results in enhanced oxygenation of the inner retina from the choroid. Another possible contributing factor is the production of a diffusible anti-angiogenesis factor by the proliferated cells in laser scars (19).

Finally, each of the three markers showed roughly proportionate variation after each of the treatments. Though this does not prove that a single factor is responsible for these activities, it at least suggests rough co-localization of responsible agents.

Purification of retinal angiogenesis factors followed by the development of antibodies will allow immunohistochemical localization. Using molecular biology techniques, Dr. Leonard Hjelmeland has already provided information on the retinal localization of two angiogenic proteins, acidic and basic fibroblast growth factors (see elsewhere in this symposium). The correlation of such antigenic localization with the biochemical localization in this study may provide some useful insights into the process of retinal neovascularization.

REFERENCES

1. Michaelson, I.C. Trans. Ophthalmol. Soc. U.K. 68:137-180, 1948.
2. Wise, G.N. Trans. Am. Ophthalmol. Soc. 54:729-825, 1956.
3. Ashton, N. Am. J. Ophthalmol. 44:7-17, 1957.
4. Kohner, E.M., Shilling, J.S. and Hamilton, A.M. Metab. Ophthalmol. 1:15-23, 1976.
5. Shimizu, K., Kobayashi, Y. and Muraoka, K. Ophthalmology 88:601-612, 1981.
6. Glaser, B.M., D'Amore, P.A., Michels, R.G., Patz, A. and Fenselau, A. J. Cell. Biol. 84:298-304, 1980.
7. Federman, J.L., Brown, G.C., Felberg, N.T. and Felton, S.M. Am. J. Ophthalmol. 89:231-237, 1980.
8. Ausprunk, D.H. and Folkman, J. Microvasc. Res. 14:53-65, 1977.

9. Gross, J.L., Moscatelli, D. and Rifkin, D.B. Proc. Natl. Acad. Sci. U.S.A. 80:2623-2627, 1983.

10. Glaser, B.M., D'Amore, P.A., Seppa, H., Seppa, S., Schiffman, E. Nature 288:483-484, 1980.

11. Noell, W.K. J. Cell Comp. Physiol. 40:25-47, 1952.

12. Schwarcz, R. and Coyle J.T. Invest. Ophthalmol. Vis. Sci. 16:141-148, 1977.

13. Lowry, D.H., Rosenbrough, N.J., Farr, A.L. and Randall, R.J. J. Biol. Chem. 193:265-275, 1951.

14. Fenselau, A. and Mello, R.J. Cancer Res. 36:3269-3273, 1976.

15. Gross, J.L., Moscatelli, D., Jaffe, E.A. and Rifkin, D.B. J. Cell Biol. 95:974-981, 1982.

16. Wallimann, T., Wegmann, G., Moser, H., Huber, R. and Eppenberger, H.M. Proc. Natl. Acad. Sci. U.S.A. 83:3816-3819, 1986.

17. Sternberg, P. Jr., Landers, M.B. III and Wolbarsht, M. Am. J. Ophthalmol. 97:788-789, 1984.

18. L'Esperance, F.A. Am. J. Ophthalmol. 68:263-273, 1969.

19. Glaser, B.M., Campochiaro, P.A., Davis, J.L. Jr. and Sato, M. Arch. Ophthalmol. 103:1870-1875, 1985.

PATHOLOGICAL CHANGES IN RETINAL VASCULATURE ASSOCIATED WITH HEREDITARY RETINAL DYSTROPHY IN RCS-RATS

E. EL.-HIFNAWI
Institute of Anatomy, Medical University of Lübeck
Ratzeburger Allee 160, D-2400 Lübeck - Federal Republic of Germany

SUMMARY

Initial changes in the retinal vasculature of RCS rats become apparent when early degenerative changes in the photoreceptor cell layer are already evident (1). Focal constricture and obstruction as well as the gradual loss of cellular elements of the vessel wall begin in the superficial capillary network and later spread throughout the retina. Coarsening of the entire capillary network ensues after the appearance of acellular channels proliferating retinal vessels invade the partially regenerated retinal pigment epithelium when the photoreceptor layer has disappeared and retinal thickness has dramatically reduced. Some endothelial cells of the invading retinal capillaries immediately adjacent to Bruch's membrane exhibit fenestration. Results suggest that factor(s) deriving from the retinal pigment epithelium may play a role in initiating neovascularization and partial fenestration of some endothelial cells

INTRODUCTION

Retinal dystrophy in the Royal College of Surgeons (RCS) rat is a recessively inherited disorder characterized by gradual loss of the photoreceptor cells. Numerous studies demonstrate a disruption in phagocytosis of discarded outer segments by the retinal pigment epithelium (RPE) (1-6). The precise extent of the role played by the dysfunctional pigment epithelium in causing degeneration of the photoreceptor cells and other factors involved remains uncertain. It is well established that the retinal vasculature is also detrimentally effected by these dystrophic processes (1,8). The primary focus of the present study has been to examine changes in the retinal vessels occuring after loss of the photoreceptor cells. Especial attention is paid to the topographical relationship between the proliferating retinal vessels and pigment epithelium as well as their atypical morphological characteristics throughout the course of the disorder.

MATERIAL AND METHODS

In this study, the retinas of 100 Royal College of Surgeons (RCS) rats ranging in age from 4 to 130 weeks were examined. Effected and control animals (Wistar rats) were kept under identical laboratory conditions. Illumination (maximally 200 Lux) alternated with 12 hours of darkness. Treatment of animals in this study conformed to the ARVO resolution on use of animals in research. Examination was done using a variety of techniques including india ink injection, trypsin digestion and corrosion cast preparations as well as transmission electron microscopy. The animals were anesthetized i.p. using Pentobarbital (Nembutal 0.1 ml/100 g body weight). Fixation for electron microscopy was done using a solution of 0.2 ml Cacodylate buffer, 3.2 % Glutaraldehyde, 2.6 % Paraformaldehyde and 0.03 % CaCl = (pH 7.3, 900 mOsm). Subsequent preparation was done according to schedules described in earlier studies. Oriented semi thin sections were stained according to Richardson et al. (1960) (9). Ultrathin sections were double stained with uranyl acetate and lead citrate (Reynolds 1963) (10). The electron-microscopic examination was done on TEM Phillips 200 and 400 and TEM Zeiss 109.

Animals being prepared for studies using the india ink injection and corrosion cast methods of demonstrating retinal vasculature were perfusion fixed with the solution described above. Further preparation for these techniques was completed according to methods described in our previous studies.

Flat preparation samples (trypsin digestion) were fixed in 4 % formalin and digested in 3 % trypsin according to the method of Kuwabara and Cogan (1960) (11) and stained with HE.

RESULTS

The development of the retinal vascular pattern has been studied extensively in man, the cat, and the rat. A similar mode of development has been found in each (12). A specific account of retinal circulatory development in the RCS rat has been given elsewhere (1). Early development, differentiation and distribution of the retinal vessels of these rats does not significantly differ from that observed in control animals. There is a basic two layered pattern in the retinal capillary bed: the deeper capillaries lying in the inner nuclear layer and forming a closer set meshwork than the superficial capillaries which occupy the ganglion cell layers and the nerve fiber (13). The techniques of india ink injection, trypsin digestion and corrosion cast preparation augment one another in making a feasibly complete and accurate analysis of the vascular morphology and its pathology in RCS rats.

Initial irregularities in the superficial capillary network in the midperiphery of the retina of RCS rats become evident in about the third postnatal week after the first pathological changes in the photoreceptor cells have become apparent (1). Flat preparations reveal focal hypocellularity of endothelial cells and pericytes in some capillaries. An unusually large number of endothelial cells can be observed in neighbouring intact vessels, especially at junctions of effected and non-effected vessels (Fig. 1a). As the disorder progresses, changes gradually spread to ever increasing areas and finally involve the entire retinal capillary network.

The progressive and gradual reduction in the number of cellular elements in effected capillaries eventually leads to the appearance of acellular channels. These consist of the basal membrane tubes of the former capillaries (Fig. 1a-d). Interestingly, at points of contact between the acellular channels and intact capillaries, funnel shaped areas containing pericytes can frequently be detected. The acellular channels can persist over long periods of time. Some have been observed in 2 1/2 year old animals. India ink injection and corrosion cast

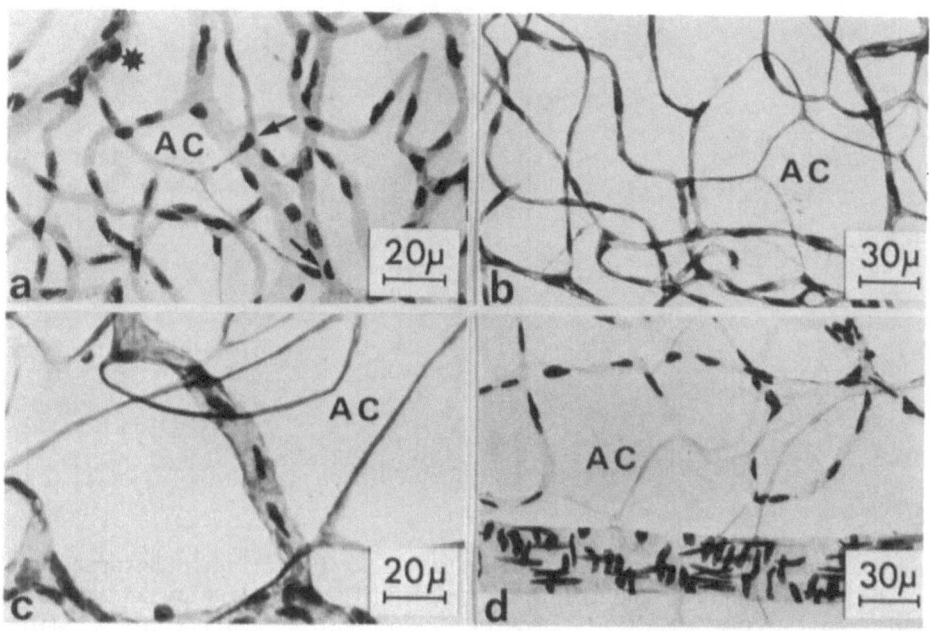

FIGURES 1. a-d Flat preparations show progressive stages of deterioration of the retinal capillary network of RCS rats at a) 4 weeks, b) 4 months, c) 6 months and d) 1 year. Arrows: Pericytes in funnel shaped transitions from intact to effected vessels. Acellular channels: (AC) Hypercellular area: (*).

preparation reveal focal constricture of some capillary lumina, to the point of obstruction in some instances. The entire capillary network coarsens as a result of the formation of these acellular channels.

The thickness of the retina decreases considerably as a result of the loss of the photoreceptors, bringing the bipolar cell layer with the remaining intact retinal capillaries into ever closer proximity to the RPE (Fig. 2). After the third month, the RPE evidences regeneration by proliferating over defective regions and becoming multilayered in some areas (Fig. 3b). Proliferation of the RPE is evident concurrent with still clearly visible signs of degeneration in some of its cells. RPE cells adjacent to Bruch's membrane appear to have lost their normally prominent basal infoldings (Fig. 3b).

At this point in time, one can find newly formed vessels embedded in the RPE, sometimes reaching as far as Bruch's membrane (Fig. 3a, b). Examination of serial semi thin sections of these fenestrated capillaries reveal the origin of these proliferating vessels in the retinal capillary bed, most of them stemming from the deeper, venous side. RPE cells surrounding the proliferating vessels extend numerous branched cytoplasmic processes to the basement membrane of these capillaries (Fig. 3b, 4). One can often find RPE cells in the dystrophic retina along the course of the proliferating retinal capillaries.

412

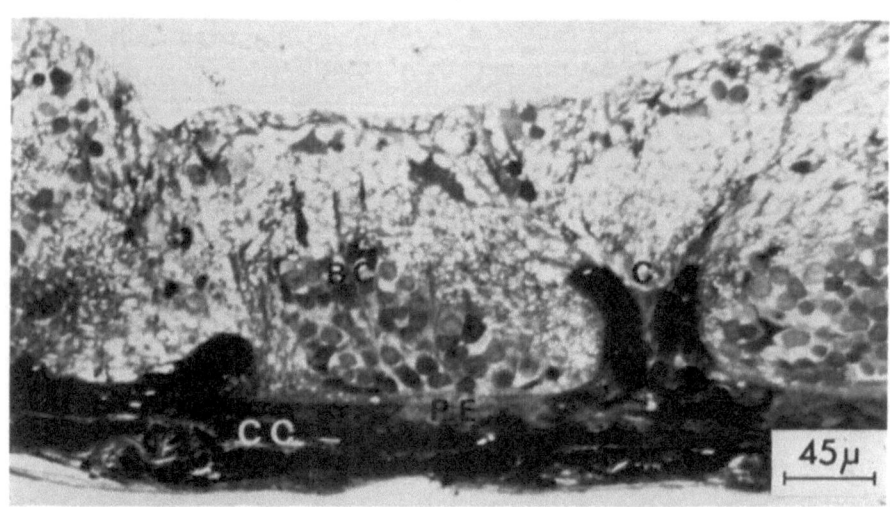

FIGURE 2. Light micrograph of 15 month old RCS rat retina. Photoreceptor layer has disappeared and bipolar cells (BC) are directly adjacent to pigment epithelium (PE). Invading retinal capillaries: (C), Choriocapillaris (CC).

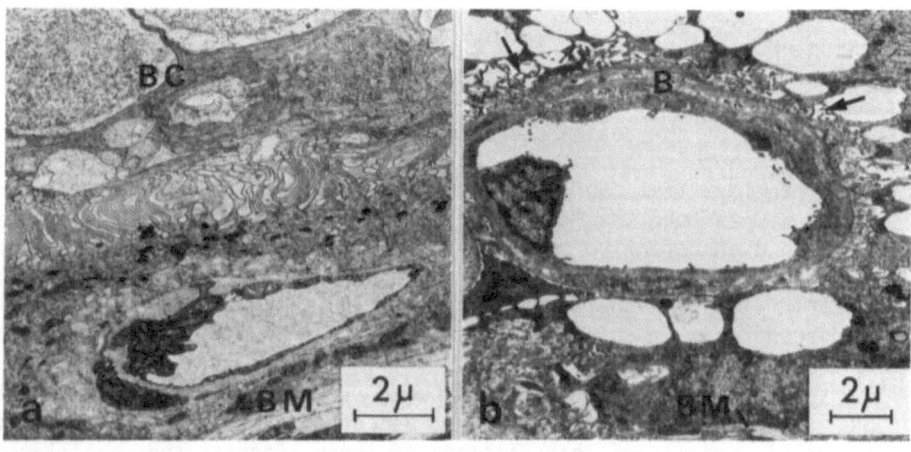

FIGURES 3. a+b Electron micrographs of proliferating RCS rat retinal vessels in the pigment epithelium at a) 6 months and b) 17 months (Note: Cell processes (arrows) extending from the encapsulating RPE toward the basement membrane of the vessel (B), Bipolar cells (BC), Bruch's membrane (BM).

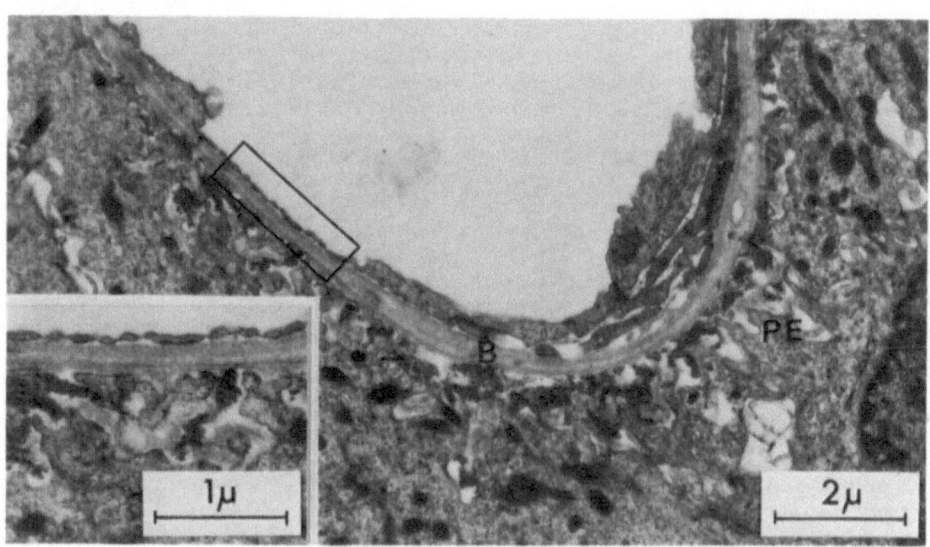

FIGURE 4. Electron micrograph of 18 month old RCS rat retina showing invading retinal capillary encapsulated by retinal pigment epithelial cells (PE). Inset: Higher magnification of enclosed area shows fenestration of endothelial cell facing Bruch's membrane.

The newly formed vessels appear to be coiled in contrast to the normal course of retinal capillaries as can be seen in corrosion cast and india ink preparations (Fig. 5a, b). The lumina of the new vessels are larger than is usual for retinal capillaries. Some endothelial cells of the invading retinal capillaries immediately adjacent to Bruch's membrane exhibit fenestration (Fig. 4). Interestingly, these fenestrae are found almost exclusively in cells facing the Bruch's membrane. It should be noted that no significant changes could be detected in the choriocapillaris in the stages examined in this study.

414

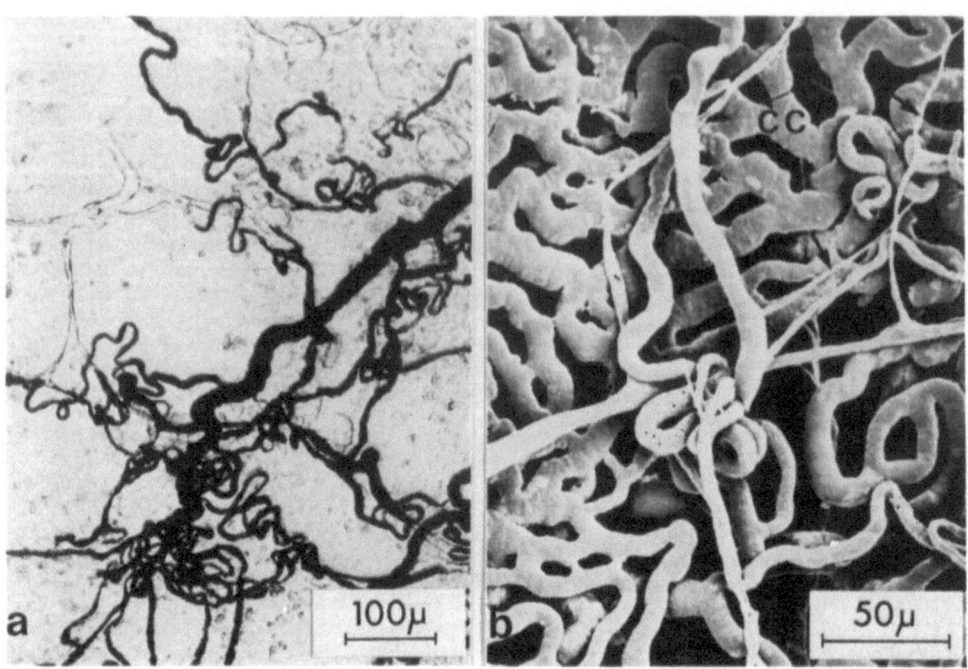

FIGURES 5. a+b   a) 2 year old injected RCS rat retina showing
proliferating vessels of the venous side. Arrows: Constricted retinal
capillaries. b) 7 month old RCS rat retina. Corrosion cast preparation
details choriocapillaris (CC) behind unusually large caliber newly formed
retinal capillaries. Note: wide mesh of retinal capillary bed and coiled
appearence of new vessels in each figure.

DISCUSSION
   Our previous findings demonstrate that pathological changes effect the
retinal vasculature beginning in the superficial capillary network in
early stage of the disorder in RCS rats (1,7). These changes emerge in
the form of focal constricture and obstruction as well as the gradual
loss of endothelial cells and pericytes leaving acellular channels and
leading to a widening of the capillary meshwork. Interestingly, initial
changes in retinal vasculature can be observed immediately subsequent to
the first detectable changes in the photoreceptor cells.
   The formation of acellular channels, which are the basement membrane
remnants of preexisting vessels, is not an unusual occurrence in the
retina, but has been observed in apparently normal retinas. A loss of
endothelial cells and later of pericytes has been observed in humans,
occurring as part of the aging process and remaining restricted to the
periphery of the retina (14, 15). In the case of phototoxin (16) and
urethane induced retinopathy, ·(17, 18) rarefication of the cellular
elements of the vessel wall becomes evident immediately subsequent to the
loss of the photoreceptor cells.

Factors responsible for the vascular retinopathy are largely unknown. The chronological succession of the dystrophic changes in the photoreceptor cells and increase in the formation of acellular channels in the retinal vasculature as documented in this and our earlier studies leads one to postulate a relationship between the degeneration of the photoreceptor cells and changes in the retinal vessels. On the basis of our results, it can be suggested that toxic byproducts of the process of photoreceptor cell degeneration could be a factor responsible for the widening of the capillary meshwork.

It has been well established that an increase in O_2 partial pressure in retinal tissue leads to vasoobliterative changes in RCS rat retinal vasculature (8). Several investigators have proposed that this is also the root of vasoobliterative changes in RCS rat retinal vasculature. In later stages of the disease, the reduced photoreceptor layer allows for unusually close proximity of the retinal vessels to the choriocapillaris which probably does lead to an increase in the O_2 tension in the retinal tissue. Our previous studies, however, indicate that the initial changes in retinal vasculature occur well before the stages in which the proximity of the retinal vessels to the choriocapillaris could produce these effects (1). Indeed, initial changes in the retinal vasculature can be observed when the neural retina is actually thicker than usual due to the accumulation of non-phagocytosed outer segment debris.

Retinal vessels proliferate into the pigment epithelium in advanced stages of the disease. Similar proliferation has been observed clinically in retinal vein occlusion (19) and diabetic retinopathy, (20) and experimentally in phototoxin (16) and urethane induced retinopathy (17, 18). In previous studies, proliferation took place in the presence of ischemic retinas. Factors deriving from the ischemic retina are thought to induce endothelial cell proliferation (21). The ischemic factor, however, cannot be the sole cause of neovascularization as proliferation begins when the photoreceptor cell layer has nearly disappeared leaving a reduced retina topographically close to the choriocapillaris. The choriocapillaris remains essentially uneffected by the disorder and is thus capable of supplying the entire retina with oxygen. On the basis of our present findings, we conclude that factors arising in the RPE initiate retinal neovascularization. Several morphological observations presented in this study support this supposition: 1) Neovascularization begins when RPE degeneration has largely ceased and regeneration has begun as signified by its proliferation. 2) The thinning of the retinal layers brings the retinal vasculature into unusually close proximity with the RPE. It is even partially enveloped by the proliferating RPE cells which would easily allow for the transfer of an inducing factor(s). 3) The enveloping RPE cells have numerous cytoplasmic processes contacting the basement membrane of the new capillaries. This strengthens the suggestion that factors could easily be transferred from the RPE to the proliferating retinal vessels.

Plasma cells have also been cited as inducers of neovascularization (22, 23). In the course of this and earlier studies we have found no plasma cells in the dystrophic retina so that we do not believe that this is the source of stimulus for the neovascularization in RCS rats. In contrast, migrating pigment epithelial cells in the dystrophically changed retina are frequently found in the region of the proliferating vessels. Similar findings have been recently reported in urethane induced retinopathy (18).

Fenestration of some retinal capillaries becomes apparent when retinal neovascularization is already well advanced. The fenestrae are almost exclusively limited to endothelial cells lying opposite Bruch's membrane in capillaries generally enveloped by proliferating pigment epithelial cells. This fenestration is possibly due to the necessarily increased metabolic exchange between the focally multilayered RPE cells and the proliferating retinal vessels.

A noticeable decrease in the number of basal infoldings of the RPE toward the choriocapillaris indicates a reduction in the free cell surface available for metabolic exchange. The newly formed vessels in the RPE may well provide its major blood supply. Based on these findings, we suggest that factors deriving from the RPE may well be responsible for neovascularization as well as fenestration of the newly formed vessels.

REFERENCES

1. El-Hifnawi, E. (1985): Pathomorphologische Untersuchungen zum Verlauf der hereditären Netzhaut-Dystrophie bei R.C.S.-Ratten. Ferdinand Enke, Stuttgart.
2. Dowling, J.E. and Sidman, R.L. (1962): Inherited retinal dystrophy in the rat. J. Cell Biol. 14, 73-109.
3. Edwards, R.B. and Szamier, R.B. (1977): Defective phagocytosis of isolated rod outer segments by RCS rat retinal pigment epithelium in culture. Science 197, 1001-1003.
4. Herron, W.L. jr., Riegel, B.W., Myers, O.E. and Rubin, M.L. (1969): Retinal dystrophy in the rat - A pigment epithelial disease. Invest. Ophthalmol. Vis. Sci. 8, 595-604.
5. Herron, W.L. jr., Riegel, B.W., and Rubin, M.L. (1971): Outer segment production and removal in the degenerating retina of the dystrophic rat. Invest. Ophthalmol. Vis. Sci. 10, 54-63.
6. Herron, W.L. jr., Riegel, B.W., Brennan, E. and Rubin, M.L. (1974): Retinal dystrophy in the pigmented rat. Invest. Ophthalmol. Vis. Sci. 13, 87-94.
7. El-Hifnawi, E. (1981): REM-Untersuchungen an Gefäßausgußpräparaten von Rattenaugen mit hereditären Netzhautdegenerationen. Verh. Anat. Ges. 75, 963-964.
8. Gerstein, D.D. and Dantzker, D.R. (1969): Retinal vascular changes in hereditary visual cell degeneration. Arch. Ophthalmol. 81, 99-105.
9. Richardson, K.C., Jarett, L. and Finke, E.H. (1960): Embedding in epoxy resins for ultrathin sectioning in electron microscopy. Stain Technol. 35, 313-323.
10. Reynolds, E.S. (1963): The use of lead citrate at high pH as an electronopaque stain in electron microscopy. J. Cell Biol. 17, 208-212.
11) Kuwabara, T., Cogan, D.G. (1960): Studies of retinal vascular patterns. Part I. Normal architecture. Arch. Ophthalmol. 64, 904-911.
12) Michaelson, I.C. (1954): Retinal circulation in man and animals. Springfield, IL, Thomas.

13) Michaelson, I.C. (1948): The mode of development of the vascular system of the retina, with some observations on its significance for certain retinal diseases. Trans. Ophthalmol. Soc. UK 68, 137-180.

14) Kuwabara, T. and Cogan, D.G. (1965): Retinal vascular patterns. VII. Acellular change. Invest. Ophthalmol. Vis. Sci. 4, 1049-1058.

15) Kuwabara, T., Carrol, J.M. and Cogan D.G. (1961): Retinal vascular patterns. Part III. Age, hypertension, absolute glaucoma, injury. Arch. Ophthalmol. 65, 708-716.

16) Bellhorn, R.W., Burns, M.S. and Benjamin, J.V. (1980): Retinal vessel abnormalities of phototoxic retinopathy in rats. Invest. Ophthalmol. Vis. Sci. 19, 584-595.

17) Bellhorn, R.W., Bellhorn, M., Friedman, A.H. and Henkind, P. (1973): Urethane-induced retinopathy in pigmented rats. Invest. Ophthalmol. Vis. Sci. 12, 65-76.

18) Shiraki, K. and Burns, M.S. (1986): Neovascularization in urethane rat retinopathy demonstrated by thymidine labelling. Curr. Eye Res. 5, 683-695.

19) Hamilton, A.M., Kohner, E.M., Rosen, D. and Bowbyes, J.A. (1974): Experimental venous occlusion. Proc. R. Soc. Med. 67, 1045-1048.

20) De Venecia, G., Davis, M. and Engerman, R. (1976): Clinicopathologic correlations in diabetic retinopathy. 1. Histology and fluorescein angiography of micoraneurysms. Arch. Ophthalmol. 94, 1766-1773.

21) Patz, A. (1982): Clincal and experimental studies on retinal neovascularization. XXXIX Edward Jackson Memorial Lecture. Am. J. Ophthalmol. 94, 715-743.

22) Saba, H.I., Hartman, R.C. and Saba, S.R. (1978): Effects of polymorphonuclear leukocytes on endothelial cell growth. Thromb. Res. 12, 397-407.

23) Wall, R.T., Harker, L.A., Quadracci, L.J. and Striker, G.E. (1978): Factors influencing endothelial cell proliferation in vitro. J. Cell Physiol. 96, 203-213.

RETINAL PIGMENT EPITHELIAL TEARS AND SUBRETINAL NEOVASCULARIZATION

G. COSCAS, F. KOENIG, G. SOUBRANE, E.BENHAMOU - CRETEIL (France)

Serous detachment of the retinal pigment epithelium is a well-recognized feature of age-related macular degeneration. The major complications of this lesion are either invasion of the subpigment epithelial space by subretinal new vessels (1, 2) or geographic atrophy of the choriocapillaris and the retinal pigment epithelium (3). An additional complication, tearing of the retinal pigment epithelium (Fig. 1), was reported in 1981 by Hoskin, Bird and Sehmi (4). Since then, other observations of retinal pigment epithelial tears have been described.

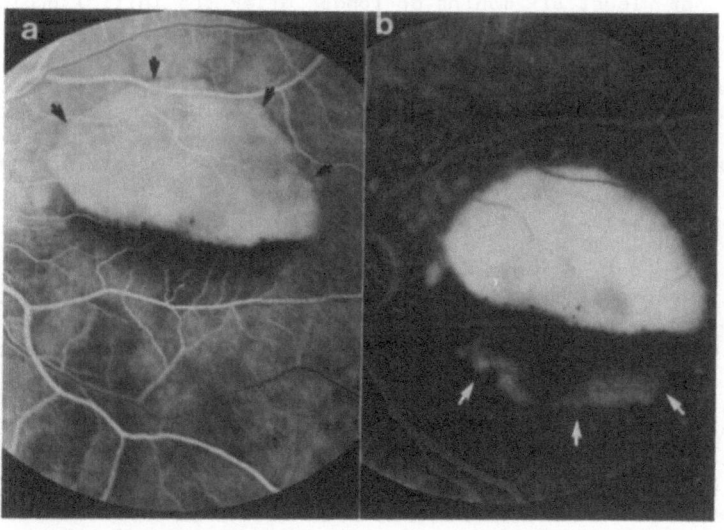

Figure 1 : Acute retinal pigment epithelial tears. A well-defined pigmented linear band separates : (1) a superior region of exposed choroïd with bare Bruch's membrane with uniform, sharply demarcated hyperfluorescence (black arrows) ; (2) an inferior remaining region of pigment epithelial elevation (white arrows). Case N.2 : (a) 19 second ; (b) 5 min.

The tears can occur either spontaneously or after the photocoagulation of a retinal pigment epithelium detachment (4-12). Several hypotheses have been developed to explain the pathogenesis of the spontaneous tears (4, 6, 8, 9, 12).

This clinical and fluorescein angiographic study of spontaneous retinal pigment epithelial tears was undertaken to assess the natural history of this lesion better, particularly its relationship with subretinal new vessels.

MATERIALS AND METHODS

Only spontaneous tears associated with age-related macular degeneration and retinal pigment epithelial detachment were considered in this retrospective study.

Included in this study were 30 eyes from 29 patients (from a total of 74 patients) with recent spontaneous retinal pigment epithelial tears who were observed in the Department of Ophthalmology of Créteil from 1981 to 1986. The follow-up period ranged from 6 to 70 months (mean, 22.5 months). The patients (8 men - 21 women) ranged in age from 56 to 84 years (average, 70.9 years).

The following data were recorded for each patient : age and sex ; duration of symptoms ; best corrected initial and final visual acuities; signs of age-related macular changes ; and size, location, and ophthalmoscopic features of the retinal pigment epithelial tear. Stereoscopic color photographs and fluorescein angiography were performed at least six months or longer after the initial angiography. Red light frames were required to delineate the area of the tear.

For each patient, the presence of a retinal pigment epithelial tear and the existence and exact location of subretinal neovascularization was checked or discussed by 3 separate observers. Follow-up with fluorescein angiography was obtained to document this neovascularization.

RESULTS

Most of our patients experienced a substantial decrease in visual acuity immediately after the tearing of the retinal pigment epithelium. Subsequently, visual outcome was very poor and did not improve during the follow-up period. Visual acuity was recorded as 20/400 or less for 86% of the patients. These patients who suffered very severe loss of vision gained no help from low vision aids. In these cases, the area of the tear involved the subfoveolar retinal pigment epithelium. In 3 cases, the outcome was less severe because the retracted retinal pigment epithelium still covered the foveolar area. These patients maintained a visual acuity of 20/200 after 16 to 32 months of follow-up. In one case, the lesion remained extra-macular with a visual acuity of 20/40 after six months.

Twenty two eyes were examined before the tear developed. The most frequently (13 of 22 eyes)noted feature was a large serous retinal pigment epithelial detachment, irregular in shape and associated with a notch, frequently on the foveal edge of the detachment (Fig 2). Fluorescein angiography of these cases revealed a delay in overall fluorescein staining. The late frames showed the filling of the retinal

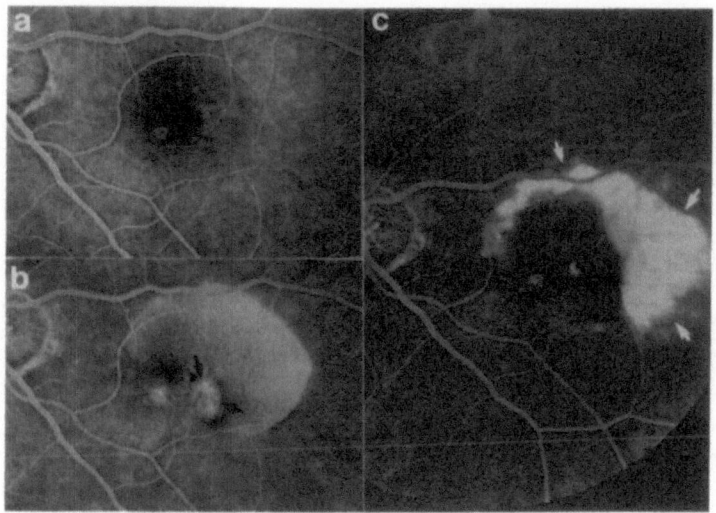

Figure 2 :Case N.16 : (A) August 10, 1984 - (b) Mars 5, 1985 - (c) Mars
29, 1985.
Pre-tear stage : Serous retinal pigment epithelial detachment
associated with a notch on the foveal edge of the detachment
(black arrows). Extensive ripping that involved 270 : at the
supra-temporal edge (white arrows).

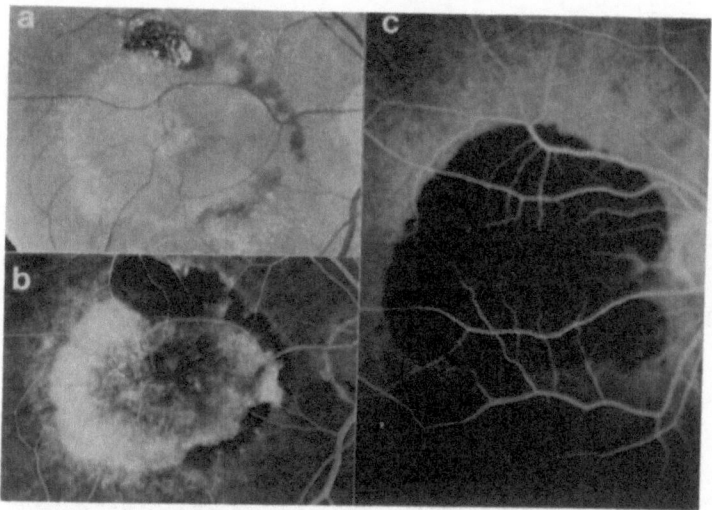

Figure 3 :(a) Case N.12 : Arciform hemorrhage underlining the retinal
pigment epithelial detachment.
(b) Case N.6 : Profuse hemorrhage blocking the background
fluorescence.

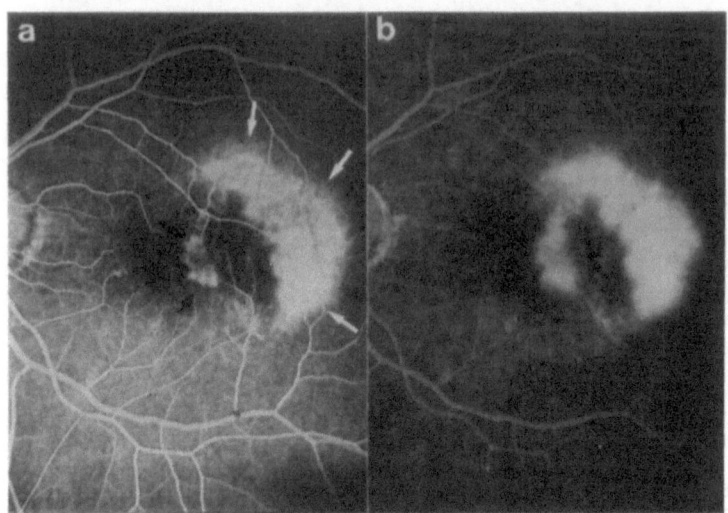

Case N.14 : Subretinal new vessels (black arrows) with typical
lacy pattern (a) and leakage (b), located opposite to the area
of bare Bruch's membrane (white arrows).

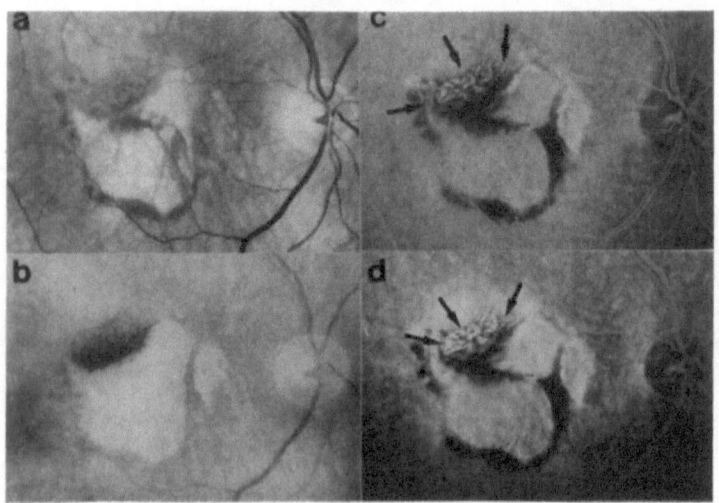

Case N.4 : Detached retinal pigment epithelium retracted with
vermiculate-like retinal pigment epithelial obliterations
(black arrows) without late leakage.
(a) red-free light frame ; (b) red light frame ; (c)
angiography early frame (37sec.) ; (d) late stage (5mn).

pigment epithelial detachment to be uneven, irregular and more dense at the periphery. Soft drusen surrounding the retinal pigment epithelial detachment were visible in 11 of 22 eyes at the pre-tear stage and in 18 of 30 eyes of the study.

In 15 of 22 eyes, the tearing was announced and accompanied by a deep subretinal hemorrhage (Fig 3). The hemorrhage was usually large and extensive, but occurred mostly in an arciform or circumferential pattern, (8 of 15 eyes) underlining the retinal pigment epithelial detachment (Fig. 3a). The hemorrhage could be very profuse and even block the hyperfluorescence in the area of the tear (Fig. 3b).

In 27 of 30 eyes, we recognized subretinal new vessels, sometimes easily as a typical lacy hyperfluorescence with leakage (11 of 27 eyes) (Fig. 4). But, more frequently (16 eyes), the new vessels were partially hidden by hemorrhages or by retracted retinal pigment epithelium. The location of the new vessels was suggested by late mottled staining surrounded by small patchy hemorrhages suggesting "occult" subretinal neovascularization.

The new vessels were usually located opposite to the area of bare Bruch's membrane (18 eyes). Although, in 9 eyes, they appeared in or progressed into the area of the tear.

Retinal pigment epithelial tears rarely (3 of 30 eyes) demonstrated no evidence of progressive and active new vessel growth during the follow-up period. New vessels, however may appear long after the tear presents : in one eye, they developed 10 months after the tear occurred.

The tear remained relatively small in four cases. The tearing involved half the circumference of the retinal pigment epithelial detachment in most cases (17 eyes). We also observed a second tearing (1 eye), or more extensive ripping, that involved more than 270° (8 eyes). In one eye, the tear even extended to 360°. In three eyes, the tearing occurred in an old fibrovascular scar, associated with a recurrence of the serous retinal detachment.

One patient presented with bilateral recent retinal pigment epithelial tear. Of 28 patients, the fellow eye exhibited at initial examination : soft drusen (4 eyes) or pigment epithelial detachment (2 eyes) or atrophic scar (1 eye) and or disciform lesion with active new vessels growth (7eyes) ; the remaining fourteen eyes presented with an old fibro-glial scar (with evidence of previous tear in six eyes).

DISCUSSION

In the natural course of a retinal pigment epithelial detachment, the following features are suggestive of the retinal pigment epithelial tearing. A well-defined pigmented linear band separates two distincts areas : a crescent - shaped region of exposed choroïd, and a remaining region of pigment epithelial elevation. In the area of bare Bruch's membrane, the filling of choroïdal vessels was already visible in the first angiographic frame, and was rapidly replaced by uniform, sharply demarcated hyperfluorescence within the first seconds. Seen stereoscopically, the dye remained at the level of Bruch's membrane. In most cases there was no leakage or accumulation of dye into the subretinal space.

The free edge of the retinal pigment epithelium was well demarcated and always visible in the red light frame. The retinal pigment epithelium appeared retracted and rolled up, thus resulting in some cases of vermiculate-like retinal pigment epithelial alteration (Fig. 5). Angiography showed streaks or spots of early fluorescence at the surface of the pigmented mound, without late leakage. The remaining area of pigment epithelial elevation filled with dye later and remained uneven and less hyperfluorescent than the area of bare Bruch's membrane.

In their initial report, Hoskin and coll. (4) postulated that these detachments of the retinal pigment epithelium in which tears occur are composed of two parts. In one segment, the retinal pigment epithelium together with its basement membrane become detached and this part of the detachment fills early with hyperfluorescence on angiography. In the other segment, the retinal pigment epithelium is detached without its basement membrane and the detachment fills with regular, even, and late hyperfluorescence. The retinal pigment epithelial tear occurs where the authors presume the retinal pigment epithelium to be detached from its basement membrane. They observed hemorrhages in a few cases (5 of 44 cases) and failed to identify with certitude any associated subretinal new vessels. These authors did not consider the new vessels to be a factor in the pathogenesis of retinal pigment epithelial tears.

Some reports (6, 8) doubt Hoskin's hypothesis that the detachment of the retinal pigment epithelium from its basement membrane is the cause of retinal pigment epithelial tears. Moreover, in these reports the association of the tear with subretinal new vessels remains unclear. One investigation noted evidence of choroidal neovascularization in 4 of 6 patients with a tear (6). Another observed subretinal and subpigment epithelial blood following the development of a large tear with a visibly rolled margin (8). However, the latter was attributed to a mechanical disruption of the choriocapillaris at the site of the tear.

For Gass (9), there is a more plausible explanation for the pathogenesis of spontaneous retinal pigment epithelial tears : (1) in the first stage, subretinal new vessels invade and grow through Bruch's membrane into the subpigment epithelial space ; (2) over a period of weeks or months, these vessels proliferate to form a fibrovascular mound that gradually elevates the basement membrane, drusen, retinal pigment epithelium, and retina and may produce no symptoms ; (3) a rapid change in the permeability of these new vessels within this occult lesion produces a serous detachment of the adjacent retinal pigment epithelium, and the drusen disappear, presumably dissolving within the serous exudate ; (4) as the pressure of fluid increases within the detachment, a breaking point is reached and a tear occurs at the junction of the attached and detached retinal pigment epithelium (Fig. 2).

Our observations show a relationship between the occurrence of retinal pigment epithelial tears and the presence of new vessels in 27 of 30 cases. These patients were suspected of or assumed to have subretinal new vessels when either on of two angiographic features was present : a directly visible neovascular network (Fig. 4) or focal hyperfluorescent spots with late "pin-points" and leakage, already described as "occult" subretinal new vessels (Fig. 4) (13, 14). Both features differed from the angiographic pattern seen in the area of the tear in the way the filling occured. Also, in the red light frame, the area of the tear always appeared clearly visible, but the subretinal new vessels did not.

Conversely, we also observed 3 cases in which we could not even suspect the presence of subretinal new vessels (Fig. 1). In these cases it is not possible to explain the occurrence of the tear by a secondary retraction after development of a fibrovascular subretinal mound.

Therefore, it appears that a tear can occur in 2 different circumstances. When new vessels are clinically present, the new vessels growth can act as a retracting focus and/or create pressure changes within the retinal pigment epithelial detachment as suggested by Gass (9). When new vessels are clinically absent, other factors must explain the occurrence of the tear, such as pressure forces within the retinal pigment epithelial detachment and possibly anatomically weak areas of the retinal pigment epithelium. This theory could explain why the site of the tear is always on the edge of the retinal pigment epithelial detachment. However, Green's observation (15) that subretinal neovascularization can exist and be undetected by clinical and angiographic methods must not be forgotten.

We noted also that the tear could occur in association with a large subretinal hemorrhage, which was always located at the edge of the retinal pigment epithelial detachment. These circumferential hemorrhages are probably caused by mechanical disruption of the choriocapillaris layer at the site of the tear, due to tractional forces. Although, a cleavage appears unlikely between the retinal pigment epithelial cells and their basement membrane.

The clinical and angiographic features that produce the retinal pigment epithelial tear including the pre-tear stage, the tear stage and late scarring illustrate that the tearing and subretinal new vessels are both manifestations of age-related macular degeneration and the underlying diffuse retinal epitheliopathy. It seems very important to be able to recognize the subtle changes that occur in the retinal pigment epithelial detachment just before the tear develops.
These changes include the arciform hemorrhage surrounding the detachment and the variations in the filling of this detachment on angiography. In these particular cases, photocoagulation should be avoided because it could precipitate the actual tearing. Of all the aspects of age-related macular degeneration, tearing of the retinal pigment epithelium is of particular interest because it challenges some long-held concepts, such as hemorrhage always being due to new vessels. In addition, the natural course of this condition is very poor, even in the absence of subfoveolar new vessels. Moreover the process leading to scar formation remains unclear in the absence of pathologic correlation.

The use of photocoagulation in the treatment of retinal pigment epithelial detachment is already controversial, and it becomes crucial to comprehend the exact pathogenesis of retinal pigment epithelial tear better to apply laser treatment more accurately.

426

REFERENCES

1.GASS J.D.M. : Pathogenesis of disciform detachment of the neuroepithelium. Am. J. Ophthalmol., 1967, 63, 573-711.
2.MEREDITH T.A., BRALEY R.E., AABERG T.M. : Natural history of serous detachments of the retinal pigment epithelium. Am. J. Ophthalmol., 1979, 88, 643-651.
3.BLAIR C.J. : Geographic atrophy of the retinal pigment epithelium. Arch. Ophthalmol., 1975, 93, 19-25.
4.HOSKIN A., BIRD A.C., SEHMI K. : Tears of detached retinal pigment epithelium. Br. J. Ophthalmol., 1981, 65, 417-422.
5.COSCAS G., QUENTEL G., SOUBRANE G. et al : Déchirure spontanée de l'épithélium pigmentaire dans la région maculaire. Bull. Soc. Ophtalmol. Fr, 1982, 82, 815-820.
6.CANTRILL H.L., RAMSAY R.C., KNOBLOCH W.H. : Rips in the pigment epithelium. Arch. Ophthalmol., 1983, 101, 1074-1079.
7.DECKER W.L., SANBORN G.E., RIDLEY M. et al : Retinal pigment epithelial tears. Ophthalmology, 1983, 90, 507-512.
8.GREEN S.N., YARIAN D. : Acute tear of the retinal pigment epithelium. Retina, 1983, 3, 16-20.
9.GASS J.D.M. : Pathogenesis of tears of the retinal pigment epithelium. Br. J. Ophthalmol., 1984, 68, 513-519.
10.GASS J.D.M. : Retinal pigment epithelial rip during Krypton red laser photocoagulation. Am. J. Ophthalmol., 1984, 98, 700-706.
11.DE LAEY J.J., RIEMS D. : Ripping of detached retinal pigment epithelium in senile macular degeneration. Bull. Soc. Belge Ophtalmol., 1984, 207, 27-35.
12.KRISHAN N.R., CHANDRA S.R., STEVENS T.S. : Diagnosis and pathogenesis of retinal pigment epithelial tears. Am. J. Ophthalmol., 1985, 100, 698-707.
13.GASS J.D.M. : Serous retinal pigment epithelial detachment with a notch. A sign of occult choroïdal neovascularization. Retina, 1984, 4, 205-220.
14.SOUBRANE G., COSCAS G., KOENIG F. et al : Natural history of occult subretinal newvessels in age-related macular degeneration. Int. Symp. on Fluorescein Angiography (ISFA), September 9, 1985. Baden-Baden (W. Germany).
15.GREEN R., MAC DONNELL P., YEO J.H. : Pathologic features of senile macular degeneration. Ophthalmology, 1985, 92, 615-627.

ABSTRACT

Spontaneous retinal pigment epithelial tears were observed in 30 eyes of 29 patients with age-related macular degeneration. 22 patients were seen at a pre-tear stage : in 70% of these cases, a large subretinal hemorrhage occurred with an arciform or circonferential pattern surrounding the pigment epithelial detachment.
Careful analysis of fluorescein angiography allowed recognition of the hyperfluorescence due to the tear or due to associated subretinal newvessels in 27 eyes. They either demonstrated the characteristic features of lacy newvessels or were partially occulted behind an hemorrhage or behind the retracted retinal pigment epithelium. Their location was usually at the opposite from the bare Bruch's membrane.
    Visual outcome was very poor and did not improve. Visual acuity was recorded as 20/400 or less for 86% of the patients except one case with extrafoveal lesion and three cases in which the retracted retinal pigment epithelium still covered the foveolar receptors.

INTERACTIONS BETWEEN THE RETINAL PIGMENT EPITHELIUM AND THE CHORIO-CAPILLARIS AFTER KRYPTON LASER PHOTOCOAGULATION

A. POLLACK,* G.E. KORTE, W.J. HERIOT, P. HENKIND
*Kaplan Hospital, Rehovot, Israel and Albert Einstein College of Medicine, Bronx, N.Y. USA

1. INTRODUCTION

Retinal diseases involving the retinal pigment epithelial (RPE) cells and the choriocapillaris (CC) have various clinical manifestations. All, however, are accompanied by at least some changes in both the RPE cells and the CC. These changes can be classified into two broad categories: the first is an atrophic form, involving atrophy of both the RPE cells and the CC, while the second is an active form characterized by the development of choroidal subretinal neovascularization. Since atrophy occurs in the RPE cells and in the CC concomitantly, and since choroidal neovascularization is not seen in areas of atrophic RPE cells, there is reason to suspect that some interactions exist between the RPE cells and the CC. However, the nature of the interactions between the RPE cells and the vascular endothelium, as well as the factors determining whether the disease will take an atrophic or an active course, are not clearly understood.

The aim of this study was to investigate the recovery of the RPE cells following krypton laser photocoagulation in the rat, with special attention to interactions between the RPE cells and the vascular endothelium during the healing process.

2. MATERIAL AND METHODS

White laser burns - considered as equivalent to therapeutically applied lesions - were applied to the superior half of the posterior pole of the retina in 40 mature pigmented rats, described elsewhere (1). The eyes were enucleated 1,2,3,4,6,7,10,14,21,28,35,39 and 50 days after lasering and processed by routine methods for light microscopy (LM) and transmission electron microscopy (TEM).

3. RESULTS

From the 10th day after lasering, three types of regenerating RPE cells (which we designated types 1,2 and 3) could be morphologically distinguished at a recovery site. Under LM, type 1 cells had a macrophage-like appearance. They stained dark and contained numerous pigmented granules (Fig. 1). TEM revealed that these cells were electron-dense and had lobulated nuclei, diffusely spread pigmented granules and lipid droplets (Fig. 2A-C). They lacked basal folds but had microvilli (Fig. 2A,2C). They also retained certain features of normal RPE cells, such as the presence of junctional complexes between cells and basal attachments to Bruch's membrane (not shown). Type 2 cells resembled normal RPE cells and were recognizable under both LM and TEM by their prominent basal folds (Figs. 1,3). TEM also revealed additional characteristics of RPE cells, such as cell polarity indicated by the presence of basal folds, apical villi and apical melanosomes (Fig. 3). Type 3 cells appeared under both

LM and TEM as large, pale cells with few or no basal folds (Figs. 1,2,4). Under TEM the cells appeared relatively hypopigmented with diffusely spread melanosomes, and their apical villi were either elongated or short and stubby (Figs. 2,4). Some of these cells appeared to be active, e.g., they contained expanded rough endoplasmic reticulum and numerous poly-ribosomes, and were associated with accumulation of extracellular matrix (Fig. 2A).

Although all three cell types could be seen at a recovery site, there was usually a predominance of one or two types in any section studied. We attempted to establish the phase of choroidal vascular recovery (described in the accompanying paper (2)) and the presence of a certain RPE cell type. We found that in foci where macrophage-like RPE cells (type 1) and normal-looking RPE cells (type 2) were predominant, recanalization and neovascularization had occurred (Fig. 1), and the normal-looking RPE cells were located close to the reformed capillaries (Fig. 3). Type 3 cells, on the other hand, were adjacent to the degenerating endothelium of neovascular fronds or to sites of CC atrophy (Fig. 4). Atrophy of the CC was also observed in areas where no RPE cells were present and Bruch's membrane had become relined with neural retinal cells (Fig. 5).

4. COMMENT

Our work supports previous observations that there is interaction bet-ween the RPE cells and the CC (3-5). In areas where RPE cells did not recover, CC was absent as well, while in foci where regenerated RPE cells were visible the choroidal vasculature had reformed. The question then arises: do the RPE cells die as a result of insufficient blood supply from the CC, or does the CC become atrophied following the loss of RPE cells? A number of authors favor an ischemic mechanism (6), while others claim evidence from clinical material that areas of RPE atrophy undergo a concomitant loss of the CC (3,7). On the basis of these observations, Henkind et al. postulated that the RPE cells have a trophic effect on the CC. Experiments have shown that primary destruction of the RPE cells is associated with CC atrophy (4,5). However, CC atrophy may occur in other circumstances as well, e.g., when the vascular endothelium is inhibited by RPE cells as described in vitro (8). The presence of morphologically heterogeneous populations of RPE cells observed here may help to resolve conflicting suggestions with regard to interrelationships between the RPE cells and the CC.

Three types of regenerated RPE cells could be morphologically disting-uished at a recovery site. Type 1 had the ultrastructural characteristics of macrophages, such as clusters of inclusion bodies. These cells were assumed to originate from proliferating RPE cells, since 1) the latter are known to be able to give rise to macrophage RPE cells (9), and 2) in many sections they displayed features of RPE cells, such as basal attach-ments to Bruch's membrane and intercellular junctional complexes, not normally seen with macrophages. Type 2 cells resembled normal RPE cells. Type 3 cells differed from the other cell types by their pale color, hypo-pigmentation, small number of basal folds and association with accumulated extracellular matrix. The reason for these morphological variations, i.e., whether they reflect different stages of cellular maturation or alternative forms of cell differentiation, has yet to be determined.

Cell types 1 and 2 were associated with growing or normal-looking capillaries. Since type 1 cells resemble RPE macrophages, and since macrophages can induce new vascular growth, these cells may promote chor-oidal subretinal neovascularization (1). Type 2 cells, like normal RPE cells, may play a role in the maintenance of viable endothelium of reformed capillaries and of choroidal subretinal neovascularization. Type 3 cells predominated at sites of endothelial degeneration, and may account for the inhibitory effect of the RPE cells (8).

The subject of RPE-CC interactions is a complex one, probably involving other components such as the extracellular matrix. However, the present observation that regenerating RPE cells can exhibit various morphologic features somewhat reminiscent of this ability in macrophages (10), may explain how the same cell can be stimulatory on the one hand and inhibitory on the other.

REFERENCES

1. Pollack A, Heriot WJ, Henkind P: Cellular processes causing defects in Bruch's membrane following krypton laser photocoagulation. Ophthalmol 93:1113-1119, 1986.
2. Pollack A, Korte GE, Henkind P: Choroidal vascular repair after krypton laser photocoagulation in the rat. Ocular Circulation and Neovascularisation, edited by Dr. D. BenEzra and Dr. S.J. Ryan, Martinus Nijhoff Publishers Nordrecht/Boston/Lancaster.
3. Henkind P, Gartner S: The relationship between retinal pigment epithelium and the choriocapillaris. Trans Ophthalmol Soc UK 103:444-447, 1983.
4. Korte GE, Reppucci V, Henkind P: RPE destruction causes chorio-capillary atrophy. Invest Ophthalmol Vis Sci 25:1135-1145, 1984.
5. Heriot WJ, Henkind P, Bellhorn RW, Burns MS: Retinal pigment epithelial specific phototoxicity. Invest Ophthalmol Vis Sci (Suppl) 26:170, 1984.
6. Weiter J, Fine BS: A histologic study of regional choroidal dystrophy. Am J Ophthalmol 83:741, 1977.
7. Sarks SH: Changes in the region of the choriocapillaris in ageing and degeneration. XXIII Concilium Ophthalmologicum, Kyoto, Shimizu K and Oosterhuis J, editors. Amsterdam, Excerpta Medica, 228-238, 1978.
8. Glaser BM, Campochiaro PA, David JL Jr et al.: Retinal pigment epithelial cells release an inhibitor of neovascularization. Arch Ophthalmol 103:1870-1875, 1985.
9. Machemer R, Laqua H: Pigment epithelium proliferation in retinal detachment (massive periretinal proliferation). Am J Ophthalmol 80:1-23, 1975.
10. Werb Z: How the macrophage regulates its extracellular environment. Am J Anat 166:237-256, 1983.

432

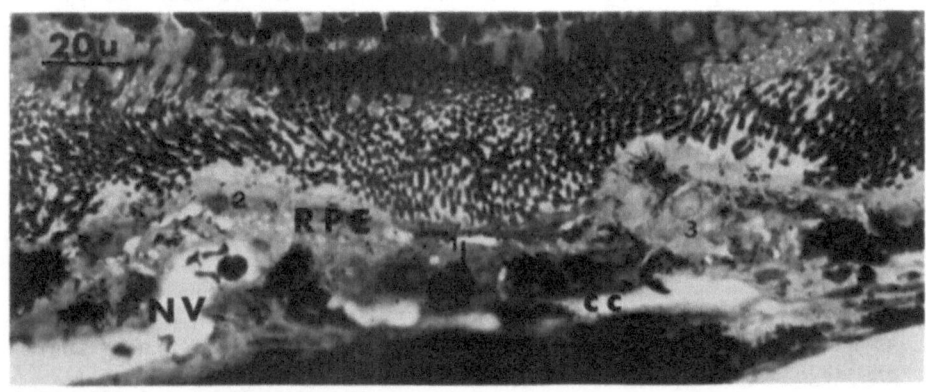

FIGURE 1. LM of a laser site with different types of regenerating RPE cells. The numbers denote the cell type. Note that cell types 1 and 2 are adjacent to patent capillaries (CC) and to choroidal subretinal neovascularization (NV). A single type 3 cell is also present. (20um=14mm).

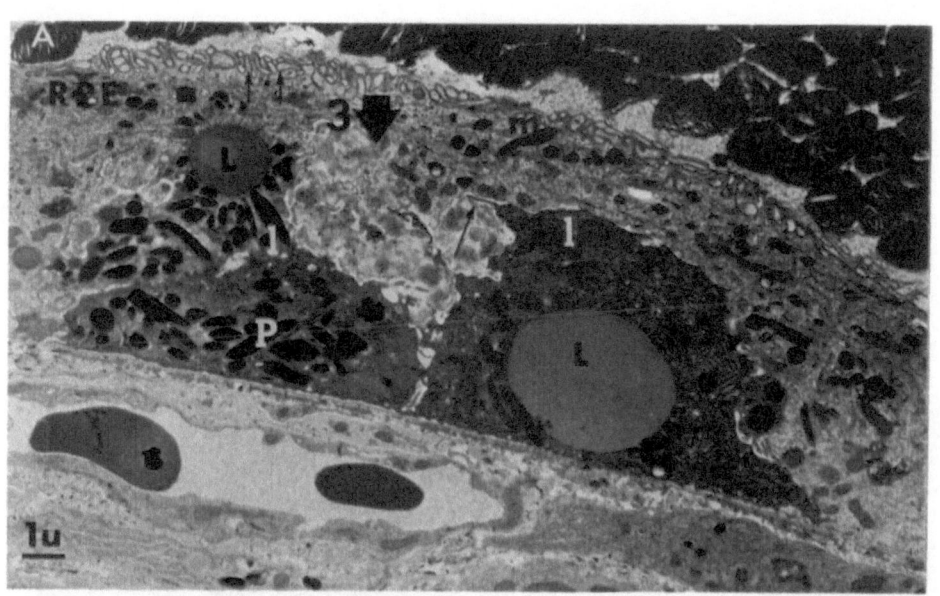

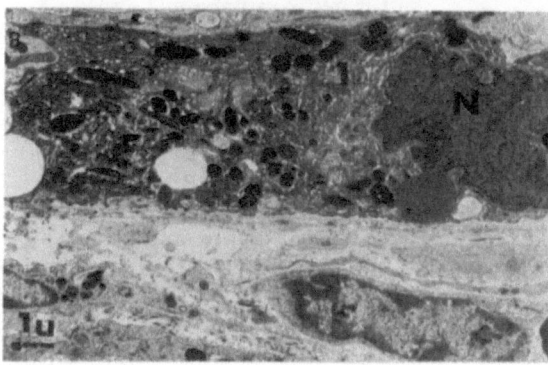

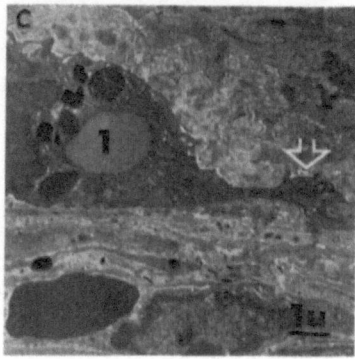

FIGURE 2A. TEM of type 1 and 3 RPE cells. Type 1 is electron-dense, and contains numerous melanolysosomes (P) and lipid droplets (L). Microvilli (narrow arrow) surround the extracellular matrix. Type 3 cells are electron-lucent, contain few melanosomes (m) and have short stubby apical villi (double arrows). An accumulation of extracellular basement membrane-like matrix can be seen between the cells (wide arrow). (1um=6mm). B, C. Serial sections of A showing some characteristics of macrophages. Note lobulated nucleus (N) in B, and cellular processes (white arrow) passing through the RPE basement membrane towards the choroid in C. (1um=5mm).

434

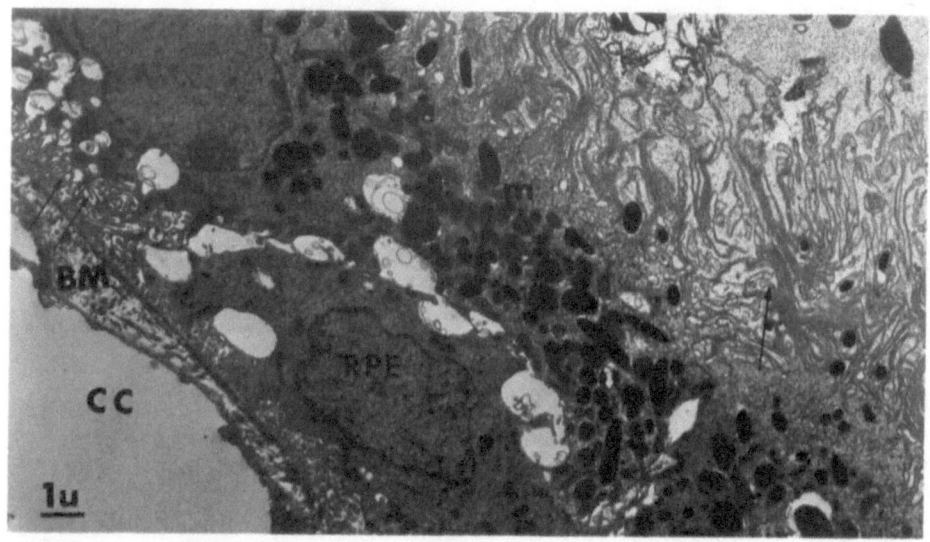

FIGURE 3. Regenerated normal-looking RPE cells (type 2) with prominent basal folds (double arrows), elongated apical villi (single arrow) and apical melanosomes (m) adjacent to a patent choriocapillary (CC). BM, Bruch's membrane. (1um=6mm).

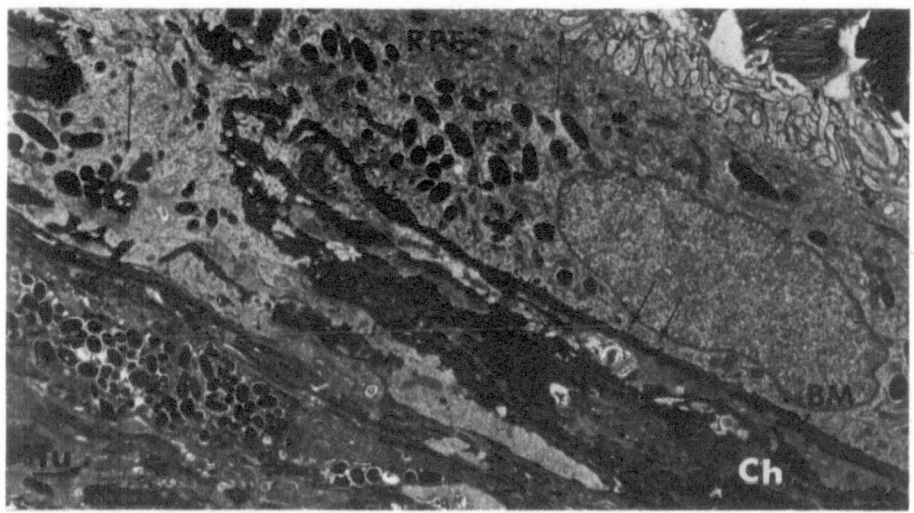

FIGURE 4. TEM of type 3 RPE cell. The cell is electron-lucent and has no basal folds (double arrows), but has stubby apical villi (single arrow). The melanosomes (m) are diffusely spread. The underlying choroid (ch) is devoid of choriocapillaries, and RPE cell processes have entered the choroid (double-headed arrow). BM, Bruch's membrane. (1um=6mm).

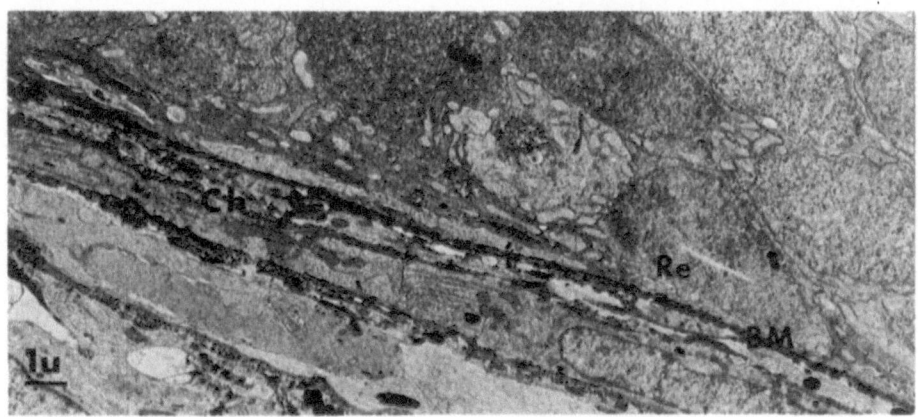

FIGURE 5. RPE is absent and neural retinal cells (Re) line Bruch's membrane (BM). The adjacent choroid (Ch) is devoid of choriocapillaris. (1um=6mm).

MECHANISMS OF LUMEN FORMATION: MORPHOLOGIC OBSERVATIONS ON EXPERIMENTAL SUBRETINAL NEOVASCULARIZATION

T. Ishibashi, H. Miller, G. Orr, N. Sorgente, S.J. Ryan

Department of Ophthalmology, University of Southern California School of Medicine, and the Estelle Doheny Eye Foundation, Los Angeles, California, USA

Abstract

Using light and electron microscopy, we studied the sequence of events that lead to the formation of new vascular lumens after laser photocoagulation of the retina and choroid of primates. Three days after photocoagulation, not only the endothelial cells in pre-existing vessels but also those in re-endothelialized vessels showed budding and lumen formation. The lumen of vessels was formed by the budding of adjacent endothelial cells that were coupled by transient intercellular junctions.

Introduction

Numerous theories have been proposed concerning the mechanisms of lumen formation in new vessels;[1-6] however, there is still no general concensus on how lumen is formed. The mechanisms of lumen formation also remain obscure in the subretinal neovascularization (SRN). We used light and electron microscopy to study the sequence of events after laser photocoagulation in a primate model that leads to the lumen formation.

Materials and Methods

SRN was induced in the macular region of cynomolgus monkeys by high-intensity laser photocoagulation, as previously described.[7,8] The eyes were enucleated at 1, 2 and 3 days after photocoagulation, opened and fixed by immersion in 2.5% glutaraldehyde and 2.0% paraformaldehyde in 0.1 M phosphate buffer (pH 7.4) for 24 hours. For light microscopy, three laser lesions from each eye were dehydrated in a graded series of alcohol and embedded in glycol methacrylate; 2.5 micron serial sections were cut and stained by periodic acid-Schiff reagent. Five laser lesions from each eye, to be studied by transmission electron microscopy, were post-fixed for 2 hours in 2% osmium tetroxide in 0.1 M phosphate buffer, pH 7.4, dehydrated in a graded series of alcohol followed by propylene oxide, and embedded in epoxy resin. Thin sections were cut on an ultramicrotome, stained with uranyl acetate and lead citrate, and viewed with an electron microscope.

Results

One day after laser photocoagulation, capillaries, venules and arterioles of the choroid were absent in the center of the laser lesion. In the area adjacent to the center of the lesion, various cellular components of the choroidal vessels had disappeared while others appeared degenerated. Thrombus formation was frequently observed in these degenerated vessels. At the periphery of the areas where thrombus formation was seen, endothelial cells in pre-existing choroidal vessels contained many ribosomes and were rich in rough endoplasmic reticulum. In some lesions between thrombotic and non-thrombotic areas, re-endothelialization began to occur, with migration of endothelial cells.

Two days after photocoagulation, re-endothelialization was completed in most of the choroidal vessels. The initial stage of endothelial cell budding was observed in pre-existing choroidal vessels at the periphery of the lesion.

Three days after photocoagulation, endothelial cell cytoplasmic processes of various shapes and lengths were present in the pre-existing venules as well as in the re-endothelialized vessels at the periphery of the laser lesions. These cytoplasmic processes were rich in ribosomes, rough endoplasmic reticulum, mitochondria, Golgi apparatuses, and microfilament bundles. The tips of the cytoplasmic processes had no basement membrane. Newly formed vascular lumens were observed in the budding portion of endothelial cells of both pre-existing and re-endothelialized vessels. The new lumens were composed of at least two budding endothelial cells that connected by intercellular junctions (Fig. 1). Progressive stages of lumen formation were observed (Figs. 2-4). The initial stage consisted of budding of two adjacent endothelial cells coupled by junction. The junction became longer with a number of short adherent regions (Fig. 2). In the next stage, adherent regions disappeared on the luminal side of the junction, resulting in the formation of a small gap between the two budding endothelial cells (Fig. 3). As the disappearance of the adherent regions took place in succession, the gap, which was apparently connected to the lumen of the parent vessel, became longer and larger (Fig. 4). The endothelial cells that covered the newly formed lumen appeared metabolically active and lacked fenestrations (Figs. 1-4). At this time mitotic figures of endothelial cells were frequently found in pre-existing as well as re-endothelialized vessels; the budding endothelial cells themselves, however, did not show mitotic figures.

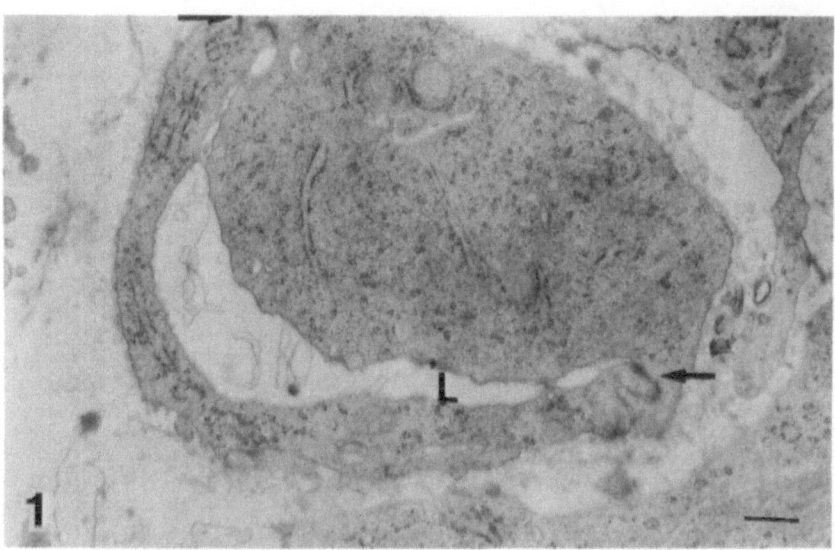

FIGURE 1. Cross section of newly formed vessel three days after photocoagulation. The newly formed lumen (L) is composed of two endothelial cells that have thickened, non-fenestrated cytoplasm with ribosomes and rough endoplasmic reticulum. Intercellular junctions (arrows) are present between these endothelial cells. (bar: 0.5 um)

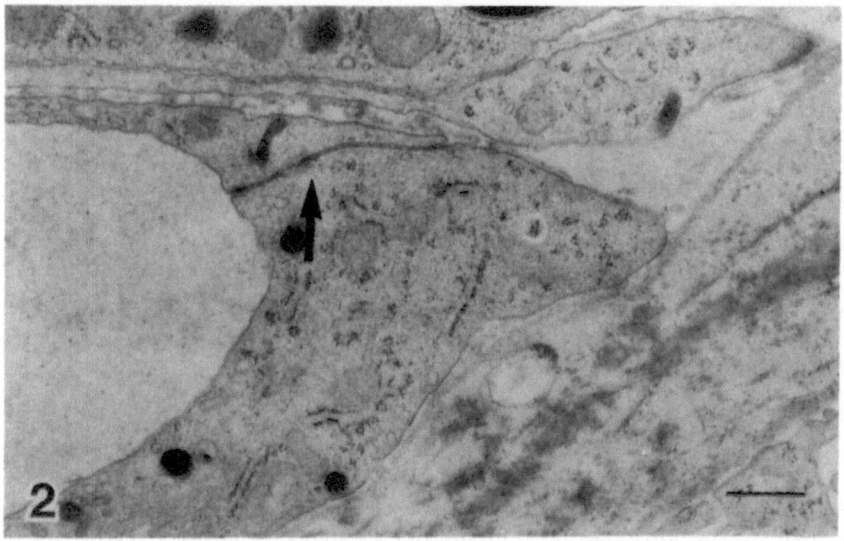

FIGURE 2. Budding endothelial cells three days after photocoagulation. Two adjacent endothelial cells coupled by intercellular junction (arrow) show budding. The junction becomes longer with short adherent regions. (bar: 0.5um)

440

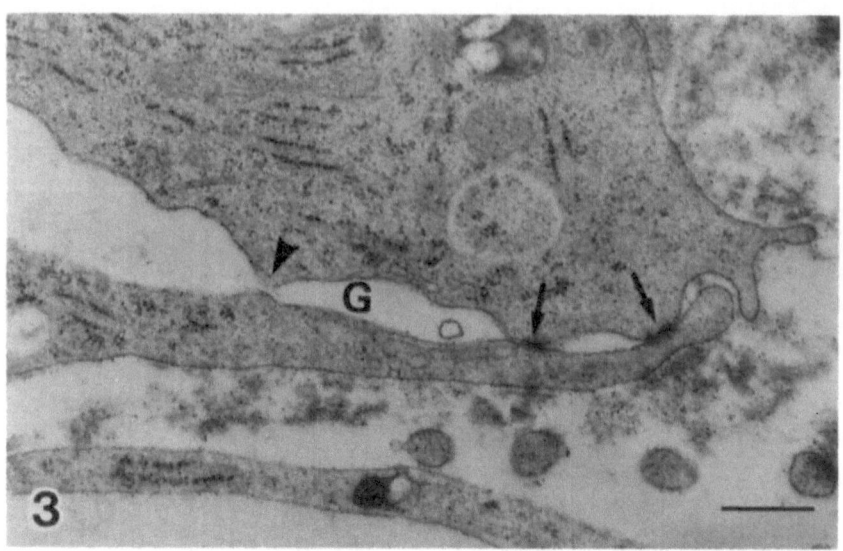

FIGURE 3. Budding endothelial cells three days after photocoagulation.
One adherent region (arrowhead) disappears on the luminal side of intercellular junction, resulting in the formation of a small gap (G). The
junction still has adherent regions (arrows) at the tip of the cell
process. (bar: 0.5um)

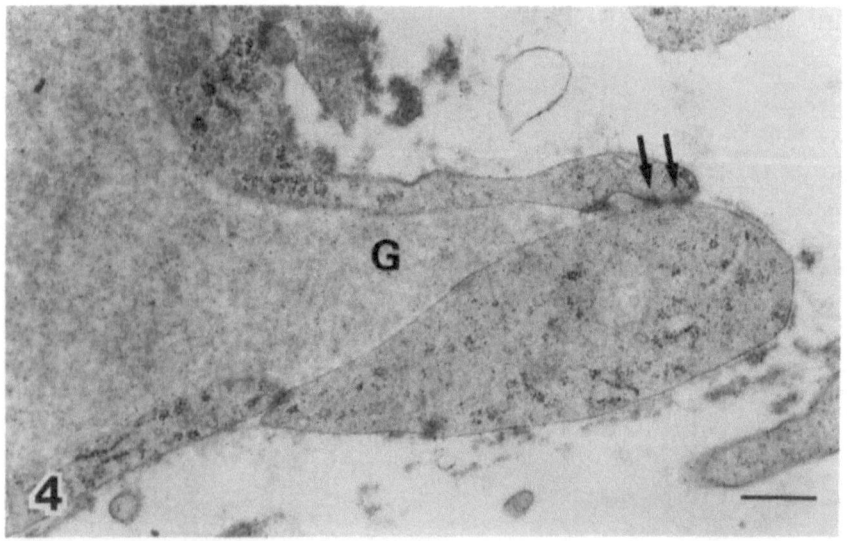

FIGURE 4. Budding endothelial cells three days after photocoagulation. A
wide gap (G) in the intercellular junction is present between two budding
endothelial cells. The junction still has adherent regions (arrows) at the
tip of the cell process. (bar: 0.5um)

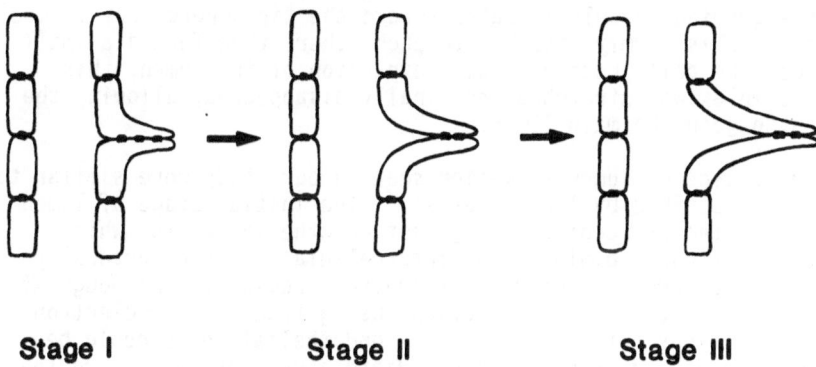

Stage I   **Stage II**   **Stage III**

5

FIGURE 5.   Schema showing the sequence of events leading to lumen formation.

Discussion

        A number of hypotheses have been advanced to account for lumen formation in new vessels;[1-6] these have been categorized by Wagner[9] as being of two basic mechanisms: an intracellular mechanism whereby vacuolization that occurs in the cytoplasm of endothelial cells leads to lumen formation, and an intercellular mechanism whereby two adjacent endothelial cell processes delimit a narrow lumen. Using cultured capillary endothelial cells, Folkman and Haudenschild[4] showed the vacuole, which seems to become a vascular lumen surrounded by an extremely thin wall of cytoplasm. In their study, basement membrane-like material was observed inside the lumen rather than on the outer surface of the endothelial cells, which suggests that the structures described were, in fact, inverted endothelial tubes. Feder et al[5] also reported the formation of inverted tubes by cultured aortic endothelial cells. Recently, Montesano et al,[6] in an in vitro study using cloned capillary endothelial cells from bovine adrenal cortex, showed that capillary-like tubes were formed by two or more cells delimiting a narrow lumen.

        We have observed lumen formation as early as three days after laser photocoagulation. The newly formed vascular lumens were always composed of at least two budding endothelial cells; we found no evidence that lumen formation resulted from vascularization within the bodies of the endothelial cells themselves.

Using a corneal model of neovascularization in the rabbit, some reports demonstrated the mechanisms of lumen formation by electron microscopy. Ausprunk and Folkman[3] showed that endothelial cells within existing venules appeared to slide past one another and enclose a portion of the vascular lumen, and then the cells on the abluminal side of the new lumen continued to migrate outward until they were completely outside the wall of the parent vessel. Inomata et al[2] showed that new endothelial cells of the growing vessels migrated toward the tip, where they formed a solid cord of cells firmly attached to each other, then formed a small lumen between the cell junction. With expansion of the lumen, this junctional complex was stretched and finally disappeared, allowing the small lumen to join the main lumen.

The processes of lumen formation seen in our study were similar to the processes described by Inomata et al.[2] The initial stage of lumen formation consisted of budding of adjacent endothelial cells, which exhibited a junctional complex. The intercellular junction gradually became longer and more open with short adherent regions. Although it is difficult to define the type of junctions using transmission electron microscopy, junctions between the budding endothelial cells could be classified as zonula adherens or intermediate junctions, which are the first junctional contacts to form both in vivo[10] and in vitro;[11] with time, the adherent region on the luminal side of the junction disappeared, as has been reported by other investigators.[12-14] A small gap was then formed between two budding endothelial cells; this gap was apparently connected to the lumen of the parent vessel. Figure 5 schematically presents a postulated sequence of events leading to lumen formation.

Our findings in this experimental model suggest that the newly formed vascular lumen of SRN is always composed of at least two budding endothelial cells (intercellular mechanism) that are coupled by transient intercellular junctions.

References

1. Schoefl GI: Studies on inflammation. III. Growing capillaries: their structure and permeability. Virchows Arch path Anat 337:97, 1963.

2. Inomata H, Smelser GK, and Polack FM: Corneal vascularization in experimental uveitis and graft rejection. An electron microscopic study. Invest Ophthal 10:840, 1971.

3. Ausprunk DH and Folkman J: Migration and proliferation of endothelial cells in preformed and newly formed blood vessels during tumor angiogenesis. Microvasc Res 14:53, 1977.

4. Folkman J. and Haudenschild C: Angiogenesis in vitro. Nature 288:551, 1980.

5. Feder J, Marasa JC, and Olander JV: The formation of capillary-like tubes by calf aortic endothelial cells grown in vitro. J Cell Physiol 116:1, 1983.

6. Montesano R, Orci L, and Vassalli P: In vitro rapid organization of endothelial cells into capillary-like networks is promoted by collagen matrices. J Cell Biol 97:1648, 1983.

7. Ryan SJ: The development of an experimental model of subretinal neovascularization in disciform macular degeneration. Trans Am Ophthalmol Soc 77:707, 1979.

8. Ryan SJ: Subretinal neovascularization: natural history of an experimental model. Arch Ophthalmol 100:1804, 1982.

9. Wagner RC: Endothelial cell embryology and growth. Adv Microcirc 9:45, 1980.

10. Hastings RA II and Enders AC: Junctional complexes in the preimplantation rabbit embryo. Anat Rec 181:17, 1975.

11. Crawford BJ: Development of the junctional complex during differentiation of chick pigmented epithelial cells in clonal culture. Invest Ophthalmol Vis Sci 19:223, 1980.

12. Revel JP, Yip P, and Chang LL: Cell junctions in the early chick embryo--a freeze etch study. Dev Biol 35:302, 1973.

13. Lane NJ and Swales LS: Dispersal of junctional particles, not internalization, during the in vivo disappearance of gap junctions. Cell 19:579, 1980.

14. Lane NJ and Swales LS: Changes in the blood-brain barrier of the central nervous system in the blowfly during development, with special reference to the formation and disaggregation of gap and tight junctions. II. Pupal development and adult flies. Dev Biol 62:415, 1978.

ANIMAL MODEL OF RPE-CHORIOCAPILLARIS INTERACTIONS: SODIUM IODATE
RETINOPATHY IN THE RABBIT

GARY E. KORTE, AYALA POLLACK AND PAUL HENKIND

INTRODUCTION: When rabbits receive intravenous injections of sodium
iodate the retinal pigment epithelium (RPE) is destroyed over large
expanses of the fundus (Noell,1953). We have shown that the choriocapillaris (CC) adjacent to the necrotic RPE atrophies, while that
adjacent to spared RPE (consistently located at the far periphery and
around the optic disc) remains normal in appearance (Korte et al.,1984).
This observation and a consideration of published reports on retinal
histopathology led us to suggest that CC depends on the RPE for its
survival, and that RPE influences some of its functionally important
structural specializations, such as numbers of endothelial fenestrae
(Henkind and Gartner,1983; Korte et al.,1984). Our initial observations
were made, however, at widely separated times after administration of
sodium iodate; primarily 1 and 11 weeks after injection. Continued examination of material obtained from 1 day to 6 weeks after sodium iodate not
only buttressed our notion that CC atrophy and RPE destruction are
linked, but suggested that RPE regeneration and CC regeneration occur in
tandem. These observations are presented here.

PROCEDURES: The observations were derived from over 40 pigmented rabbits
that received sodium iodate intravenously as previously described (Korte
et al.,1984). One day to 6 weeks later the animals were processed for
routine transmission electron microscopy, some of them receiving
horseradish peroxidase intravenously 15 minutes prior to euthanasia. The
tracer was localized by the diaminobenzidine procedure, as detailed in
other reports (Korte et al.,1983). Animals used in our initial report
were also used in this study to obtain tissue at 11 or more weeks after
administration of sodium iodate.

RESULTS: As early as one day after administration of sodium iodate the
correlation between RPE destruction and CC atrophy reported at 1 week
after iodate was apparent. This was seen by comparing the RPE-CC interface at the far periphery or optic disc, where RPE was spared, with the
midperiphery, where a fulminant necrosis of RPE occurred. The CC adjacent
to spared RPE remained normal in appearance (Fig. 1) while that adjacent
to necrotic RPE showed evidence of atrophy. The endothelium had thickened
and lost fenestrae (Fig. 2). Endothelial necrosis was seen 3-5 days
after iodate (Fig. 3).

    By 1 week after iodate a mixture of atrophic and regenerating CC was
apparent (Figs. 4,5). By this time the RPE necrosis had been resolved by
macrophagic activity and the denuded Bruch's membrane was being re-covered
by macrophagic cells, Muller cell processes and regenerating RPE.

Up to approximately 6 weeks after iodate the regenerating CC was seen adjacent to regenerating RPE as well as scar tissue formed by Müller cell processes. Beyond this time, however, regenerating CC profiles became less numerous adjacent to scar tissue and appeared restricted to two sites: areas where RPE was spared and areas where RPE had regenerated. This suggested that a process of secondary atrophy might mold the regenerating CC so that its geographic extent matched that of the RPE. Evidence for this was found in two observations: one, regenerating CC adjacent to scar tissue began to lose its permeability to HRP, the profiles showing this change having a thickened endothelium and no fenestrae (Fig. 6). Second, scattered examples of degenerating endothelium similar to that illustrated in Fig. 3, only in immature CC, were seen. These two changes occurred only adjacent to scar tissue and were not seen adjacent to regenerating RPE.

DISCUSSION: These observations have further confirmed that CC atrophy occurs when and where RPE is destroyed, and suggest that RPE and CC regeneration occur in tandem.

Linkage of CC Atrophy and Destruction: The examination of tissue obtained during the first week after administration of sodium iodate shows the rapidity with which the CC response can occur. As early as one day after damaging the RPE the adjacent CC endothelium had thickened and lost fenestrae. We assume permeability changes would occur also, as seen in regenerated capillaries undergoing secondary atrophy and in which the same pattern of changes -- endothelial thickening and loss of fenestrae -- occurred. We speculate that CC may respond within hours of RPE damage; or, that subtle changes in RPE function may elicit changes in CC permeability as part of the homeostasis acting at the RPE-CC interface.

Tandem Nature of RPE and CC Regeneration: An interesting finding was the way in which secondary atrophy of regenerating CC molds the geographic extent of the capillary plexus to match that of regenerated RPE. This process, acting during the first several weeks after iodate administration, produces the striking correlation between RPE and CC extent described in the later stages of the retinopathy (Korte et al., 1984). We suggest that the secondary atrophy is a result of the absence of a proximate RPE. We envision that CC growth is robust enough to initially outstrip RPE regeneration. But by doing this it exceeds the distance by which RPE can exert the trophic effect suggested by the correlation between CC atrophy and RPE destruction. When this occurs the regenerating CC atrophies and dies back to match the RPE in extent. This is further evidence that RPE and CC work as a unit. It will be most interesting to determine if a similar interaction occurs during development or during retinal disease.

In so far as these processes cannot yet be studied in vitro, it is clear that animal models such as rabbits with the sodium iodate retinopathy and rats with phototoxic and urethane retinopathies (see Korte et al., this volume) have a lot to offer in helping us understand the biology of the RPE-CC interface.

ACKNOWLEDGEMENT: Supported by grants from the NEI and Research to Prevent Blindness, Inc.

REFERENCES:

1. Henkind P and Gartner S: The relationship between retinal pigment epithelium and choriocapillaris. Tr. Ophthalmol. Soc. U.K. 103:444. 1983.
2. Korte GE, Bellhorn RB and Burns MS: Ultrastructure of blood-retinal barrier permeability in rat phototoxic retinopathy. Invest. Ophthalmol. Vis. Sci. 24:962. 1983.
3. Korte GE, Reppucci V and Henkind P: RPE destruction causes choriocapillary atrophy. Invest. Ophthalmol. Vis. Sci. 25:1135. 1984.
4. Noell WK: Experimentally induced effects on structure and function of visual cells and pigment epithelium. Am. J. Ophthalmol. 36:103. 1953.

FIGURES:

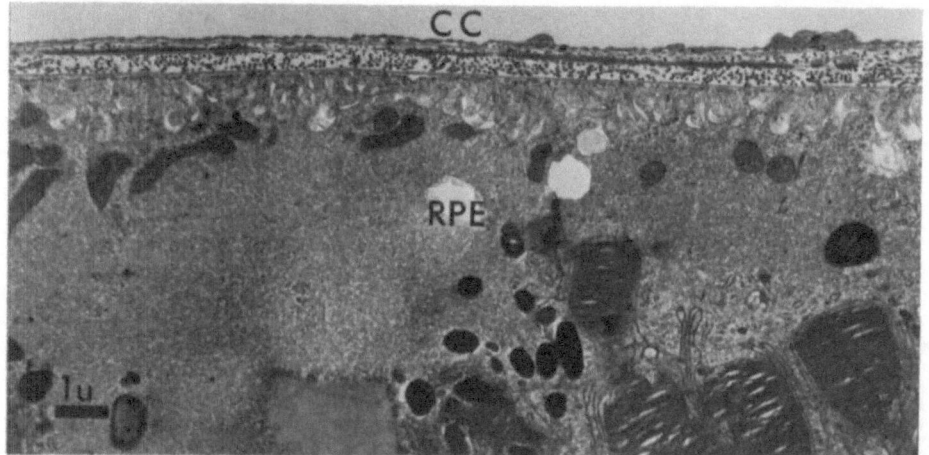

Figure 1: RPE near optic disc, 1 day after iodate administration. RPE and CC appear normal. The latter has a thin endothelium and is highly fenestrated.

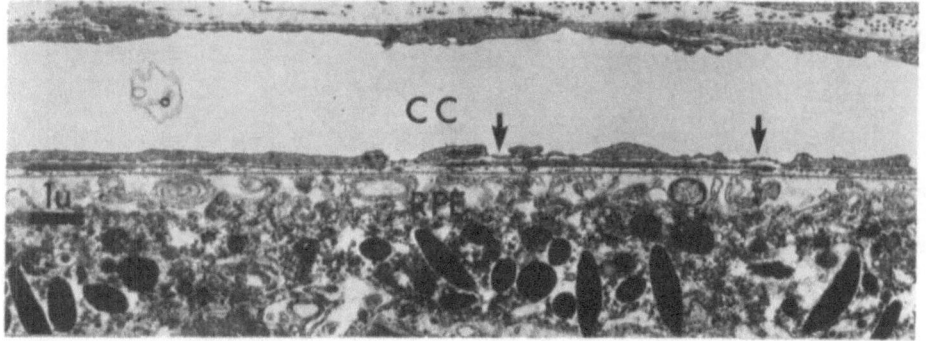

Figure 2: From same eye as Fig. 1, but at mid-periphery. RPE is necrotic and CC endothelium has thickened and lost fenestrae; they are restricted to small patches (arrows).

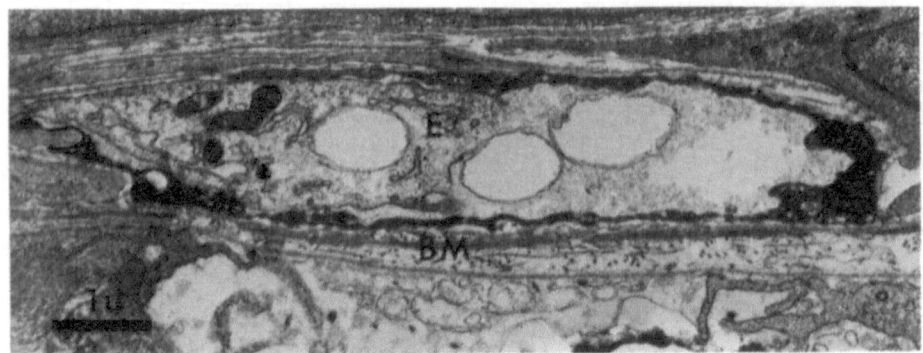

Figure 3: Five days after iodate administration there is necrotic endothelium (E) in the choriocapillaris. BM denotes Bruch's membrane.

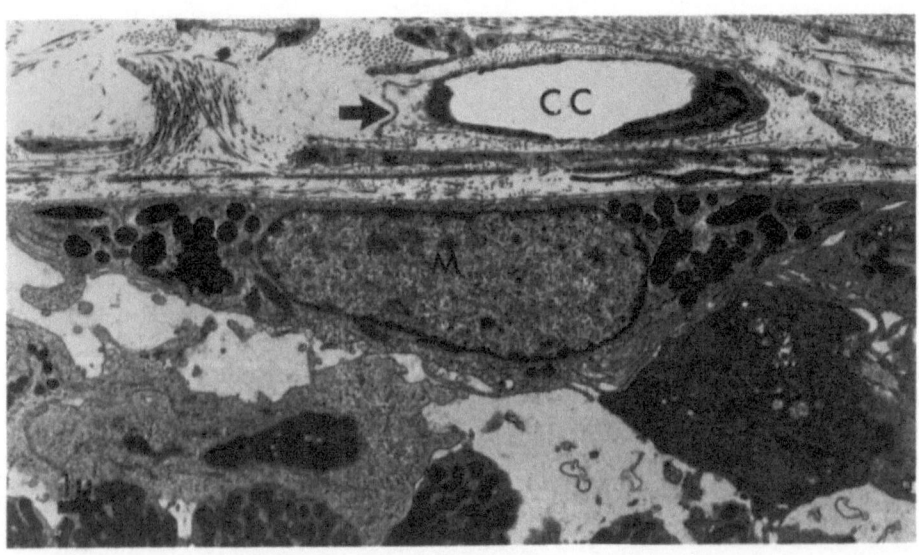

Figure 4: One week after iodate administration remnant CC is seen within
a loose sleeve of redundant basement membrane (arrow). Necrotic RPE has
been replaced by macrophagic cells (M).

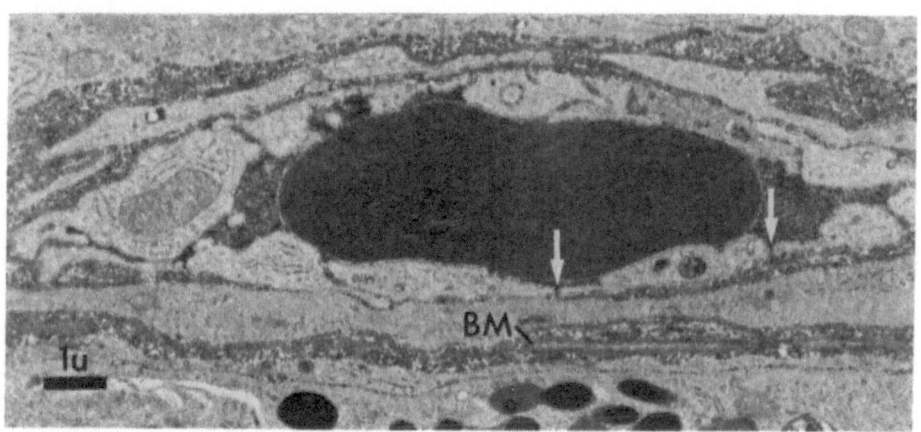

Figure 5: HRP leakage at regenerating CC. The leakage probably occurs at fenestrae, located at arrows but obscured by reaction product. BM denotes Bruch's membrane.

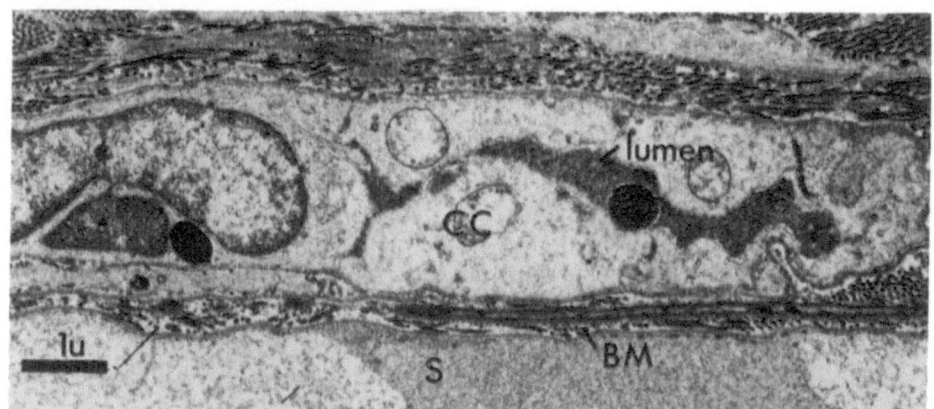

Figure 6: HRP does not leak out of immature CC that is undergoing secondary atrophy. This is seen as endothelial thickening and loss of fenestrae. Note Bruch's membrane has no tracer deposit it it, unlike the regenerating CC seen in Fig. 5. S denotes scar formed by Müller cell processes.

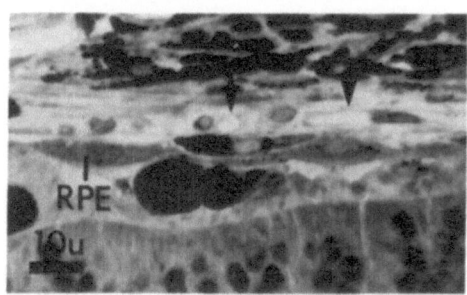

Figure 7: Regenerating RPE with regenerating CC (arrows) next to it.

CHOROIDAL NEOVASCULARIZATION AND THE RETINAL PIGMENT EPITHELIUM

MASANOBU UYAMA, M.D., HIROSHI OHKUMA, M.D., TAKASHI ITAGAKI, M.D.,
KAZUYA YAMAGISHI, M.D., TETSUYA NISHIMURA, M.D., KANJI TAKAHASHI, M.D.
DEPARTMENT OF OPHTHALMOLOGY, KANSAI MEDICAL UNIVERSITY,
FUMIZONOCHO, MORIGUCHI, OSAKA, 570 JAPAN

1. INTRODUCTION

Senile disciform macular degeneration is increasing as a cause of blindness in elderly aged people. It is well known senile disciform macular degeneration is caused by development of choroidal neovascularization.

To clarify pathophysiology of choroidal neovascularization (ChN), we have studied on experimentally produced ChN in the monkey eye according to Ryan's experimental model[1,2,3]. In the previous studies [4,5,6], we showed natural course of experimental ChN, occurrence, development and spontaneous regression of ChN following laser photocoagulation (LPC). From our histopathological observations on natural course of experimentally produced ChN, we have noticed the retinal pigment epithelium (RPE) has contributed greatly to development and regression of ChN.

To confirm our thought, we have used drugs, which have been known to damage RPE selectively, ornithine[7] and sodium iodite[8,9]. By administration of these drugs at different stages of development of ChN, ChN changed their natural courses. From our results[10,11] we could suggest the possibility of the RPE behaving in a different manner at different stages of the process.

2. MATERIALS AND METHODS
2.1. Experimental model of ChN

Macaque monkeys (Macaca irus) weighing 1.5~2.5 Kg were used.

Intensive laser photocoagulations were applied at the posterior pole of the retina in grid pattern by Krypton red laser (Cohrent Radiation System 910), according to Ryan's experimental model[1,2] (100 μm in spot size, duration of 0.1 seconds, and power of 200 mW). Following LPC, the fundi were checked by ophthalmoscopy, fundus camera and fluorescein angiography, at defferent intervals through 23 weeks after LPC.

After enucleation of the eyes, ChN were observed histopathologically by light and electron microscopy in usual procedure. ChN of some eyes were observed under scanning electron microscope on choroidal vascular cast preparations using Mercox resin infusing through the carotid artery.

2.2. Ornithine administration

A phisiological saline solution of 0.05 ml containing l. ornithine hydrochloride (1 mol/l, pH 7.2) were given intravitreously through pars plana by 27 gaze needle, immediately after LPC (nine eyes of 5 monkeys). The same amount of the physiological saline solution without ornithine were given in the same manner for control study.

2.3. Sodium iodite administration

A physiological saline solution containing 2.5 % of sodium iodite (NaIO$_3$) were givin intravenously in 25 mg/kg at each time.

Times of administration were followings:

2.3.1. Before LPC : Sodium iodite were given in 3 times at 3, 2 and 1 week before LPC (6 eyes of 3 monkeys).

2.3.2. The same time at LPC : Sodium iodite were given once immediately after LPC (2 eyes of 2 monkeys).

2.3.3. After LPC : Sodium iodite were given once at 3 weeks before LPC and twice at 1 and 2 weeks after LPC (6 eyes of 3 monkeys).

3. RESULTS

3.1. Natural course of choroidal neovascularization

3.1.1. Clinical course. By ophthalmoscopy and fluorescein angiography, choroidal neovascularizations appeared in 1 to 2 weeks after LPC at photocoagulation spots. Ophthalmoscopically, they associated flat serous detachment of the retina and vascular nets were revealed by fluorescein angiography. Incidence of ChNs for each lasered spots as about 50 % in the controls. In 2 to 3 weeks after LPC, neovascularization spreaded widely and serous retinal detachment became remarkable.

Thereafter, ChNs had gradually regressed in 4 to 8 weeks after LPC. The lasered sites became atrophic scarring and serous retinal detachment disappeared. So, almost all of ChN regressed spontaneously within 8 weeks after LPC. In this paper, persistence of ChN means ChN lasted over 8 weeks after LPC and spread beyond 1 disc diameter in width by fluorescein angiography. Rate of persistance of ChN for each lasered spots as 9 % in control animals.

3.1.2. Histopathology of natural course. In histopathological observations on natural course of experimental ChN, we found that at the growing process of newly formed vessels from the choroidal vessels into the subretinal space, in 1 to 2 weeks after LPC, ChNs always developed accompaning with reactively migrated or proliferated RPE cells. Migrated RPE cells were usually found beside the newly formed vessels in the subretinal space (Fig. 1). And moreover, electron microscopy revealed ChN situated at the basel side of the RPE cells (Fig. 2).

At the stage of clinical spontaneous regression, ChNs had existed in the subretinal space, however, they had been enveloped by a layer of the proliferated RPE cells and had been sealed off from the sensory retina (Fig. 3).

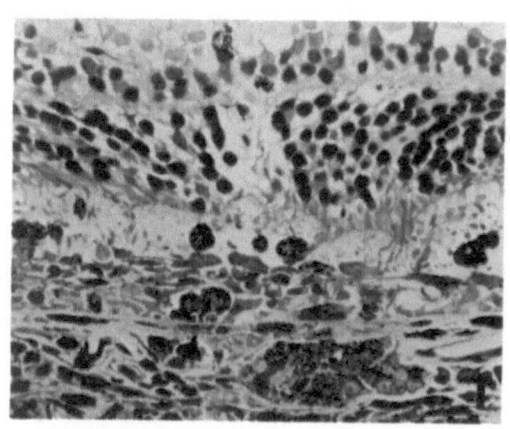

Fig. 1. One week after laser photocoagulation (LPC). At the stage of development of ChN, at lasered area, many reactively proliferated and migrated RPE cells, and developed neovascularization from the choroidal vessels were found.

Fig. 2. Electron micrograph of the subretinal space in Fig.1. Choroidal neovascularization (Nv) was immature and situated at the basal side of RPE cell.

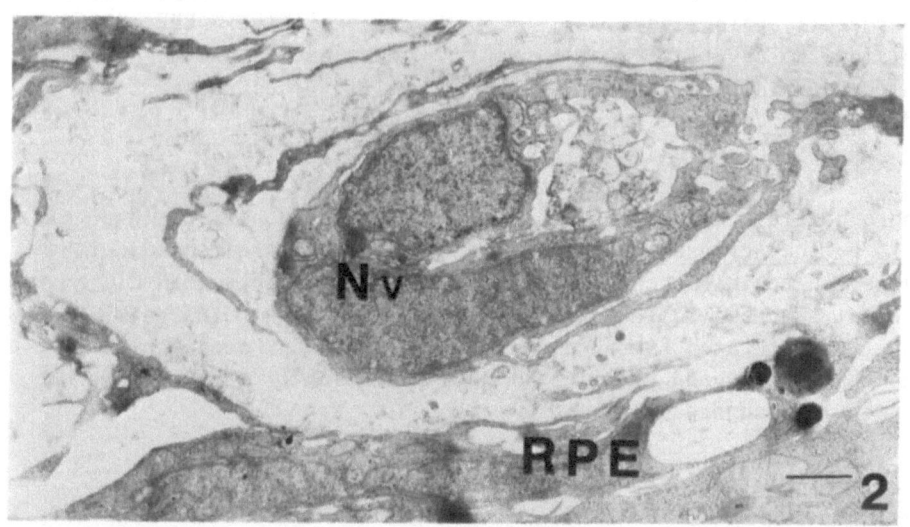

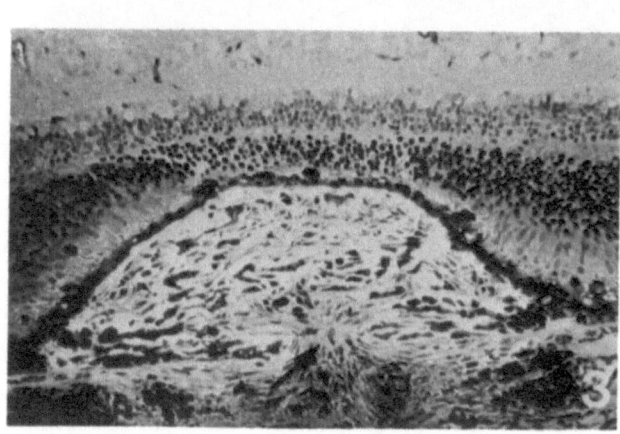

Fig. 3. Four weeks after LPC. At the stage of spontaneous regression of ChN, at lasered area, ChN existed, but were enveloped by a sheet of proliferated RPE cells and sealed off from the sensory retina.

454

3.2. Intravitreal administration of ornithine

3.2.1. Retinal damage by ornithine.
Following an intravitreal injection of a small amount of 1. Ornithine, in a week edema of the deep retina and slight pigment mottling of the RPE were found ophthalmoscopically, and diffuse marked hyperfluorescence on background were seen in fluorescein angiography.

In 2 weeks after administration, RPE layer showed marked mottling of pigmentation ophthalmoscopically, and fine granular hyperfluorescence of window defect of RPE layer were seen in fluorecsein angiography.

On histopathology, in a week after ornithine administration, RPE were markedly degenerated and necrotic, and in 2 weeks RPE were markedly atrophic. But the sensory retina

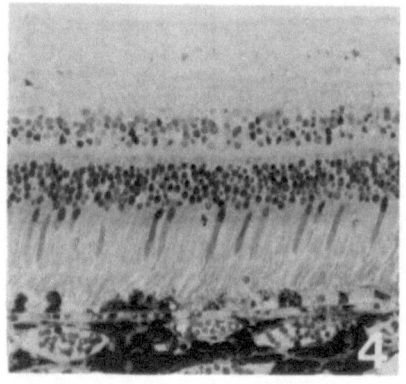

Fig. 4. Two weeks after intravitreous injection of 1. ornithine. RPE cells were markedly damaged selectively, destructed and degenerated.

and choroid were remained almost intact during these periods (Fig. 4).

3.2.2. Following laser photocoagulation.
In eyes pretreating with ornithine, in ophthalmoscopy and fluorescein angiography, ChN did not occurred at any area following LPC (Fig. 5). Histopathologically, some layers of proliferated fibroblsts were found, but any neovascularization was not seen and proliferation or migration of RPE cells were few at the lasered areas (Fig. 6).

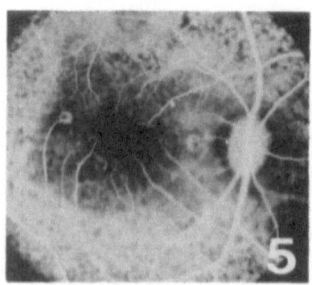 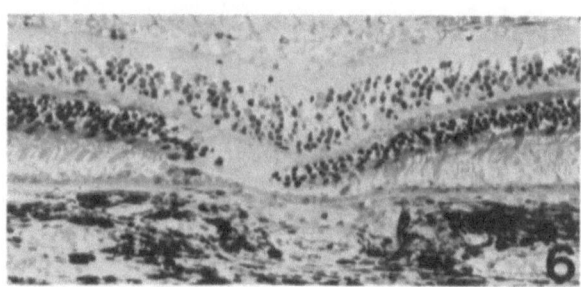

Fig. 5. Two weeks after LPC and intravitreous injection of ornithine, Fluorescein angiography. RPE showed fine granular hyperfluorescens of window defect. ChN did not appear from any lasered spot.
Fig. 6. Histology of Fig.5. ChN and proliferation of RPE were not seen at lasered area.

3.3. Intravenous administration of sodium iodite

3.3.1. retinal damage by sodium iodite.

Following intravenous administration of sodium iodite, in 1 to 2 weeks fundus showed mottled appearance of pigmentation at RPE, and bull's eye appearance at the macula. Fluorescein angiography revealed fine granular hyperfluorescens of window defect on choroidal fluorescences.

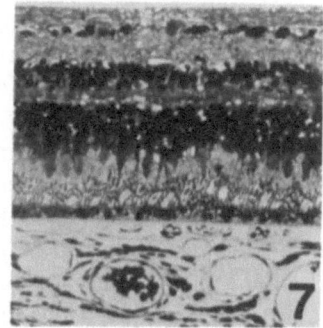

Fig. 7. Two weeks after intravenous injection of sodium iodite. RPE was injured selectively and degenerated.

On histopathology, RPE showed moderate degeneration and slight disappearance of melanin granules, and no necrosis was found in RPE (Fig. 7). The outer segments of the photoreceptors were slightly degenerated, but the sensory retina had remained intact.

3.3.2. Following laser photocoagulation.

In the eyes which iodite was given before LPC, ChN did not occur clinically at any lasered area (Fig. 8). Histopathologically, neovascularization was not seen in the subretinal space, and the RPE also did not proliferate nor migrate at the lasered site (Fig. 9). By cast preparations of these eyes we had confirmed no development of ChN at any lasered area.

In the eyes which iodite was given immediately after LPC, ChN did not occur clinically and histopathologically.

In animals in which sodium iodite were given in 2 weeks after LPC, clinically ChNs developed markedly at each lasered area and associated widespread serous detachment of the retina and lasted over 8 weeks

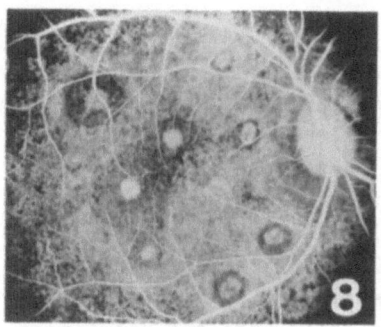
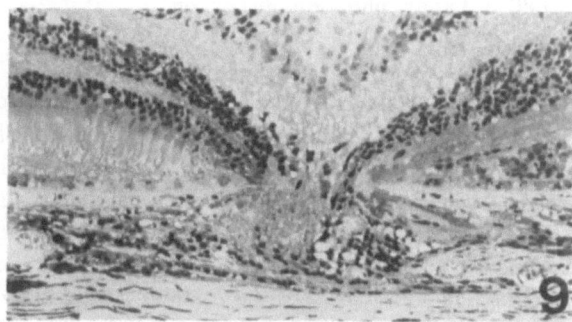

Fig. 8. Two weeks following LPC after 2 weeks of sodium iodite administration. ChN did not occur at lasered areas, and RPE showed fine granular hyperfluorescens of window defect.

Fig. 9. Histology of Fig.8. ChN was not seen and no proliferation of RPE was found.

after LPC (Fig. 10), and did not show tendency towards spontaneous regression. In these eyes, fluorescein angiography revealed well developed ChN and marked extravascular leakage from these vessels (Fig. 11). Histopathologically, in these eyes there were a lot of well developed ChNs in the subretinal space, and no enveloping nor sealing off by proliferation of RPE was seen (Fig. 12). Cast preparations showed development of sea-fun like ChNs at each lasered areas (Fig. 13). ChNs in these eyes were large and wide in caliber.

In eyes post-treating with iodite, ChNs occurred in 50 % of lasered areas, and half of them developed actively and lasted over 8 weeks. Some of them have lasted for 24 weeks, actively. Rate of persistance of ChN was 25 % in these eyes.

3.4. Incidence and persistence of ChN

Rate of incidence of ChN and rate of persistance of ChN from each lasered spot were summarized in Table 1.

TABLE 1. Incidence and durability of ChN

	Rate of Incidence	Rate of Persistence
Control	50 %	9 %
Ornithine		
immediately after LPC	0	0
Sodium iodite		
before LPC	0	0
Immediately after LPC	0	0
after LPC	50	25

Persistence : ChN lasting actively over 8 weeks after LPC
ChN : Choroidal neovascularization
LPC : Laser photocoagulation

4. DISCUSSION

In the experimental model of ChN, which occurred after intensive laser photocoagulation at the posterior pole of the monkey retina, we found at the stage of growing of ChN, ChN had developed always associating with reactively proliferated and migrated RPE in the subretinal space. And ChN was always found at the basal side of RPE keeping anatomical situation of both cells in normal condition. These results suggestedd RPE may act to induce the development of ChN[4] . At the stage of clinical involution of ChN, histologically ChNs had not disappeared, but existed. However, they had been completely enveloped by a sheet of proliferated RPE cells, which had sealed off them from the sensory retina. These results suggested RPE may play to regress ChNs by proliferating to cover them[5, 6]. In ocurrence of ChN, it is well known degeneration and damage in Bruch's membrane is most important

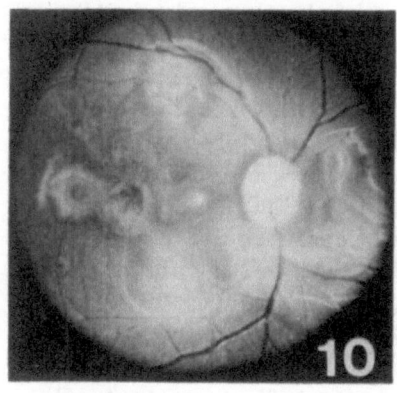 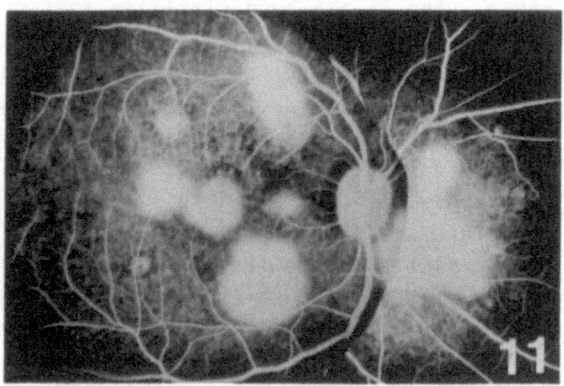

Fig. 10. Eight weeks following LPC. Sodium iodite were given 3 weeks
before LPC, and 1 and 2 weeks after LPC. ChN developed markedly from
lasered areas and associated with serous detachment of the retina.
Fig. 11. Fluorescein angiography of the case of Fig.10. Marked extra-
vascular leakages in the subretinal space from well developed   ChN
were seen.

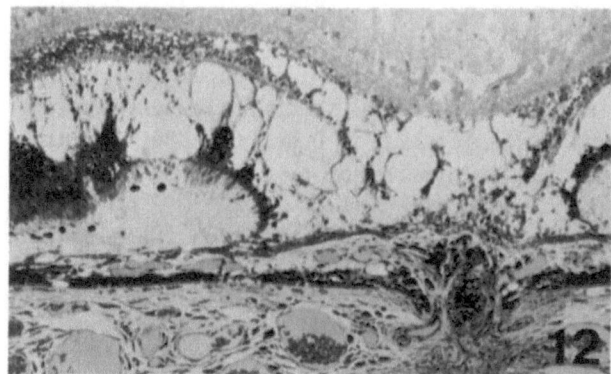

Fig. 12. Histology of
a lasered area of the
case of Fig.10,11.
There were many well
developed ChN and no
enveloping by prolifer-
ation of RPE.

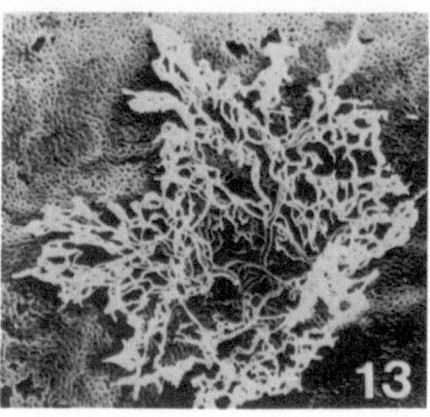

Fig. 13. Scanning electron microscopy of cast preparation of the
choroidal vessels of the case of
Fig.10,11,12. ChN developed
markedly and lasted over 8 weeks.

cause. And it has been clarified that process of development of ChN from the choroidal vessel to subretinal space, and it wes discussed factors to induce or inhibit growth of ChN. Among them, importance of endothelial cells, macrophages as well as inflamrmatory responce in the subretinal space was mentioned (Ryan, Millers, and Ishibashi). However, a little was known about the relationship of RPE cells to development of ChN[12, 13, 14] . Henkind[12] suggested that RPE modulates structure and function of the choriocapillaris, and also RPE may liberate a factor induce the vascular growth, and he suggested roll of RPE in growing of ChN. As above mentioned, our previous results[4, 5, 6] showed there are close interactions between RPE and ChN in the natural course of experimental ChN.

It was known that administration of sodium iodite[8, 9] or ornithine[7] damages RPE acutely. In our present experiments, we confirmed, intravitreal injection of a small amount of l. ornithine, or intravenous administration of sodium iodite injured RPE selectively and produced degeneration of RPE in the monkey eye.

To confirm our previous results about role of RPE in experimental ChN, we treated RPE by these drugs. When RPE has already been degenerated by administration of sodium iodite, ChN did not occur at all, following LPC. When RPE was damaged by l. ornithine or sodium iodite immediately after LPC, ChN did not appear also. In these experiments, RPE did not show any reactive proliferation or migration and any new vessels were not found at lasered areas following LPC. These results suggested that in the process of development of ChN after LPC, healthy and proliferated RPE was necessary to growing of new vessels in the subretinal space.

When RPE was damaged after growing of neovascularization, ChN lasted for a long duration and developed markedly, without enveloping by reactively proliferated RPE. This results suggested that in the process of regression of ChN, proliferation of RPE was necessary to sealing off ChN from the sensory retina.

From our present experiments, we could confirmed in the process of development and regression of choroidal neovascularization, the retinal pigment epithelial cells induced the development of ChN in the early stage, and contributed the regression of ChN in the late stage. And it seemed that these rolls of RPE in the process of ChN will be added as a newly recognized function of RPE among its various functions. These long lasting ChNs will be available for a experimental model to test effect of laser therapy on senile disciform macular degeneration.

This study was supported by Grants-in-Aid for Scientific Research (B 59480354, B61480371) from the Ministry of Education, Science and Culture, Japan.

REFERENCES

1. Ryan SJ: Development of an experimental model of subretinal neovascularization in disciform macular degeneration. Tr. Am. Ophthalmol. Soc. 77:707-745, 1979.
2. Ryan SJ: Subretinal neovascularization, natural history of an
   experimental model. Arch. Ophthalmol. 100:1804-1809, 1982.
3. Ohkuma H and Ryan SJ: Experimental subretinal neovascularization
   in the monkey. Permeability of new vessels. Arch. Ophthalmol.
   101:1102-1110, 1983.
4. Itagaki T, Ohkuma H, Kato N and Uyama M: Studies on experimental
   subretinal neovascularization. I. Development. Acta Soc. Ophthalmol. Jap. 89:600-610, 1985.
5. Itagaki T, Ohkuma H, Kato N, Uyama M: Studies on experimental
   subretinal neovascularization. II. Regression of new vessels.
   Acta Soc. Ophthalmol. Jap. 89:941-948, 1985.
6. Miki K, Ryan SJ, Ohkuma H, Uyama M: Choroidal neovascularization
   studied with fluorescein angiography and cast preparation. Acta
   Soc. Ophthalmol. Jap. 90:749-756, 1986.
7. Kuwabara T, Ishikawa Y, Kaiser-Kupfer MI: Experimental model of
   gyrate atrophy in animals. Ophthalmology. 88:331-334, 1981.
8. Noell WK: Experimentally induced toxic effects on structure and
   function of visual cells and pigment epithelium. Am. J. Ophthalmol. 33:103-115, 1953.
9. Nilsson SEG, Knave B, Persson HE: Changes in ultrastructure and
   function of the sheep pigment epithelium and retina induced by
   sodium iodite. Acta Ophthalmol. 55:1007-1026, 1977.
10. Itagaki T, Ohkuma H, Yamagishi K, Takahashi K, Uyama M: Studies on
    experimental subretinal neovascularization, relationship between
    new vessels and retinal pigment epithelium. Therapeutic Research.
    5:665-670, 1956.
11. Yamagishi K, Ohkuma H, Itagaki T, Kato N, Uyama M: Relationship
    between subretinal neovascularization and the retinal pigment
    epithelium. Folia Ophthalmol. Jap. 37:1154-1157, 1986.
12. Henkind P, Gartner S: The relationship between retinal pigment
    epithelium and the choriocapillaris. Trans. Ophthalmol. Soc. U.K.
    103:444-446, 1983.
13. Korte GE, Reppucci V, Henkind P: RPE destruction causes chorio-
    capillary atrophy. Invest. Ophthalmol. Vis. Sci. 25:1135-1145,
    1984.
14. Glaser BM, Camplchiaro AO, Davis JC, Sato M: Retinal pigment
    epithelial cells release an inhibitor of neovascularization. Arch.
    Ophthalmol. 103:1870-1875, 1985.

EXPERIMENTAL EVIDENCE THAT CAPILLARIES INFLUENCE RPE POLARITY.

GARY E. KORTE, ROY BELLHORN AND MARGARET BURNS

INTRODUCTION: When rats are exposed to fluorescent light or receive subcutaneous injections of urethane the photoreceptors degenerate and retinal capillaries move into the retinal pigment epithelium, or RPE (Bellhorn et al.,1973,1980). Here they become inserted between the lateral plasma membranes of adjacent RPE cells. This membrane, normally flat and undifferentiated, responds to the presence of the intraepithelial capillaries by developing structures and assuming functions that are normally restricted to the basal plasma membrane, i.e., that facing the choriocapillaris. In this article the changes in the lateral plasma membrane are described and presented as evidence that capillaries influence the structural and functional polarization of RPE cells. With our previous observation that the capillary segments apposed to RPE respond by losing their "retinal" characteristics (the endothelium thins, develops fenestrae and becomes permeable to horseradish peroxidase; they become choriocapillaris-like: Bellhorn et al.,1973,1980; Korte et al., 1983) these observations show that RPE and capillaries interact. These interactions probably contribute to homeostasis at the RPE-choriocapillaris interface in the normal retina. An upset in these interactions may contribute to the development of retinal disease, e.g., by permitting neovascularization or altering the blood-retinal barrier.

PROCEDURES: Foci of intraepithelial capillaries were produced in the RPE by exposing albino or pigmented rats to fluorescent light or urethane, as previously described (Bellhorn et al.,1973,1980). Rats were prepared for routine transmission electron microscopy 7-12 months later. Some animals received an intravenous injection of horseradish peroxidase (HRP) 15 minutes prior to euthanasia, as previously described (Korte et al., 1983,1984).

RESULTS: Similar observations were made in phototoxic and urethane treated rats. In either case the photoreceptor layer was destroyed, leaving the inner retina in apposition to the RPE (Fig. 1). The RPE remained normal where intraepithelial capillaries did not develop; the basal plasma membrane bore numerous folds and intracytoplasmic tubules (described by Korte,1984) and basement membrane attachment sites (described by Miki et al.,1975). These are seen in Fig. 2 from an animal that received HRP (in which the tracer advantageously outlines the surface) and in Fig. 3 from an animal that did not receive HRP. Where intraepithelial capillaries do not occur the lateral plasma membrane remains flat and unspecialized, as in normal rats.

Where intraepithelial capillaries occur, however, the lateral plasma
membrane undergoes profound changes. In Figs. 4 and 5 the lateral RPE
plasma membrane facing intraepithelial capillaries has formed numerous
folds. In Fig. 6 one can also see attachment sites, coated pits and
coated vesicles, which are rare or absent at lateral membrane that does
not face intraepithelial capillaries. The coated pits are sites of HRP
endocytosis; in Fig. 7 a coated pit is seen filling with HRP, and in
Fig. 5 tracer-filled coated vesicles are seen in the adjacent cytoplasm.
Apparent basement membrane deposition in seen in Fig. 6. Pockets of
lateral plasma membrane are filled with material similar to that forming
the basement membrane of the capillary, and vesicles bearing similar
material are seen in the adjacent cytoplasm of the RPE cell. These
vesicles appear to originate from the Golgi apparatus. Both of these
functions -- endocytosis and basement membrane secretion -- are rare or
absent on the lateral plasma membrane that does not face an intraepithelial
capillary.

As described previously (Bellhorn et al.,1973,1980; Korte et al.,
1983,1984) the endothelium of intraepithelial capillaries also undergoes
striking changes. It thins, develops fenestrae and becomes permeable to
intravenously injected HRP (Fig. 7).

DISCUSSION: It has been known for some time that intraepithelial capillaries in phototoxic rats, rats treated with urethane and in rodents with
genetic dystrophies undergo profound changes in the structure and function
of their endothelia (see Burns et al.,1986 for review). These include
thinning of endothelium, development of fenestrae, and attendant
permeability to HRP. Based on these and other observations it has been
suggested that capillaries respond to changes in their environment and to
the presence or absence of RPE (Bellhorn et al.,1980; Bellhorn,1980; Korte
et al.,1984; see article by Korte et al. in this volume).

In this report we show, however, that it is more accurate to speak of
interactions between RPE and capillaries; and, by extension, between RPE
and choriocapillaris. The response of the lateral RPE plasma membrane
abutting intraepithelial capillaries shows that the RPE can rearrange
its structural and functional polarity in response to the presence of one
or more capillary components: endothelium, pericyte and basement membrane.
Which of these components influences the described changes in RPE plasma
membrane conformation and function is speculative at this time (see
Korte et al.,1986 for discussion). In vitro experiments of the type
described by several investigators in this volume will help solve this
problem.

REFERENCES:
1. Bellhorn RW: Control of blood vessel development. Tr. Ophthal. Soc.
U.K. 100:328. 1980.
2. Bellhorn RW, Bellhorn MS , Friedman AH and Henkind P: Urethane
induced retinopathy in pigmented rats. Invest. Ophthalmol. Vis. Sci.
12:65.1973.
3. Bellhorn RW, Burns MS, Benjamin JV: Retinal vessel abnormalities
of phototoxic retinopathy. Invest. Ophthalmol. Vis. Sci. 19:584,1980.
4. Burns MS, Bellhorn RW, Korte GE and Heriot WJ: Plasticity of the
retinal vasculature. Prog. Retinal Res. 5:253,1986.
5. Korte G: New ultrastructure of rat RPE cells: basal intracytoplasmic
tubules. Exp. Eye Res. 38:399. 1984.

6. Korte GE, Bellhorn RW, Burns MS: Ultrastructure of blood-retinal barrier permeability in rat phototoxic retinopathy. Invest. Ophthalmol. Vis. Sci. 24:962. 1983.

7. Korte GE, Bellhorn RW and Burns MS: Urethane induced rat retinopathy. Plasticity of the blood-retinal barrier in disease. Invest. Ophthalmol. Vis. Sci. 25:1027. 1984.

8. Korte GE, Bellhorn RW and Burns MS: Remodelling of the retinal pigment epithelium in response to intraepithelial capillaries: evidence that capillaries influence the polarity of epithelium. Cell Tissue Res. 245:135. 1986.

9. Korte GE, Reppucci V and Henkind P: Retinal pigment epithelial destruction causes choriocapillary atrophy. Invest. Ophthalmol. Vis. Sci. 25:1135. 1984.

FIGURES:

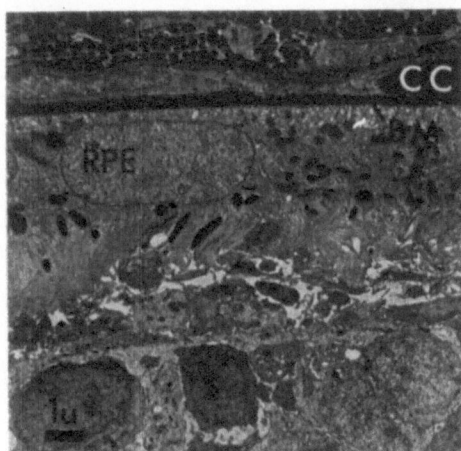

Fig. 1: RPE from an area with no intraepithelial capillaries. Cells appear normal, as detailed in Fig.2. BM, Bruch's membrane. CC,choriocapillaris. Note absence of photoreceptors.

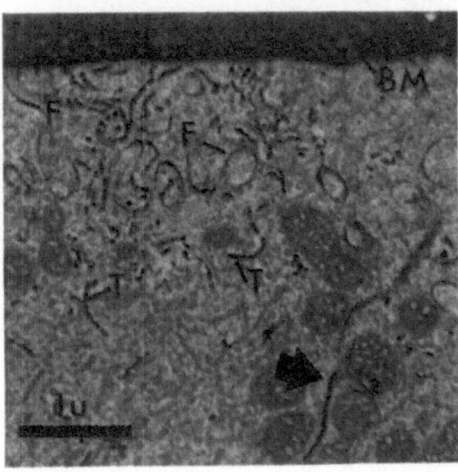

Fig. 2: Basal folds (F) and tubules (T) arise from basal RPE plasma membrane facing Bruch's membrane (BM). HRP reaction product outlines the folds and tubules and tinctures Bruch's membrane. Note lateral membrane (arrow) is flat and undifferentiated.

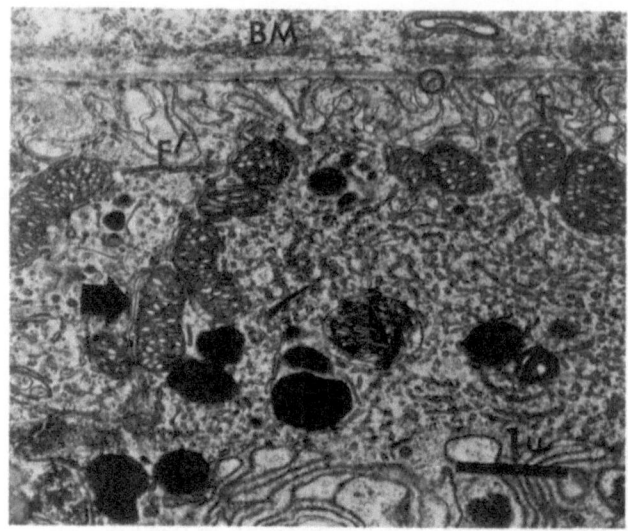

Fig. 3: Basal and lateral RPE plasma membrane from a rat that did not receive HRP, also from a site where no intraepithelial capilaries occur. Folds (F) and tubyles (T) occur on the basal membrane but the lateral membrane (arrow) is flat. Attachment sites that stud the basal membrane are encircled. BM, Bruch's membrane.

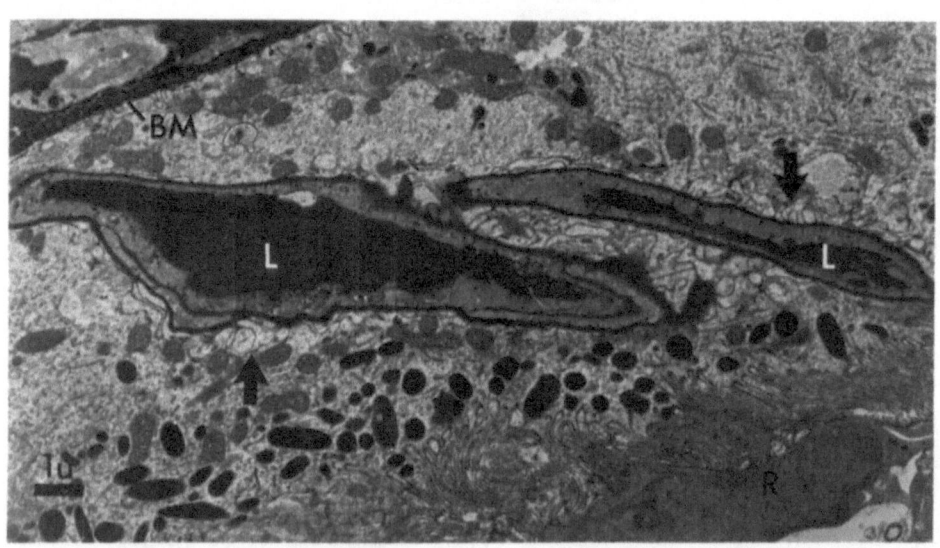

Fig. 4: RPE at focus of intraepithelial capillaries in a rat that received HRP. Capillary lumena (L) are filled with tracer. RPE lateral membrane has formed folds facing them (arrows), seen at higher magnification from another animal in Fig. 5. BM, Bruch's membrane. R, remnant inner retina.

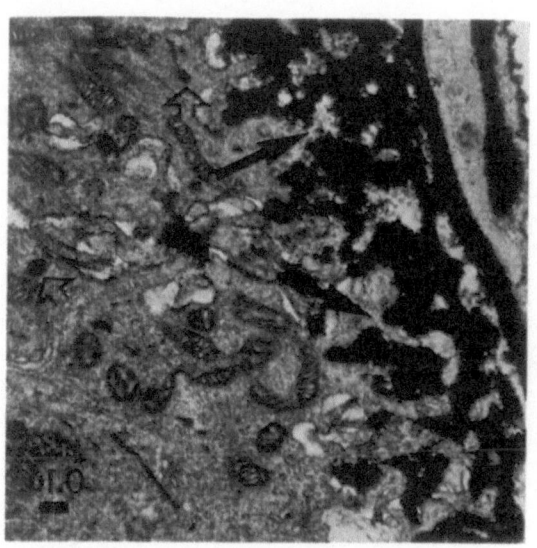

Fig. 5: Lateral RPE plasma membrane facing an intraepithelial capillary, its endothelium at left. HRP reaction product fills the pericapillary space, which is bordered by folds (arrows) newly formed by the RPE. Tubules described by Korte (1984) also form at this membrane but are not illustrated here. Arrowheads denote HRP-labelled endocytic vesicles.

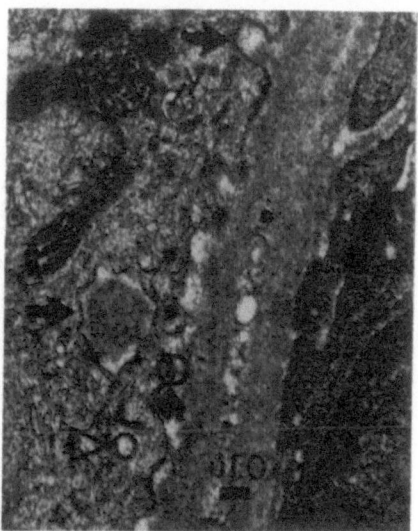

Fig. 6: Lateral membrane at an intraepithelial capillary, at left. Presumed basement membrane secretion in RPE occurs at pockets (arrows). V denotes vesicles with basement membrane like material. Arrowhead denotes a coated vesicle or tangentially cut coated pit. Attachment sites (encircled) have formed facing the basement membrane.

Fig. 7: Lateral membrane at an intraepithelial capillary (L its lumen) from an animal that received HRP. Black arrow denotes coated pit filled with tracer. White arrow is at fenestra site in endothelium. The fenestra itself is obscured by reaction product.

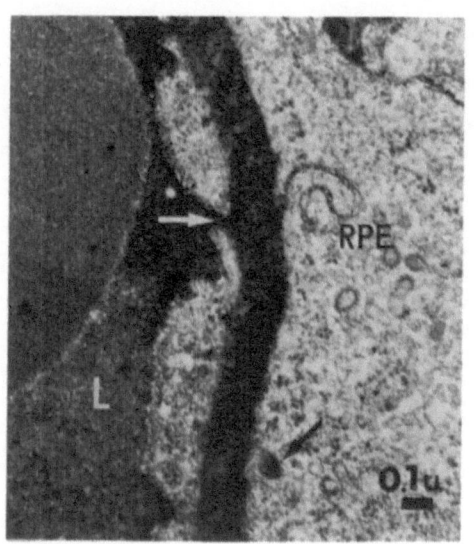

INVOLUTION OF SUBRETINAL NEOVASCULARIZATION

HEDVA MILLER[1], BENJAMIN MILLER[2], TATSURO ISHIBASHI[3] AND STEPHEN J. RYAN[4]

1. Faculty of Medicine and the Rappaport Family Institute for Research in the Medical Sciences, Technion, Haifa, Israel.
2. Department of Ophthalmology, Rambam Medical Center, Haifa, Israel.
3. Department of Ophthalmology, Kyushu University 60, Fukuoka, Japan.
4. Department of Ophthalmology, USC and Doheny Eye Foundation, Los Angeles California, USA.

1. INTRODUCTION

Subretinal neovascularization (SRN) is a pathologic feature of many eye diseases (1). For example, it accounts for more than 80% of severe visual loss associated with macular degeneration (2). The newly formed vessels proliferate from the choroid into the subretinal space and are diagnosed by fluorescein leakage during angiography (3,4). In both humans (4) and animal models of subretinal neovascularization (5) this leakage persists for only a certain period of time, after which it diminishes gradually until it disappears completely and staining of the scar only is seen on the angiogram. This process is defined as involution of the subretinal membrane.

In a previous study of our primate model of subretinal neovascularization we showed that the cessation of leakage is not a result of degeneration and disappearance of the subretinal vessels but rather results from disappearance of fluid pooling in the subretinal space, between the vessels and the sensory retina, in which the dye collected (6). In the present communication we will demonstrate that the disappearance of the subretinal fluid cannot be attributed to changes in the ultrastructural features of the subretinal vessels with maturation, but rather results from changes in the subretinal milieu around the vessels, more specifically from retinal pigment epithelial (RPE) cells proliferation around the subretinal vessels, that eventually totally envelope the vessels and probably absorb the fluid that separated the vessels from the overlying retina.

2. MATERIALS AND METHODS

Choroidal neovascularization was induced in cynomolgus monkeys by intense laser photocoagulation. Eight high-intensity laser burns were applied at and around the macula of one eye of each monkey, as previously described (5). The lesions were monitored once a week by fluorescein angiography for up to 10 weeks; one monkey was followed for 10 months.

On the basis of the angiographic findings, the laser lesions were divided into two groups: 1) leaky lesions, those that leak fluorescein profusely and pool dye in the subretinal space; 2) involuted lesions, those that no longer leak and pool dye in the subretinal space but show staining of the scar only. The eyes were enucleated at 2, 3, 7 and 10 weeks and at 10 months after photocoagulation, opened and fixed overnight by immersion in 2% paraformaldehyde and 2.5% glutaraldehyde in 0.1M phosphate buffer, pH 7.4. Each laser lesion was resected in a triangular block so that orientation of the lesion with respect to the fovea was maintained(6). The lesions to be studied by LM were dehydrated and embedded in glycol-methacrylate; 3-micron serial sections were cut and stained by periodic acid-Schiff. The lesions to be studied by TEM were postfixed with 1% osmium tetroxide for 2 hours at room temperature, dehydrated in a series of graded alcohols followed by propylene oxide, and embedded in plastic. Thin sections were taken at various planes of the laser lesions (e.g. the periphery of the scar, middle of the scar), stained by uranyl acetate and lead citrate and viewed by a Zeiss 106 TEM at 60 kV.

3. RESULTS

The eight standard laser lesions are demonstrated by fluorescein angiography in Fig. 1. Two weeks after laser photocoagulation lesions 1-5 demonstrate for the first time variable amounts of fluorescein leakage and pooling in the subretinal space; these lesions are defined as leaky lesions. We have previously demonstrated that in our experimental model (like in the clinical situation) the leakage persists for a variable period of time (1-12 weeks) after which it diminishes gradually until staining of the scar only is seen during angiography (5), i.e. the lesion has completed its involution process.

Light microscopy of the leaky lesions at the early stage of development revealed that when the first signs of leakage appeared on angiography, the newly-formed fibrovascular tissue had already proliferated into the subretinal space around the center of the scar (defined by the break in Bruch's membrane), and fluid, assumed to come from the newly-formed subretinal vessels, had accumulated in the subretinal space (Fig. 2). At this early stage of the neovascular membrane development, proliferating retinal pigment epithelial (RPE) cells were found at the periphery of the scar around the break in Bruch's membrane, between the membrane and the newly-formed subretinal vessels, and also in some areas between the newly formed subretinal vessels and the sensory retina.

At the end of the involution process, i.e. when the lesions stopped demonstrating fluorescein leakage and showed staining of the scar only, serial light microscopy revealed a tube of RPE cells completely ensheathing the newly formed subretinal vessels (Fig. 3). These vessels were connected to the choroidal vasculature through the center of the scar (where the break in Bruch's membrane occurred) and were spread in the subretinal space around the break in Bruch's membrane. The RPE cells were arranged around the vessels in a papillary pattern (Fig. 3a). The RPE envelope seemed to end at the edges of the break in Bruch's membrane; the center of the lesion consisted of a chorioretinal scar (Fig. 3a). No fluid was present between the enveloped vessels and the sensory retina.

Electron microscopy of the laser lesions revealed that the newly formed subretinal vessels had similar ultrastructural features at both their early and late stages of development: they had wide lumens formed by thin endothelial cells that contained many diaphragmed fenestrations (Fig. 4). The only ultrastructural difference between the subretinal vessels of the early leaky stage and of the late involuted stage lay in their interendothelial junctions: at the early leaky stage the vessels had open interendothelial clefts with short adherens regions (Fig. 5), while at the late involuted stage the junctional complexes were highly convoluted and contained longer adherens regions with focal fusion points between the outer leaflets of plasma membranes of opposing cells (Fig. 6).

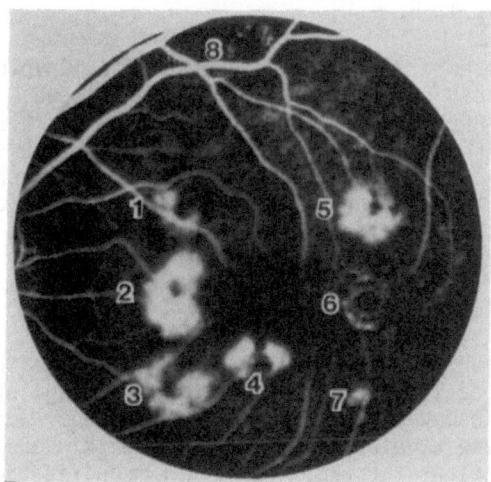

FIGURE 1. Late phase fluorescein angiogram of cynomolgus monkey macula with eight laser lesions (1 to 8) two weeks after laser photocoagulation. Lesions 1 to 5 demonstrate variable amounts of fluorescein leakage and pooling and are defined as leaky lesions.

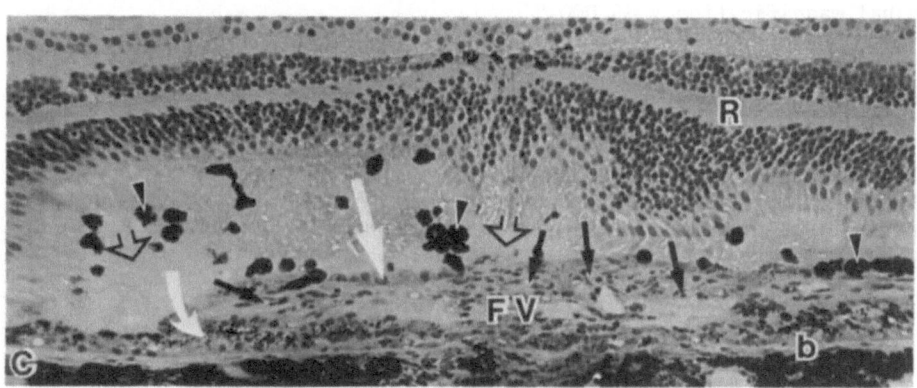

FIGURE 2. Light micrograph of a laser lesion demonstrating first signs of leakage on angiography two weeks after photocoagulation. Newly formed subretinal vessels (black arrows) have spread into the periphery of the lesion where bruch's membrane (b) is intact. Note the double layer of retinal pigment epithelial (RPE) cells (white curved arrow) between Bruch's membrane and the subretinal vessels. Note also the short area in which a monolayer of RPE cells (long white arrow) is separating the fibrovascular tissue (FV) from the overlying fluid (open arrows).
Arrowheads = macrophages. C = choroid. R = retina.
Original magnification x 200.

LEGENDS TO FIGURES 3, 4, 5, 6.

FIGURE 3. Two representative serial sections of an involuted lesion.
A. The edge of the scar center (open arrow) can be seen. Note the papillary arrangement of RPE cells (white arrow) around the vessels (arrowhead)
and the absence of RPE cells (black arrow) between Bruch's membrane (b)
and the subretinal vessels in the area approaching the center of the scar.
B. The periphery of the lesion. A tight envelope of RPE cells (white
arrows) around the subretinal vessels (arrowheads) can be seen. No fluid
is present in the subretinal area throughout the lesion. Original
magnification x 250.

FIGURE 4. A newly formed subretinal vessel from the lesion in Figure 3.
The eye was enucleated 10 months after laser photocoagulation, long after
fluorescein leakage stopped; staining only of the scar was seen. The
lumen (L) is wide, the endothelial cells (E) are thin and contain many
diaphragmed fenestrations (arrows). Original magnification x 56,000.

FIGURE 5. An interendothelial junction of a subretinal vessel from a leaky
lesion. The eye was enucleated 7 weeks after laser photocoagulation when
the lesion was still actively leaking and pooling fluorescein in the
subretinal space. The junction (arrows) is open except for a short
adherent region (curved arrow) in which the junctional membranes show
increased electron density. The cytoplasm immediately adjacent to the
membranes has finely filamentous material and the interendothelial matrix
a tenuous condensation. E = endothelial cell; L = lumen; E = erythrocyte.
Original magnification x 85,000.

FIGURE 6. An interendothelial junction of a newly formed blood vessel
from an involuted lesion. The eye was enucleated 10 weeks after laser
photocoagulation when the lesion was no longer demonstrating fluorescein
leakage. Note the long adherent region of the junction (curved arrow)
with its focal fusion point (arrow). Crystal Bodies (CB) are frequently
found in the endothelial cells (E) of the subretinal vessels. L = lumen.
Original magnification x 88,000.

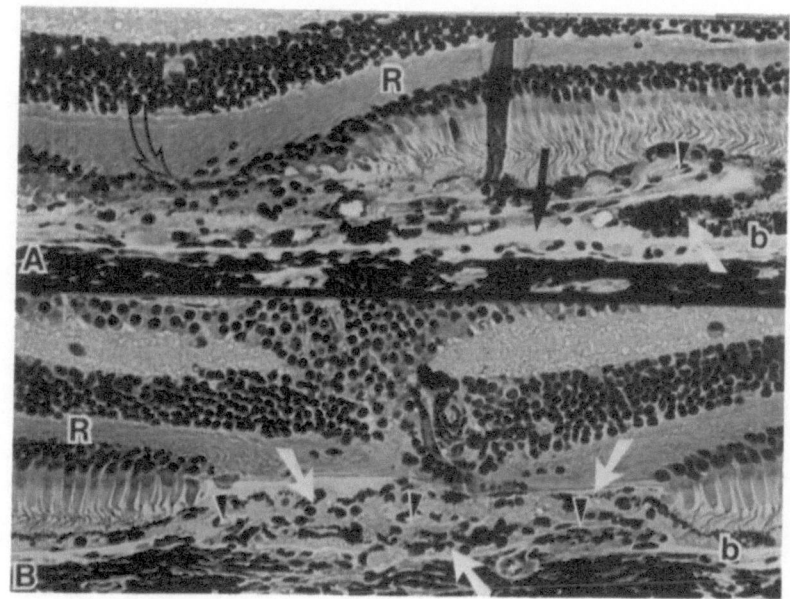

FIGURE 3.

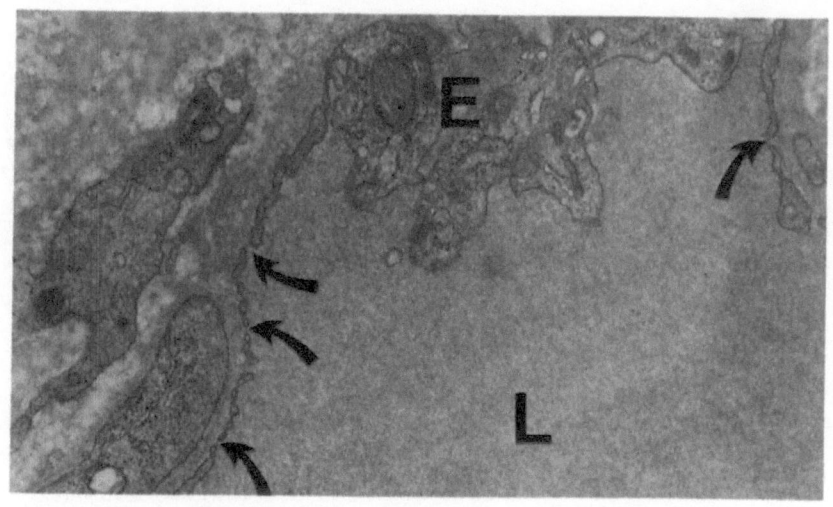

FIGURE 4.

472

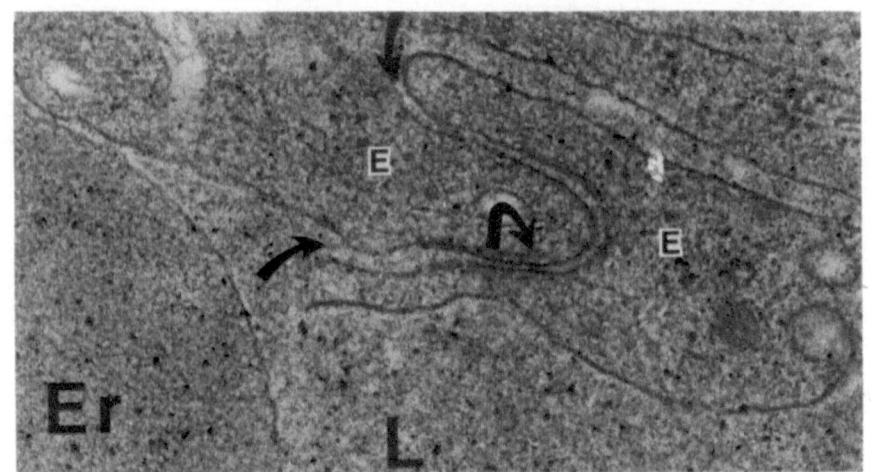

FIGURE 5.

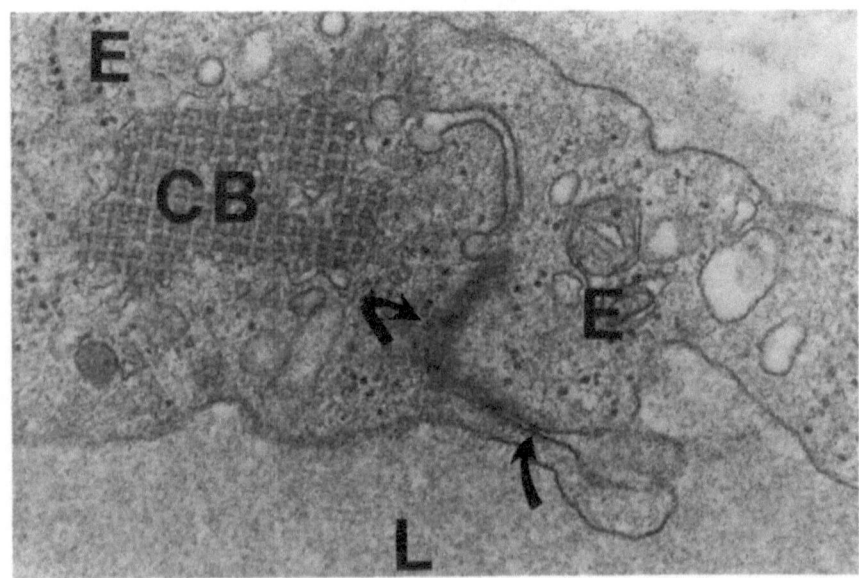

FIGURE 6.

4. DISCUSSION

The results presented in this communication show that the involution of laser induced choroidal subretinal neovascularization, ie. the cessation of dye leakage and pooling that accompanies the maturation of the neo-vascular membrane, cannot be attributed to changes in the ultrastructural features of the subretinal vessels with maturation, but rather results from RPE proliferation around the subretinal vessels. As RPE proliferation progresses, the subretinal fluid diminishes. At the end of the involution process RPE totally envelops the subretinal vessels and no fluid separates the vessels from the sensory retina.

From our results it appears that RPE proliferation starts at the peri-phery of the injury, probably with RPE cells that have not been severely damaged, and proceeds in a papillary pattern around the subretinal vessels (Fig. 3). With maturation of the neovascular membrane, RPE cells continue to envelope the newly-formed subretinal vessels. As these vessels have fenestrated endothelial walls and permeable interendothelial junctions at all stages of their development (Figs. 4 - 6), as long as the RPE does not form a tight barrier around them fluid can leak from the vessels and accumulate in the subretinal space. The maturation of the interendothelial junctions from open to focal tight junction cannot explain the decrease in leakage, as focal tight junctions are permeable to fluorescein.

At the end of the involution process the RPE forms a continuous tube of cells around the subretinal vessels. As RPE cells are known to actively transport fluid from the subretinal space into the choroid (7,8), they are probably responsible for the absorption of the accumulated subretinal fluid during involution.

Furthermore, although the subretinal vessels retain their "leaky" mor-phology once a tight barrier of RPE cells is formed around them, their potential to leak fluorescein cannot be demonstrated as there is no space in which the dye can accumulate and therein be visible on angiography. It seems, therefore, that in our experimental model, and perhaps also in human cases of subretinal neovascularization with leakage of fluid into the subretinal space, there is a normal healing process that involves RPE proliferation around the newly-formed subretinal vessels, with subsequent total envelopment of the vessels. The newly-formed RPE barrier may be responsible not only for pumping out the previously accumulated subretinal fluid, but also for blocking further passage of fluid from the vessels into the subretinal space.

Based on these experimental observations we have tried to enhance the involution process of leaking and pooling subretinal neovascular lesions, by stimulating RPE proliferation around the lesions with mild laser appli-cations - first in nonhuman primates and later in selected human subfoveal lesions (unpublished data 1986). Our results were encouraging enough to suggest further investigation into this possible alternative to the current destructive treatment of macular subretinal neovascularization.

5. REFERENCES

1. Yannuzzi LA, Gitter KA and Schatz H: The Macula: A Comprehensive Text and Atlas. Baltimore, The Williams & Wilkins Co. 1978, pp 180-201.
2. Hyman LG: Senile macular degeneration: an epidemiologic case control study. Baltimore, Maryland: Johns Hopkins University 1981. PhD disser-tation.
3. Teeters VW and Bird AC: A clinical study of the vascularity of senile disciform macular degeneration. Am J Ophthalmol 75:53, 1973.

4. Gass JDM: Pathogenesis of disciform detachment of the neuroepithelium. IV. Fluorescein angiographic study of senile disciform macular degeneration. Am J Ophthalmol 63: 645, 1967.
5. Ryan SJ: Subretinal neovascularization: Natural history of an experimental model. Arch Ophthalmol 100: 1804, 1982.
6. Miller H, Miller B and Ryan SJ: Correlation of choroidal subretinal neovascularization with fluorescein angiography. Am J Ophthalmol 99: 263, 1985.
7. Miller SS, Hughes BA and Machen TE: Fluid transport across retinal pigment epithelium is inhibited by cyclic AMP. Proc Natl Acad Sci USA 79: 2111-2115, 1982.
8. Pederson JE and MacLellan HM: Experimental retinal detachment. I. Effect of subretinal fluid composition on reabsorption rate and intraocular pressure. Arch Ophthalmol 100:1150, 1982.

CHOROIDAL VASCULAR REPAIR AFTER KRYPTON LASER PHOTOCOAGULATION IN THE RAT

A. POLLACK,* G.E. KORTE, P. HENKIND
*Kaplan Hospital, Rehovot, Israel and Albert Einstein College of Medicine,
Bronx, N.Y., USA

1. INTRODUCTION

Choroidal subretinal neovascularization occurs in a large number of
fundus disorders (1) and experimental models (2,3). However, neither its
pathogenesis nor its regression is clearly understood. Of particular
interest is the response of choroidal subretinal neovascularization to
laser photocoagulation, resulting in the growth of new vessels as well as
their obliteration (4,5). In order to better understand this dual
response, we studied the restoration of the choroidal vasculature following krypton laser photocoagulation in the retina of the rat.

2. MATERIALS AND METHODS

Our main aim was to investigate the effect in the rat of laser photocoagulation at a level comparable with therapeutic levels used in human
patients. Laser burns which cause whitening of the retina were considered
as equivalent to moderate intensity therapeutic lesions.

Small lesions were formed by applying individual krypton laser burns
(100μ), as described elsewhere (6), to the superior nasal quadrant of the
retina in 40 mature pigmented rats. Large lesions were formed in the
temporal quadrant by the application of six confluent burns of the same
beam size. The nonirradiated inferior hemisphere served as an internal
control. The eyes were enucleated 1,2,3,4,6,7,10,14,21,28,35,39 and 50
days after lasering and processed by routine methods for light microscopy
(LM) and transmission electron microscopy (TEM).

3. RESULTS

Twenty-four hours after irradiation, vascular occlusion by clumped red
blood cells or thrombi, as previously described for moderate lasering
intensities, was seen (7). Endothelial necrosis was observed in the center
of some lesions, especially the large ones.

Seven to ten days after lasering, the capillaries at the periphery of
the lesions had open lumina, were devoid of occlusive thrombi and contained
monocytes and intraluminal endothelial sprouts (Fig. 1). Extraluminal
cellular processes similar to the intraluminal sprouts were also visible
(Fig. 1). They were either continuous or discontinuous with the endothelial cells and some were surrounded by basement membrane (Fig. 1).

From the 21st day onward, normal-looking choriocapillaries were visible
at the periphery of all lesions (Fig. 2). In the case of large lesions,
well developed choroidal subretinal neovascularization entering Bruch's
membrane towards the retina could also be seen (Fig. 3). At the center of
all the lesions, areas without capillaries were filled with fibrous tissue
(Fig. 2). At the junctional zone between the center of the lesion and its
periphery, some endothelial cells of patent capillaries showed signs of
degeneration such as dark or swollen vacuolized cellular organelles and

membranous debris in the capillary lumen (Fig. 4). Similar signs of degeneration were observed in the extraluminal endothelial sprouts and in the choroidal subretinal neovascularization (Fig. 5).

4. COMMENT

The main immediate effect of moderately intense krypton laser photo-coagulation on the choroidal vessels is their occlusion by thrombogenesis (7). These thrombi may however resolve, leading to re-opening of the occluded vessels (8). Indeed, seven to ten days after lasering the capillaries were devoid of occlusive thrombi and contained intraluminal sprouts; these findings are consistent with fibrinolysis and recanalization (8). Also observed at this time were extraluminal endothelial sprouts budding off the reforming capillaries at the periphery of the lesions, as the first steps of neovascularization (9). At the center of the lesions, where endothelial necrosis was noted in the first 24 hours after lasering, the capillaries did not reform and became atrophied.

From the 21st day onward the center of all the lesions was replaced by fibrous tissue, and recanalized capillaries were visible at the periphery. In the large lesions new vessels were also present at the periphery. However, some of the endothelial cells in the new vascular fronds showed signs of degeneration, such as the presence of vacuolized cellular organelles. We concluded that these new vessels had become involuted. Similar signs of cell death were found in the endothelial cells at the junctional zone between the center of the lesion and its periphery. We assume that this atrophy developed as a secondary process after recanalization, since 1) it occurred in an area where at an earlier stage of recovery we had observed patent capillaries with active endothelial cells bearing expanded rough endoplasmic reticulum, and 2) the changes occurred in both intra- and extraluminal endothelial sprouts. We would therefore apply the term "primary atrophy" to the capillary degeneration occurring in the center of the lesions and already visible within the first ten days, and "secondary atrophy" to that which developed after the third week of follow-up and occurring in new vascular fronds or recanalized capillaries.

The development of secondary atrophy may in part explain the beneficial effect of laser photocoagulation. Although the thrombosed vessels can reopen and even give rise to neovascularization initially, the mechanism of secondary atrophy may result in permanent vascular obliteration.

REFERENCES

1. Henkind P: Ocular neovascularization. The Krill Lecture. Am J Ophthalmol 85:287-300, 1978.
2. Ryan SJ: The development of an experimental model of subretinal neovascularization in disciform macular degeneration. Trans Am Ophthalmol Soc 77:707-745, 1979.
3. Archer DB, Gardiner TA: Electron microscopic features of experimental choroidal neovascularization. Am J Ophthalmol 91:433-457, 1981.
4. Macular Photocoagulation Study Group: Recurrent choroidal neovascularization after argon laser photocoagulation for neovascular maculopathy. Arch Ophthalmol 104:503-512, 1986.
5. Coscas G, Soubrane G: The effect of red krypton and green argon laser on the foveal region. A clinical and experimental study. Ophthalmol 90:1013-1023, 1983.

6. Pollack A, Heriot WJ, Henkind P: Cellular processes causing defects
    in Bruch's membrane following krypton laser photocoagulation.
    Ophthalmol 93:1113-1119, 1986.
7. Thomas EL, Apple DJ, Swartz M, et al.: Histopathology and ultra-
    structure of krypton and argon laser lesions in a human retina-
    choroid. Retina 4:22-39, 1984.
8. Robbins SL, Cotran RS, Kumar V: Fluid and hemodynamic derangements.
    In Robbins SL, Cotran RS, Kumar V (eds): Pathologic Basis of
    Diseases, 3rd ed. Philadelphia, WB Saunders; 100-102, 1984.
9. Kalebic T, Garbisa S, Glaser B, Liotta LA: Basement membrane
    collagen: degradation by migrating endothelial cells. Science
    221:281-283, 1983.

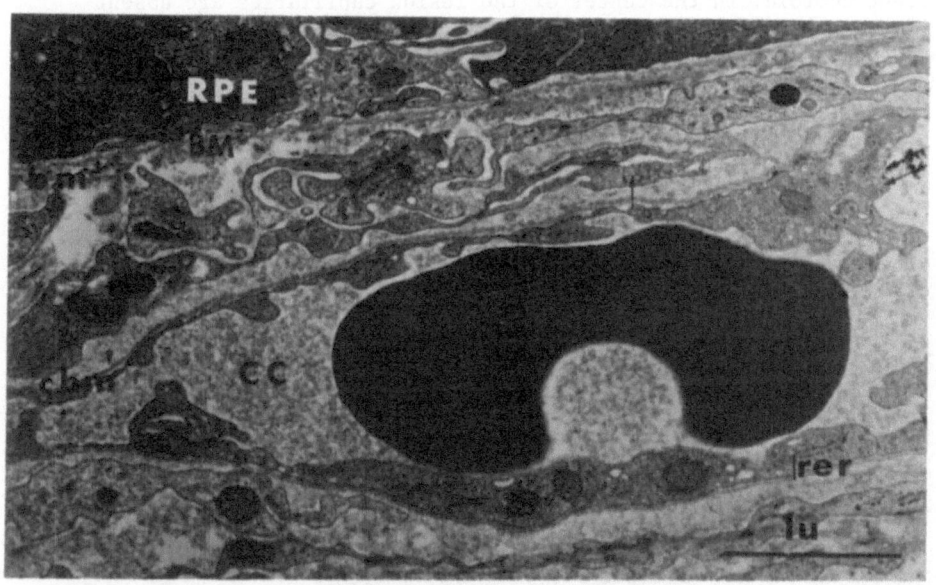

FIGURE 1. TEM of the choroidal vascular repair ten days after lasering.
A choriocapillary (CC) without occlusive thrombi shows signs of activation,
i.e., expanded rough endoplasmic reticulum (rer), and contains intraluminal
endothelial sprouts (double arrows). Similar extraluminal endothelial
processes (arrow) are visible between the CC basement membrane (cbm) and
the retinal pigment epithelial basement membrane (rbm). (1um=32mm).

478

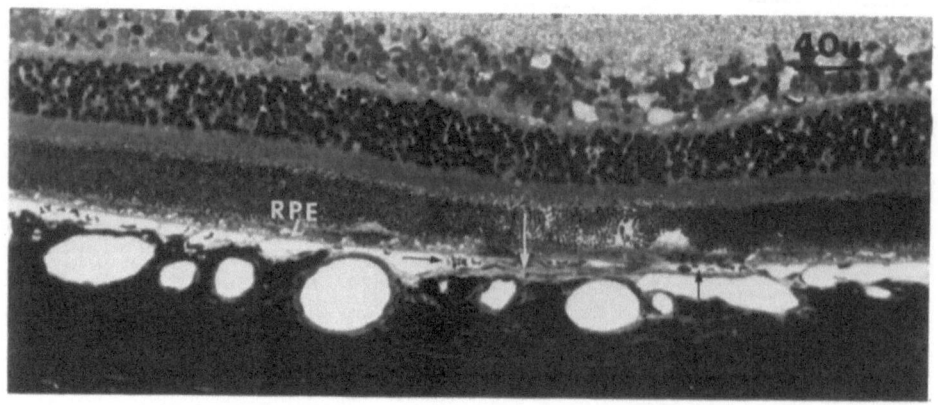

FIGURE 2. LM of healed laser lesion covered with RPE cells. At the adjacent choroid, in the center of the lesion capillaries are absent (white arrow), while normal-looking capillaries can be seen at the periphery (black arrows). (20um=6mm).

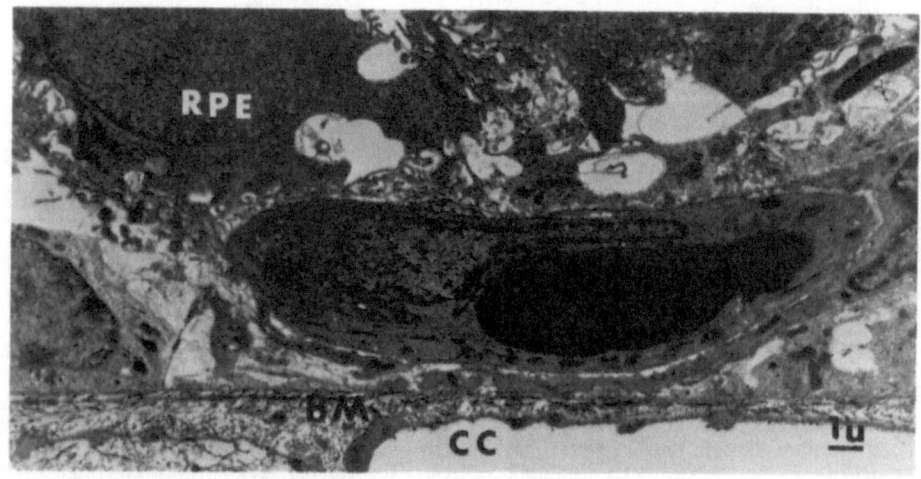

FIGURE 3. TEM of new vessels (*) lying on the retinal side of Bruch's membrane (BM) and among RPE cells. CC, choriocapillary. (1um=6mm).

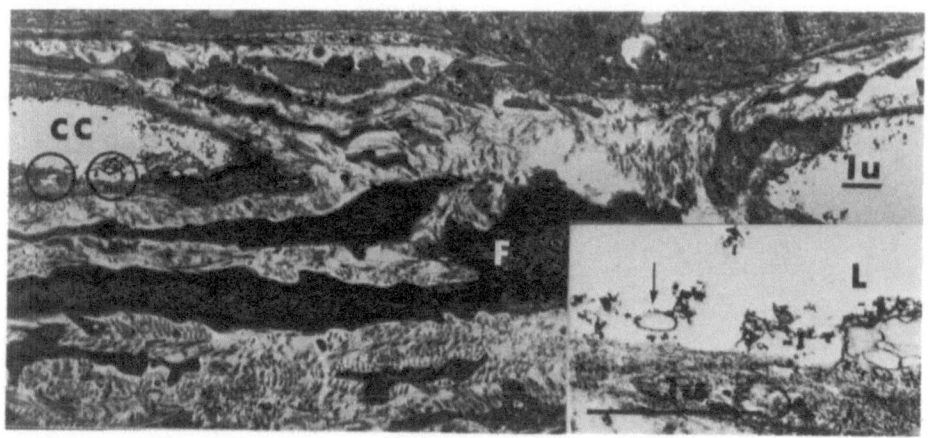

FIGURE 4. TEM of a junctional zone between the center of a lesion and its periphery. Swollen cell organelles (encircled, left) are seen in the endothelial cell, and membranous debris (encircled, right) is present in the lumen (see inset). (1um=6mm). Inset, high magnification of a serial section of encircled area showing membranous debris in the lumen (arrow). (1um=28mm).

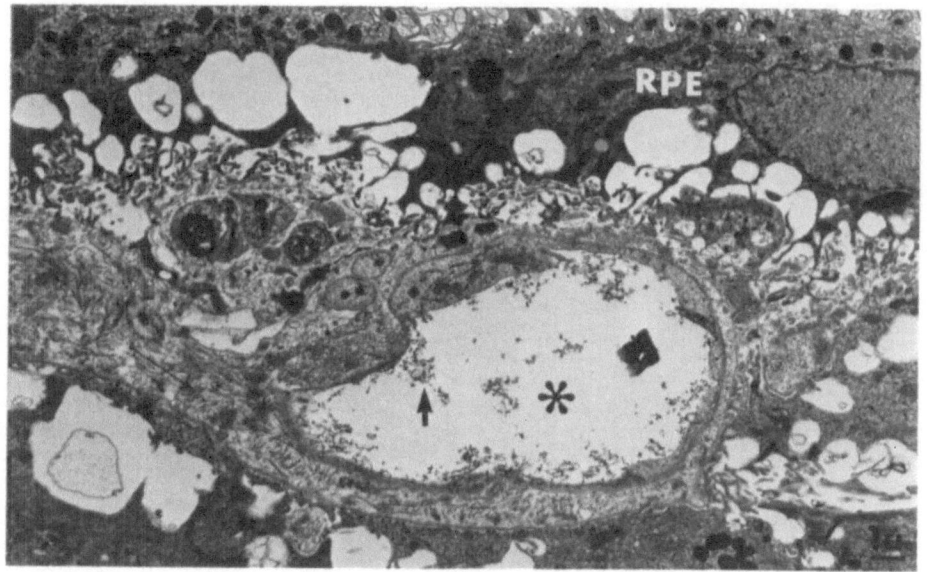

FIGURE 5. Choroidal neovascularization (*) surrounded by connective tissue matrix (narrow arrow) and embedded between RPE cells shows signs of degeneration such as membranous debris in the capillary lumen (wide arrow). (1um=5mm).

GROWTH CHARACTERISTICS OF RETINAL MICROVASCULAR CELLS IN CULTURE

Hong Chai Wong, Mike Boulton, John Marshall and Peter Clark.
Institute of Ophthalmology, London WC1, England.

INTRODUCTION.

Pre-retinal neovascularisation is a common cause of blindness in the U.K.[1] Although retinal ischaemia, inflammation and neoplasia commmonly precede pre-retinal neovascularisation [2], the mechanism of new vessel formation is unknown. Investigation of factor(s) controlling the growth of pre-retinal new vessels have been impeded by the lack of a reproducible animal model. Another approach to this problem is to use cultured vascular endothelial cells to seek out the factors controlling their growth. Though in vitro growth conditions of endothelial cells are different to those in vivo, studies of their proliferation in vitro can be reproduced for quantitative analysis. This allows us to begin to determine the factor(s) which may play a part in neovascularisation in vivo.

The main obstacle to in vitro studies of retinal capillary endothelial cells has been the difficulty to establish longterm cultures. Busney [3] used sarcoma conditioned medium (SCM) to enhance the growth of bovine retinal capillary endothelial cells (BRCEC). However, BRCEC which have been cultured in the presence of SCM may not be suitable for studies of pre-retinal new vessel formation since the major cause of pre-retinal neovascularisation is retinal ischaemia and not neoplasia. This problem was addressed in a study [4] which omitted SCM and instead used a growth medium containing retinal derived growth factor and platelet poor plasma. In our laboratory this method has produced inconsistent results in sustaining endothelial cell growth. This report describes a novel technique for the rapid growth of BRCEC without the use of SCM.

PRIMARY ISOLATION OF RETINAL MICROVESSELS

The isolation procedure was developed from previous published methods [3-5]. Bovine eyes were transported on ice to the laboratory. The retinas were aseptically removed and placed in cold Eagle's minimal essential medium (MEM) supplemented with 30mM HEPES at pH7.4. They were homogenised in cold MEM using a rotary teflon-glass homogeniser. The homogenate was centrifuged at 400g for 10 minutes and the resultant pellet was resuspended in 10ml of calcium and magnesium free Dulbecco's phosphate buffered saline (PBSA). Microvessels were trapped on an 83 micron nylon mesh and transferred to a petri dish containing an enzyme cocktail [6]. They were incubated at 37°C on a rotatory shaker and enzyme treated. For isolation of pericytes this was usually between 15 to 20 minutes at which time the majority of pericytes remained adherent to the microvessels. For isolation of BRCEC this was between 20 to 30 minutes of incubation when at least 50% of microvessels were devoid of pericytes, The resultant vessel fragments were trapped on a 53 micron mesh, washed with cold MEM and centrifuged at 400g for 5 minutes, the pellet was resuspended in MEM and recentrifuged. The pellet was finally resuspended in growth medium for culture of either BRCEC or pericytes.

CULTURE OF PERICYTES

The resultant pellet from the primary isolation was resuspended in Dulbecco's modified Eagle's medium (DMEM) supplemented with 20% foetal calf serum (FCS) and antibiotics. 5ml aliquots were pipetted into 25cm^2 plastic tissue culture flasks (Falcon) and the cultures incubated at 37°C in a 95% air/5% CO_2 atmosphere. Confluent cultures were passaged by detaching the cells with 0.25% trypsin and 0.02% EDTA in PBSA and plated at a split ratio of 1:3.

PRODUCTION OF FRESH MEDIUM (FM) AND PERICYTE CONDITIONED MEDIUM (PCM)

Confluent and post confluent pericyte cultures between the 2nd and 4th passage were first washed twice with 5 ml of PBSA prior to the production of PCM. 8 ml of fresh DMEM supplemented with 7.5% human platelet poor plasma [7], 2.5 ug/ml transferrin (Sigma), 5 ug/ml ascorbic acid (BDH), antibiotics (designated as FM) was added to each flask of confluent pericytes. After 2 days the PCM was collected and stored at -20°C.

CULTURE OF BRCEC

Endothelial cell growth medium (EGM) consisted of a 1:1 mixture of PCM and FM. This mixture was supplemented with 20 ul/ml retinal crude extract [4], 90 ug/ml heparin [8] and 0.2 ug/ml Insulin. EGM was added to the primary isolation pellet and plated onto gelatinised 60mm tissue culture dishes (Falcon). Thereafter the media was changed every 3 to 4 days. BRCEC were detached with 0.05% trypsin and 0.02% EDTA [3] at preconfluence; and subcultured at a split ratio of 1:3.

PRODUCTION OF BOVINE TENON'S FIBROBLAST CONDITIONED MEDIUM

Fibroblasts from bovine Tenon's capsule were cultured in DMEM + 20% FCS. Conditioned medium from post confluent cultures was prepared in ident, al manner as for PCM. A mixture of 1:1 ratio by volume of FM and conditioned medium from bovine Tenon's fibroblast was designed as BTFCM.

PROLIFERATIVE ASSAYS

A. Using cultures of BRCEC between 2nd and 4th subculture. 2×10^4 BRCEC in one ml of EGM containing retinal crude extract, heparin and insulin (see "Culture of BRCEC") were seeded into each gelatinised well of a 24 multiwell dish. After a period of 2 days to allow for attachment and initial growth, 6 wells in each multiwell dish were processed for cell counts. The cells were washed twice with PBSA, trypsinised and counted using a haemocytometer. The mean count of these 6 wells was designated the "initial count" for that dish. The remaining wells were each washed with 1ml of DMEM. 1 ml of the test media was added to each of 6 wells and a number of different test media were studied (Fig. 3). After 3 days in test media, the cells counts were determined and designated as the "final count". Each experiment was performed on two occasions.

B. Using microvessels from primary isolation. In order to see whether insulin had a mitogenic effect on microvessel fragments in primary culture 2 x 10^5 microvessel fragments in 0.5 ml in FM were added to each gelatinised multiwell. 0.5 ml of test media containing either PCM or FM, each supplemented with or without insulin (80 ng/ml) was also added. Thus when insulin was present the final concentration would have been diluted to 40 ng/ml. After an initial period of 2 days for attachment, the multiwells were washed with PBSA and identical fresh test media were added. On the 5th day after isolation each well was processed for cell counts in an identical manner as for the proliferative assays of BRCEC and pericytes.

STATISTICAL ANALYSIS OF PROLIFERATIVE STUDIES

For the assays using BRCEC, the growth rate of the test medium in each well was expressed as the ratio of the "final count" to "initial count" of that multiwell dish. Analysis of variance, t-test and Newman Keuls analysis[9] were used on the logarithim of this ratio to assess the significance of any differences between types of test growth media. For the assays using microvessel, the final cell count on the 5th day of the assay was subjected to analysis of variance and Newman Keuls.

RESULTS

Pericytes could be seen to migrate and proliferate from the attached microvessels on the 3rd day after isolation in DMEM + 20% FCS. These pericytes were factor VIII negative and could be routinely passaged up to 12 times. Their morphology was polygonal and stress fibres could be seen within the cells (Fig. 1a). When allowed to grow to a post confluent state they typically formed heaped up islands of cells.

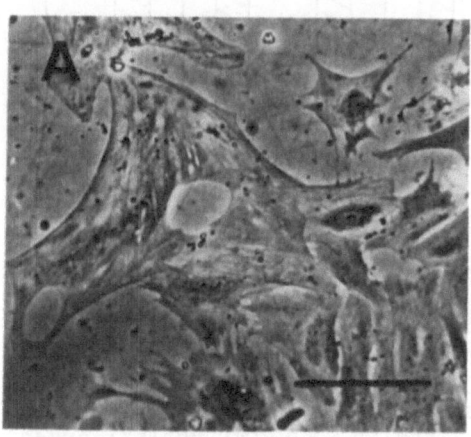 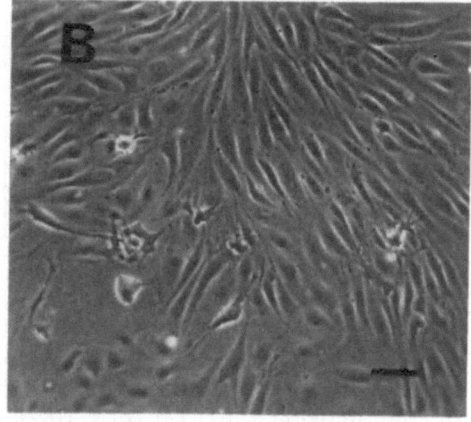

Figure 1. Light micrographs of primary cultures of a) pericytes; note the presence of stress fibres and b) BRCEC at confluence in EGM with insulin, retinal crude extract and heparin. Bar marker 100u.

484

Using EGM, BRCEC grew out from attached microvessels to form islands of spindle shaped cells by the 2nd day after isolation. Primary cultures of BRCEC grown in EGM supplemented with retinal crude extract, heparin and insulin regularly reached confluence as a monolayer by the 5th or 6th day (Fig. 1b) and could be routinely passaged up to 8 times. Primary cultures grown in FM supplemented with full factors rarely reached confluence and could not be passaged without the emergence of a large number of contaminating pericytes in the resultant subculture. BRCEC between the primary and 5th subculture were Factor VIII positive. By the 7th or 8th subculture senescent cells were seen, typified by cellular enlargement and pleomorphism.

The proliferative assays (Fig.2a) showed that the growth rate of BRCEC in EGM (containing PCM) was significantly greater than that of FM. When retinal crude extract, heparin and insulin were added alone or in combination (Fig.2b) enhancement of cell growth by EGM was still present. EGM had significantly greater mitogenic activity than FM without additional factors or when supplemented with insulin alone, heparin alone or a combination of heparin and retinal crude extract (Table 1). All test media containing retinal crude extract had significantly greater mitogenic effect than media without retinal crude extract ($P < 0.01$). Insulin or herapin alone at a concentration of 0.2 ug/ml and 90 ug/ml respectively in FM or EGM did not have a mitogenic effect.

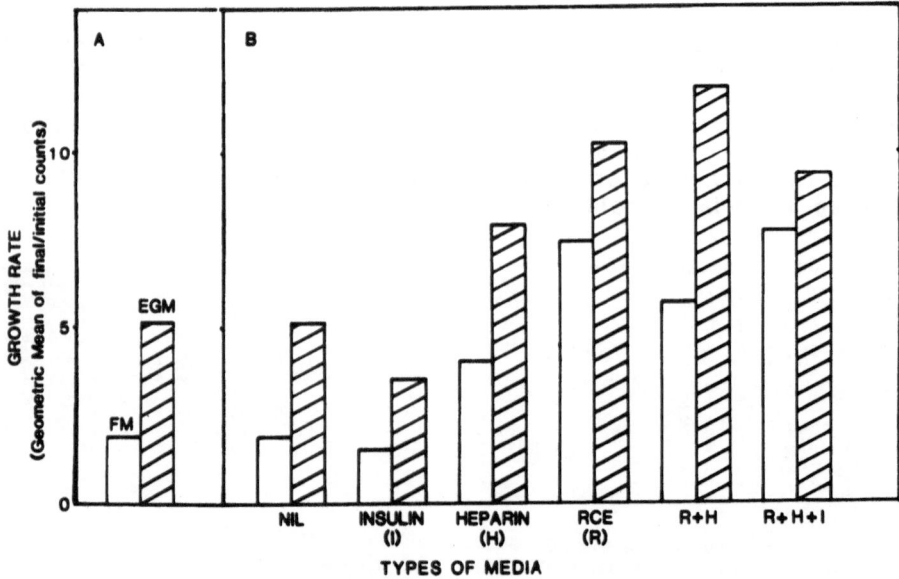

Figure 2. Comparison of BRCEC growth rates in fresh medium (FM-open bar) versus EGM (shaded bar). a) in the absence of factors and b) in the presence of factors (0.2ug/ml insulin, 20ul/ml retinal crude extract and 90ug/ml heparin, nil is in the absence of factors).

Table 1.   Statistical Analysis of the growth rates of BRCEC in
Endothelial Growth Medium (EGM) versus Fresh Media (FM)[*].

Types of factors in EGM or FM	Ratio of growth rate of EGM to FM	Ratio needed for EGM FM (P<0.01)
No factors present	2.74	1.40
I (Insulin)	2.30	1.49
H (Heparin)	1.97	1.49
R (Retinal Crude Extract)	1.38	1.49
R+H	2.09	1.40
R+H+I	1.21	1.49

[*] See fig.3 for concentrations of the factors used.

Post confluent cultures of pericytes and Tenon's fibroblasts between the 2nd and 4th subculture contained on average $3-5 \times 10^5$ and $1-1.5 \times 10^6$ cells respectively in a $25cm^2$ flask. Both EGM and BTFCM had significantly greater mitogenic activity than FM.(fig.3).

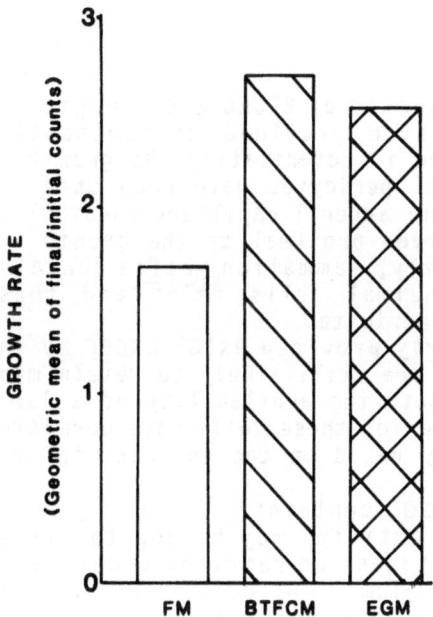

Figure 3. A comparison of BRCEC growth rates in FM, EGM and BTFCM (bovine tenon fibroblast conditioned medium).

Proliferative assays (fig. 4) using microvessel fragments showed that EGM had greater mitogenic activity than FM. However insulin at a concentration of 40 ng/ml had significant mitogenic effect only in the presence of FN.

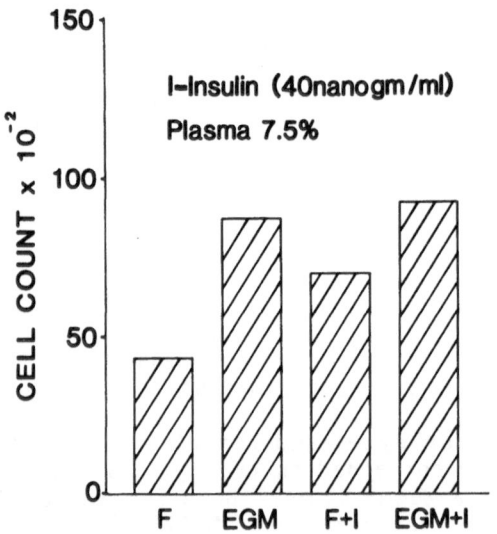

Figure 4. The mitogenic effect of insulin on primary microvessels.

DISCUSSION

The use of PCM to enhance the growth of BRCEC was prompted by three independant observations which provided circumstantial evidence that pericytes were involved in potentiating the growth of capillary endothelial cells. Adrenal pericytes have been used for the enhancement of growth of bovine adrenal capillary endothelial cells [10]. Pericytes have been observed proximal to the growth tip of a pre-retinal new vessel [2]. Lastly, mammalian retina contains potent growth factors for endothelial cells [11-13] and these factor(s) could be derived from the pericyte.

Our culture method has regularly provided 9×10^6 BRCEC by the 2nd passage at which time the BRCEC are still likely to retain many of their in vivo characteristics. Both the availability of a large number of BRCEC and the rapid turnover of these cells have permitted the development of a mitogenic assay based on the increase in cell numbers over three days.

The assays demonstrated that EGM containing PCM had greater mitogenic activity than FM. This activity may be due to either pericytes secreting endothelial mitogens or removing endothelial inhibitors from the unconditioned medium. The concept of pericyte induced endothelial mitogenic activity may appear to be paradoxical in diabetic retinopathy where their degeneration precedes proliferative retinopathy [15]. The resolution of this paradox is complex, but may relate to a decrease of total number of pericytes and to an increase of production of growth factor by pericytes in the neighbourhood of the new vessel as pericytes have been found to invest preretinal new vessels in diabetic proliferative retinopathy [16].

The mitogenic assays confirmed previous findings that retinal crude extract stimulated proliferation of BRCEC [4]. Since the effect of retinal crude extract was not enhanced by heparin it either meant that heparin has no effect on the mitogenic activity of retinal crude extract or that retinal crude extract was already at optimal concentration. The observation that heparin alone had no effect on BRCEC agreed with the findings of Azizkhan [17] using adrenal capillary endothelial cells.

That insulin did not show a mitogenic effect on BRCEC between the 2nd and 4th subculture would appear to be contrary to previous data [18]. This may be due to differences in culture and assay methods. King [18] cultured BRCEC in physiological concentrations of insulin prior to testing the growth effect of insulin on BRCEC. In this study, the insulin concentration in EGM was 5-10 times that of normal human plasma. Thus the number of insulin receptors on BRCEC would have decreased by down regulation and thus accounted for the lack of response. This is substantiated by the results of microvessel assays (fig. 4) which showed that insulin in FM alone had a mitogenic effect on microvascular cells in primary culture.

BTFCM also had a significant growth effect on BRCEC demonstrating that this activity was not specific to PCM. This confirmed the report by Folkman et al [10] who found conditioned media derived from a variety of cell types were capable of supporting the growth of adrenal capillary endothelial cells. Though the effect of PCM is non cell specific, the demonstration of this activity from the pericyte with its proximity to retinal capillary endothelial cell is important since it does not exclude that this effect may be operative in vivo. Furthermore the mitogenic effect derived from 3-5 $\times 10^5$ pericytes was about the same as from 1-1.5 $\times 10^6$ bovine Tenon's fibroblasts. Therefore pericytes appeared to have greater growth activity per number of cells than Tenon's fibroblasts.

IN CONCLUSION

Longterm cultures of bovine retinal capillary endothelial cells have been established using pericyte conditioned medium. The mitogenic activity of PCM was not cell specific since fibroblast conditioned medium also had significant activity. The activity was not significantly enhanced by heparin though it was additive to that of retinal crude extract.

ACKNOWLEDGEMENTS

This study was supported by the Francis and Renee Hock Foundation; Moorfields Eye Hospital Endowment Fund; The Mason Medical Foundation; Smith Kline and French Foundation; Lasertek Ltd.; The Help to Hospitals Charity. The authors are indebted to David McLeod of the Vitreoretinal Unit, Moorfields Eye Hospital for moral and technical support, Stephen Rothery and Meryl Bayly for their technical assistance and Corinne White for secretarial assistance.

REFERENCES
1. Medical Research Council Medical Party. Diseases of the eye: a report submitted to the MRC's Neurobiology and Mental Health Board. London: Medical Research Council. 1983.
2. Archer D B. Retinal neovascularisation. Trans Ophthal Soc UK 103:2-27, 1983.
3. Busney S M et al. Retinal vascular endothelial cells and pericytes. Invest Ophthalmol Vis Sci 24:470-480, 1983.
4. Gitlin J D, D'Amore P A. Culture of retinal capillary endothelial cells using selective growth media. Microvascular Res 26:74-80, 1983.
5. Bowman P D et al. Primary culture of microvascular endothelial cells from bovine retina. In Vitro 18:626-632, 1982.
6. Banda J M et al. Isolation of a nonmitogenic angiogenesis factor from wound fluid. Proc Natl Acad Sci USA 79:7773-7777, 1982.
7. Pledger W J et al. Induction of DNA synthesis in BALB/c3T3 cells by serum components: Reevaluation of the commitment process. Proc Natl Acad Sci USA 74:4481-4485, 1977.
8. Thornton S C et al. Human endothelial cells: use of heparin in cloning and long-term serial cultivation. Science 222:623-625, 1983.
9. Winer J B. Statistical principles in experimental design. New York: McGraw-Hill. 1971.
10. Folkman J et al. Long-term culture of capillary endothelial cells. Proc Natl Acad Sci USA 76:5217-5221, 1979.
11. Elstow S F et al. Bovine retinal angiogenesis factor is a small molecule (molecular mass 600). Invest Ophthalmol Vis Sci 26: 74-79, 1985.
12. Kissun R D et al. A low-molecular-weight angiogenic factor in cat retina. Br J Ophthalmol 66:165-169, 1982.
13. Baird A et al. Retina- and eye- derived endothelial cell growth factors: partial molecular characterisation and identity with acidic and basic fibroblast growth factors. Biochemistry 24: 7855-7860, 1985.
14. Glaser B M at al. Demonstration of vasoproliferative activity from mammalian retina. J Cell Biol 84:298-304, 1980.
15. Addison D J et al. Degeneration of intramural pericytes in diabetic retinopathy. Br Med J 1:264-266, 1970.
16. Wallow I H C and Geldner P S. Endothelial fenestrae in proliferative diabetic retinopathy. Invest Ophthalmol Vis Sci 19:1176-1183, 1980.
17. Azizkhan R G et al. Mast cell heparin stimulates migration of capillary endothelial cells in vitro. J Exp Med 152:931-944, 1980.
18. King G L et al. Differential responsiveness to insulin of endothelial and support cells from micro- and macrovessels. J Clin Invest 71:974-979, 1983.

STORAGE OF HEPARIN-BINDING ENDOTHELIAL CELL GROWTH FACTORS IN THE CORNEA: A NEW MECHANISM FOR CORNEAL NEOVASCULARIZATION

Israel Vlodavsky[1], Michael Klagsbrun[2,3] and Judah Folkman[2,4]
Department of Oncology, Hadassah-Hebrew University Hospital, Jerusalem, Israel, [2]Department of Surgery, Children's Hospital and Departments of [3]Biological Chemistry and [4]Anatomy, Harvard Medical School, Boston.

ABSTRACT

While the cornea is normally avascular, injury to Descemet's membrane can induce intense neovascularization. This suggested to us that Descemet's membrane could contain sequestered angioenic factors. Bovine corneas were dissected into three layers. The inner layer comprising almost pure Descemet's membrane was found to contain readily releasable angiogenic heparin-binding growth factors for capillary endothelial cells. These factors appeared to be structurally related to basic fibroblast growth factor (FGF) and were similar to growth factors extracted from the Descemet's membrane-like extracellular matrix deposited in <u>vitro</u> by bovine corneal endothelial cells. When the three corneal layers were subjected to more extensive extraction conditions, heparin binding basic FGF-like growth factors were released also from the middle (stromal) and outer (epithelial) portions of the cornea, albeit at smaller amounts as compared with Descemet's membranes.

These findings indicate that Descemet's membrane and to a lesser extent, other parts of the cornea may serve as a physiological depot for storage of angiogenic molecules. Abnormal release of these factors could be responsible for a variety of different types of pathological corneal neovascularization.

INTRODUCTION

Neovascularization of the cornea can result from trauma and from cellular infiltrates induced by a variety of inflammatory, immunologic and neoplastic processes (1,2). Macrophages have been shown to induce angiogenesis in the cornea (3) and in a healing wound (4). However, it is not clear how corneal neovascularization is triggered by injuries that do not recruit heavy infiltrates of inflammatory cells. For example, it has long been known that intralamellar surgery may induce intense corneal neovascularization if Descemet's membrane is injured. Yet, neovascularization usually does not occur if the injury is limited to the outer third of the cornea. For example, an incision into the corneal stroma does not induce neovascularization, nor does the intralamellar insertion of an inert polymer pellet (5). Similarly, the insertion of a large hydrogel implant for the correction of myopia usually does not cause neovascularization (6).

Recently, a breakthrough in the purification of angiogenic endothelial cell growth factors was reported based on their unusually high affinity for heparin (7). This finding led to the identification of two classes of heparin-binding angiogenic growth factors that are structurally and functionally related to either acidic or basic fibroblast growth factor (FGF) (8-11). The availability of these purified endothelial cell growth factors has permitted the elucidation of their complete amino acid sequence and gene structure (11-13). Heparin-binding growth factors have been isolated from various tumors (7,14) as well as many normal tissues including brain hypothalamus, eye, retina, corpus luteum, placenta and macrophages (8-13,15). The fact that capillary endothelial cells are usually not actively proliferating in normal tissues indicates that these potent angiogenic endothelial mitogens must somehow be stored in an inactive state within normal non-growing tissues. However, the potential sites of this storage remain to be elucidated.

Heparin-like molecules (e.g., heparan sulfate proteoglycans) that are present within extracellular matrices and basement membranes could serve as sites for storage of endothelial cell growth factors which have the property of heparin affinity. In fact, the Descemet's membrane-like extracellular matrix (ECM) layed down by cultured bovine corneal endothelial cells has been shown to replace the requirement that various cell types have for FGF in order for them to proliferate and express their differentiated functions (16,17). This supportive role of ECM on cell proliferation has been attributed to changes in cell shape dictated by structural components of the ECM because ECM treated so as to inactivate growth factors still supports cell growth (18,19). However, the possibility that ECM contains highly stable growth factors has not been ruled out. In support of this possibility are recent observations on the potentiation and stabilization of endothelial cell growth factors by heparin (20,21). In this report we show that heparin-binding growth factors for capillary endothelial cells are secreted by cultured corneal endothelial cells into the subendothelial ECM and that in vivo these factors are stored in the ECM of the bovine cornea, mainly in Descemet's membrane.

MATERIALS AND METHODS
Cell Cultures: Bovine capillary endothelial cells were cloned from adrenal cortex and cultured as previously described (22). Cultures of bovine corneal endothelial cells were established from steer's eyes as described (23) and maintained in Dulbecco's modified Eagle's medium (DMEM, 1 mg/ml glucose) supplemented with 10% calf serum and antibiotics. Cells were dissociated weekly with 0.05% trypsin/0.02% EDTA in PBS and subcultured at a split ratio of 1:5.
Stimulation of DNA Synthesis and Cell Proliferation: Growth factor activity was determined as previously described by measuring the ability of samples to stimulate the incorporation of [H^3]thymidine into the DNA of confluent quiescent BALB/3T3 cells (10,14), and to stimulate the proliferation of bovine capillary and aortic endothelial cells seeded at low and clonal cell densities (10,19,24).
Extraction of ECM Derived Growth Factors from Dishes Coated with ECM: Bovine corneal endothelial cells were plated at an initial density of 10^6 cells per 10 cm tissue culture dishes and maintained under the conditions described above. Six to eight days after reaching confluency, the cell layer was dissolved by 2-3 min exposure to 0.5% Triton X-100 and 20mM NH$_4$OH in PBS followed by four washes in PBS (16,17). Alternatively, the endothelial cells were removed by exposure (10-20 min) to 1M urea in DMEM, a procedure which exposes the subendothelial ECM without lysing the cells (18). In order to extract growth-promoting activity from the ECM, the matrix coating 10 cm culture dishes (100-200 dishes) was incubated for 2 h at 37°C with 50 μg/ml collagenase in PBS. Insoluble material was removed by centrifugation (5000 x g, 20 min) and the supernatant applied to a column of heparin-Sepharose (25). Heparin Sepharose chromatograhpy was performed as previously described (7,14).

<u>Isolation of Descemet's Membrane from Other Components of the Cornea:</u>
Bovine eyes were obtained fresh from the slaughterhouse and maintained at
4°C. The eyes were washed with cold saline. Under sterile conditions a
transverse incision was made across the cornea through approximately one-
third its depth. The outer corneal layer containing the epithelium was
dissected away and removed from the corneal stroma with a corneal spatula.
The central stromal layer of the cornea was similarly dissected away.
Finally, the innermost layer of cornea, which is comprised almost entirely
of Descemet's membrane was then excised. The procedure was carried out
under 2.5X operating binocular loupes. Histologic sections confirmed the
level of dissection of each layer (26).

<u>Extraction of Growth Promoting Factors from Bovine Corneas:</u> The three
corneal layers (from 20 eyes) were respectively collected into 3 tubes
containing 2-3 ml serum-free tissue culture medium (RPMI) supplemented
with 25 mM Hepes, 50 U/ml penicillin and 50 μg/ml streptomycin at 4°C. At
various times (20-180 min) of incubation at either 4°C or 37°C, aliquots
(1-30 μl) of the incubation medium were tested for growth factor activity
on 3T3 and capillary endothelial cells. Extraction of growth factors in
preparation for heparin-Sepharose chromatography was performed by mincing
the tissue (outer, middle and inner corneal layers, each separately) with
opposing scalpel blades followed by 1 hour incubation at 37°C with 50
μg/ml collagenase in RPMI, two cycles of freezing and thawing and 1 min
sonication at 4°C. The extract was then centrifuged (25,000 g, 30 min) and
the supernatant applied to a column (5ml) of heparin-Sepharose.

<u>Electrophoretic Transfer (Western) Blots:</u> Proteins were separated by
electrophoresis on sodium dodecyl sulfate/15% polyacrylamide gels and
transferred into nitrocellulose paper at 40 volts overnight at 4°C. The
nitrocellulose paper was either stained for protein with Aurodye colloidal
gold reagent or incubated with anti-basic FGF antisera prepared by
immunizing rabbits with synthetic peptides corresponding to positions 1-15
(amino terminal) and positions 33-43 (internal) of basic FGF (14,27).
Immuno-reactivity was visualized by successive incubations with
biotinylated goat anti-rabbit antibodies, peroxidase-conjugated
strepavidin, and 4-chloro-naphthol substrate (14,27).

RESULTS
I. Subendothelial extracellular matrix in vitro
<u>Extraction of Basic FGF - like Growth Factor from the Subendothelial ECM:</u>
Cultured corneal endothelial cells secrete ECM in a polar fashion
exclusively underneath the cell layer (16-19). Unlike tissue culture
plastic (Fig.1a1) subendothelial ECM supports the growth of aortic
endothelial cells seeded at clonal cell densities (17). A similar result
was obtained when 2M NaCl extract of ECM was added to cells seeded on
tissue culture plastic (Fig.1a2), suggesting that growth factors might be
involved in ECM induction of cell proliferation (25). The ability of 2M
NaCl-extracted ECM to be still mitogenic for endothelial cells suggested
that more growth factor might be present within the ECM that could not be
extracted with 2M NaCl. Accordingly, ECM was extracted with collagenase
and the yield of ECM-derived growth factor was found to be increased from
about 5-10% to about 30% of that found in the corresponding endothelial
cell lysate. To verify that the matrix-derived growth factor was not an
artifact of intracellular growth factor release occurring when cells were
lysed by the Triton/NH$_4$OH treatment, endothelial cells were removed intact
from culture dishes with 1M urea, a procedure that exposes subendothelial
ECM with little or no cell lysis (18). Extraction of ECM after urea

treatment yielded about 100 units of growth factor activity per 10cm ECM coated dish, an amount similar to that obtained after the Triton/NH$_4$OH treatment. These results suggested that most of the matrix derived growth factor represented growth factor deposited by viable endothelial cells into ECM rather than by lysed cells.

Biochemical Characterization of Matrix Derived Growth Factor: We have recently demonstrated that bovine aortic and corneal endothelial cells synthesize heparin-binding growth factors that are structurally and functionally releated to basic FGF (25).

When extracts of subendothelial ECM were analyzed by heparin-Sepharose affinity chromatography, one single peak of growth factor activity for both 3T3 fibroblasts and capillary endothelial cell eluted at about 1.5 M NaCl (Fig.1a) and co-migrated with hepatoma and brain derived basic FGF. More conclusive evidence that the matrix derived growth factor was a form of basic FGF was obtained by using specific anti-FGF antibodies in electrophoretic transfer blots (Fig.1b). Antibodies to synthetic peptides corresponding to both the amino terminal (not shown) and internal regions (Fig.1b, lane 1) of pituitary and brain FGF cross-reacted with an 18,400 molecular weight polypeptide doublet purified from subendothelial ECM by heparin-Sepharose affinity chromatography. The combination of heparin affinity elution profiles, electrophoretic transfer blots and stimulation of endothelial cell proliferation suggested strongly that the same basic FGF-like growth factor was found intracellularly in endothelial cells (25) and in the subendothelial ECM.

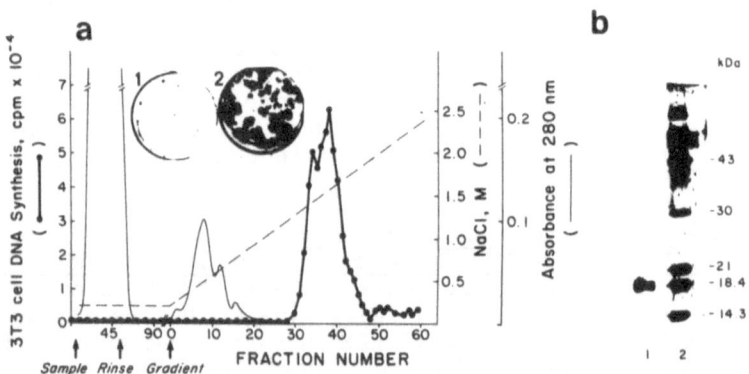

Figure 1. Heparin-Sepharose chromatography, mitogenic activity and electrophoretic transfer blot of the endothelial cell matrix derived growth factor. (a): Heparin-Sepharose chromatography. Insert: Mitogenic activity. Bovine aortic endothelial cells were seeded at a clonal density in the absence (1) or presence (2) of a dialyzed NaCl extract of ECM.(b): Electrophoretic transfer blot. Active fractions eluted from heparin-Sepharose were dialyzed, lyophilyzed and electrophoresed on SDS-PAGE. Proteins were transferred to nitrocellulose and stained with antibodies directed against basic FGF (Lane 1). Lane 2, molecular weight markers.

II.Descemet's membrane in vivo

Endothelial Cell Growth factors in the Cornea: When specimens of bovine
corneas containing almost pure Descemet's membrane were incubated in RPMI
medium at 4°C, growth promoting activity for both 3T3 fibroblasts (20-40
units/cornea) (Fig.2) and capillary endothelial cells (Fig.3) was released
into the medium. The middle layer corresponding to the corneal stroma also
released mitogenic activity for both cell types, albeit to a much lesser
extent as compared with Descemet's membrane (Fig.2). In contrast, medium
incubated with the outer corneal layer exhibited a toxic effect and
inhibited cell proliferation (Fig.3A). Preliminary studies on the nature
of this inhibitory activity indicated that it is a heat stable, low
molecular weight, dialyzable substance (26). By applying more extensive
extraction conditions rather than mere incubation in RPMI at 4°C, a growth
promoting activity was found to be present also in the outer corneal
layer, although at a lower quantity as compared with the middle and inner
layers. These extraction conditions included incubation (2-3h) at 37°C
rather than at 4°C, (Fig. 3B), 2-3 cycles of freezing and thawing of the
tissue specimens or enzymatic digestion of minced tissue fragments with
collagenase and heparitinase.

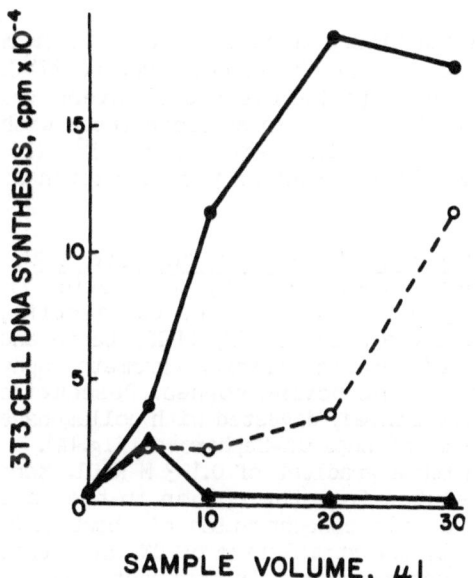

Figure 2. Growth promoting activity
released at 4°C from bovine
corneas. Bovine corneas (15) were
dissected into three layers: inner
(mostly Descemet's membrane) (●),
middle (○), and outer (▲); which
were collected into separate tubes
and each incubated with 3 ml RPMI
medium at 4°C for 2 h. Aliquots (5-
30 μl) were then tested for their
effect on ³H-thymidine
incorporation into the DNA of 3T3
cells.

Since the growth promoting activity detected in the outer portion of
the cornea could originate from the outer layers of corneal epithelial
cells which lyse upon freezing and thawing or enzymatic digestion, various
treatments were applied to remove the epithelial cells prior to extraction
of growth factors. These included exposure of the outer corneal layer to
either 0.02% EDTA/0.05% trypsin, 0.5% Triton X-100/20mM NH₄OH (16), or to
1M urea in RPMI (18). The tissue specimens were then washed with RPMI
medium and subjected to 3 cycles of freezing and thawing. Only about 20-
30% reduction in growth factor activity was obtained as compared to

494

specimens containing corneal epithelial cells. The same result was obtained with the Descemet's membrane portion of the cornea, suggesting that the corneal-derived growth factors are associated mainly with the ECM rather than with the epithelial or endothelial cells (26).

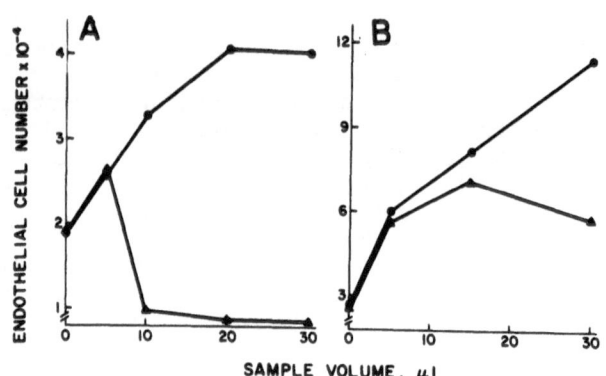

SAMPLE VOLUME, μl

Figure 3. Growth promoting and growth inhibitory activities released from the inner and outer layers of bovine corneas at 4°C as compared to 37°C. Inner (endothelial side) (●) and outer (epithelial side) layers (▲) dissected from bovine corneas were incubated (3 hr) in separate tubes with RPMI medium (about 0.2 ml per cornea) at either 4°C (A) or 37°C (B). Aliquots (1-30μl) were then tested for their effect on proliferation of bovine capillary endothelial cells.

Descemet's Membrane - Derived Growth Factor is Related to Basic FGF: Because different growth factors differ in their affinity to heparin (7), heparin-Sepharose affinity chromatography has been used to identify, resolve or purify a number of growth factors such as EGF, PDGF, basic and acidic FGF (9). Accordingly, we employed heparin affinity chromatography to analyse the growth factor content of the bovine cornea. Descemet's membranes dissected from 25 corneas were minced, digested with collagenase and the supernatant applied to a column of heparin-Sepharose (Fig.4A).

Growth factor activity was eluted with a gradient of 0.1-3 M NaCl. More than 90% of the applied protein was eluted from the column in the void volume followed by a protein peak at a salt concentration of about 0.4M. No growth promoting activity, measured by the stimulation of DNA synthesis in 3T3 cells, was detected in these protein peaks. In contrast, growth factor activity and no detectable protein was eluted from the column as a single peak at a salt concentration of about 1.7 M (Fig.4A). The active fractions were highly mitogenic for bovine aortic and capillary endothelial cells (26). When a sample from this peak was analyzed by electrophoretic transfer blot, anti-FGF antisera cross-reacted with a polypeptide doublet of about 18,400 (Fig.4B, lane 2) suggesting that the Descemet's derived growth factor was a form of basic FGF.

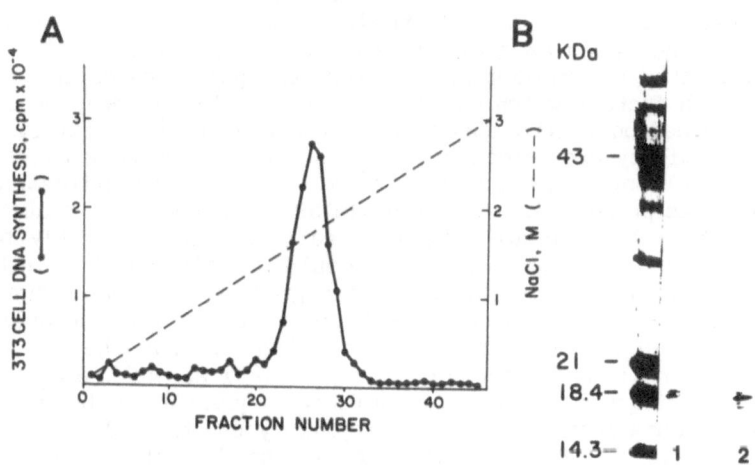

Figure 4. Heparin-Sepharose chromatography (A) and electrophoretic transfer blot (B) of growth factors extracted from Descemet's membranes. A. Inner layers dissected from 30 corneas and suspended in RPMI were minced and digested with collagenase. The tissue digest was centrifuged and the supernatant applied to a column of heparin-Sepharose (●). B. Active fractions eluted from heparin-Sepharose and extracted from Descemet's membranes (lane 2) or from the outer portion of bovine corneas (lane 1) were dialyzed, lyophilized and electrophoresed on on SDS PAGE. Proteins were transferred to nitrocellulose paper and stained with antibodies directed against basic FGF.

Localization of basic FGF in the bovine cornea using affinity-purified antibodies directed against two different sequences of basic FGF revealed identical patterns of staining within the subendothelial portion of Descemet's membrane (26). The inner two thirds of Descemet's membrane that remained apposed to corneal stroma appeared to be relatively free of staining as did adjacent stroma.

DISCUSSION

This study shows that a readily releasable growth factor for capillary endothelial cells is stored mainly in Descemet's membrane of the bovine cornea. This factor was found to be structurally and functionally related to basic fibroblast growth factor (FGF) as demonstrated by:(i) high affinity binding to heparin-Sepharose, eluting at about 1.7 M NaCl; (ii) molecular weight of about 18,400; (iii) cross-reactivity with antibodies directed against two different sequences of pituitary basic FGF, and (iv) potent mitogenic activity for capillary endothelial cells and fibroblasts. Immunofluorescence studies utilizing affinity-purified antibodies to basic FGF demonstrated intense and preferential staining of Descemet's membrane (26). An identical heparin-binding basic FGF purified from tumor, was previously shown by us to be highly angiogenic in the chick embryo and in the rat cornea (28). Lesser concentrations of the same factor are found in the middle (stromal) and outer (epithelial) parts of the cornea and are not as readily released as from Descemet's membrane. Analysis of the corneal extracts by heparin-Sepharose chromatography revealed that of the different growth factors which can be resolved by this method, Descemet's membrane contained only basic FGF-related growth promoting activity.

Mitogenic activity was released from Descemet's membrane even after removal of overlying corneal endothelium. This finding indicates that growth factor was present in the extracellular compartment and that it was in a form that could be readily dissociated (i.e., not covalently bound). It is possible that some growth factor could be released from cells or matrix as a result of the accummulation of degradative enzymes between the time of sacrifice and surgical dissection or during incubation in the tissue culture medium. However, demonstration that endothelial growth factors can be released from ECM in vitro (25) as well as in vivo suggests that angiogenic factors may normally be present in the ECM.

A low molecular weight inhibitor of capillary endothelial and 3T3 cell proliferation was released under mild conditions from the outer corneal layer. This factor also inhibited angiogenesis in the chick embryo (data not shown). Purification and further characterization of this inhibitor is being carried out currently. Taken together, these results indicate that there is a gradient of angiogenic activity decreasing toward the epithelial layer of the cornea and a gradient of anti-angiogenic activity decreasing toward Descemet's membrane (26).

The work reported here suggests a mechanism for the corneal neovascularization induced by injury to Descemet's membrane, namely that this layer of ECM acts as a large storage depot of a potent heparin-binding growth factor for capillary endothelial cells. Lack of spontaneous angiogenesis in the normal cornea implies that the basement membrane may act to physically separate these potent mitogens from their sites of action (i.e., receptors on capillary endothelial cells which are located in the limbal edge). On the other hand, damage to Descemet's membrane by trauma or by various cell-derived degradative enzymes may release these factors and induce angiogenesis from the limbal vessels.

It is unclear how these mitogenic peptides are stored in ECM without being inactivated or degraded, yet are capable of being released in a biologically active form when the matrix itself is damaged. We propose that the high binding affinity of these peptides for heparin may also immobilize them to heparan sulfate. Heparan sulfate, which is structurally related to heparin, is the major glycosaminoglycan in basement membranes including Descemet's membrane (29,30). Since heparin has been shown to stabilize (21) the activity of growth factors for vascular endothelial cells, this property could permit the long-term storage and protection from degradation of heparin-binding growth factors. The affinity of these angiogenic factors for heparin may also serve as a means for their deposition into the ECM. For example, one could speculate that heparin-binding growth factors could form an intracellular high-affinity complex with heparan sulfate proteoglycans prior to their secretion from the basal surface of the cell into the basement membrane. We have recently demonstrated that growth factors can be released from corneal endothelial

ECM in vitro by treatment with soluble heparin or heparan sulfate as well
as by exposure to heparanase (31). In a similar fashion, certain types of
corneal neovascularization could be caused by release of angiogenic
factors from Descemet's membrane following mechanical injury, release of
heparin by mast cells (32), or as a result of elaboration of matrix-
degrading enzymes by inflammatory cells (33).

Based on the studies reported here, we can now appreciate that various
inflammatory and immunologic cells which infiltrate the cornea may induce
neovascularization either directly, by secreting their own angiogenic
factors, and/or indirectly, by causing angiogenic factors to be released
from the ECM, mainly Descemet's membrane. For example, the
neovascularization sometimes associated with corneal transplantation, may
begin because of injury to Descemet's membrane, but be sustained by an
infiltrate of immune cells.   If the results of these studies apply to
the ECM of other tissues, then a general mechanism of storage of
angiogenic factors may provide an indirect pathway for induction of the
angiogenic response by cells capable of releasing the matrix-sequestered
angiogenic factors. For example, heparanase activity in certain tumor
cells which correlates with their ability to invade and metastasize
(33,34), is likely to be indirectly involved in the induction of tumor
angiogenesis. If these ideas hold up, experimental study of the cornea
will again have enlarged our understanding of the phenomenon of tumor
angiogenesis (35).

REFERENCES

1. Cogan, D..G., (1962) Invest. Opthalmol. 1:253.
2. Burger, P.C., Chandler, D.B. and Klintworth, G.K. (1983) Laboratory
    Investigation, 48:169.
3. Polverini, P.J., Cotran, R.S., Gimbrone, M.A. and Unanue, E.R. (1977)
    Nature, 269:804.
4. Hunt, T.K., Knighton, D.R., Thakral, K.K., Goodson, W.H. and Andrews,
    W.S. (1984) Surgery, 96:48.
5. Langer, R. and Folkman, J. (1976) Nature, 263:797.
6. Binder, P.S. (1983) Current Eye Research, 2:435.
7. Shing, Y., Folkman, J., Sullivan, R., Butterfield, C., Murray, J. and
    Klagsbrun, M. (1984) Science, 223:1296.
8. Maciag, T., Mehlman, T., Friesel, R. and Schreiber, A.B. (1985)
    Science, 225:932.
9. Lobb, R., Sasse, J.,Shing, Y., D'Amore, P., Sullivan, R., Jacobs, J.
    and Klagsbrun, M. (1986) J. Biol. Chem. 261:1924.
10. D'Amore, P.A. and Klagsbrun, M. (1984) Biochemical and Biological
    Similarities. J. Cell Biol. 99:1545.
11. Esch, F., Baird, A., Ling, N., Ueno, N., Hill, F., Denoroy, L.,
    Klepper, R., Gospodarowicz, D., Bohlen, P. and Guillemin, R. (1985)
    Proc. Natl. Acad. Sci. USA. 82:6507.
12. Abraham, J.A., Mergia, A., Whang, J.L., Tumolo, A., Friedman, J.,
    Hjerrild, K.A., Gospodarowicz, D. and Fiddes, J.C. (1986) Science,
    233:545.
13. Jaye, M., Howk, R., Burgess, W., Ricca, G.A., Chiu, I.M., Ravera,
    M.W., O'Brien, S.J., Modi, W.S., Maciag, T. and Droham, W.N. (1986)
    Science, 233:541.
14. Klagsbrun, M., Sasse, J., Sullivan, R. and Smith, J.A. (1986) Proc.
    Natl. Acad. Sci. USA. 83:2448.
15. Gospodarowicz, D., Neufeld, G. and Schweigerer, L. (1986) Cells and
    Differentiation, 19:1.

16. Gospodarowicz, D., Delgado, D. and Vlodavsky, I. (1980) Proc. Natl. Acad. Sci. USA. 77: 4094.
17. Gospodarowicz, D., Vlodavsky, I. and Savion, N. (1980) J. Supramol. Struct. 13: 339.
18. Gospodarowicz, D., Gonzalez, R. and Fujii, D.K. (1983) J. Cell. Physiol. 114:191.
19. Fridman, R., Ovadia, H., Fuks, Z. and Vlodavsky, I. (1985) Exptl. Cell Res. 157:181.
20. Thornton, S.C., Mueller, S.N. and Levine, E.M. (1983) Science 222:623.
21. Gospodarowicz, D. and Cheng, J. (1986) J. Cell. Physiol. 128:475.
22. Folkman, J., Haudenschild, C.C. and Zetter, B.R. (1979) Proc. Natl. Acad. Sci. USA. 76:5217.
23. Gospodarowicz, D., Mescher, A.L. and Birdwell, C.R. (1977) Exp. Eye Res. 25:75.
24. Connolly, D.T., Knight, M.B. Harakas, N.K., Wittwer, A. and Feder, J. (1986) Analytical Biochemistry, 152:136.
25. Vlodavsky, I., Folkman, J., Sullivan, R., Fridman, R., Ishai-Michaeli, R. Sasse, J. and Klagsbrun, M. (1986) Submitted.
26. Folkman, J., Klagsbrun, M., Sasse, J., Wadzinsky, M., Ingber, D. and Vlodavsky, I. (1986) Submitted to: Invest. Ophthamol & Visual Science.
27. Wadzinski, M., Folkman, J., Sasse, J., Ingber, D., Devey, K. and Klagsbrun, M. (1986) Clin.Physio. Biochem. In press.
28. Shing, Y., Folkman, J., Haudenschild, C., Lund, D., Crum, R. and Klagsbrun, M. (1985) J. Cell. Biochem. 29:275.
29. Hassell, J.R., Gehron Robey, P., Barrach, H.J., Wilczek, J., Rennard, S.I. and Martin, G.R. (1980) Proc. Natl. Acad. Sci. USA. 77:4494.
30. Robinson, J. and Gospodarowicz, D. (1983) J. Cell. Physiol. 117:368.
31. Vlodavsky, I., Sullivan, R., Fridman, R., Sasse, J., Folkman, J. and Klagsbrun, M. (1986) J. Cell Biology. In press (abstract).
32. Folkman, J. (1985) Biochemical Pharmacology, 34:905.
33. Vlodavsky, I., Fuks, Z., Bar-Ner, M., Yahalom, J., Eldor, A., Savion, N., Naparstek, J., Cohen, I.R., Kramer, M. and Schirrmacher, V. (1985) In: Extracellular Matrix: Structure and Function, UCLA Symposia on Molecular and Cellular Biology (A.H. Reddi, ed.) 283-308.
34. Nakajima, M., Irimura, T., DiFerrante, N. and Nicolson, G.L. (1984) J. Biol. Chem. 259:2283.
35. Folkman, J. (1985) Perspectives in Biology and Medicine 29:10.

Acknowledgements

This work was supported by National Cancer Institute grants CA 30289 to I.V. , CA 37392 to M.K., and CA 14019 to J.F. I.V. is a Leukemia Society of America Scholar.

THE NONTUMOR PERSPECTIVE: ANGIOGENESIS AND GEOMETRY IN GROWTH CONTROL

N.G. MAROUDAS, A. FUCHS AND E.S. LINDENBAUM

Faculty of Medicine, Technion-Israel Institute of Technology, Haifa, Israel

1. INTRODUCTION

Morphometry and mathematics have recently become guiding principles in growth control. Precise measurements of cell shape have shown that geometry is a major stimulus of growth and differentiation. Calculations of diffusion gradients pinpointed the importance of microcirculation. We have shown the power of morphometry to demonstrate gradients of growth near capillaries and to locate the site of angiogenesis in human pregnancy. It is not by coincidence that the proponents of geometric growth control were also driven to look for angiogenesis factors. Newly induced blood-vessels form striking geometric patterns, that literally point towards the source of diffusible factor.

The increasing availability of pure angiogenins presents an unprecedented challenge for morphometrists. Can geometrical factors such as diffusion and stretch really predict the observed patterns of angiogenesis? We have made a start by trying to explain the classical radial pattern of angiogenesis in the CAM ("Spokewheel") by a growth-and-stretch mechanism.

2. ANGIOGENESIS, A BRIDGE BETWEEN COORDINATE AND LOCAL CONTROL

The recent discovery of peptide hormones which powerfully stimulate the local growth of capillary bloodvessels (1,2) stems from 20 years of work on tumors by Prof. Judah Folkman and associates at Harvard. The free availability of pure angiogenins would have fundamental implications for many fields of biomedical science, because the fundamental laws of physico-chemical hydrodynamics dictate that most bodily metabolic, communication and repair processes depend on transport through the microcapillary net-work. Thus angiogenesis may be said to constitute a bridge between coordinate i.e. overall, and local growth control processes in the body. The connection between angiogenesis and tissue structure is shown not only by the parallel collagenolytic activity (Weiss, this volume) but by reports of accelerated repair process with stimulated migration of connective tissue as well as capillary cells (2).

Since the connective tissue matrix is the extracellular medium through which local (and some coordinate) mechanical and diffusional signals are transmitted, this may be a good time to recall the "nontumor" perspective on angiogenesis. Thus we shall review that theoretical framework which Folkman has called "Geometry in Growth Control" (3). The idea of physical, coordinate determinants of development goes back to D'Arcy Thompson's "Growth and Form" (4) but Thompson was unable to demonstrate any actual detailed testable mechanisms for linking geometry to gene products - or vice versa. It was precisely through Folkman's development of the now classical HEMA method for linking cell shape to cell growth (5) as much as by his relentless pursuit of chemically defined factors to link up with the diffusion problem, that Folkman formed a bridge between the earlier, formal descriptive developmental theory and modern, gene product mechanisms.

As a result of this type of experiment, by a relative handful of workers over the past decade, we now know that cells respond directly to mechanical deformation. Also, that a large class of growth factors are consumed by their target cell and thus liable to steep diffusion gradients.

3. DIFFUSION DEPTH OF PENETRATION

Folkman and Greenspan (3) base their argument on the well known "oxygen penetration depth" which for most tissues is about 1mm, this being the greatest distance that deeper cells can be sited away from a bloodvessel without risking anoxia. However, it is not generally realized that the same arguments apply to growth factors. The fact that serum's "multiplication stimulating activity" appeared to be consumed by cells in vitro led to the prediction of a general growth control mechanism through "Shortrange Diffusion Gradients" (6). It may be worth here presenting the updated calculations, which have not been previously published, in the light of modern data on the insulin-related growth factors (EGF, FGF, NGF etc). Their MW is about 15,000; they are active at very low concentration, 10 picomolar; and they bind to receptors and are then destroyed at the rate of about 10 molecules per cell per second. If we calculate for cells that are about 30 micron apart (0.03mm) and assume a diffusion coefficient about 1/10th that of water (ie, one millionth sq cm per sec) then we can insert these data into our previous equation for penetration of hormone across an empty medium into a flat sheet of cells (6,7).

From Fick's first law:
$$L = D.C.d.d/Q$$
where   L is the hormone penetration depth, cm
           D is its diffusion coefficient, sq cm per sec
           C is its concentration in bulk fluid, molecules per cc
           Q is its consumption rate, molecules per cell per sec
           d is the intercellular distance, cm

whence $L = 60$ micron (0.06mm).

This is a very steep gradient, even steeper than was thought before (6,7) because at that time it was not known how low were the active concentrations of "multiplication stimulating" factors, nor how fast their receptors were turning over. Further, we have since looked for experimental evidence of growth gradients in vivo (8). In this case, the cells are distributed normal to the flux of solute, and Fick's second law applies. The continuum penetration depth, 1, is given by:

$$1 = sqrt\ 2.L.d$$

where sqrt is the square root symbol and other symbols have the significance above. On this basis,

$$1 = L = 60\ micron.$$

In this case it does not seem to matter whether the cells are a flat sheet or a distributed continuum. Either way, the hormone penetration depth is very restricted - only a couple of cells deep. Almost "contact" distance (7).

Experimentally, we have measured the gradients of nuclear activation near the capillaries of pregnant rat mesometria (8) and found them to be even steeper than predicted - about 30 micron (0.03mm) from the capillary wall. Thus, both theoretic and experimental evidence has been adduced for the existence of very short range growth gradients near the capillaries and this case is not restricted to tumor growth. These results not only confirm Folkman's insistence on the critical importance of microvasculature - in fact, they emphasise it. Hence, we asked whether similar angiogenic factors might not be found in the pregnant uterus, whose growth is actually faster and larger than that of most tumors.

4. UTERINE ANGIOGENESIS FACTOR

In our search for the likely site of angiogenesis factors in the pregnant human uterus (9) we were likewise guided by morphometric reasoning, based on our previous studies of human uterine neovasculature (10,11). The new bloodvessels were obviously oriented toward the site of implantation (10) and it was in that site (ie in the decidua rather than in placenta or fetus) that we looked for and found the highest angiogenic activity (9).

For comparison, the richest tumor source is a rat chondrosarcoma (1). A subsequent human nontumor source is placenta (12). Compared to decidua, both sources are relatively lean. Typically, they yield less than a microgram per gm of source tissue: only enough to treat half a dozen eggs or a few cc of skin. We find that one gm of decidua yield enough activity to produce strong angiogenesis in 1000 eggs. This is an almost incredible amount - equivalent to 100 microgram of pure factor - but we are somewhat reassured to learn that activated macrophages are similarly potent sources, per gm wet weight (see Knighton, this volume). Interestingly, decidual cells also are thought to have a bone marrow origin and share the Kb antigen with macrophages (13).

At present we fractionate HUAF by molecular filtration and heparin column. The ultrafiltrate, F1, is a 500 times enriched product compared to the unfiltered decidual homogenate, but retains most of the activity. It is convenient that most of the soluble proteins are above 30,000MW. The ultrafiltrate F1 is directly usable for animal trials. It is strongly angiogenic on the CAM test at 0.5 to 1 microgm per egg. Criteria of "strong" angiogenesis are as published (9), i.e. one cm diam spokewheel, 40 to 100 radially oriented bloodvessels and a d50 dose which induces strong positives in 2 eggs out of 3 with larger doses scoring up to 9 eggs out of 10 tested. F1 is about 50 times more potent, and obtainable at 50 times higher yield per gm of source tissue, than the partially purified factor from animal cartilage, which Klagsbrun's group has used to enhance wound repair in rats (2).

The second step after ultrafiltration is a heparin-Sepharose column (1, 14). Only 10% of the activity is bound by the column, and this is eluted with a 0.5 to 2M salt gradient to yield a product E1. The E1 fraction is strongly active at 50 to 100ng per egg, and represents a 100,000 fold purification relative to initial homogenate. This is the highest potency fraction that we have thus far obtained, and compares well, as regards d50 dose per egg, with more highly purified angiogenic factors (1, 2, 14).

Further biochemical trials are in progress, to improve the yield and purity of the column eluate E1, and to characterize the non-heparin-binding fractions.

5. MECHANISM OF ANGIOGENESIS IN THE CAM

There seems to be a difference between angiogenesis in the chick chorioallantoic membrane, which is actually a developing embryonic system, and angiogenesis in the rabbit cornea, which is a relatively avascular connective tissue. At first, we regarded the "spokes" in the CAM as being equivalent to the "sprouts" in the cornea - ie, as evidence of chemotactically directed migration of capillaries towards a central source of diffusible angiogenic factor. However, it bothered us that the radial bloodvessels were appearing so fast on the CAM. Whereas the sprouts in the cornea take a sedate 15 days to migrate 2mm, the spokes of the CAM appear to cover 6mm in 48 hrs! Also, we first thought that the spokes arose by growth, as the sprouts do - and it bothered us too. Because, one has to allow 24-36 hours between the first reception of a mitotic stimulus and the actual mitosis. This does not leave much time out of the 48 hours of the actual CAM assay, for 100 new bloodvessels, 6mm long and several hundred micron across, to suddenly grow out of an apparently empty field - less than 12 hours for all that growth! Then there were physicochemical bothers. The spokes appear in the ordinary dissecting microscope (X10 for assay purposes) as having closed ends or tips: so how was the blood circulating through them? Also, some of these tips appeared to be pointing away from the centre - which did not make sense in terms of a chemotactic gradient!

Finally, for what it is worth, there was the bother about the range of the diffusion gradient. All our previous work had been at pains to show the existence of very short range gradients (6,7,8). Yet here we were apparently confronted with a soluble factor whose influence appeared to diffuse a distance of 6mm in only 48 hours. Now there is a rough-and-ready criterion of penetration time, namely:

$$t = L.L / D$$

where L is 0.6cm and D is 1 millionth of a sq cm per sec. From this equation, t works out to be about 100 hours - rather longer than the time of the assay! Of course the calculations are not accurate, and perhaps the capillary cells were switched on by the arrival of just the first few molecules of factors - like moths with pheromones?

However, by examining the CAM with a higher power dissecting scope, a physically more realistic picture emerged. Firstly, the spokes are not true capillaries. The real capillary bed can be observed in a good scope at X40 magnification, as a network of bloodflow between adjacent tips of the spokes. The structure of this capillary network was then made manifest by application of the corrosion-cast technique, as in our previous studies on uterine bloodvessels (10,11). This network answered two of our queries: how the blood flowed between tips, and how the angiogenic factor managed to spread so quickly.

But the problem about rapid spoke growth remained, as did the orientation of some tips away from the centre. However, the spokes can be shown, with a dissecting needle, to be not in the plane of the membrane: they are actually free-floating venules and arterioles, anchored at their tips to the CAM proper. We postulate that the spokewheel arises as a result of expansion of the CAM, under the mitotic influence of the angiogenic factor. This expansion of the capillary bed tenses the underlying arterioles and venules. Hence, these are pulled up to the surface and outwards. This explains why some of the spokes were pointing away from the centre. We call it "the umbrella model" (17). Measurements of

time-lapse photos of the CAM show an increasing distance between bloodvessels with time, which agrees with the idea of an expansive, mitotic
action of angiogenesis. Also, histological sections of decidual tissue
in contact with the CAM show a local thickening of the tissue, as well as
migration of bloodvessels. This is similar to the findings of Klagsbrun's
group - connective tissue growth and recruitment of fibroblasts as well as
capillary endothelial cells (2). Finally, the existence of an extensive
reservoir of endothelial cells in the true capillary bed of the CAM
removes some of the puzzle about where all that rapid mitosis is coming
from, a problem that had so plagued us in the beginning when we were
still thinking of the "spokes" in the CAM as though they were the same as
the "sprouts" in the cornea.

6. CONCLUSIONS

The application of physical and geometric reasoning can lead to some
valid conclusions in morphogenesis. The study of mechanical effects on
cell growth and differentiation is in progress (15,16). The study of
diffusion gradients, more slowly (18). The spectacular isolation of pure
factors mobilizing the microcirculation will, inevitably, serve to focus
attention on coordinate mechanisms of growth control. A recent mathematical model of tumor-induced capillary growth includes parameters to
define: diffusion, density of capillary sprouts, rate of elongation of
tips and rate of appearance of new tips - all of which are tied to local
concentration of factor (19). Our results suggest that the elongation of
pre-existing bloodvessels, and local expansion of tissue, should be
included in future mathematical models.

REFERENCES

1. Shing Y, Folkman J, Sullivan R, Butterfield C, Murray J and Klagsbrun M:
    Heparin affinity: purification of a tumor-derived capillary endothelial
    cell growth factor. Science 223: 1296-1298, 1984.
2. Davidson JF, Klagsbrun M, Hill KE, Buckley A, Sullivan R, Brewer PS
    and Woodward SM: Accelerated wound repair, cell proliferation and
    collagen production, are produced by a cartilage derived growth factor.
    J Cell Biol 100: 1219-1227, 1985.
3. Folkman J and Greenspan H: Influence of geometry on control of cell
    growth. Biochem Biophys Acta 417: 211-236, 1975.
4. Thompson DW: On Growth and Form. Dover, USA, 1942.
5. Folkman J and Moscona A: The role of cell shape in growth control.
    Nature 273: 345-349, 1978.
6. Maroudas NG: Short-range diffusion gradients. Cell 3:217-219, 1984.
7. Maroudas NG: Diffusion control of growth. Correspondence. Nature
    274: 722, 1978.
8. Maroudas NG and Wray S: Nuclear activation of chromatin in stretch-
    dependent growth of tissues. Connective Tissue Res 13:217-225, 1985.
9. Fuchs A, Lindenbaum ES and Maroudas NG: Location of the angiogenic
    activity in the pregnant human uterus. Acta Anatomica 124:241-244,1984
10. Lindenbaum ES, Brandes JM and Itskovitz J: Ipsi- and contra-lateral
    anastomosis in the uterine arteries. Acta Anatomica 102: 157-161, 1978.
11. Itskovitz J, Lindenbaum ES and Brandes JM: Arterial anastomosis in the
    pregnant human uterus. Obstet Gynec 55: 67-71, 1980.

504

12. Moscatelli D, Presta M and Rifkin DB: Purification of a factor from human placenta that stimulates capillary endothelial cell protease production, DNA synthesis and cell migration. Proc Nat Acad Sci USA 83: 2091-2095, 1986.
13. Kearns M and Lala P: Bone marrow origin of decidual cell precursors in a pseudopregnant mouse uterus. J Exptl Med 155: 1537-1554, 1982.
14. Sullivan R and Klagsbrun M: Purification of a cartilage-derived growth factor by heparin affinity chromatography. J Biol Chem 260: 2399-2403, 1985.
15. Ben-Ze'ev A, Farmer SR and Penman S: Protein synthesis requires cell-surface contact while nuclear events respond to cell shape in anchorage dependent fibroblasts. Cell 21: 365-372, 1980.
16. O'Neill CH, Jordan P and Ireland G: Evidence for two distinct mechanisms of anchorage stimulation in freshly explanted and 3T3 Swiss mouse fibroblasts. Cell 44: 489-496, 1986.
17. Fuchs A and Lindenbaum ES: The two and three dimensional structure of the microcirculation of the chick chorioallantoic membrane (CAM). (Submitted) 1986.
18. Dunn GA and Ireland GW: New evidence that growth in 3T3 cell cultures is a diffusion limited process. Nature 312: 63-65, 1984.
19. Balding D and McElwain DLS: A mathematical model of tumor-induced capillary growth. J Theor Biol 114: 53-73, 1985.

ACKNOWLEDGEMENT
   Supported by the Samuel Neaman Foundation.

ANGIOGENESIS AND INTERLEUKINS

Itzhak Hemo, David BenEzra, Genia Maftzir and Viviane Birkenfeld, Immuno-Ophthalmology and Laboratory of Ocular Angiogenesis, Department of Ophthalmology, Hadassah University Hospital, Jerusalem, Israel

INTRODUCTION

Vascularization of tissues is a normal event during embryogenesis and healing-repair processes. In the eye, early vascularization of the vitreous cavity by the hyaloid system is later replaced by the definite retinal/choroidal vessels. The former system involutes (1) leaving the vitreous cavity and lens clear and devoid of direct vascularization. In various pathological conditions, however, neovascularization of avascular ocular tissues is triggered (2). In an attempt to elucidate the basic mechanisms involved in ocular angiogenesis, the possible role of leukocytes and leukocyte products were investigated. Early on, it became evident that cellular and humoral factors of immune reactions could stimulate neovascular processes (3-5). Following these findings, a panel of purified compounds was examined and the possible regulating role of prostaglandins in angiogenesis unveiled (6,7). Although early studies indicated that lymphokines and/or monokines are involved in the stimulus of neovascularization (4,5,8), the lack of purified isolates prevented further clarification. Recently, recombinant interleukin-1 (IL-1) and interleukin-2 (IL-2) became available. In this study, we are reporting our findings on the effect of IL-1 and IL-2 on angiogenesis of ocular tissues.

MATERIALS AND METHODS

Interleukins: Recombinant human interleukin-1 (IL-1) obtained from Collaborative Research, Inc. (Lexington, MA) and recombinant human interleukin-2 (IL-2) from Cetus Corporation (Emeryville, CA) were used throughout the study.

Assessment of angiogenic capacity: Interleukin-1 was incorporated into Elvax-40 and implants sequestering 1 to 20 half-maximal units were prepared as described previously (6). Implants of interleukin-2 were similarly prepared to sequester one to 200 units. IL-1 and IL-2 containing implants as well as "empty" implants used as controls were inserted in the mid-stroma of rabbit corneas at a distance of 2.0 mm from the corneoscleral limbus. Eyes were examined every day under slit lamp and/or operating microscope. The progress of new blood vessels from the limbus toward the implant was measured and recorded. Photographs were taken every 48 hours. At various intervals after implantation, eyes were enucleated and the corneas subjected to

506

histological examinations.

RESULTS

Interleukin-1 is a very potent stimulator of neovascularization. Inconsistent angiogenesis is observed with as little as one half-maximal unit per implant. At a concentration of 5 half-maximal units, all implants were positive (Table 1).

Table 1: Corneal neovascularization induced by IL-1

1/2 max. units	No. expts.	No. Positive	Surface Neo*
0	6	0	0
1	3	2	1.0
5	7	7	4.5

* Mean surface of neovascularization (in mm^2) of all experiments calculated as half the multiplication of leading vessel length by length of active base at the limbus.

Implants sequestering IL-1 induced engorgement of limbal vessels that was prominent 24 hours after implantation. On the second day, new vessels directed toward the implant were observed. These advanced steadily, reached the implant by day 7 and continued to proliferate around it (Figure 1).

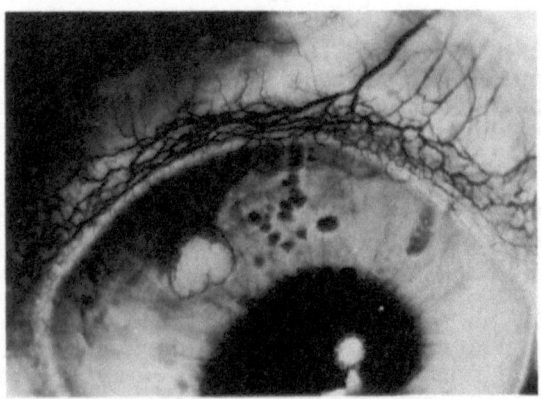

Figure 1. Vessels growing toward implant sequestering 5 half-maximal units of recombinant IL-1.

Interleukin-2 was a less potent stimulator. Implants sequestering as much as 200 units by seven days showed only corneal edema and engorgement of the limbal vessels. After one week, initial neovascularization could be observed.

Histology of the rabbit corneas with implants sequestering IL-1 showed that the corneal structures were well preserved. New blood vessels grew toward the implant. This process was not accompanied by any significant inflammatory cell infiltrates (Fig. 2 and 3).

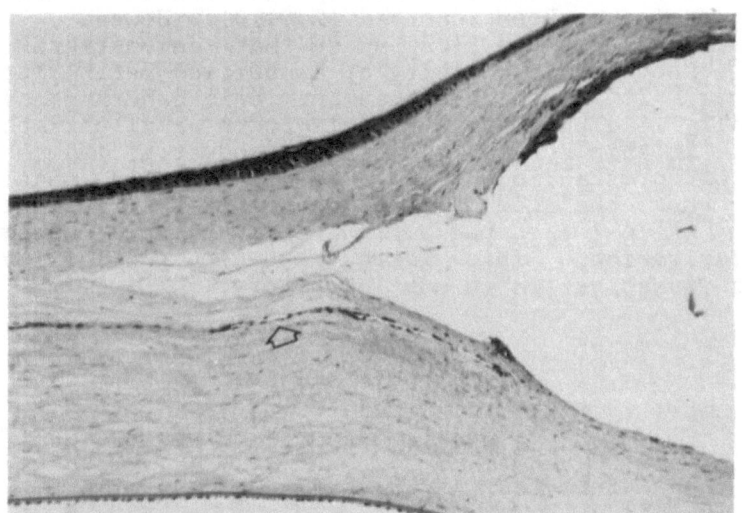

Figure 2. New vessels (arrow) invade the mid stroma and reach the IL-1 implant by day 7.

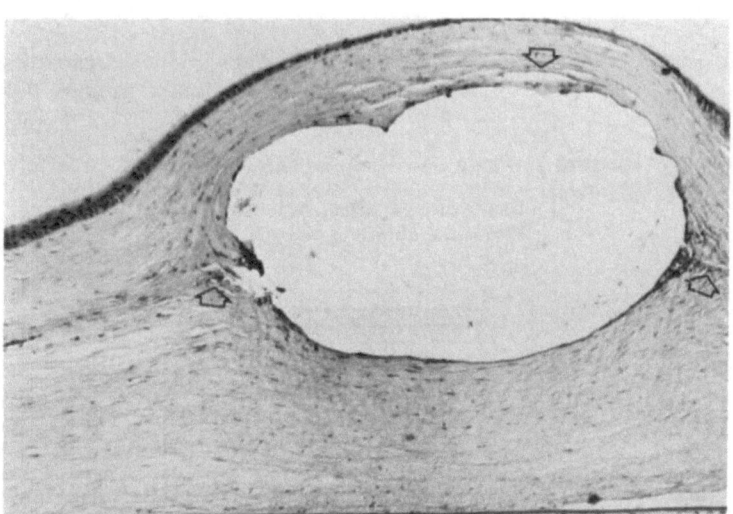

Figure 3. Angiogenic stimulus induces vessel proliferation around the implant (arrows).

508

DISCUSSION

The strong and rapid angiogenic potential of IL-1 and the delayed and relatively weaker angiogenesis observed with IL-2 could be interpreted as an indication for a direct role of IL-1 in this process, while IL-2 may be only an intermediary substance. The latter could stimulate the generation of IL-1 by affecting the macrophages (or other cells) activity. While IL-2 is a specific product of the lymphocytes (9), Interleukin-1 can be produced by a variety of cells (10). The role of macrophages and their products in angiogenesis has been reported (2,8,10). However, to our knowledge, this is the first study that demonstrates the potential neovascular activity of a purified metabolite of macrophages. It is possible that IL-1 only generates events that finally lead to the new vessel growth as illustrated in figure 4. In this scheme, macrophage product(s) induces the release of prostaglandins (6). It is equally possible, however, that the role of prostaglandins is to promote the secretion of IL-1 from the various cell tissue undergoing neovascularization. This latter appealing possibility is now under investigation in our laboratory.

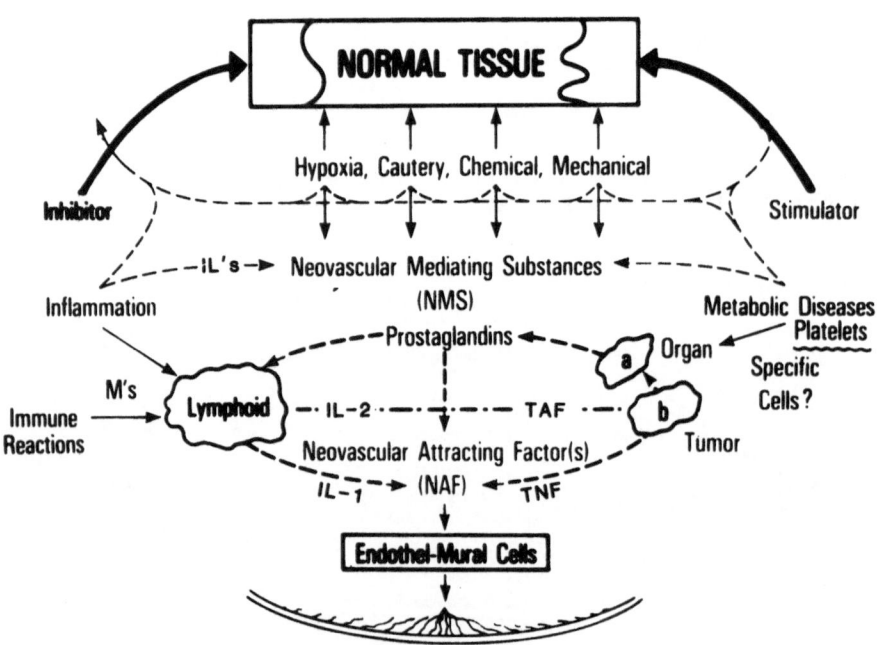

Figure 4. Schematic representation of possible events that could determine the extent of angiogenesis.

REFERENCES
1. Michaelson IC: Retinal Circulation in Man and Animals. Springfield, Charles C Thomas, 1954.
2. BenEzra D: Neovasculogenesis. Triggering factors and possible mechanisms. Surv. Ophthalmol. 24:167, 1979.
3. Sidky YA, Auerbach R: Lymphocyte-induced angiogenesis in tumor bearing mice. Science 192:1237, 1976.
4. BenEzra D: Mediators of immunological reactions and neovascularization. Presented at the Jerusalem Conference on Impaired Vision in Childhood, Jerusalem, May 1977.
5. BenEzra D: Mediators of immunological reactions. Function as inducers of neovascularization. Metabolic Ophthalmol 2:339, 1978.
6. BenEzra D: Neovasculogenic ability of prostaglandins, growth factors and synthetic chemoattractants. Am J Ophthalmol 86:455, 1978.
7. BenEzra D: Neovascularization, a unitarian phenomenon. Docum Ophthalmol Proc Series 25:125, 1981.
8. Polverini PJ, Cotran RS, Gimbrone MA, Unanue ER: Activated macrophages induce vascular proliferation. Nature 269:804, 1977.
9. Hess AD: Effect of interleukin 2 on the immunosuppressive action of cyclosporin. Transplantation 39:62, 1985.
10. Gery I, Lepe-Zuniga JL: Interleukin-1: Uniqueness of its production and spectrum of activities. Lymphokines 9:109, 1984.
11. Knighton DR, Hunt TK, Schenenstuhl H, Halliday BJ, Werb Z, Banda MJ: Oxygen tension regulates the expression of angiogenesis factor by macrophages. Science 221:1283, 1983.

THE ROLE OF LACTIC ACID IN THE MECHANISM OF NEOVASCULARIZATION

G. IMRE

It is known that hypoxic tissues generally vascularize. The late professor Michaelson /1948/ was one of the firsts to suppose that his X-factor may be released in hypoxic tissues and since then we have known that in the pathogenesis of a proliferative retinopathy the retinal areas of closed capillaries are essential. Neovascularization begins on the border of these areas. So the starting point of my investigations was hypoxy 24 years ago. In hypoxic tissues anaerobic glycolysis prevails and if the venous circulation deteriorates which is a very important conditions of neovascularization, lactic acid the end product of the anaerobic glycolysis accumulates. The possibility that an increased lactic acid concentration may have an important role in the mechanism of neovascularization was confirmed by the fact that the corneal vascularization was a typical sign in riboflavin deficiency, so I began my experiments.

The important role of an increased lactic acid concentration is shown by the following data:
1. Lactic acid concentration is increased in vascularizing tissues. There are several indirect data proving this, but in connection with corneal vascularization there are direct proofs, too /Levene et al., 1963; Chernova, 1968/. In our experiment on rabbit corneas a severe alkali burn was inflicted. After vascularization had begun both the avascular part of the burnt corneas and an identical part of control corneas were excised, dried and the lactic acid concentration was determined by the enzymatic method described by Hohorst /1962/. The lactic acid concentration of the avascular part of alkali burnt vascularizing corneas was significantly increased.

TABLE 1.   Lactate concentration on the 8th day

μg/mg dry weigth, mean $\pm$ SD /No. of corneas/

Alkali burned	6.49 $\pm$ 2.44 /7/
Control	2.76 $\pm$ 0.43 /7/

$p < 0.01$

In cases of rubeosis iridis we found a significant increase in lactic acid concentration in the aqueous humour.

TABLE 2.   Lactate concentration of the aqueous humour
mean ± SD

Rubeosis iridis /11 eyes/	Control eyes /10/
10.68 ± 2.47mM/L	7.68 ± 2.08mM/L

$p < 0.01$

But the aqueous lactic acid concentration can definitely increase only if the rate of aqueous flow decreases and in cases
of rubeosis iridis the rate of aqueous flow is in fact decreased.

TABLE 3. Tonographic values of 28 eyes with rubeosis iridis
mean ± SD

C:0.09 ± 0.09	F:0.61 ± 0.72 μl/Min
in 20 eyes 0.15	in 21 eyes 1.0
in 8 eyes 0.15	in 7 eyes 1.0

This was determined by the tonographic method on 28 eyes affected by rubeosis iridis and the mean was found to be 0.61 μl/min
which has to be accepted as a decrease in spite of the errors
of the method.

2. Increasing the lactic acid concentration of avascular
tissues leads to vascularization, e.g. the vascularization of
the cornea began earlier and was significantly more intensive
after intracorneal lactic acid injections than after injections
of other solutions which caused a more serious corneal damage.

TABLE 4. Length of vascularization on the 6th day
mm, mean ± SD /No. of corneas/

2 intra-	Lactic acid	1.34 ± 0.35 /5/
corneal	Sodium hydroxide	1.00 ± 0.10 /5/[x]
inj.	Acetic acid	0.58 ± 0.23 /5/[xx]
0.05 ml, 0.1%	Hydrochloric acid	0.46 ± 0.23 /5/[xx]

[x]$p < 0.05$,   [xx]$p < 0.01$

The intravitreal injections of lactic acid in 0.1% concentration caused in 8 from 16 kitten eyes a preretinal neovascula-

rization /Imre, 1964/. Originally this was my first experiment and I was lucky because it was difficult to inject the solution into the vitreous into the very same place near to the retina several times. Later Cunha-Vaz /1978/ proved that one single intravitreal injection of lactic acid may cause venular endothelial proliferation, the first step of retinal neovascularization. This was observed also after puncture of the lens /Deem et al., 1974; Heffernan et al., 1978/ and we found a significantly increased lactic acid concentration in the vitreous after posterior lens puncture /Imre and Pálfalvy, 1977/.

TABLE 5. The lactic acid concentration of the vitreous
mM/L mean $\pm$ SD /No. of eyes/

control	after posterior lens puncture
7.65 ± 2.41 /9/	13.61 ± 6.51 /9/

$p < 0.05$

3. L-lactate produced by the organism induces more intensive corneal vascularization than D-lactate does, a compound foreign to the organism.

TABLE 6.   Length of vascularization on the 6th day
mm, mean $\pm$ SD /No. of corneas/

2 intra-corneal inj. 0.05 ml, 0.1%		
	D-lactate	0.23 ± 0.40 /11/
	L-lactate	0.47 ± 0.38 /11/

$p < 0.02$

4. Prolonged swelling of the cornea is an important condition for its vascularization. The compactness of the cornea and that of some other tissues seems to prevent their vascularization. Swelling of the cornea, however, is not always accompanied by vascularization. In cases of experimentally produced avascular swelling the lactic acid concentration of the cornea was significantly decreased.

TABLE 7.   Lactate concentration on the 14th day
μg/mg dry weight, mean $\pm$ SD /No. of corneas/

Avascular swelling	1.78 ± 0.15 /6/
Control	2.97 ± 0.90 /6/

$p < 0.02$

Avascular swelling was induced by filling the anterior chamber of rabbit eyes with silicon oil.

5. Lactic acid promotes the proliferation of mesenchymal cells as has been proved in fibroblast cultures /Castor and Yuron, 1969; Comstock and Udenfriend, 1970; Kittlick and Neupert, 1972/ but lactic acid stimulates the proliferation of cultured aortic endothelial cells, too. In our last experiment aortic endothelial cells were obtained from 4-7th subcultures of a Minnesota mini pig cell culture. All cell cultures were grown in plastic tubes in Dulbecco's modified MEM containing 10% foetal calf serum. Lactic acid was added in different concentration to the series of tube cultures. Cell number was determined on the 4th day of cultivation. Lactic acid in 10^{-2} mol/l concentration was toxic for the endothelial cells, but in 10^{-3} mol/l concentration significantly increased the proliferation of the endothelial cells.

TABLE 8. Endothelial cell number in thousands

on the 4th day of cultivation

mean $\pm$ SD

Control	101.5 ± 24.3	
10^{-2}M lactic acid	toxic	
10^{-3}M lactic acid	144.4 ± 35.9	p<0.01
10^{-4}M lactic acid	124.3 ± 24.5	N.S.

According to these results, a prolonged increase in lactic acid concentration caused by increased glycolysis and drainage difficulties of metabolites seems to be the most important condition for neovascularization.

But how does lactic acid stimulate the endothelial cells? Lactic acid like other organic anions diffuses through the endothelial cells, too, into the blood. If in a tissue there is an increased lactic acid concentration its effect depends on the venous circulation. If the venous circulation is intact, the blood leads the lactic acid away and there is no neovascularization. If there is a total venous obstruction, the lactic acid reaches toxic concentration within the endothelial cells too, resulting in cell death and there is no neovascularization as there is no retinal neovascularization in cases of central retinal vein occlusion. Chan and Little /1979/ proved that in cases of a total obstructio of the vein there is a widespread endothelial cell death, no endothelial cells will remain to build up new vessels. But if there is only a deteriorated venous flow and the intracellular lactate concentration slowly increases the endothelial cells are compelled as a defence to use up the lactic acid and hereby they will be activated and they will proliferate forming new vessels.

It is probable that other factors are also influencing the

mechanism of neovascularization. So e.g. prostaglandins and different mitogen and growth factors can play a role, too, in addition to the increased lactic acid concentration. It is possible that these other factors may play a role by increasing the lactic acid concentration. If there are fibroblasts or macrophages growing into a hypoxic tissue the metabolism of these cells may increase the lactic acid concentration further on. In malignant tumours there is an increased aerobic glycolysis. The vascularization of these tissues can be explained not only with the TAF but with the increased lactic acid production, as well.

REFERENCES

1. Castor CW, Yuron M: Leukocyte-connective tissue cell interaction II. The specificy duration and mechanism of interaction effects. Arthr.Rheum. 12, 374-386, 1969.
2. Chan CC, Little HL: Infrequency of retinal neovascularizations following central retinal vein occlusion. Ophthalmology 96, 256-262, 1979.
3. Chernova AA: The effect of some conservative methods of treatment on the lactic acid content in an alkali burnt cornea. Vestn. Oftal. /Mosk./ Nr. 3., 28-32, 1968.
4. Comstock JP, Udenfriend S: Effect of lactate on collagen proline hydroxylase activity in cultured L-929 fibroblasts. Proc. Nath. Acad. Sci. 66, 552-557, 197o.
5. Cunha-Vaz J: Physiopathogenesis of retinitis proliferans and new vessel formation. In: 5th Congr. Europ.Soc.Ophthal. Hamburg 1976. Ed. J. François, pp. 247-253, Stuttgart, Enke, 1978.
6. Deem CW, Futterman S, Kalina RE: Induction of endothelial cell proliferation in rat retinal venules by chemical and indirect physical trauma. Invest. Ophthal. Visual Sci. 13, 58o-585, 1974.
7. Heffernan JT, Futterman S, Kalina RE: Dexamethasone inhibition of experimental endothelial cell proliferation in retinal venules. Invest. Ophthal. Visual Sci. 17,565-568, 1978.
8. Hohorst HJ:In: Methoden der enzymatischen Analyse. Ed. H.V. Bergmeyer, pp. 266, Chemie, Weinheim, 1962.
9. Imre G: Studies on the mechanism of retinal neovascularization. Role of lactic acid. Brit. J. Ophthal. 48,75-82,196l
10. Imre G, Pálfalvy M: Lactate concentration of the vitreous after lens puncture. Data relating to the mechanism of neovascularization. IRCS Med. Sci. The Eye, 5, 231, 1977.
11. Kittlick PD, Neupert S: Experimentelle Beeinflussung der Synthese saurer Mucopolysaccháride /Glycosaminoglycose/ in Fibroblastkulturen. V. Über den Einfluss von D,L-Lactat auf die Synthese der sauren Mucopolysaccharide unter alkalischen und sauren Kulturbedingungen. Exp. Path. 7,125-136, 1972.
12. Levene R, ShapiroA, Baum J: Experimental corneal vascularization.Arch.Ophthal./Chicago/ 7o,242-252, 1963.
13. Michaelson IC: The mode of development of the vascular

system of the retina, with some observations on its significance for certain retinal diseases. Trans. Ophthal. Soc. U.K.
<u>68</u>, 137-180, 1948.

KINETICS OF ACTIVATION OF PROCOLLAGENASE BY A LOW MOLECULAR WEIGHT MASS, NON PROTEIN ANGIOGENIC FACTOR

JACQUELINE B. WEISS, B. McLAUGHLIN and C.M. TAYLOR
Department of Rheumatology, University of Manchester Medical School, Manchester, M13 9PT

INTRODUCTION

We have identified a low molecular mass factor (M_r approximately 400), from a variety of tissue sources, which is angiogenic in vivo tests and which is also able to stimulate capillary endothelial cells in culture to proliferate (1,2). In vivo testing has been on the chick chorioallantoic membrane, the rabbit cornea and on sponge implants into skin wounds of rats.

Stimulation of endothelial cells in culture by this factor is specific for capillary cells and the factor has no activity towards either adult or foetal aortic endothelial cells. Additionally, the conditions of culture for the capillary cells are important. For a proliferative response, the cells must be grown on a substratum of either collagen or fibronectin (we have used type I collagen gels). The use of gelatin or plastic as substrata is ineffective.

The most interesting activity (aside from its angiogenic potential) of this small molecule, which we have called endothelial cell stimulating angiogenesis factor (ESAF), is its ability to activate latent forms of mammalian collagenase (3). That is to say both procollagenase itself, which is the inactive precursor of collagenase (4), and active collagenase which has been inhibited by a tissue inhibitor of metalloproteinases (TIMP) (5,6). TIMP is present throughout the matrix and is thought to inhibit any active collagenase or neutral metalloproteinases which may be present in the tissues. Until now this inhibition has been thought to be irreversible.

Apart from the interest in the physiological behaviour of ESAF as an angiogenesis factor which this property confers, on a more mundane level, it has enabled us to quantify it and to relate these biochemical results to its biological properties.

In this paper we will present studies on the kinetics of activation of procollagenase by ESAF and the action of ESAF in reactivating collagenase inhibited by TIMP. We will also show that the ability to activate procollagenase is quantitatively related to its in vivo potential as an angiogenic factor as well as to its efficiency as a capillary cell mitogen.

We will also describe the potentiating effect of heparin on the procollagenase activation by ESAF (7).

This paper is dedicated to the memory of the late Dr. S.F. Elstow who was tragically killed in a road traffic accident in December, 1985.

ACTIVATION OF PROCOLLAGENASE

Procollagenase was prepared from tissue culture medium conditioned by human skin fibroblasts using standard techniques (8). ESAF was extracted from bovine retina (9). An amount of ESAF extracted from approximately three retinas was used to activate procollagenase. The results can be seen in Table 1. As can be seen ESAF had no effect on

Table 1: EFFECT OF ESAF ON SKIN FIBROBLAST PROCOLLAGENASE

PROCOLLAGENASE ALONE	0.7 ug collagen degraded/hr	
PROCOLLAGENASE + ESAF	9.37 ug "	" "
PROCOLLAGENASE + MERSALYL	7.3 ug "	" "

Blank 1180 cpm
Clostridiopeptidase 10121 cpm

collagenase itself. Mersalyl (an organic mercurial) was used as a control as this chemical is known to be able to activate procollagenase. ESAF was a more effective activator. Higher quantities of mersalyl than those used begin to inactivate the liberated enzyme, presumably because of the toxic effects of mercury on the enzyme. Heparin, when added to amounts of ESAF not able to fully activate the enzyme, potentiated the effect (Table 2). Heparin was obtained from Sigma chemical company (UK)

Table 2: POTENTIATING EFFECT OF HEPARIN ON ESAF ACTIVATION OF SKIN FIBROBLAST COLLAGENASE

Procollagenase alone	0.68 ug collagen degraded/hr	
Procollagenase + ESAF	4.6 " "	" "
Procollagenase + ESAF + Heparin	8.9 " "	" "

and was from pig mucosa. Before use it was fractionated by gel filtration on a column of Biogel P10 (BioRad, UK) and the 16,000 M_r fraction was used. The amount of heparin required for potentiation was small, approximately 10 pM and this is in the physiological concentration of heparin.

KINETIC STUDIES OF ACTIVATION OF PROCOLLAGENASE BY ESAF

The activation of procollagenase by ESAF was shown to be linear and this enabled Michaelis-Menton kinetics of the reaction to be obtained. Activation of procollagenase at different concentrations of ESAF with and without the addition of heparin was determined and the results expressed using a double reciprocal plot of substrate (collagen) concentration against the release of products of the reaction (collagen fragments) according to the method of Lineweaver and Burk (10). The assay for collagenase was according to the method of Weiss et al (11). In order to determine the amount of heparin to be used a constant amount of ESAF was added to procollagenase and varying concentrations of heparin (0-50 pM) were added. The results are shown in Fig. 1. It

Figure 1:

Effect of heparin on
the activation by ESAF
on procollagenase. Note
that the figures represent
values above the maximum
activation achieved by
ESAF alone.

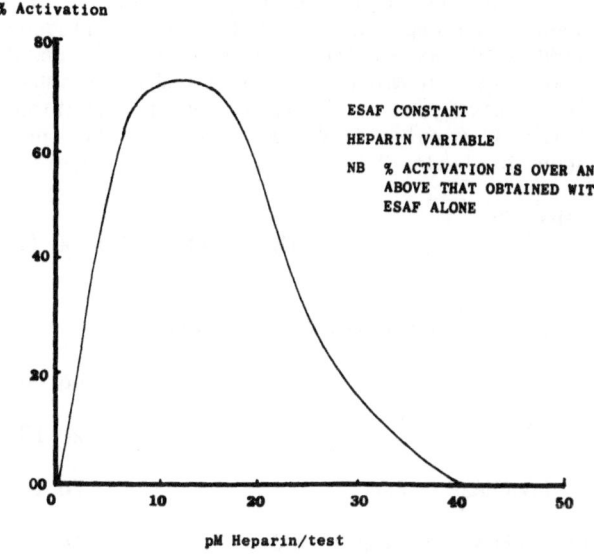

% Activation

ESAF CONSTANT

HEPARIN VARIABLE

NB % ACTIVATION IS OVER AND
ABOVE THAT OBTAINED WITH
ESAF ALONE

pM Heparin/test

can be seen that an increase of nearly 100% over the original
activation by ESAF was obtained when 5-10 pM heparin was added. At
higher concentrations the potentiating effect was diminished. Kinetics
of activation were studies using ESAF alone or with 6.5 pM heparin. It
can be seen from Fig. 2 that the kinetics of activation of
procollagenase by ESAF alone are not linear. However, when heparin was
included in the reaction mixture a linear reponse was obtained. These
results suggest

Figure 2:

Double reciprocal plot of
substrate concentration
against velocity of reaction
for ESAF and Procollagenase
and ESAF + 6.5 pM heparin
and procollagenase. The
maximum velocity is the
same for both reactions but
the K_m (substrate affinity)
is lower when heparin is added
indicating an increased affinity
of the enzyme for the substrate.

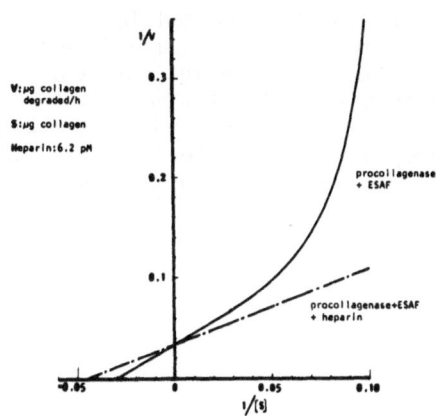

1/v

V:μg collagen
degraded/h

S:μg collagen

Heparin:6.2 pM

procollagenase
+ ESAF

procollagenase+ESAF
+ heparin

1/[s]

that the effect of heparin with ESAF is a co-operative one.

ACTIVATION OF INHIBITED COLLAGENASE

In addition to its ability to activate procollagenase, ESAF has also been shown capable of reactivating collagenase inhibited by TIMP. The TIMP used was a kind gift from Dr. T. Cawston, Addenbrokes Hospital, Cambridge. An amount of TIMP capable of inhibiting approximately 90% of the activity of a fully active preparation of collagensae was used. After 30 minutes ESAF was added to the incubation mixture. As can be seen in Table 3, ESAF was able to reactivate the enzyme inhibitor

Table 3:

ANGIOGENESIS FACTOR (ESAF)

EFFECT ON TIMP INHIBITED COLLAGENASE

	ug collagen degraded/hr
COLLAGENASE ALONE	20.13 ± 0.166
COLLAGENASE + ESAF	20.14 ± 0.172
COLLAGENASE + TIMP + ESAF	18.25 ± 0.108

30 minute incubation

complex. The amounts of ESAF used in these experiments was too small to be estimated.

RELATIONSHIP BETWEEN IN VIVO AND IN VITRO EFFECTS OF ESAF

ESAF as its name implies is able to stimulate capillary endothelial cells to proliferate and also to give a positive response on the chick chorioallantoic or yolk sac membranes. We have used the activity of ESAF in activating procollagenase as a quantitative measure to relate the amounts of ESAF needed in each of these assays. We have observed that in order to obtain a positive response on the chick membrane (Fig 3), we need an amount of ESAF able to activate sufficient procollagenase to the active form of the enzyme that will degrade 10 ug collagen in 1 hour. To obtain a maximal stimulation of a culture of capillary endothelial cells commencing at 5,000 cells per well, an amount sufficient to activate enough enzyme to degrade 0.7 ug collagen is needed.

Figure 3:

A Positive Response
to ESAF on the
Chicken Yolk Sac
Membrane

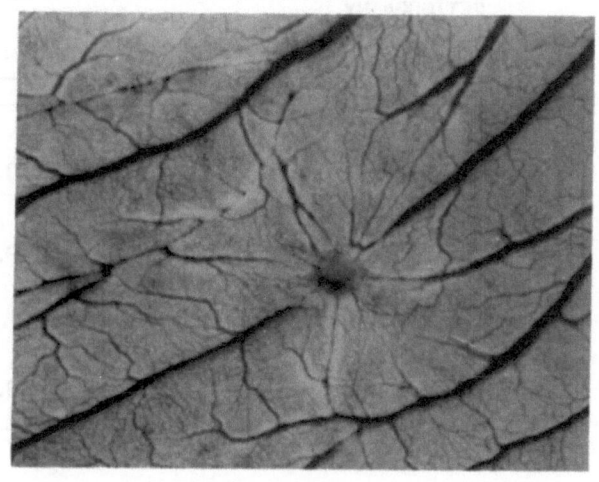

SOURCES OF ESAF

ESAF is a ubiquitous factor found in nearly all tissues and in serum. It is particularly evident in the retina but the amounts vary both with species and with disease (14).

ESAF IS NOT A PROSTAGLANDIN

Prostaglandin E_1 has been shown to provoke a positive angiogenic response in the cornea (12,13). However, we have not been able to demonstrate an angiogenic response for PGE_1 in the chick chorio-allantoic membrane. Neither can we show it to be able to activate procollagenase. Furthermore, preparations of ESAF have been tested for the presence of PGE_1 but none has been detected.

DISCUSSION

The article, in this volume, by Professor Alec Garner indicates the importance of ESAF in experimentally induced retrolental fibroplasia. We have also found elevated amounts of ESAF in vitrectomy samples from patients with diabetic retinopathy (Taylor, Weiss, Kissun and Garner unpublished results) (Table 4). The increase in amounts of ESAF present

522

Table 4:   ACTIVATION OF PROCOLLAGENASE BY EXTRACTS OF VITREOUS OBTAINED FROM PATIENTS WITH DIABETIC RETINOPATHY

1	Pro Enzyme	(procollagenase) alone	0.7
2	Pro Enzyme	+ organic mercurial activator	19.3
3	Pro Enzyme	+ Low molecular mass angiogenic factor from human vitrectomy samples	29.3

in tissues undergoing proliferative vascularisation suggests an important role for ESAF in the angiogenic process. Its ability to activate latent forms of collagenase is unique. No naturally occurring non protein activator of procollagenase has been previously described. However, more important from a physiological point of view, is that until now the enzyme inhibitor complex of TIMP and collagenase has been thought of as being resistant to any form of reactivation. As collagen is the stabilising fibre of the vitreous gel, activation of inhibited forms of collagenolytic enzymes by a small freely diffusible molecule may be a cause of liquefaction of the vitreous.

We hope shortly to be able to report the chemical structure of ESAF.

REFERENCES

1.   Schor AM, Schor SL, Weiss JB, Brown RA, Kumar S and Phillips P, Br. J. Cancer, 41, 790 (1980).
2.   Weiss JB, Elstow SF, Hill CR, McLaughlin B, Davidson EM, Schor A and Ayad SR, Prog. Appl. Microcirc. 4, 76 (1984).
3.   Weiss JB, Hill CR, Davis RJ and McLaughlin B, Agents and Actions, 15, 107 (1984).
4.   Harris ED, Welgus HG and Krane SM, Collagen and Rel. Res., 4, 493 (1984).
5.   Aggeler J, Engvall E and Werb Z, Biochem. Biophys. Res. Commun., 100, 1195 (1981).
6.   Mercer E, Cawston TE, De Silva M and Hazleman BL, Biochem. J, 231, 505 (1985).
7.   Weiss JB, Hill CR, McLaughlin B and Elstow S, FEBS Letters, 163, 62 (1983).
8.   Stricklin GP, Eisen AZ, Bauer EA and Jeffrey JJ, Biochemistry, 17, 2331 (1978).
9.   Elstow SF, Schor A and Weiss JB, Invest. Ophthalmol. Vis. Sci, 26, 74 (1985).

10. Lineweaver H and Burk D, J. Amer. Chem. Soc. 56, 658 (1934).
11. Weiss JB, Hill CR, Davis RJ, McLaughlin B, Sedowofia KA and Brown RA, Bioscience Reports, 3, 171 (1983).
12. Ben Ezra D. Amer. J. Ophthalmol. 86, 455 (1978).
13. Form DM, Sidky YA, Kubai L and Auerbach R. Prostaglandins and Cancer p 685, Alan Liss, New York (1982).
14. Taylor CM, Weiss JB, Kissun RD and Garner A, Br. J. Ophthamol, 70, 162 (1986).

RETINAL PIGMENT EPITHELIAL CELLS INHIBIT VASCULAR ENDOTHELIAL CELLS INVASION

Bert M. Glaser and John L. Davis

INTRODUCTION

New blood vessels generally form as sprouts from existing vessels[1]. One of the first steps to occur during sprout formation is the localized dissolution of the extracelluar matrix (ECM) surrounding an existing vessel[2,3,4]. The disruption of the ECM permits the migration of vascular endothelial cells from the wall of the existing vessel to form a new vessel sprout. The dissolution of ECM is thought to proceed via the action of locally acting proteases[5]. Plasmin, generated via the activation of plasminogen, may be a crucial protease in this process. This is supported by the fact that plasmin formation is localized to the advancing tips of newly forming blood vessels in the developing retina[6]. Furthermore, angiogenic factors from a variety of sources, including tumors and retina, stimulate vascular endothelial cells to release plasminogen activators resulting in the generation of plasmin[7]. The action of plasminogen activators is confined to their ability to catalyze the conversion of plasminogen to plasmin. On the other hand, plasmin acts on a wide variety of substrates important to the structure of the ECM. For instance, plasmin degrades ECM glycoproteins such as fibronectin and laminin[8]. In addition, plasmin can activate tissue collagenase which are often secreted in latent form[7]. In neovascularization during wound healing, the ability of plasmin to degrade fibrin has an important role. The generation of plasmin via the activation of plasminogen has been implicated in a number of other biological systems requiring controlled local proteolysis including tumor metastasis and growth, macrophage function, neuroontogenesis, and ovulation[9].

Based upon the observation that photocoagulation induced chorioretinal scars protect against the development of neovascularization in diabetic retinopathy we have proposed the novel theory that the chorioretinal scars may release an inhibitor or inhibitors of new blood vessel formation[10]. Since plasminogen activators are associated with the early stages of new blood vessel formation it would be of interest to determine if the cellular constituents of chorioretinal scars can release inhibitors of plasminogen activation. Chorioretinal scars are mainly composed of astrocytes, RPE, and possibly fibroblasts[11]. We therefore, have tested the ability of these cells to release inhibitors of plasminogen activators and plasmin. We have found that human RPE in culture, but not astrocytes or fibroblasts release an inhibitor of plasminogen activator. The release of the pigment epitheilal-derived protease inhibitor(PEPI) is abolished by inhibitors of RNA and protein synthesis.

Protamine, a cationic, arginine rich protein, has been found to inhibit neovascularization in vivo[12]. The mechanism of this inhibition is not fully known. Protamine does not inhibit vascular endothelial cell migration or proliferation in response to tumor-derived angiogenic factors (unpublished data). However, protamine is a potent inhibitor of vascular endothelial cell-derived plasminogen activators (unpublished data). In spite of significant effort, little is known about the mechanism of action of naturally occurring inhibitors of neovascularization derived from avascular tissues such as cartilage[13], vitreous[14], and lens[15]. This is due to the fact that only limited quantities of inhibitor can be extracted from these sources. The fact that the inhibitor described in the current report is continuously synthesized by cells in culture will permit the large scale production of inhibitor and allow investigators to overcome a major obstacle impeding research in this area.

Photocoagulation not only inhibits the development of neovascularization in diabetic retinopathy but also induced the regression of the most newly formed vessels[16]. We have recently shown that RPE conditioned media causes new blood vessels of the chick embryonic yolk sac to regress[10]. In contrast, media conditioned by astrocytes or fibroblasts did not cause regression[10]. The way in which new blood vessels regress is not well understood. Histologic examination of regression of new blood vessels shows that the earliest discernible event is the formation of intravascular clots [17]. Plasminogen activators are central elements of the fibrinolytic system and are likely to play a crucial role in preventing thrombogenesis. This is probably especially important in newly formed blood vessels since the endothelial cells composing these vessels are often separated by intracellular gaps that allow the blood stream to be exposed to the thrombogenic surfaces of the surorunding extracellular matrix[3]. These intraendothelial cell gaps have been found in new vessels of the cornea, in wounds, and in membranes from eyes with proliferative diabetic retinopathy. Therefore, the release of PEPI by RPE in chorioretinal scars may induce vascular regression via its ability to alter the thrombogenic balance within the new blood vessel.

The release of PEPI is dependent upon pigment epithelial cell density. PEPI released by RPE in confluent cultures is less than by RPE in subconfluent cultures. Several days after RPE reach confluence the release of PEPI once again increases. Corresponding to the increase in PEPI release the RPE begin to overgrow the monolayer to form localized regions with multiple cell layers. The decrease in PEPI release when RPE reach confluence is not related to decreased cell division since inhibition of DNA synthesis by hydroxyurea does not inhibit PEPI release. The effect of cell density on PEPI release is likely to depend upon the cell-cell relationships and associated cellular morphology. The RPE in subconfluent and superconfluent cultures do not maintain the RPE monolayer in the normal eye. Alterations in the highly ordered RPE monolayer that occur in chorioretinal scars and that are possibly mimicked in superconfluent and subconfluent RPE cultures may result in the enhancement of PEPI release. The resultant release of PEPI into the adjacent retina and vitreous may account for the effect of photocoagulation induced chorioretinal scarring in preventing neovascularization in diabetic retinopathy.

The identification of a protease inhibitor released by human RPE in culture raises interesting questions regarding a possible role under normal physiologic conditions. It is conceivable that RPE normally releases small amounts of PEPI that are incorporated into Bruch's membrane to serve as a biochemical barrier to new blood vessel invasion in addition to whatever physical barriers exist. That a biochemical barrier to new blood vessel invasion of Bruch's membrane might exist is suggested by the fact that vascular endothelial cells can readily release a variety of proteases capable of degrading Bruch's membrane[5,7]. Perhaps RPE in the macular region of eyes with senile macular degeneration lose some of their ability to produce PEPI and thereby the biochemical barrier to blood vessel invasion is reduced. Blood vessel formation may be induced by a variety of normally occurring events such as phototoxic stimuli or mild trauma but could not progress in the presence of a normal biochemical barrier. With an altered biochemical barrier, as might occur in SMD, these relatively minor stresses could induce significant neovascularization. Furthermore, laser photocoagulation of sub-RPE neovascularization nets may not only function to destroy new blood vessels but may also serve to inhibit regrowth by producing chorioretinal scars composed, in part, of RPE with altered morphology and therefore, better able to release protease inhibitors. This possible scenario is interesting in view of the fact that tissue destruction occurring in the aftermath of photocoagulation would seem to be an ideal environment for the further formation of new blood vessels. In view of our recent findings, the above sequence of events is certainly plausible but more importantly, provides a framework for future experiments to further elucidate RPE-endothelial cell interactions and their role in various ophthalmic disorders.

In summary, we have described a pigment epithelial-derived protease inhibitor (PEPI). The discovery of this protease inhibitor raises several interesting possibilities that require further investigation. Under normal conditions the RPE and Bruch's membrane are positioned as a barrier between the highly vascular choriocapillaris and the avascular outer retina. The ability for RPE to release a protease inhibitor may provide the biochemical mechanism by which the barrier functions. Since cell-cell relationships seems to alter PEPI released by RPE, photocoagulation and subsequent chorioretinal scarring may function by altering the local architecture and morphology of the RPE so that increased levels of the inhibitor may be achieved in the surrounding retina and vitreous, thereby, inhibiting vessel formation in proliferative diabetic retinopathy. Most important, further study of the interaction between RPE and the vasculature is likely to be fruitful in improving our understanding of neovascularization and suggesting new approaches to its treatment.

528

REFERENCES
1. Clark ER. Microscopic observations on the growth of blood capillaries in the living mammal. Am J Anat 64:251-301, 1939.
2. Ausprunk DH and Folkman J. Migration and proliferation of endothelial cells in performed and newly formed blood vessels during tumor angiogenesis. Microvasc 14:53-65, 1978.
3. Schoefl GI. Studies on inflammation. III. Growing capillaries: Their structure and permeability. Virchows Arch 337:97-141, 1963.
4. Yamagami I. Electromicrscopic study on the cornea. I. The mechanism of experimental new vessel formation. Jpn J Ophthalmol 14:41-42, 1970.
5. Kalebic T, Garbisa S, Glaser BM and Liotta L. Basement membrane collagen: Degradation by migrating endothelialcells. Science 221:281-283, 1983.
6. Pandolfi M. Localization of fibrnolytic activity in the developing rat eye. Arch Ophthalmol 78:512-519, 1967.
7. Gross JL, Moscatelli D, Jaffe EA, Rifkin DB. Plasminogen activator and collagenase production by cultured capillary endothelial cells. J Cell Biol 95:974-981, 1982.
8. Liotta LA, Goldfard RH, Brundage R, Siegal GP, Terranova V and Garbisa S. Effect of plasminogen activator (urokinase), plasmin, and thrombin on glycoprotein and collegenous components of basement membrane. Can Res 41:4629-4636, 1981.
9. Christman JK, Silverstein SC, Acs G. Plasminogen activators. In Proteinases in Mammalian Cells and Tissues, ed. Barrett A. Elsevier/North-Holland Biomedical Press, New York, NY, 1977, pp. 91-149.
10. Glaser BM, Campochiaro PA, Davis JL and Sato M. Retinal pigment epithelial cells release an inhibitor of neovascularization. Arch Ophthalmol 103:1870-1875, 1985.
11. Wallow IHL and Davis MD. Clinicopathologic correlation of xenon arc and argon laser photocoagulation procedure in human diabetic eyes. Arch Ophthalmol 97:2308-2315, 1979.
12. Taylor S and Folkman G. Protamine is an inhibitor of angiogenesis. Nature 297:307-312, 1982.
13. Brem H and Golkman J. Inhibition of tumor angiogenesis mediated by cartilage. J Exp Med 141:427-439, 1975.
14. Lutty GA, Thompson DC and Gallup JY. Vitreous: An inhibitor of retinal-extract induced neovascularization. Invest Ophthalmol 24:52-56, 1983.
15. Williams GA, Eisenstein R and Schumacher B. Inhibitor of vascular endothelial cell growth in the lens. Am J Ophthalmol 97:366-371, 1984.
16. Doft BH and Blankenship G. Retinopathy risk factor regression after laser penretinal photocoagulation for proliferative diabetic retinopathy. Ophthalmol 91:1453-1457, 1984.
17. Ausprunk DH, Falterman K and Folkman J. The sequence of events in the regression of corneal capillaries. Lab Invest 38:284-294, 1978.

A MITOGENIC FACTOR OR FACTORS PRODUCED BY CULTURED HUMAN RETINAL PIGMENT EPITHELIAL CELLS

Mike Boulton, Hong Chai Wong, Peter Clark and John Marshall
Institute of Ophthalmology, London.

INTRODUCTION

Two observations concerning the interactions of retinal pigment epithelial (RPE) cells and microvascular elements in the posterior globe have prompted this study. The first is that large numbers of RPE cells are destroyed by pan photocoagulation in the treatment of proliferative diabetic retinopathy and regression of new vessels occurs remote from the site of photocoagulation. The second is that in end stage retinitis pigmentosa, retinal vascular attenuation is associated with loss of RPE cells. The aim of this study was to determine if RPE cells can influence the retinal microvasculature.

Folkman et al (1979) demonstrated that tumor conditioned medium enhanced the proliferation of cultured capillary endothelial cells. However, this effect was not cell specific since conditioned medium from other cell types such as aortic smooth muscle cells and fibroblasts had similar activity. The effect of RPE conditioned medium (RPE-CM) on the proliferative ability of vascular endothelial cells is at present confused. Bryan and Campochiaro (1986) have demonstrated that serum free RPE-CM has stimulatory activity on corneal fibroblasts, astrocytes and RPE cells themselves; but did not have any significant affect on aortic endothelial cells. However, it was observed by Glaser et al (1985) that serum free RPE-CM inhibited the growth effect of retinal crude extract on bovine aortic endothelial cells. Due to the possible interactions between the RPE and the retinal vasculature we investigated the effect of human RPE-CM on cultured retinal capillary endothelial cells.

To determine the specificity of human RPE-CM it was tested on a variety of cell types namely bovine tenon fibroblasts, pericytes, aortic smooth muscle cells and retinal capillary endothelial cells. Furthermore, to determine if this effect was restricted to RPE cells, conditioned medium was produced from bovine tenons fibroblasts.

CELL CULTURE

Human RPE cells were grown in Ham's F10 medium supplemented with 20% foetal calf serum as previously described by Boulton et al (1983). All cultures used were between the third and sixth passage.

RPE-CM was prepared by washing confluent or post-confluent RPE cultures grown in 75 cm^2 Falcon flasks twice with phosphate buffered saline. 24 ml of either a) Dulbecco's Modified Eagle's Medium (DMEM) plus 7.5% human platelet poor plasma or b) plasma free DMEM were added to each flask for 2 days. The conditioned medium was then removed and stored at -20°C until required.

Bovine aortic smooth muscle cells, tenon fibroblasts and pericytes were routinely grown in DMEM plus 20% foetal calf serum. Tenon fibroblast conditioned medium (BT-CM) was produced as described for RPE cells.
Bovine retinal capillary endothelial cells (BRCEC) were routinely grown on a gelatin substrate in DMEM plus 7.5% human platelet poor plasma: pericyte conditioned medium (1:1) supplemented with retinal crude extract, heparin and insulin as described by Wong et al (this volume).

MITOGENIC ASSAY

At day 0, cells were plated at either 1 or 2×10^4 cells per 17mm multiwell in their respective growth media. In the case of BRCEC the multiwells were gelatin coated. At day 1, cells were detached with trypsin from a number of the wells and cell counts made using a haemocytometer. These counts were designated the initial cell count. The remainder of the wells had the growth media removed and replaced with test media which consisted of either:

a)   7.5% plasma conditioned medium : fresh unconditioned 7.5% plasma media (1:1).

or   b)   plasma free conditioned medium : fresh unconditioned 7.5% plasma media (1:1) - giving a final concentration of 3.75% plasma in the test media.

or   c)   respective control media for a) and b).

At day 4 a final cell count was made on BRCEC, tenon fibroblast and smooth cells. However, because of the slow growth rate of pericytes intermediate cell counts were made at day 5 and final counts were determined on day 7. The level of significance of any differences between the various test media was determined by analysis of variance and Neuman-Keuls (Winer 1971).
It can be seen from Figure 1 that RPE-CM significantly enhanced the proliferation of smooth muscle cells, tenons fibroblasts, pericytes and BRCEC when tested in 7.5% plasma. In the case of smooth muscle cells and tenon fibroblasts this was also true when the test was carried out in 3.75% plasma. This effect was not specific to RPE-CM since BT-CM also showed stimulatory activity for BRCEC (Fig. 1d). RPE-CM also enhanced the proliferation of tenon fibroblasts in the presence of retinal crude extract (Fig. 2). Furthermore, preliminary data indicates that RPE-CM also enhances the proliferation of BRCEC in the presence of retinal crude extract.
When the mitogenic activity of RPE-CM was compared between confluent and post-confluent cultures it was observed that when tested in 7.5% plasma, RPE-CM derived from confluent cultures had a more potent mitogenic activity for BRCEC than that produced from post-confluent cultures (Fig.3). This was surprising since there was a greater number of cells present in the post-confluent cultures. However, when tested in 3.75% plasma RPE-CM had no significant effect on the proliferation rate of BRCEC (Fig. 3).
Since the biological response of subcultured BRCEC may not relate to the in vivo situation we decided to examine the effect of RPE-CM on freshly isolated microvessels. Microvessels were prepared as described above and between 1 to 2×10^4 plated out in 1ml of test media in 17mm gelatin coated multiwells. Two days post-plating the

media was replaced with a further 1ml of test media and after a

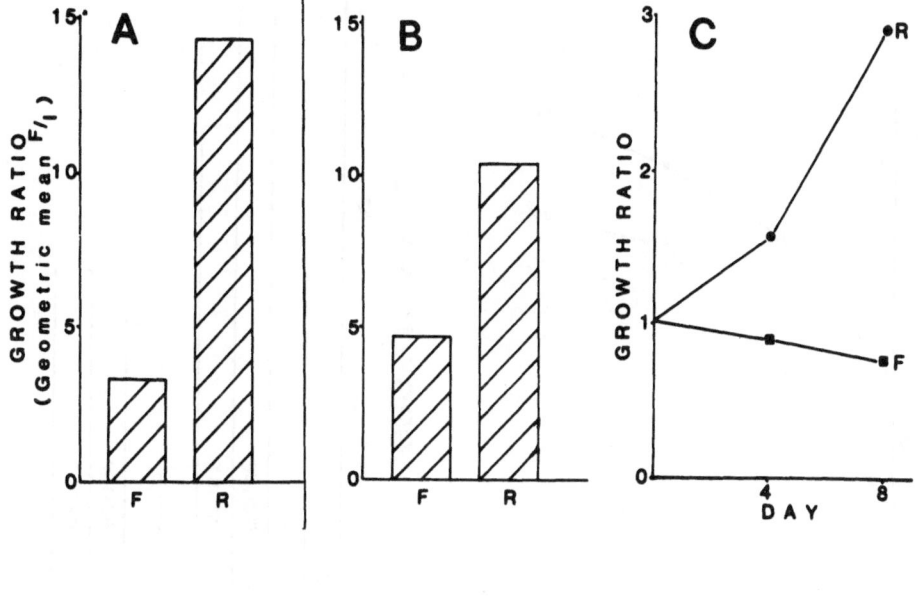

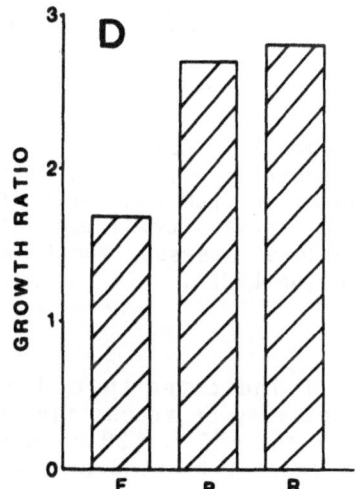

Figure 1. Comparison of the effect of RPE-CM (R) versus fresh medium (F) on a) aortic smooth muscle cells, tenon fibroblasts, c) retinal pericytes and d) BRCEC; tenon conditioned medium (B) was also tested against BRCEC.

further 3 days the cell numbers were determined. Results demonstrated that RPE-CM significantly stimulated the outgrowth and proliferation of microvascular cells (Fig. 4), the morphology of which was predominantly that of endothelial cells. The addition of 40nanogram/ml of insulin produced an additional stimulatory effect over and above that of RPE-CM on BRCEC.

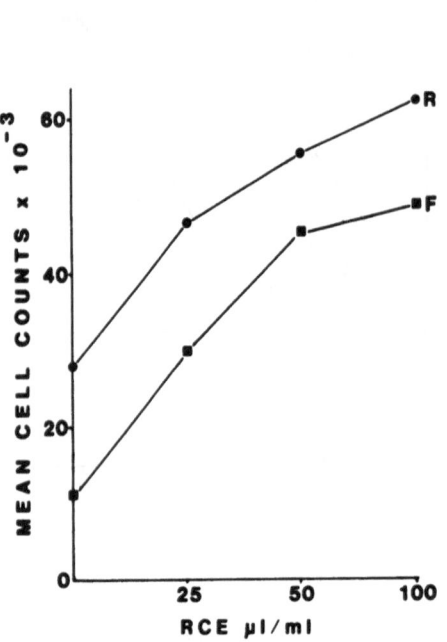

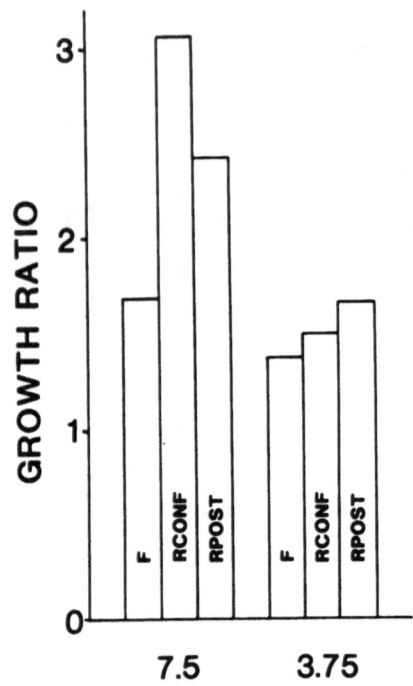

Figure 2. Graph showing the effects of different concentrations of retinal crude extract (RCE) on the growth rates of tenons fibroblasts in RPE-CM (R) and fresh medium (F).

Figure 3. Comparison of the mitogenic effect of RPE - CM obtained from confluent (RCONF) and post - confluent (RPOST) cultures versus fresh medium (F) on BRCEC.

Initial characterisation of RPE-CM indicated that there was approximately a 42% loss of mitogenic activity on tenons fibroblasts when the conditioned medium was heated to $56^{\circ}C$ for 30 minutes and that 95% of the mitogenic activity was lost by heating at $100^{\circ}C$ for 3 minutes. Further, greater than 65% of the activity was dialysable using tubing with a 10,000 to 12,000 Mwt cut off.

DISCUSSION

From our data it may well be that plasma concentration is a determining factor in the mitogenic response. This is in agreement with Gitlin and D'Amore (1983) who also showed that the mitogenic activity on BRCEC is dependant on the plasma concentration used in the assay. This observation may possibly explain the differences observed between the data presented in this paper and that of the observations of Glaser et al (1985) who reported that RPE-CM was inhibitory to the mitogenic response of bovine aortic endothelial cells to retinal crude extract when tested in serum free medium.

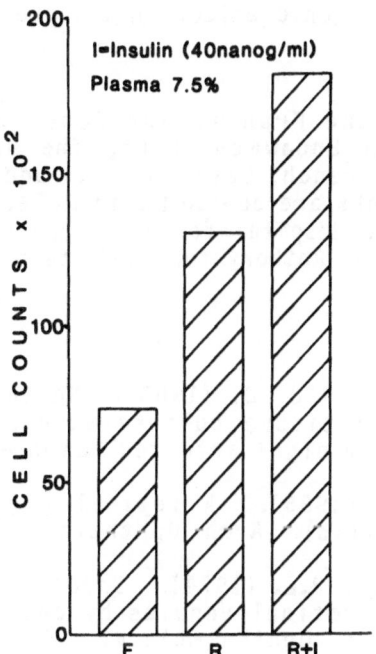

Figure 4. A comparison of the mitogenic effects of RPE-CM (R), RPE-CM + insulin (R+I) and fresh medium on primary microvessels.

Care should be taken in interpreting results as capillary endothelial cell mitogenesis whether demonstrated experimentally in vivo or in vitro is not the same as new vessel formation in vivo. This has been exemplified by Deem et al (1974) and Marshall et al (1983) who showed that chemical or physical injury to the adult retina induced tritiated thymidine uptake and hence cell division in retinal venous and capillary cells. Surprisingly this resulted in no new or pre-retinal vessels. Furthermore, Marshall et al (1983) used laser photocoagulation to induce this endothelial cell turnover; a technique which is used clinically to regress retinal new vessels.

In neovascularisation other components to that of mitogenesis i.e. basement membrane breakdown and migration, or even other steps may be the controlling events. Mitogenesis may well be a secondary prerequisite of new vessel formation. This is exemplified by the observations that there is a significant level of endothelial mitogens in the normal adult retina where no new vessel formation occurs.

SUMMARY
1. RPE-CM is mitogenic for both microvessels and BRCEC. This is a non-cell specific conditioning effect as both tenon fibroblast-CM and pericyte-CM (Wong et al, this volume) showed similar mitogenic activities.
2. RPE-CM is not specific for BRCEC since it is also mitogenic for tenon fibroblasts, smooth muscle cells and pericytes.

3. Mitogenic activity of RPE-CM appears to be dependant on plasma concentration.

4. Insulin produces an additional mitogenic effect in the presence of RPE-CM.

ACKNOWLEDGEMENTS
        This study was supported by the Francis and Renee Hock Foundation, Moorfields Eye Hospital Endowment Fund, The Mason Medical Foundation, SmithKline and French, Lasertek Ltd. and the Help the Hospitals Charity. Our thanks are due to David Mcleod of the Vitreoretinal Unit, Moorfields Eye Hospital for his support and are indebted to Meryl Bayly and Stephen Rothery for their technical assistance.

REFERENCES

BOULTON, M.E., MARSHALL, J. and MELLERIO, J. (1983). Retinitis pigmentosa: A preliminary report on tissue culture studies of retinal pigment epithelial cells from eight affected human eyes. Exp. Eye Res. 37; 307-313.
BRYAN, J.A. and CAMPOCHIARO, P.A. (1986). A retinal pigment epithelial cell-derived growth factor(s). Arch. Ophthalmol. 104; 422-425.
DEEM, C.W., FUTTERMAN, S. and KALINA, R.E. (1974). Induction of endometrial cell proliferation in rat retinal venules by chemical and indirect physical trauma. Invest. Ophthalmol. Vis. Sci. 13; 580-585.
FOLKMAN, J., HAUDENSCHILD, C.C. and ZETTER, B.R. (1979). Long-term culture of capillary endothelial cells. Proc. Natl. Acad. Sci. USA 76; 5217-5221.
GITLIN, J.D. and D'AMORE, P.A. (1983). Culture of retinal capillary cells using selective growth media. Microvasc. Res. 26; 74-80.
GLASER, B.M., CAMPOCHIARO, P.A. and DAVIS, J.L. (1985). Retinal pigment epithelial cells release an inhibitor of neovascularisation. Arch. Ophthalmol. 103; 1870-1875.
MARSHALL, J., CLOVER, G. and ROTHERY, S. (1984). Some new findings on retinal irradiation by krypton and argon lasers. In Docum. Ophthal. Proc. Series (Ed. Birngruber, R. and Gabel, V.P.), Vol. 36; 21-37. Dr W. Junk, The Hague.
WINER, J.B. (1971). Statistical Principles in Experimental Design. McGraw-Hill, New York.

RETINAL PIGMENT EPITHELIAL CELLS RELEASE INHIBITORS OF NEOVASCULARIZATION

B.M.Glaser, P.A. Campochiaro, J.L. Davis, Jr., and J.A. Jerdan

INTRODUCTION

Neovascularization plays a crucial role in the pathogenesis of several important human disorders including diabetic retinopathy, retinopathy of prematurity, choroidal neovascularization (age-related macular degeneration, histoplasmosis, etc.), sickle cell retinopathy, tumor growth, and rheumatoid arthritis. The possibility that controlling neovascularization will aid in the treatment of these disorders has prompted an extensive search for inhibitors of new blood vessel formation (1). Most inhibitors of neovascularization so far identified have been extracted from tissues that are avascular, ie. cartilage (2-5), vitreous (6,7), and lens (8). Unfortunately, the study of these inhibitors is severely limited by the fact that only small quantities of active material can be extracted from these sources (9).

It has been suggested that diabetic intraocular neovascularization is less likely to occur in eyes with chorioretinal scars (10). This has led to the widespread use of argon laser and xenon photocoagulation to therapeutically induce chorioretinal scar formation. The production of these scars often results in the rapid regression of intraocular neovascularization in eyes with proliferative diabetic retinopathy (10,11). Regression occurs even when photocoagulation and resultant chorioretinal scarring are located in areas remote from the new blood vessels (10-15). Retinal pigment epithelial cells (RPE) are one component of these scars. We now show that human RPE cells in culture release a substance (or substances) that causes the regression of new blood vessels on the chick embryonic yolk sac and inhibits vascular endothelial cell proliferation in vitro.[33]

Matherial and methods

Cell cultures

Retinal pigment epithelial cells (RPE), neonatal rat brain astrocytes, bovine corneal fibroblasts and fetal bovine aortic endothelial cells (FBAE) were cultured as previously described.[33]

Human retinal microvessel endothelial cells were also cultured as previously described.[34]

Conditioned media

Retinal pigment epithelial cell conditioned medium (RPE-CM), astrocyte conditioned medium (Astro-CM), and

MEM/10 containing 0.004 uCi 14C-thymidine/ml for 4 days as
described by Eckel and Fujimoto (27). The prelabeled cells
were then trypsinized and plated in 24 well plates at a
concentration of 45,000 cells/well as described above.
after 16 hours, the wells were rinsed with MEM/0 and filled
with MEM/0 or various concentrations of RPE-CM diluted with
MEM/0. All wells received RE diluted 1:20. The plates
were reincubated at 37°C and 5% CO_2 for an additional 24
hours. At this time 1 uCi of 3H-thymidine was added to
each well and the plates reincubated for 2 hours. 14C-
thymidine or 3H-thymidine content of cells was determined
as previously described (20).

Results

Discs of filter paper soaked in media conditioned by
RPE cells (RPE-CM) placed on the surface of the
vascularized yolk sac caused regression of adjacent
capillaries resulting in a localized avascular zone (Figure
1a). In contrast, media conditioned by either astrocytes
(Astro-CM) or bovine corneal fibroblasts (Fibro-CM) did not
affect the adjacent vasculature (Figure 1b).

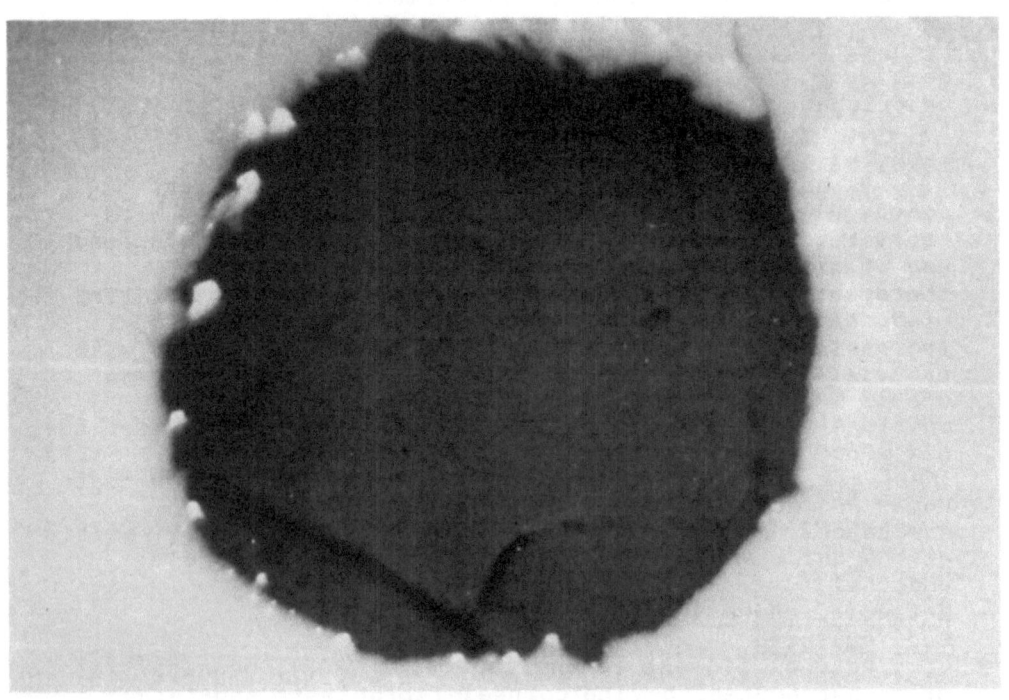

FIGURE 1. a) Yolk sac vasculature within central cutout of filter disc
soaked in RPE conditioned medium (magnification x27). Regression of vessels
within central cutout of filter disc, with no vessels in this area perfused. (cf. control photograph in Figure 1b).

fibroblast conditioned medium (Fibro-CM) were prepared by plating each cell type in 75 cm^2 tissue culture flasks at a density of 6.6 x 10^5 cells in 20 ml of either MEM/20 for RPE or MEM/10 for astrocytes and fibroblasts. Media were changed every 3 days. After 6 days, all cultures had reached confluence. The media were then removed and replaced with 10 ml of Eagle's minimal essential medium without serum (MEM/0). Forty-eight hours later, the conditioned media were removed, centrifuged, and the supernatant stored at -20°C for later use. RPE were also grown in MEM/10 prior to transfer to MEM/0 with identical results.

Alternatively, to determine the effect of cell density, media were conditioned 3 to 4 days after plating the cells for experiments using subconfluent cultures and 10 to 12 days after plating for experiments using superconfluent cultures.

Inhibition of new blood vessels on the chick embryonic yolk sac

The effect of conditioned media on the vasculature of the chick embryonic yolk sac was evaluated using a modification of the technique described by Taylor and Folkman (25). Three day old fertilized White Leghorn chicken eggs were opened and their contents carefully placed in a hammock of plastic wrap suspended in a small plastic drinking cup so that the chick embryo and vascularized yolk sac were fully exposed. The eggs were incubated at 37°C for 6 hours. The various conditioned media were concentrated 5-fold by ultrafiltration using an Amicon YM10 filter (molecular weight cut off = 10,000 daltons). Filter discs (13 mm diameter; HATF 01300; Millipore, MA) had a 4 mm circle punched out of their central portion and were soaked for 1 hour in the various concentrated conditioned media. The filter discs were then placed on the vascularized yolk sacs. Twenty-four hours later, the yolk sac vasculature within the central cutout of the filter disc was observed for signs of regression using a Zeiss operating microscope (Mag=260x). The effects of conditioned media on the yolk sac vasculature within the central cutout of the filter disc were graded as to whether there was (+) or was not (-) regression of blood vessels. Regression was considered present if at least 75% of the area within the central cutout of the filter had become avascular.

FBAE cell proliferation and survival

Fetal bovine aortic endothelial (FBAE) cell proliferation was determined as previously described.[33] Retinal extract (RE) was prepared as previously described.[20] RE stimulates neovascularization in vivo as well as FBAE proliferation in vitro. The loss of ^{14}C-thymidine was used to estimate cell death after the addition of RPE-CM (27). FBAE were cultured as described above. Cells were plated into 75 cm^2 flasks at a concentration of 2 X 10^6 cells/ flask and incubated with

538

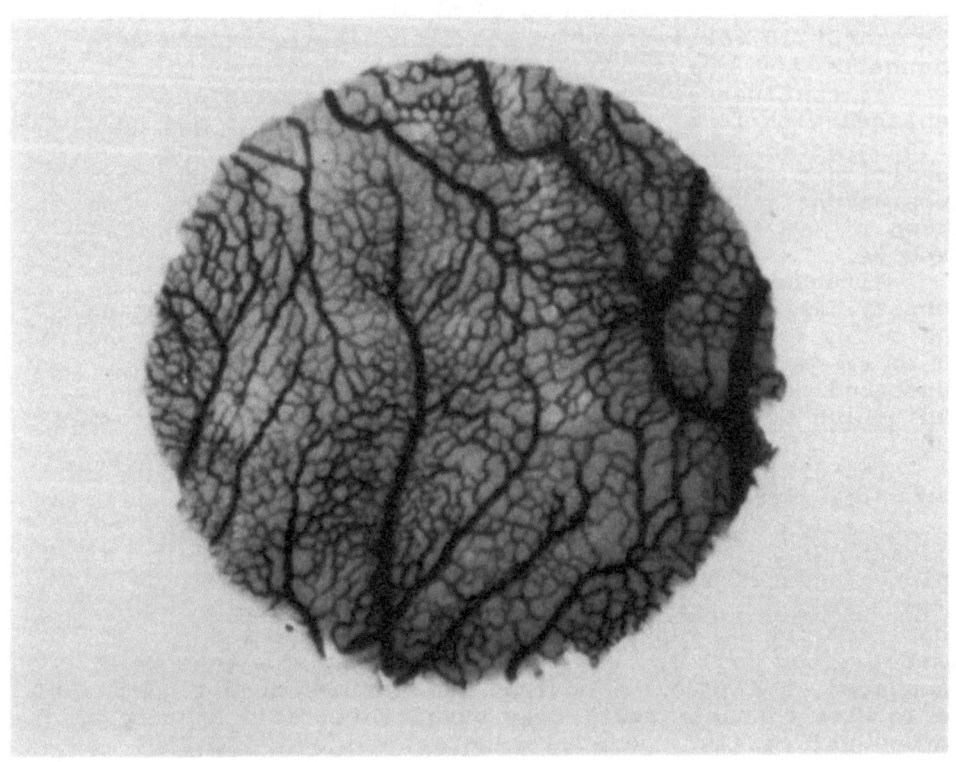

FIGURE 1. b) Yolk sac vasculature within central cutout of filter disc soaked in fibroblast conditioned medium (magnification x27). The vasculature is unaffected.

As previously demonstrated (20) an extract of adult bovine retina stimulated proliferation of FBAE in culture. RPE-CM inhibited the proliferative response of FBAE to retinal extract. Interestingly, RPE-CM did not inhibit the baseline cell growth in MEM/0 without retinal extract. In contrast, Astro-CM and Fibro-CM not only failed to inhibit FBAE proliferation in response to retinal extract but slightly enhanced the proliferative response. Furthermore, Astro-CM itself stimulated FBAE proliferation. The ability of RPE-CM to inhibit FBAE proliferation in response to retinal extract is enhanced by pretreating the FBAE with RPE-CM for 24 hours prior to adding the retinal extract. Pretreatment of FBAE with Astro-CM or Fibro-CM did not inhibit proliferation. Removal of RPE-CM restored the rate of FBAE proliferation to that of control cultures growing without RPE-CM. Therefore, the inhibitory effect of RPE-CM is reversible. In another series of experiments, we studied the effect of RPE-CM on FBAE prelabeled with ^{14}C-thymidine. The loss of ^{14}C-thymidine from prelabeled cells provides an estimate of cell death (27). The addition of

RPE-CM to FBAE did not result in the loss of 14C-thymidine but did inhibit cell proliferation as indicated by a decrease in ^{3}H-thymidine uptake. In a similiar manner, RPE-CM inhibited retinal extract induced proliferation of human retinal microvessel endothelial cells.

In contrast to its effect on vascular endothelial cells, RPE-CM alone caused a marked stimulation of fibroblast proliferation.

In all experiments described so far, RPE-CM was harvested from confluent cultures. Therefore, we next looked at the effect of RPE cell density on the release of inhibitor of FBAE proliferation. Confluent RPE produce significantly less inhibitor than subconfluent RPE. When the RPE are allowed to remain in culture for 4 to 5 days after they reach confluence (superconfluent cultures) the inhibitory activity of the conditioned media increases once again. Corresponding to this increase in inhibitory activity the RPE begin to overgrow the monolayer and form localized regions with multiple cell layers. Media conditioned by fibroblasts and astrocytes at comparable levels of confluency still did not inhibit FBAE proliferation.

Comments

Chorioretinal scars are mainly composed of astrocytes, RPE, and possibly fibroblasts (28-30). In our experiments, human RPE in culture, but not astrocytes nor corneal fibroblasts, released a substance (or substances) that caused the regression of new blood vessels on the chick embryonic yolk sac. Vessels appear in the chick embryonic yolk sac at 48 hours and grow rapidly over the next 6-8 days (25). Therefore, the vasculature of the 4-5 day old embryos used in our studies was in an actively developing or "neovascular" mode. Inhibitors of neovascularization derived from cartilage (32), aorta (24), and lens (8) also inhibit vascular endothelial cell proliferation. We have found that RPE-CM, but not Astro-CM nor Fibro-CM, inhibited retinal extract (RE) induced proliferation of FBAE and human retinal microvessel endothelial cells. The effect of RPE-CM on FBAE human microvessel endothelial cells proliferation was reversible and was not associated with FBAE death. In contrast, RPE-CM enhanced the proliferation of fibroblasts in culture.

The inability of rat brain astrocytes and bovine corneal fibroblasts to release detectable levels of substances that cause regression of new blood vessels and inhibit vascular endothelial cell proliferation demonstrates the relative uniqueness of human RPE in this regard. However, it does not indicate that other cell types, cells from other species, or cells under other conditions might not release similar substances. These possibilities are currently being addressed in our laboratory.

Cell-cell interactions play an important role in a large number of biologic processes including those occurring during development, wound healing, and tumor growth and spread. The establishment and control of an adequate blood supply has a role in all of these processes. Therefore, cell-cell interactions are also likely to be involved in controlling new blood vessel formation and regression during these processes. The ability of RPE to inhibit vascular endothelial cell proliferation and to induce the regression of new blood vessels may be important during ocular development where the RPE lies between the extremely vascular choroid and the avascular outer retina. RPE in a laser induced chorioretinal scar may release the same substance into the vitreous cavity to cause regression of intraocular new blood vessels. Previous studies (20) have shown that retina, under certain conditions, can release a stimulator of neovascularization. It is therefore of significant interest that RPE cells, although derived from the same neuroectoderm as the remainder of the retina, release inhibitors of neovacularization.

The release of the inhibitor of vascular endothelial cells proliferation is dependent upon RPE cell density. Inhibitor release by RPE in confluent cultures is less than by RPE in subconfluent cultures. Several days after RPE reach confluence, the release of inhibitor once again increases. Corresponding to the increase in inhibitor release, the RPE begin to overgrow the monolayer to form localized regions with multiple cell layers. The effect of cell density on inhibitor release possibly depends upon the cell-cell relationships and associated cellular morphology. The RPE in subconfluent and superconfluent cultures do not maintain the highly ordered cell-cell relationships present within the RPE monolayer in the normal eye. Alterations in the highly ordered RPE monolayer that occur in chorioretinal scars and that are possibly mimicked in superconfluent and subconfluent RPE cultures may result in the enhancement of inhibitor release. This may occur in spite of the fact that some RPE are destroyed by the photocoagulation since it is the remaining cells that can then undergo alterations in morpholology. The resultant enhancement in the release of inhibitor into the adjacent retina and vitreous may play a role in the effect of photocoagulation induced chorioretinal scarring on the regression and prevention of neovascularization in diabetic retinopathy. Further studies of the relationship between inhibitor release and RPE morphology and environment are underway in our laboratory.

Other inhibitors of neovascularization so far studied have their effect on actively proliferating vessels but do not cause regression of established vessels (25). Therefore, inhibitors potentially released by normal RPE would not be expected to cause regression of the nonproliferating, established capillary bed of the choroid. However, small amounts of RPE-derived inhibitor may prevent any inadvertent new blood vessel formation from the choriocapillaries. In senile macular degeneration, one might speculate that the RPE may suffer a biochemical defect, even in the absence of morphologic alterations, so that the level of inhibitor production is reduced and new blood vessel invasion from the choriocapillaries becomes more likely.

In summary, we have described, for the first time, a pigment epithelial-derived substance (or substances) that stimulates the regression of new blood vessels on the chick embryonic yolk sac and inhibits FBAE and human retinal microvessel endothelial cell proliferation. This discovery raises several interesting possibilities that require further investigation. Under normal conditions RPE and Bruch's membrane are positioned as a barrier between the highly vascular choriocapillaris and the avascular outer retina. The ability of RPE to release an inhibitor of vascular endothelial cell proliferation may provide the biochemical mechanism by which the barrier functions. Since cell-cell relationships seem to alter inhibitor release by RPE, photocoagulation and subsequent chorioretinal scarring may function by altering the local architecture and morphology of the RPE so that increased levels of the inhibitor may be achieved in the surrounding retina and vitreous, thereby inhibiting vessel formation in proliferative diabetic retinopathy. Most importantly, further study of the interaction between RPE and the vasculature is likely to be fruitful in improving our understanding of neovascularization and suggesting new approaches to its management.

Acknowledgement: We are deeply grateful to Dr. Arnall Patz for his helpful discussions and enormous support.

REFERENCES

1. Folkman J. Tumor Angiogenesis: Therapeutic Implications. **New Eng J Med 285:1182-1186, 1971.**
2. Eisenstein R, Sorgente N, Soble LW, et al. The resistance of certain tissues to invasion. Penetrability of explanted tissues by vascular mesenchyme. **Am J Pathol 73:765-774, 1973.**
3. Sorgente N, Kuettner KE, Soble LW, et al. The resistance of certain tissues to invasion II. Evidence for extractable factors in cartilage which inhibit invasion by vascularized mesenchyme. **Lab Invest 32:217-222, 1975.**
4. Brem H and Folkman J. Inhibition of tumor angiogenesis mediated by cartilage. **J Exp Med 141:427-439, 1975.**
5. Langer R, Brem H, Falterman K, et al. Isolation of a cartilage factor that inhibits tumor neovascularization. **Science 19:70-72, 1976.**
6. Brem S, Preis I, Langer R, et al. Inhibition of neovascularization by an extract derived from vitreous. **Am J Ophthalmol 84:323-328, 1977.**
7. Lutty GA, Thompson DC, Gallup JY, et al. Vitreous: An inhibitor of retinal-extract induced neovascularization. **Invest Ophthalmol 24:52-56, 1983.**
8. Williams GA, Eisenstein R, Schumacher B, et al. Inhibitor of vascular endothelial cell growth in the lens. Am. J. Ophthalmol 97:366-371, 1984.

9. Lee A and Langer R. Shark cartilage contains inhibitors of tumor angiogenesis. **Science 221:1185–1187, 1983.**

10. Beetham WP, Aiello LM, Balodimos MC, et al. Ruby-laser photocoagulation of early diabetic neovascular retinopathy: Preliminary report of a long-term controlled study. **Trans Am Ophthalmol Soc 67:39–67, 1969.**

11. Doft BH and Blankenship G. Retinopathy risk factor regression after laser panretinal photocoagulation for proliferative diabetic retinopathy. **Ophthalmology 91:1453–1457, 1984.**

12. Diabetic Retinopathy Study Group. Photocoagulation treatment of proliferative diabetic retinopathy: The second report of diabetic retinopathy findings. **Ophthalmology 85:82–106, 1978.**

13. Weiter JJ and Zuckerman R. The influence of the photoreceptor-RPE complex on the inner retina. An explanation for the beneficial effects of photocoagulation. **Ophthalmology 87:1133, 1980.**

14. Foulds WS. The role of photocoagulation in the treatment of retinal disease. **Trans Ophthalmol Soc N Z 32:82–90, 1980.**

15. Stefansson E, Landers MB, and Wolbarsht ML. Oxygenation and vasodilation in relation to diabetic and other proliferative retinopathies. **Ophthalmic Surgery 14:209–226, 1983.**

16. Vidaurri-Leal JS, Hohman R, and Glaser BM. Effect of vitreous on retinal pigment epithelial cell morphology: A new approach to the study of proliferative vitreoretinopathy. **Arch Ophthalmol 102:1220–1223, 1984.**

17. McCarthy KD and deVellis J. Preparation of separate astroglial and oligodendroglial cell cultures from rat cerebral tissue. **J Cell Biol 85:890–902, 1980.**

18. Raff MC, Fields KL, Hakamori SI, et al. Cell-type-specific markers for distinguishing and studying neurons and the major classes of glial cells in culture. **Brain Res 174:283–308, 1979.**

19. Parks DR, Bryan VM, Oi VT, et al. Antigen-specific identification and cloning of hybridomas with a fluoroscence activated cell-sorter. **Proc Nat'l Acad Sci USA 76:1962–1966, 1979.**

20. Glaser BM, D'Amore PA, Michels RG, et al. Demonstration of vasoproliferative activity from mammalian retina. **J Cell Biol 840:298–304, 1980.**

21. Rifkin DB, Gross JL, Moscatelli D, et al. Proteases and anginogenesis: Production of plasminogen activator and collagenase by endothelial cells. In: Pathobiology of the Endothelial Cell HL Nossel and JH Vogel, Eds. (Academic Press, New York,) pp. 191–197, 1982.

22. Glaser BM, Kalebic T, Garbisa S, et al. in: Development of the Vascular System, Ciba Foundation Symposium 100, J Nugent and M O'Connor, Eds (Pitman, London,) pp. 150–162, 1983.

23. Kalebic T, Garbisa S, Glaser BM, et al. Basement

membrane collagen: Degradation of migrating endothelial cells. **Science 221:281–283, 1983.**

24. Goren SB, Eisenstein R, and Chromokos E. The inhibition of corneal vascularization in rabbits. **Am J Ophthalmol 84:305–309, 1977.**

25. Taylor S and Folkman J. Protamine is an inhibitor of angiogenesis. **Nature 297:307–312, 1982.**

26. Lowry OH, Rosebrough NJ, Farr AL, et al. Protein measurement with the Folin phenol reagent. **J Biol Chem 193:265–275, 1951.**

27. Eckel RH and Fujimoto WY. Quantification of cell death in human fibroblasts by measuring the loss of [^{14}C] thymidine from prelabeled cell monolayers. **Biochem 114:118–124, 1981.**

28. Wallow IHL, Tso MOM, and Fine BS. Retinal repair after experimental xenon arc photocoagulation.I. A comparison between rhesus monkey and rabbit. **Am J Ophthalmol 75:32–52, 1973.**

29. Wallow IHL and Tso MOM. Repair after xenon arc photocoagulation 3. An electron microscopic study of the evolution of retinal lesions in rhesus monkeys. **Am J Ophthalmol 1973; 75:957–972, 1973.**

30. Wallow IHL and Davis MD. Clinicopathologic correlation of xenon arc and argon laser photocoagulation procedure in human diabetic eyes. **Arch Ophthalmol 97:2308–2315, 1979.**

31. Ausprunk DH, Falterman K, and Folkman J. The sequence of events in the regesssion of corneal capillaries. **Lab Invest 38:284–294, 1978.**

32. Eisenstein R, Kuettner KE, Neopolitan C, et al. The resistance of certain tissues to invasion III. Cartilage extracts inhibit the growth of fibroblasts and endothelial cells in culture. **Am J Pathol 81:337–348, 1975.**

33. Glaser BM, Campochiaro PA, Davis JL, and Sato M. Retinal pigment epithelial cells release an inhibitor of neovascularization. Arch. Ophthmol. 1985; 103: 1870–1875.

34. Del Vecchio PJ, Sharuk GS, Mac Elroy KF isolation and culture of cells from human retinal microvessels. Invest Ophthal. 1984: V 25 p 247.

INHIBITION OF NEOVASCULAR STIMULI

David BenEzra and Genia Maftzir, Immuno-Ophthalmology, Hadassah University Hospital, Jerusalem, Israel

INTRODUCTION

Clinical and experimental observations regarding the conditions under which ocular neovascularization is triggered led us to postulate that angiogenic factors are most probably normal tissue metabolites (1). These metabolites are produced in high levels under certain stress conditions of the affected tissues. When the concentration reaches a stimulating level, neovascularization is induced (1,2). Corneal neovascularization stimulated by controlled cauterization of the corneal tissue could be affected by the administration of steroids during the process (3). Furthermore, indomethacin, an inhibitor of prostaglandin synthesis, decreased significantly the extent of neovascularization induced by epidermal growth factor (EGF), fibroblast growth factor (FGF), lipopolysaccharide (LPS) and prostaglandin (PGE1). However, in most cases indomethacin did not abolish completely the angiogenic stimulus even in very high concentrations (4). More recently, tumor and corneal vascularization have been inhibited using a combination of heparin and cortisone (5,6). We report herein our observations regarding the effect of various antimetabolites, steroids/indomethacin and aqueous humor on various angiogenic stimuli.

MATERIALS AND METHODS

Inhibitors: The following were assayed: 5-fluoruracyl (5FU), Cyclophosphamide (Endoxan), Abiplatin, Cyclosporin A (CsA), Prednisolone and allogeneic aqueous humor. These were used as daily subconjunctival injections (5FU, Cyclophosphamide, Abiplatin), eye drops (Prednisolone), or incorporated into Elvax-40 to form a slow-release device (indomethacin, CsA). Allogeneic aqueous humor was obtained from a pool of paracentesis taps from the anterior chamber of 20 normal rabbit eyes. Inhibitory effects were studied after incubating the activated leukocytes in aqueous humor for a few hours.

Stimulators: Electrical cauterization of the cornea was performed as described previously (3). Activated lymphocytes were obtained after 48 hours incubation of rabbits' peripheral leukocytes (mainly mononuclear cells) with 10 ug of Concanavalin A (Con A). Elvax-40 implants were prepared as previously reported (1). Within the Elvax-40, various concentrations of prostaglandin E1, epidermal growth factor (EGF), fibroblast growth factor (FGF) and lipopolysaccharide (LPS) were sequestered.

Assessment of extent of neovascularization: This was
performed   by   daily   observations   under   the   operating
microscope   or slit lamp.   The length of the leading vessel
progresing   from   the limbus to the implant and   the   length
of   the active base of the limbus were recorded.   The   data
are   presented   as   the   surface   of   the   neovascular   tuft
calculated   as a triangle.   If not stated   otherwise,   data
recorded   on   day 6 after initiation of   the   stimulus   are
presented.

RESULTS
Table   1   illustrates   the   effects   of   various
antimetabolites   and   Cyclosporin A   on   the   extent   of
neovascularization   induced   by   activated   leukocytes   or
cautery.   The antimetabolites had no effect on the extent of
angiogenesis,   while   only   a minimal inhibitory effect   was
observed with Cyclosporin A.

Table 1:   Effect of antimetabolites and CsA on angiogenesis

Tested drug	Dose (mg)	Activated L's	Cautery
None	0	9.2*	6.1
5FU**	0.5	9.0	5.8
Cyclophosphamide**	1.0	10.1	7.5
Abiplatin**	1.0	8.7	6.0
CsA***	0.1	7.1	5.0

*   Average surface of neovascularization of 4 experiments
**   Daily subconjunctival injections
*** CsA was incorporated in Elvax-40

Indomethacin   and   prednisolone had a more   significant
effect on the extent of neovascularization induced by growth
factors,   LPS, PGE1 and cautery (Table 2).   As one can seen,
the   inhibitory   effect is more marked when both   substances
(indomethacin   sequestered   within   the   implant   and
prednisolone drops) are used simultaneously.

Table 2: Effect of indomethacin and prednisolone on corneal angiogenesis

Stimulant	ug per implant	Without Inhibitors	With Inhibitors Indometh*	Pred**	Ind+Pred
PGE1	5	16.2***	6.9	14.0	3.1
	10	20.8	13.8	19.1	7.2
EGF	10	3.2	1.6	3.4	0.0
	20	6.8	3.0	6.9	1.8
FGF	10	1.5	0.0	1.0	0.0
	20	2.9	1.2	3.9	0.0
LPS	1	18.6	8.1	20.6	6.2
	5	25.2	16.8	25.8	12.9
Cautery	---	6.5	3.9	6.0	2.1

*   Indomethacin (40 ug) was sequestered into the implant along with the tested material.
**   Prednisolone phosphate 1% eye drops solution was instilled 8 times daily.
***   Numbers designate the mean surface of neovascularization calculated from the recorded data of 4 to 8 experiments.

Allogeneic aqueous humor had an inhibitory effect on the capacity of activated leukocytes to induce angiogenesis (Table 3). Most significant inhibition was observed when the cells were incubated for a period of 8 hours before their injection into the cornea.

Table 3: Effect of allogeneic aqueous humor on angiogenesis induced by activated leukocytes

	Time of incubation (hrs)	Surface of neovascularization
Aqueous humor	0*	8.5**
	4	4.9
	8	2.5
Culture medium	0	9.0
	4	8.0
	8	7.5

*   Cells were resuspended in saline phosphate buffer 0.0067M pH 7.2
**   Average of 3 experiments

548

DISCUSSION

In debating the ways and means to inhibit neovascularization, one is always tempted to search for explanations looking into the naturally occurring avascular tissues, e.g. cornea, lens, vitreous, cartilage. Experiments have been carried out demonstrating the "inhibitory" capacity of these tissues and their potential to decrease the extent of experimental neovascularization (7,8). As suggested earlier (1), we believe that for every tissue, inhibitory and stimulatory factors are taking place, reaching a steady state characteristic for each specific organ. As depicted in the following scheme, an imbalance of the steady state would trigger the sequence of events that could lead to vascularization of an avascular tissue. The steady-state situation of a given tissue is probably dependent on its interactions with the surrounding tissues and not only on its intrinsic characteristics. In our study, we have shown that the normal aqueous humor inhibits the angiogenic capacity of activated lymphocytes. These findings may have some relevance regarding the trigger of corneal neovascularization or the regression of new vessels. Indeed, we have shown earlier that the aqueous humor may be responsible for the inhibition of neovascularization of the deeper layers of the cornea (2).

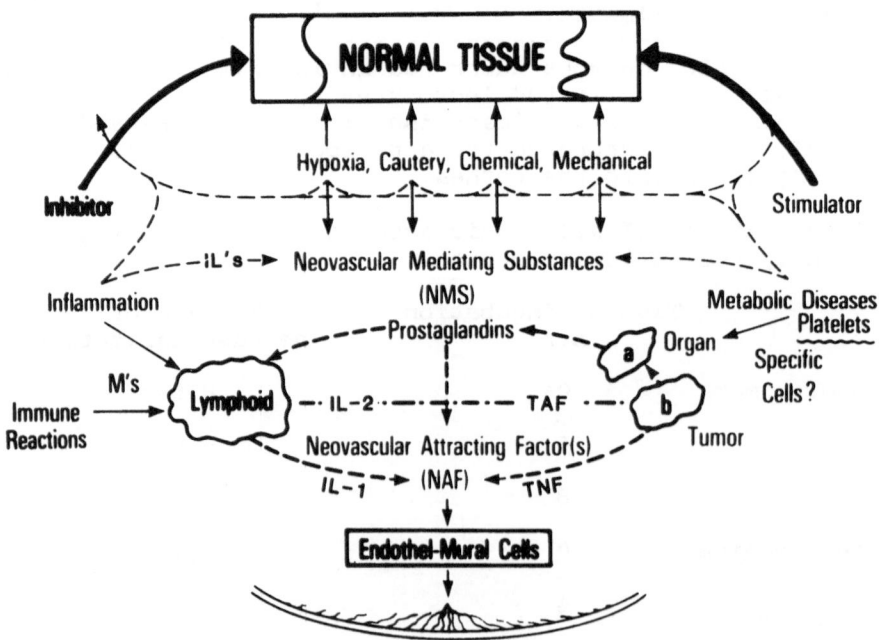

Figure 1. Schematic interpretation of interactions that may take place during tissue angiogenesis.

In the above scheme, prostaglandins play a central role as regulatory intercellular messengers. Indomethacin (an inhibitor of the enzyme oxycyclogenase responsible for the generation of prostaglandins) and steroids (inhibitors of the lipoxygenase, a crucial enzyme in the second cycle for prostaglandin generation) inhibit the extent of vascularization. Moreover, the two preparations were found to be synergistic. These findings reinforce our surmise regarding the pivotal role of prostaglandins in angiogenesis. Nonetheless, the possibility that other metabolites are also crucial for this process cannot be ruled out.

Interleukins or other lymphokines may well be adequate candidates for the regulating role. IL-1 can be secreted by a variety of cells, especially macrophages and endothelial cells (9,10). Our newer findings regarding the angiogenic potential of IL-1 (see also chapter on "Angiogenesis - Multiple Factors") would support this latter possibility. Furthermore, the feedback mechanism of regulation that exists between prostaglandins and IL-1 production in immune reaction (11) and between tumor necrosis factor (TNF) and IL-1 in their interaction with endothelial cells (12) may also take place during neovascularization. If the generation of interleukins plays a role in the regulation of angiogenesis, CsA should have a marked influence on the process. In our study, however, only a negligible inhibition was observed with relatively high doses of CsA.

REFERENCES
1. BenEzra D: Neovasculogenic ability of prostaglandins, growth factors and synthetic chemoattractants. Am J Ophthalmol 86:455, 1978.
2. BenEzra D: Neovasculogenesis. Triggering factors and possible mechanisms. Survey Ophthalmol 24:167, 1979.
3. Michaelson IC: Effect of cortisone upon cornea vascularization produced experimentally. Arch Ophthalmol 47:459, 1952.
4. BenEzra D: Neovascularization, a unitarian phenomenon. Docum Ophthalmol Proc Series 25:125, 1981.
5. Folkman J, Langer R, Lindhorst RJ, Handenschmild C, Taylor S: Angiogenesis inhibition and tumor regression caused by heparin in the presence of cortisone. Science 221:719, 1983.
6. Nikolic L, Friend J, Taylor S, Thoft R: Inhibition of vascularization in rabbit corneas by heparin: cortisone pellets. Inves Ophthalmol Vis Sci 27:449, 1986.
7. Lee A, Langer B: Shark cartilage contains inhibitors of tumor angiogenesis. Science 221:1185, 1983.
8. Garner A: Ocular angiogenesis. Int Rev Exp Pathol 28:249, 1986.
9. Dinarello CA: Interleukin-1. Rev Inf Dis 6:51, 1984.
10. Gery I, Lepe-Zuniga JL: Interleukin-1: Uniqueness of its production and spectrum of activities. Lymphokines 9:109, 1984.

11. Goodwin JS, Bankhurst AD, MEssner RP: Suppression of human T-cell mitogenesis by prostaglandins. Existence of a prostaglandin-producing suppressor cell. J Exp Med 146:1719, 1977.
12. Nawroth PP, Bank I, Handley D, Cassimeris J, Chess L, Stern D: Tumor necrosis factor/cachectin interacts with endothelial cell receptors to induce release of interleukin-1. J Exp Med 163:1363, 1986.

ALEC GARNER
Department of Pathology, Institute of Ophthalmology, University of London,
United Kingdom.

During the course of this meeting we have been reminded that
retinopathy of prematurity (ROP) is, once again, a problem in the management of babies born before term. The disease has not, as was hoped after
the crucial studies of Ashton and Patz showing the association with
hyperoxia, been relegated to a footnote in the history of ophthalmology.
To a considerable extent the present resurgence is linked with an increase
in the number of babies of exceptionally low birth weight (500-750 g) but
the precise mechanism remains to be demonstrated.

As several contributors to this conference have shown, hyperoxia
continues to be a major hazard but other risk factors, such as hypercarbia
and acidosis, have also been shown to be important. Moreover, it has been
recognised that a primary hypoxia related to persistent pulmonary
dysfunction can itself be a stimulus to proliferative changes.

Several speakers referred to the spindle-shaped cells which constitute a 'vanguard' in front of the emergent network of capillaries as the
vaso-formative 'rearguard' advances from the optic disc. What is the
nature of these cells? Thought for many years to be mesenchymal precursors of the definitive vascular endothelium, it has recently been
suggested that they are the cause of the arrested intraretinal angiogenesis in ROP, a source of the angiogenic factor responsible for the
extravascular proliferation, a source of energy by virtue of their
considerable glycogen content, and perhaps of astrocytic origin. Further
study involving histochemical cell markers, electron microscopy and, if
possible, tissue culture could be informative.

The kitten model of ROP has been criticised because, contrary to
the human situation, the preretinal vascular proliferation is not followed
by retinal detachment. A seemingly inevitable accompaniment of contractile
fibroblastic cells in the human situation and their complete absence in the
kitten is almost certainly a vital factor in the profoundly different
behaviour patterns, and it is important to discover both where the fibroblasts come from and what stimulates their activity. If these cells represent a metaplasia of the proliferating endothelium, what provokes this
change in function and why doesn't it occur in the feline retina? Kittens
do not have spindle cells: is this a clue?

ROP of minor degree commonly regresses spontaneously but it would
be valuable to identify the factors responsible for the reversal if only to
recognise those babies at risk of further progression. Cryopexy of the
avascular peripheral retina has been tried on the assumption that such

tissue is the principal source of the angiogenic factor associated with the extraretinal fibrovascular response. But results have been variable. Is this because the assumption is mistaken or is it because the extent of the tissue ablation is not always adequate? Controlled clinical study is needed.

Will it be possible in due course to treat the proliferative manifestations of ROP (and of other vascular retinopathies) pharmacolog-ically? If the nature of the angiogenic and fibrogenic factors can be identified it is conceivable that competitive inhibitors or other anti-dotes can be developed which would be suitable for intravitreal injection.

These are just some of the problems surrounding ROP that are waiting to be investigated. There are many others not touched upon in this conference including, for instance, the precise character of the vascular injury which precedes the clinical manifestations of ROP, but the way is now open for at least some of these basic issues to be addressed.

Arnall Patz

The Wilmer Institute, Johns Hopkins Medical Institutions, Baltimore, MD, USA.

I'd like to amplify very briefly on what Dr. Garner mentioned, namely that those of us, and there are very few here, who were old enough to be working in the 1950's, felt that retrolental fibroplasia (RLF) was going to be a dead disease very quickly. But we were so wrong, as is quite apparent. It was pointed out during the meeting, and it's obvious, we're dealing with a new disease. There's a population of immature infants, namely those with an extreme low birth weight, under 1000 grams, who are living today who, back in the epidemic of the 1950's, would not have lived long enough to develop ROP. Today, there is approximately a 5- to 6-fold increase in survival in that extremely low birth weight group. We're indeed faced with a new challenge. The questions regarding the type of treatment are most appropriate, because we are faced with active, proliferative ROP that in the '50's, once oxygen was incriminated, was rarely seen.

The new international classification of ROP, which was recently introduced, is helping to address this new epidemic of ROP. This classification probably will do the same as the classification of diabetic retinopathy did for the Diabetic Collaborative Retinopathy Study in the 1970's. Indeed it will not only foster the ability to compare results from different clinics and institutions, it will certainly provide the opportunity to standardize collaborative studies when multiple centers are using the same methodology.

In the presentations, I found the prevalence and natural history studies from Denmark and from Beersheba in Israel extremely interesting and informative. The observation from Beersheba regarding the different racial incidence of ROP raises several interesting questions that if answered during the coming years could enhance significantly our understanding of the pathogenesis in ROP. An excellent update was presented by the Philadelphia group on the use of large doses of Vitamin E. Recently, the Institute of Medicine in the U.S. evaluated very carefully and critically all of the published studies on the effect of vitamin E in preventing the sequelae of ROP and brought together the key investigators, including Dr. Quinn who is here, who have been involved in the controlled clinical trials. The agreed conclusion drawn from the meeting was that the status of vitamin E in the prevention of ROP is still unresolved. Therefore, it was recommended that a multi-center trial be considered to further evaluate the role of vitamin E.

The last part of the session dealing with cryotherapy
in ROP was the most interesting and indeed challenging.
There were individual reports suggesting a definite benefit
and others questioned the benefit of this approach. In
order to verify these controversies, a collaborative
clinical trial of 24 centers is going on now in the U.S.
Namely, the centers were willing to test this particular
form of treatment because it does appear promising. There
are reports, just as we heard here, that suggested a
benefit. But, on the other hand, recognizing the high rate
of spontaneous regression, there is a need for a very large
sample size in order to draw significant conclusions. I'm
hopeful that by three years from now, when the next
symposium is held, these studies as well as other ongoing
investigations will provide a definitive answer on the role
of cryotherapy in ROP.

In closing, I want to tell you how grateful we are in
Baltimore that your committee has selected that city for the
next, the second international, symposium on ocular
circulation and neovascularization. This coincides with the
100th anniversary centennial celebration of Johns Hopkins
Medical Institutions. So we're very pleased and
appreciative that you've made that choice. On behalf of Bert
Glaser and Bob Murphy, I want to thank you for that.

G. SOUBRANE – CRETEIL (France)

This last session was built to summarize the recent approaches to neovascularization and to precise the possible future goals for clinical research. Treatment methods, mainly photocoagulation, have become available in the major vascular diseases.

Evidence is now acquired that laser photocoagulation is efficient in reducing the risk of visual loss due to preretinal neovascularization in ischemic retinopathies. The role of ischemia in relation to new vessels growth was widely emphasized. The modality of the effect of laser photocoagulation remains still partially unclear.

There is also evidence that photocoagulation is beneficial for preserving visual loss due to macular edema secondary to branch vein occlusion and diabetic retinopathy. Focal coagulation of leaking abnormalities showed to be efficient not only anatomically but also functionnally.

Although more is known about subretinal neovascularization, there are numerous gaps in our knowledge, even in their natural history. If the animal model available provides some clues in well defined subretinal new vessels, occult SRNV remain a challenging diagnosis. When associated with a pigment epithelial detachment, the features of SRNV are even more subtle to analyse. In these difficult clinical situations, no experimental model is available. Moreover, there is actually no experimental approach for the understanding of age-related macular degeneration.

Blue green argon laser had demonstrated its value on visual acuity in well defined SRNV. The specific effect of the different wavelengths now available have to be precised. But we still do not know the goal we want to achieve when performing photocoagulation of SRNV in human. Is our goal to achieve direct obliteration of the neovascular membrane ? Is it to destroy the choroid from which the new vessels arise ? Do we want the pigment epithelium to proliferate in order to induce the involution of the neovascular tufts ? What is the possible benefit of destroying damaged pigment epithelium cells and to replace them by rejuvenated cells ? More questions remain unsolved and especially on the preferential critical location of not only the recurrences but also of the original neovascular membrane in the vicinity of the avascular zone.

We, clinicians, can only suspect some of the factors concerned, but, obviously the response will be the result of the cooperation with basic researchers. To stimulate our thoughts, I would remind to each of us that laser photocoagulation is and remains a destruction of the tissue we want to protect : the retina.

ROBERT B. NUSSENBLATT, M.D.
LABORATORY OF IMMUNOLOGY, NATIONAL EYE INSTITUTE,
NATIONAL INSTITUTES OF HEALTH, BETHESDA, MD

Intra-ocular inflammatory disorders (uveitis) represent a large array of conditions, many of which have profound effects on the ocular vasculature. It is often these sequelae of the inflammation that lead to irreversible sight-threatening problems. It will be the attempt of this short report to review some of the more classic vasculature alterations noted with uveitis, the potential role of the vascular endothelium in uveitis, and the effects of newer immunomodulating agents on this specific aspect of the disease.

Uveitic conditions leading to profound vascular alterations in the eye:

Sarcoidosis: This disorder of a putative autoimmune nature characteristically presents with a granulomatous uveitis. Neovascularization is not infrequently seen in the course of posterior pole involvement, with retinal and optic nerve head neovascularization medically treatable. However, subretinal neovascular membranes in the macula must be aggressively looked for, and treated (1).

Behcet's Disease: This multi-system disorder frequently leads to recurrent explosive posterior uveitic episodes, with the final outcome often being severe visual handicap. In this disorder, neovascular disorders, both of the anterior and posterior segments can be seen. The severe, explosive, inflammatory episodes typical of this disorder can mask the neovascular retinal lesions which require immediate evaluation and treatment. In addition, areas of capillary dropout and venous shunts may very often be noted in these patients, leading to severe retinal ischemia, with resultant neovascular glaucoma.

Presumed Ocular Histoplasmosis Syndrome: This disorder is particularly prevalent in a broad band that sweeps through the mid-section of the United States. It is characterized by an absence of inflammatory cells in the vitreous, but with focal areas of choroiditis, seen as multiple white, cream colored spots. These lesions, if seen in the macula, will have a marked propensity to develop subretinal neovascularization with a resultant fall in visual acuity.

Pars Planitis: This entity can produce several alterations to the ocular vasculature. Within the snowbank, neovascular lesions extending into the vitreous can be noted, particularly in younger patients. In extreme cases, the neovascularization can even extend onto the back surface of the lens. Neovascular lesions can also be seen and can be the source of recurrent vitreal hemorrhages. However, cystoid macular edema is the most common ocular vascular alteration noted in patients with this entity, and frequently leading to a decrease in visual acuity.

Possible Mechanisms by Which Intra-Ocular Inflammation Affects the Ocular Vasculature:

As noted above, these intra-ocular inflammatory disorders all can induce profound retinal and choroidal vascular alterations. The major underlying mechanism is not thought to be hypoxia, but rather the inflammatory disease itself. Recent evidence would suggest that the vascular endothelium may be responsive to factors produced by various arms of the immune system, and it would be worthwhile to review some of the points that support this argument.

It is clear that factors produced by immune cells, particularly T-cells have an effect on non-immune elements. T-cell products have been extensively studied and shown to alter fibroblast growth and mobility (2,3). This effect may have real import in the eye. By stimulating fibroblast growth, vitreal traction may be enhanced. This phenomenon may lead to "scaffolding", permitting neovascular growth into the vitreous. Alternatively, the increased traction may pull already existing new vessels leading them to bleed, leading to vitreal hemorrhage.

More direct effects on the vascular endothelium by immune products have been noted. BenEzra has demonstrated the effective induction of new vessel growth in the eye (4) by prostaglandins and other lymphoid products (5). Further, more recent evidence strongly demonstrates that vascular endothelial cells express Ia antigens, a critical membrane protein required for antigen processing and the transfer of immune information to T-cells that ultimately leads to this cell's activation (6). Ia activation is classically induced by either interferon or tumor necrosis factor (7). We have looked at Ia activation in the eye during retinal S-antigen induced experimental autoimmune uveitis. Ia activation of the endothelial cells occurs at the very early stages of the disease, before there is overt destruction of the retina, or large numbers of immune cells present (8). Since vascular endothelial cells not from the eye have been shown to be capable of presenting antigen to T-cells (6), it is tempting to speculate that similar phenomenon is occurring here as well. It may be that these activated vascular endothelial cells act as localizing sign posts for primed, antigen specific T-cells, leading to an organ specific inflammatory response.

Leung and colleagues have recently demonstrated the presence of circulating IgM antibodies directed against only Ia+ vascular endothelial cells in patients with Kawasaki's disease (9). Initial results would suggest that a similar antibody may be present in patients with pars planitis, though this still needs to be fully confirmed (Dr. Leung, personal communication). If this is indeed the case, it is tempting to speculate that those patients with pars planitis and CME have this problem because of combined T-cell and humoral mechanisms.

Immunotherapy for Vascular Alterations Due to Uveitis:

Some of the more severe intra-ocular inflammatory conditions with prominent vascular complications are not adequately treated with corticosteroid therapy. However, corticosteroids are known to have a wide range of effects on cells at the end organ where the inflammation is occurring. It is certainly known that neovascular lesions due to sarcoid will regress with corticosteroid therapy, and the effect on the immunopotentiators as well as the responder endothelial cell leads to regression. Newer immunosuppressive agents such as cyclosporine have a profound effect in interrupting putatively T-cell mediated diseases. These include disorders with a marked retinal vascular component, such as pars planitis and Behcet's disease (10). However, it has been our observation that the neovascularization, once it occurs, does not appear to be favorably altered by the administration of this medication. The implication of these findings would be that it permits the initiation of the neovascular event may be driven by immune system products, but that the ongoing process seems self contained, which permits the resultant hypoxia being the continuing driving force.

REFERENCES

1. Nussenblatt RB: Macular thickening and visual acuity: measurement in patients with cystoid macular edema. Ophthalmology (in press).
2. Schmidt JA, Liver CN, Lepe-Zuniga JL, Green I, Gery I: Silica-stimulated monocytes release fibroblast proliferation factors identical to interleukin 1. J Clin Invest 73:1462-1472, 1984.
3. Wahl SM, Malone D, Wilder R: Spontaneous production of fibroblast-activating factors by synovial inflammatory cells. J Exp Med 161:210-222, 1985.
4. BenEzra D: Neovasculogenic ability of prostoglandins, growth factors, and synthetic chemoattractants. Am J Ophthalmol 86:455-461, 1978.
5. BenEzra D: Mediators of immunological reactions: Function as inducers of neovascularization. Metab Ophthalmol 2:339-341, 1978.
6. Roska AK, Kipsky PE: Dissection of the functions of antigen-presenting cells in the induction of T-cell altivation. J Immunol 135:2953-2961, 1985.
7. Chang RJ, Lee SH: Effects of interferon-gamma and tumor necrosis factor-gamma on the expression of an Ia antigen on a murine macrophage cell line. J Immunol 137:2853-2856, 1986.
8. Fujikawa LS, Chan CC, McAllister C, Gery I, Hooks JJ, Detrick B, Nussenblatt RB: Activation of endothelial cells in experimental autoimmune uveitis expressed by the appearance of fibronectin and the Ia antigen. Invest Ophthal Vis Sci (Suppl) 26:97, 1985.
9. Leung DYM, Collins T, Lopierre LA, Geha RS, Pober JS: Immunoglobulin antibodies present in the acute phase of Kawasaki syndrome lyse cultured vascular endothelial cells stimulated by gamma interferon. J Clin Invest 77:1428-1435, 1986.
10. Nussenblatt RB, Palestine AG, Chan CC: Cyclosporine therapy in the treatment of intra-ocular disease resistant to systemic corticosteroids or cytotoxic agents. Amer J Ophthal 96:275-282, 1983.

M. YANOFF

Department of Ophthalmology, Scheie Eye Institute, University of
Pennsylvania, Philadelphia, PA, USA.

The last 10 to 20 years have shown a marked information explosion. We are
now at the point where over 7,000 articles are published each day in the
academic journals throughout the world. The information base in academe
doubles roughly every 10 years. In the biomedical sciences information
increases at a 4% compound rate annually.[1] No question exists, therefore,
that an enormous amount of information has been, and is being, produced.
The purpose of information is to acquire knowledge in order to obtain wisdom. It is clear that the research in our area is generating lots of
information, but I respectively submit that we have not generated much
wisdom. Why is this?

A friend of mine who is a plaintiff attorney is one of the most successful
trial lawyers in the country. I asked him what was the secret of his success. He said that early in his career he realized that there was very
little difference in the amount of work necessary to prepare a case worth
$10,000 against preparing a case worth $100,000. He, therefore, concluded
that he would only accept cases worth at least $100,000. It seems to me
that our research consists of too many "$10,000 cases". If we look through
the Table of Contents of most prestigious journals, we all agree that it
is filled with articles that are of little, lasting value. It would seem
that we are asking the wrong questions.

It reminds me of a group of researchers looking out upon a field of grass.
The first researcher decides to perform a study. He counts all the blades
of grass in the field and reports it. The second researcher then does a
study and confirms the count. The third researcher states that the first
two researchers were not on target and what is important is the number of
plants, not the blades of grass. So she then counts the individual plants
and reports it. The fourth researcher, of course, confirms the findings of
the third researcher. But no one asks the question, "Why are the plants
growing?"

I overheard two people yesterday speaking at the break. One said to the
other, "That's an interesting question, not earth shattering but
interesting. Lets collaborate and answer the question." I think that it is
time to ask the earth shattering questions and answer them.

At the next International Symposium on Ocular Circulation and
Neovascularization, I would like to know the following:

What is the histochemistry and the function of the spindle cells that are
found in the retina in retinopathy of prematurity? What animal retinas
contain these cells?

What is the exact biochemical configuration of the retinal angiogenic factor or factors and of the antiangiogenic factor or factors?

What turns on the system that causes retinal neovascularization, and what turns it off?

How does panretinal photocoagulation work?

I believe it is time to stop counting blades of grass and find out why plants grow.

REFERENCES

1. Lancaster FW, Smith LC: Science, scholarship and the communication of knowledge. Library Trends 27:367-388, 1979.

Stephen Ryan

Department of Ophthalmology, USC School of Medicine, Los Angeles, CA, USA.

I'd like to focus on the question of subretinal neovascularization (SRNV) and some aspects regarding its pathogenesis. We don't have, as yet, an answer to the basic issue of why there exists such a predilection for SRNV in the macular area. What is it that seems to be different about that particular area? Surely there are lots of different causes for speculation: RPE, retinal characteristics, foveal structure, etc. Many theories have been proposed. But, at present, I don't think the evidence is there. What's the pathogenesis in clinical conditions? What's the role of the macrophage? What's the role of the RPE? What's the role of the endothelial cells? And how can we influence this process so as to cause involution? The concept that we favor is the possible involvement of many cells with complicated extracellular environment. We know that we are dealing with an area where the retinal receptors are deriving their nutrition from the choriocapillaris, across the PE, functioning as a unit. It is very important that we keep in mind that whenever we divide this unit in order to try to better understand the phenomenon, it is somewhat artifactual. We, among others, grow RPE cells or endothelial cells and we get hints and we get clues, but it's very important that we keep an open mind regarding the possible interpretations of our observations. Clearly, in vivo experiments or clinical research are more informative complicated but not always easy to evaluate. I firmly believe that the ultimate answers lie in a better understanding of cell biology at the molecular level and more efforts should be made in this direction.

The point that I'd like to stress is that when we do clinical trials or experimental models of a system that by definition is variable, we have to know exactly what's the natural course versus what's our therapeutic effect of whatever trial or whatever we do to try to alter pathogenesis. I think that good clinical trials are fundamental to our understanding of the basic pathological processes. We can never lose sight of the fact that we, as clinicians, have to try and maintain patients' vision as long as we can. We know and share the discouragement that was presented as to the long-term recurrences when you treat age-related macular degeneration (ARMD), along with the fact that we are dealing with older patients. Yet, we also believe that if we buy those people time, that's a worthwhile endeavor. I can't overemphasize that for me, thinking of the laboratory, experimental models or the clinical situation, it's a balance of factors, and I suspect it's a very delicate balance. Can RPE be causing stimulation at one time and inhibition at another time? Is it possible that we are altering the balance? Is the cell performing differently at different phases of its life cycle and/or under different conditions? Clearly, all of this is quite possible and I expect that it is probably happening.

There are three types of cells which may have crucial, still unveiled roles in angiogenesis: the RPE, the capillary endothelial cells and the macrophages. In my opinion, a better understanding of the various functions of these cells should be our prime goal in future research.

Bert M. Glaser

Center for Vitreoretinal Research, The Wilmer Institute, Johns Hopkins Medical Institutions, Baltimore, MD, USA.

Dr. Michaelson's "Factor X" is in many ways the source of the sort of research that I am doing, so it is a pure honor for me to be able to summarize my concept of future trends in neovascularization. It has been a very exciting meeting for me and I've gotten a great deal out of it.

What I'd like to do in the way of summary is to stress two things: One is, I think we are on the dawn of a new era. We're beginning to recognize, more and more, that when we treat with the laser, we're not just knocking out cells, but we're treating balances, changing balances between cells, shifting balances, etc. The other thing I'd like to talk about is that in terms of the balances, we've been spending a lot of time talking about proliferation. And it's no question that proliferation is part of what's going on. In future trends and the next time we come together, we'll probably be talking about other steps in these "proliferative processes" that maybe are as important or even more important. We need to keep in mind that proliferations are important but there are many other things going on besides the end stage of cell multiplications.

The cell-cell interactions between RPE cells and endothelial cells are important phenomena. Dr. Korte talked about the possible influence of RPE cells which, perhaps, polarize endothelial cells and cause fenestrations to form. This "normal situation" may be the delicate balance that we want to reestablish with our treatments. The treatments, perhaps, change these balances.

Again, it's the concept of these balances that may help us understand some of our empirical observations. When membranes are formed and progress, we treat them and hope to induce their involution. We believe now that we're not just doing something instantaneously with the laser and the story's over, but we're shifting balances, one way or another, hopefully towards the resolution side.

Proliferation is the end result most easily observed. But it's only one step. There probably exist many other steps. One of the earliest steps that's been identified so far is the ability of endothelial cells to degrade the surrounding extracellular matrix. This has been alluded to in several of the talks. Dr. Weiss has talked about her very elegant work with collagenases. Early histological electron micrograph studies of neovascularization have shown that endothelial cells send out small pseudopodia. Dissolution of basement membrane near the pseudopodia along with dissolution of some of the extracellular matrix were also observed. These, in my opinion, are very early steps in the initiation of neovascularization.

There are data indicating that the endothelial cells are able to release procollagenases, plasminogen activators, and probably other enzymes that degrade proteoglycans. These enzymes loosen the extracellular matrix so that the endothelial cells then have a space through which they can begin to migrate.

This phenomenon brings us to another point that Dr. Michaelson has pioneered and in which he has been a source for my own personal thinking. This is the question of the disorderly invasive process of vascular endothelial cells. When they're first beginning to form new vessels and invading a non vascular tissue, many of the actual enzymes they produce are similar and in many cases identical to enzymes produced by tumor cells that are invasive. So, these endothelial cells are transiently invasive as tumor cells often are invasive. The question that arises, and which was addressed by Prof. Michaelson, is to what extent Bruch's membrane, is a physical barrier or is it a biochemical barrier. And that's a very good question and I think we're going to find out that it probably fulfills both roles. I believe that when we meet in 1989 we'll have many more specifics about this.

As I mentioned, vascular endothelial cells can release all of the types of collagenases and plasminogen activators and several other enzymes that can actively degrade Bruch's membrane. These enzymes are released when endothelial cells are stimulated by angiogenic substances.

Ayala Pollack in her very elegant studies has shown that indeed light laser treatment does not cause "holes" in Bruch's membrane. Endothelial cells can be observed "making their way" through "intact" Bruch's membrane. Presumably they use these enzymes to do it. So a pre-existing break within Bruch's membrane, although it may occur in many cases, is not absolutely necessary for the invasive process of endothelial cells. Therefore, if they can go through, what's normally stopping them? Again, could it be the RPE, could these cells be part of the biochemical barrier that may add to the physical barrier of Bruch's membrane? These are the crucial questions to which we should be looking for answers.

We started off looking at one of the enzymes the endothelial and tumor cells produce when they're invading. It is a plasminogen activator. Why is it important? Plasminogen activator converts plasminogen to plasmin. Plasmin can degrade fibronectin and laminin, both components of Bruch's membrane; it can activate Type I and Type IV collagenase. It can also stimulate the complement systems that may be involved in some of the white cell responses as well. Dr. Weiss has shown that stimulators of angiogenesis seem to stimulate procollagenase activity or procollagenase transformation to collagenase. We're looking at plasminogen activator and we found that RPE cells can inhibit plasminogen activators. Astrocytes and fibroblasts do not inhibit plasminogen activators. I believe that these findings may have a great implication for our understanding of the cell balances mentioned earlier.

There are two types of plasminogen activator (PA): tissue type PA, which only works when there is fibrin around, and urokinase-type PA, which is independent of the presence of fibrin. Endothelial cells seem to produce the first enzyme at very low levels all the time. Apparently, these low levels of PA protect the body from inadvertent fibrin formation throughout the circulation and are less associated with invasion than with general hemostasis. Endothelial cells do not make urokinase-type plasminogen activator for the most part, except when they're actively forming new blood vessels. Furthermore, as mentioned earlier, the activity of this latter enzyme is not dependent upon fibrin being present. Many invasive tumors also produce this type of plasminogen activator in association with their invasive capacity.

When we looked at the inhibitor of plasminogen activator released by human retinal pigment epithelial cells, it did not inhibit tissue plasminogen activator. It only inhibited this urokinase PA, the one that seems to be associated with the invasive process without influence on the PA that is generally involved and necessary for hemostasis. So there is some specificity that we're beginning to unveil. The amount of inhibitor produced by the PE is increased dependent upon cell morphology. It is possible that specific cells may have different activities associated with the conditions influencing their shape, geometry and morphology. Therefore, an effective treatment might be that which induces the "right" morphologic changes.

Again, when we're thinking about treatment modalities, we need to think not only of using the laser to actually destroy the vessels. The subsequent change in the cells' environments and their morphology will induce changes not just in terms of proliferation but in terms of other cell functions.

Perhaps when subretinal neovascularization occurs, there's some disease in the retinal pigment epithelial cells that causes them to reduce any inhibiting substance that they may be producing. Alternately, there could also be an increase of stimulators. Whether one or the other of these processes is taking place is probably dependent on the specific cell-to-cell interactions about which more information should be gathered. Hopefully, we may have some answers for the next meeting in Baltimore in 1989.

Let me leave you with the two concepts that I'd like to emphasize in my summary: The cell-cell interactions and our treatments altering the established balances. In terms of neovascularization, we must not only think of proliferation but also of the other steps and functions involved.

David BenEzra

Immuno-Ophthalmology and Laboratory of Ocular Angiogenesis, Department of Ophthalmology, Hadassah University Hospital, Jerusalem, Israel

During the last 40 years, our understanding of the neovascular stimuli has evolved through various phases:
1. Michaelson's postulation of an X-factor of angiogenesis in 1948 (1) remained little-noticed and unchallenged for more than two decades.
2. The demonstration of a tumor angiogenic factor (TAF) by Folkman and his group in 1971 (2) followed by the findings of a leukocyte neovascular activating factor (NAF) by BenEzra (3) and a macrophage derived angiogenic factor (MDAF) by Polverini and colleagues (4) are milestones in the search for specific factors. During the following years, a myriad of additional factors have been identified. Most widely reported are: basic and acidic fibroblast growth factors (FGF), epidermal growth factor (EGF), heparin binding growth factor (HGF), retina derived growth factor (RDGF), corneal epithelium angiogenic factor (CETAF), human uterine angiogenic factor (HUAF), endothelial cell growth factor (ECGF), tumor necrosis factor (TNF) and interleukins. All of the above factors are large peptides with a molecular weight in the range of 20,000 daltons. Additionally, a few other small molecular weight factors have been suggested. Among these, the prostaglandins, lactic acid, and endothelial stimulating angiogenesis factor (ESAF) have been studied. The multitude of angiogenic factors and their possible effect on capillary endothelial cells are schematically represented in Figure 1.
3. At present, we are on the verge of closing the cycle initiated by Michaelson's X-factor. It is becoming more and more evident that there exists a great similarity and numerous pathways of interaction among the above identified factors. Thus, interleukin 1 (IL-1) is produced by activated leukocytes and is probably associated with NAF and MDAF. The latter is apparently identical to FGF, which may be associated with TAF, RDGF and ECGF. Furthermore, the findings of amino acid sequence homologies between FGF and IL-1 (5) reinforce my postulation made in 1978 regarding the possible identity between TAF, NAF, MDAF and Michaelson's X-factor (6).
Many tissues have been investigated for their angiogenic potential. In most, factors capable of inducing neovascularization have been detected. Cartilage, lens, cornea, and vitreous are normally devoid of blood vessels and have been found to harbor inhibitors of neovascularization. However, it was demonstrated that in

certain conditions, these tissues are able to induce strong angiogenic activity.

ANGIOGENIC STIMULI

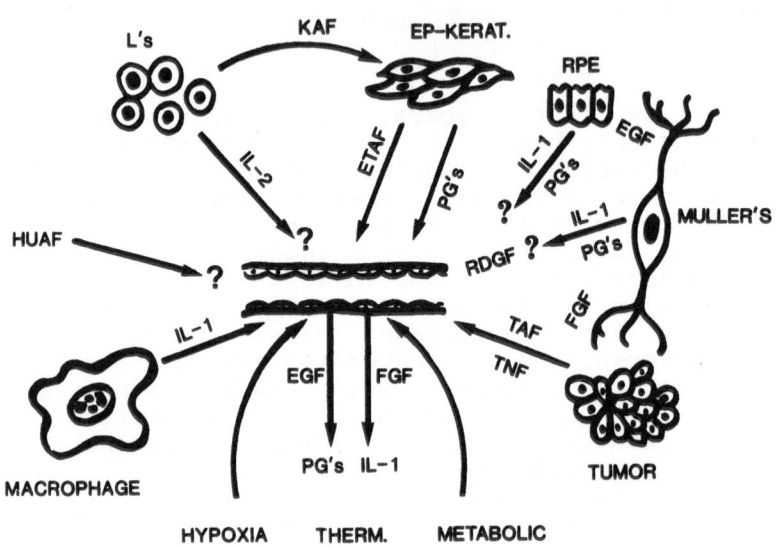

Figure 1. The multitude of possible angiogenic stimuli.

Earlier, I suggested that in every tissue, stimulating and inhibiting neovascular factors are constantly interacting, reaching a "steady state" specific for each tissue (6). Various insults may interfere with the steady state either by activating "dormant" neovascular factors or by interfering with the inhibitors' activity. Moreover, as demonstrated during this meeting, cells (like retinal pigment epithelium) which may be involved in the angiogenic process release inhibitory (Dr. Glaser) or stimulatory (Dr. Boulton) substances. A schematic representation of possible pathways of activation of the neovascular process stimulation is illustrated in Figure 2.

Neovascularization of the ocular tissues is a widespread phenomenon observed in most chronic conditions which interferes with the normal metabolic activity of the involved tissue. It is the end result of many pathological conditions (diabetes, vein occlusion, ROP, ARMD) which, as a group, are the most common causes of blindness in developed countries.

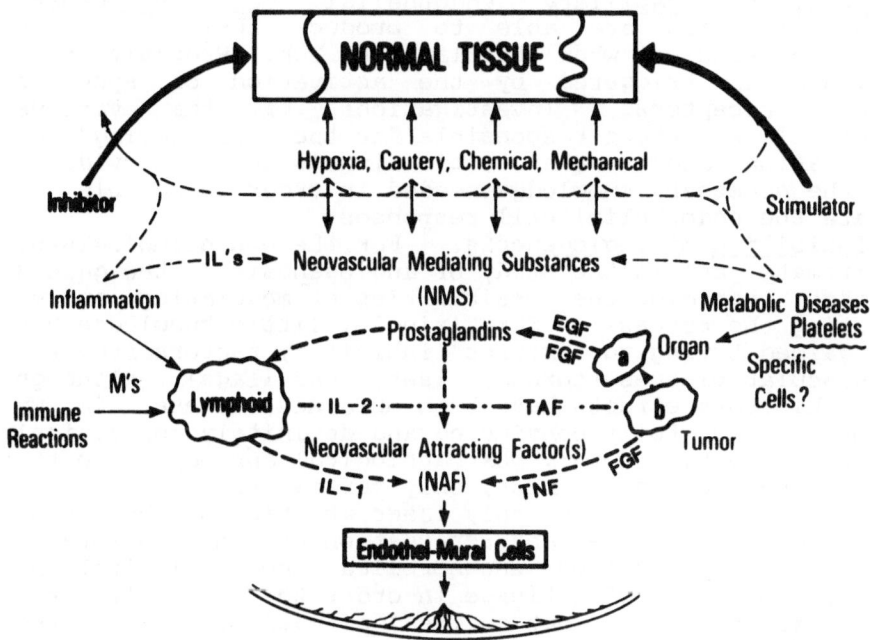

Figure 2. Possible pathway for angiogenic stimuli and probable interactions that may take place.

In order to increase our knowledge and enhance the prospects for possible future modes of therapy, there are, in my opinion, four major fields that should be intensively investigated:

A model: At present, angiogenic factors are evaluated using the rabbit, rat and mouse cornea or iris, or the chick chorio-allantoic membrane. Although my concept of neovasculogenesis has been of a "unitarian phenomenon" essentially identical in all tissues (7), direct evidence for this surmise is still lacking. There is no doubt that the in vitro models can add information to our knowledge at the cellular level. However, it should be clear that proliferation and/or chemotaxis of endothelial cells in vitro may not bear any significance regarding the in vivo neovascular processes. Therefore, concentrated efforts should be directed toward the development of a reproducible and reliable model for angiogenesis of the retina and choroid.

Histological studies: Knowledge regarding the cellular metabolic activity and/or morphological changes occurring at the site of neovascularization during its early phases is lacking. Efforts should be directed toward the understanding of the histopathological changes taking place and preceding the development of new vessels which follow different triggering stimuli.

572

Specific capillary endothelial cell receptors: Endothelial cells are able to produce IL-1 (a potent angiogenic stimulus) when stimulated by TNF. Probably, this phenomenon is triggered by the activation of specific membrane receptors. Investigations of the various endothelial receptors responsible for the "triggering" of proliferation and/or chemotactic signals should provide us with the necessary knowledge needed in order to be able to modulate the endothelial cell responses.

Inhibition of angiogenesis: For the ophthalmologists, the ultimate goal in the study of angiogenesis is the gained knowledge regarding the possibilities of modulating and/or inhibiting the process. Surprisingly, little knowledge has been gained trying to "extract" inhibitory factors from the few avascular tissues (cornea, lens, cartilage). Although some inhibitory effects have been obtained, these, in my opinion, are not fully convincing and definitely impractical for clinical use. So far, pharmacological approaches to the problem have yielded, at best, only partial success.

In clinical practice, only laser ablation of the retina has brought some relief and retardation of the inexorable blindness that follows uncontrolled neovascularization. However, ablation of a tissue in order to "save" it from neovascularization is not an ideal situation, to say the least. Future prospects for a better understanding of the basic mechanisms of angiogenesis should provide some insight into possible pharmacological therapies. At present, combinations of Indomethacin and steroids or steroids and heparin appear to influence the extent of neovascularization in experimental models. It remains to be seen whether these findings could have any therapeutical effects in clinical practice. The observation that IL-1 is a potent angiogenic factor is, in my view, most exciting because of the vast basic knowledge available on this substance. Although our initial attempts to inhibit neovascularization using a potent inhibitor of interleukin release (Cyclosporin A) have been disappointing, better treatment modalities might in future yield the long-awaited therapeutical effects.

REFERENCES
1. Michaelson IC: The mode of develoment of the retinal vessels and some observations of its significance in certain retinal diseases. Trans Ophthalmol Soc UK 68:137, 1948.
2. Folkman J, Minder E, Abernathy C, Williams G: Isolation of a tumor factor responsible for angiogenesis. J Exp Med 133:275, 1971.
3. BenEzra D: Mediators of immunological reactions. Function as inducers of neovascularization. Metabolic Ophthalmol 2:239, 1978.
4. Polverini PJ, Cotran RS, Gimbrone MA, Unanue ER: Activated macrophages induce vascular proliferation. Nature 269:804, 1977.

5.   Abraham JA, Mergia A, Whang JL, Tumolo A, Friedman J, Hjerrild KA, Gospodarowicz D, Fiddes JC: Nucleotide sequence of a bovine clone encoding the angiogenic protein, basic fibroblast growth factor.   Science 233:545, 1986.
6.   BenEzra D: Neovasculogenic ability of prostaglandins, growth factors and synthetic chemoattractants.   Am J Ophthalmol 86:455, 1978.
7.   BenEzra D: Neovascularization: A unitarian phenomenon.   Docum Ophthalmol Proc Series 25:125, 1981.